PRINCIPLES AND PRACTICE OF
HOMEOPATHY

of related interest

Homeopathy and Autism Spectrum Disorder
A Guide for Practitioners and Families
Mike Andrews
ISBN 978 1 84819 168 6
eISBN 978 0 85701 128 2

Passionate Medicine
Making the transition from conventional medicine to homeopathy
Edited by Robin Shohet
ISBN 978 1 84310 298 4
eISBN 978 1 84642 129 7

Methodologies for Effectively Assessing Complementary and Alternative Medicine (CAM)
Research Tools and Techniques
Edited by Mark J. Langweiler, BA, DC, DAAPM, and Peter W. McCarthy, BSc, PhD
Foreword by Kenneth A. Leight, PhD
ISBN 978 1 84819 251 5
eISBN 978 0 85701 197 8

The Compassionate Practitioner
How to create a successful and rewarding practice
Jane Wood
ISBN 978 1 84819 222 5
eISBN 978 0 85701 170 1

Getting Better at Getting People Better
Creating Successful Therapeutic Relationships
Noah Karrasch
ISBN 978 1 84819 239 3
eISBN 978 0 85701 186 2

PRINCIPLES AND PRACTICE OF
HOMEOPATHY

The Therapeutic and Healing Process

Edited by

Dr David Owen MBBS FFHom Homeopathic Physician
Co-founder of the Homeopathic Professionals Teaching Group, Oxford
Principal Clinical Teaching Fellow, School of Medicine,
Southampton University
Past President of the Faculty of Homeopathy, UK

Forewords by
Bob Leckridge
Peter Fisher

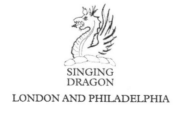

SINGING
DRAGON
LONDON AND PHILADELPHIA

This edition published in 2015
by Singing Dragon
an imprint of Jessica Kingsley Publishers
73 Collier Street
London N1 9BE, UK
and
400 Market Street, Suite 400
Philadelphia, PA 19106, USA

www.singingdragon.com

First published by Churchill Livingstone, Elsevier, London, UK, 2007

Library of Congress Cataloging in Publication Data
Owen, David K., author.
  Principles and practice of homeopathy : the therapeutic and healing process / David Owen.
      p. ; cm.
  Originally published: Philadelphia : Churchill Livingstone Elsevier, 2007.
  Includes bibliographical references and index.
  ISBN 978-1-84819-265-2 (alk. paper)
  I. Title.
  [DNLM: 1. Homeopathy. WB 930]
  RX76
  615.5'32--dc23
                            2014045614

British Library Cataloguing in Publication Data
A CIP catalogue record for this book is available from the British Library

ISBN 978 1 84819 265 2
eISBN 978 0 85701 213 5

Printed and bound in Great Britain

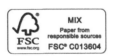

ENDORSEMENTS

At last, the first comprehensive modern homeopathy textbook in English since Herbert Roberts in 1936 and George Vithoulkas in 1978, and it surpasses them both. Despite being a textbook it is exciting and innovative with time and space for reflection and personal growth. The inspired choice of authors for some of the chapters (Sherr, Norland and Curtin, for example) crosses boundaries and enlivens the discussions. Read this and your practical understanding of the theories of homeopathy will grow. It is equally suitable for experienced medical and professional homeopaths, and for students on all qualification courses.

Francis Treuherz MA RSHom FSHom
Registered Homeopath, Homeopathic Private Practitioner, London and Letchworth, UK

A tour de force, from basic homeopathy, through practical application to the more esoteric boundaries of holistic thought. Something for everyone. David Owen's style of interactive teaching is reflected in this comprehensive work – if you want to be both educated and challenged to broaden you horizons, then read this book.

John Saxton BVet Med VetFFHom Cert. IAVH MRCVS President, Faculty of Homeopathy Homeopathic teacher, author and veterinary homeopathic referral practitioner, UK

One of the confusing aspects of homeopathic practice has been the apparently random focus of different prescribers on varying aspects of a particular case. David Owen presents a theoretical background from within which to understand and work with this phenomenon. From the outset he makes it clear that this book should bring the reader to ask and meditate on questions, as much as it may provide some answers.

This is not another study of materia medica. It is primarily a study into the concepts that lie behind, and the process of case analysis, developed in a way and to a degree that I have not met before. It will be a very useful textbook for students, and offer experienced practitioners a source for reflection and further development of their understanding of and competency with their work.

Starting from a study of different models of health, the book takes us through the themes involved in simpler case presentations on to those in difficult cases. Whilst being primarily a theoretical discussion, case examples are frequently used for illustration and avenues provided to assist with the many obstacles in the way of the homeopath.

Dr Nick Goodman MbBS MFHom FACNEM
General Practitioner and registered homeopath, Sydney, Australia

This is the most comprehensive book there is on the principles and practice of homeopathy. The beauty of this book is that its breadth is matched in equal measure by its depth. No aspect of homeopathy is neglected, from local prescribing to Sankaran's sensations and miasms.

The style is at once practical and profound, and honours the many different ways that homeopathy is practised. I am particularly impressed by Dr Owen's numerous insights into the psychodymamics of the homeopathic history, and his emphasis on the homeopath's own personal evolution. In his own words, by reading this book the student's work is transformed 'from being a necessary task to being an opportunity for growth'.

Dr Philip Bailey MBBS MFHom
Private Practitioner and author of Homeopathic Psychology (North Atlantic Books, Berkeley, California), Fremantle, West Australia

This book drips holism and there is wisdom here aplenty. Speaking as someone who has wrestled with homeopathy for 30 years, David's book touches on concerns and connections that any serious practitioner will share. I predict it will become a classic.

Professor David Peters
School of Integrated Health, University of Westminster, London, UK

This exceptional book gathers, reflects on, and deeply enquires into, the evolving principles of homeopathy in a way that encourages any practitioner to develop themselves, their understanding and their art.

Written with an approach that invites reflective pause, the reader is supported, encouraged and challenged to review issues of health, self, illness, caring and treatment. This weave is practical and accessible, rooted in clinical practice and examples, yet tackles at the same time the profound issues and questions which homeopathic practice and training raises. This is an important step forward in homeopathic textbooks that I would recommend whatever your current level of practice.

David Reilly
Consultant, Glasgow Homeopathic Hospital; Researcher and Teacher, Glasgow Homeopathic Academic Centre

THE 'FIVE THEMES'

There are five themes which run across the sections and chapters of the book. These are represented by small, stylised icons within the text to help highlight and connect the themes.

Philosophy

The principles and key concepts that provide the conceptual framework on which the clinical practice of homeopathy is based. Allowing the student and practitioner to address the practical and theoretical challenges of contemporary homeopathic practice.

Materia Medica

The materia medica of remedies is central to understanding how homeopathy is practised. How the remedy pictures are developed and the different ways the pictures are expressed provide the foundation and building blocks that allow the homeopath to both understand the patient and to prescribe rationally. The many different ways the remedy pictures can be expressed informs the very way a homeopath thinks and is able to perceive a patient.

The Case

The homeopathic case puts the relationship between the homeopath and patient at the heart of the therapeutic process. It is more than a record of the consultation as case skills facilitate what can happen in a consultation, it determines what the patient chooses to reveal, the level at which the consultation takes place and the depth to which the homeopath perceives.

Case Analysis

Case analysis allows what is perceived of the patient to be matched with what is known of the remedies; according to homeopathic principles. It governs the order, pattern and interpretation that emerge in the healing process. The variety of case analysis strategies and methodologies available to the homeopath is a major factor that determines the breadth of their clinical competence.

Case Management

The prescription of a homeopathic remedy is only one part of the therapeutic and healing process. In each case the illness, the patient, the homeopath and the effect each has on the other needs to be considered. Case management brings together the science of the homeopathic therapeutic system with the artistry of the caring and healing clinician. Focussed on the process of cure and care of the patient.

CONTENTS

CONTRIBUTORS

Helen Beaumont MB ChB DRCOG MRCGP MFHom
Homeopathic Physician and General Practitioner, UK

Iris Bell MD PhD
Professor, Department of Family and Community Medicine, USA

Maggie Curley MB ChB DRCOG MFHom
Homeopathic Physician and General Practitioner, UK

David Curtin MBBS MFHom PCH MCH(hon)
Homeopathic Physician and General Practitioner, UK

Philip Edmonds HND DSH RSHom
Homeopath, UK

Peter Gregory BVSc VetFFHom Cert. IAVH MRCVS
Veterinary Surgeon, UK

David Lilley MBChB(Pret) FFHom(London)
Homeopathic Physician, South Africa

Misha Norland RSHom FSHom
Homeopathic Physician, UK

Tony Pinkus BPharm MRPharms LFHom
Homeopathic Pharmacist, Director (Ainsworths), UK

Jeremy Sherr FSHom MCH Bac
Homeopath, UK

It is not easy to write a different book about homeopathy. This book manages to be different. Health care needs something to change. Chronic diseases are increasing throughout the world and health services in every country are straining under the burgeoning demands of people who are suffering. No government seems to be able to put sufficient resources into health care to stem the tide. The Faculty of Homeopathy, under David Owen's Presidency, developed a 25-year plan in the year 2000. The plan was firmly based on the foundation of our recognition of two important points. Firstly, that there is a desperate need for a new kind of medicine for the 21st Century. The existing model is just not good enough. Secondly, that homeopathic medicine is ideally placed to contribute to the creation of exactly the kind of medicine that the 21st Century world needs.

The structure of this book is founded on that first recognition. What might a new kind of medicine look like, and how will it relate to the current model? The five models of health laid out in the introductory chapter and which are then used as the entire framework of this text are, firstly, the pathogenic model – this is the predominant model of health underpinning the dominant biomedical model. It is highly reductionist and fundamentally based on a machine-like metaphor where parts become damaged or broken and need to be replaced or fixed. Arthur Frank, in his excellent *The Wounded Storyteller*, describes this as the 'Restitution Narrative' – 'I'm broken/ my xxx is broken...please fix me'. The second model is the biological model. This model has developed from the pathogenic model as understandings from complexity science have illuminated the processes of systems rather than only of components. As a model, it is more complex and more accurate than the pathogenic model but it is still really the same reductionist, 'fix me'

kind of approach. The third model is the holistic model and this has already become a mainstream view in undergraduate medicine, and especially in postgraduate general practice training. It is sometimes referred to as a 'biopsychosocial model' and as such represents a significant advance on the 'biomedical' one. It refuses to be reductionist and places the patient as a person at the centre of the care process. The holistic model focuses on the whole of the patient's suffering rather than solely on their pathology. Eric Cassell in *The Healer's Art* reflects this as a move away from a focus on disease to a focus on illness. These three models bring us up to the current state of the art in the practice of medicine. Inspiringly, David Owen goes on to outline two further models which chart a path to a future, better, more effective medicine. The holographic model is really unknown in the the biomedical and even biopsychosocial models. Indeed, it is only rarely mentioned by those who claim to practise holistically. I know of only one therapy which really understands it and which uses this model in daily practice – homeopathic practice. The idea that when a patient presents their suffering; everything is connected and every symptom, every area of disturbance reveals the same underlying problems and issues is fundamental to the homeopathic approach. For a doctor, such an approach is very, very exciting. It means that all the patient's symptoms can be understood to reveal the fundamental, underpinning disorder. But more than that, it also reveals the exact, best, unique therapeutic intervention for that patient. It is the antithesis of the one-size-fits-all approach of modern pharmacology. This would be enough. The vision of the holographic model would give us plenty to explore, research and develop to create a new 21st Century medicine. However, there is yet another model here too – the relational model. This, again, builds on strands and developments of recent years. Balint groups from the 1950s introduced general practitioners to ways of understanding the significance of the doctor–patient relationship and showed them how to be aware of their own responses to patients and even how to use this awareness therapeutically. Sadly, the Balint movement has been washed away by an approach based on targets and box-ticking. Medicine NEEDS these new models of health to be developed and widely disseminated.

You would think that all this would be quite enough. It is exciting and it is visionary and it should provoke any doctor to think more deeply about their practice. However, this particular book does even more than this because it lays out extremely clearly the way to practise

homeopathy. Homeopathic medicine does already use all these five models of health and any health care professional would find that their work would be enhanced and their rewards increased if they learned how to integrate homeopathy into what they already do. This book is not just about theory and models, it lays out the 'how to' of homeopathy.

I hope you enjoy this book. I am very sure that reading it has the potential to change your professional life.

Bob Leckridge BSc MB ChB MFHom
Specialist in Homeopathic Medicine
2006

FOREWORD

By his choice of title, David Owen has set himself in a proud tradition, for his *Principles and Practice of Homeopathy* is far from being the first book of this, or similar, title. Illustrious antecedents include Richard Hughes' slim volume of the same title, now over a century old. Herbert Roberts' *Principles and Art of Cure by Homoeopathy*, published in 1936. ML Dhawale's *three*-volume *Principles and Practice of Homeopathy* published in 1967 and Ernest Roberts' recent *Homoeopathy: principles and practice*. But best known to contemporary British homeopaths is Charles Wheeler's classic *Introduction to the Principles and Practice of Homoeopathy* which went through *three* editions between 1919 and 1948. Many British homeopaths of recent generations were brought up on 'Wheeler and Kenyon' (Douglas Kenyon became co-author for the third edition).

The comparison between David Owen's book and Wheeler and Kenyon is a gauge of how homeopathy has evolved over the last 60 or so years. The older book has a bare 50 pages of principles, followed by 300 of materia medica and a mini-repertory. Each medicine monograph starts with an account of the nature of the substance, followed by its toxicology and pharmacology before describing its homeopathic uses. By contrast, Owen's book contains no systematic materia medica, but the text is interspersed with numerous clinical vignettes, giving the flavour of clinical practice. It also reflects the burgeoning diversity of the contemporary homeopathic scene.

The great and unique strength of *Principles and Practice of Homeopathy* is its multi-faceted nature: between no other pair of book covers will you find the breadth of approach, by authors who know their topic in depth, distilled with such brevity and clarity. No one author can claim the depth of expertise in all areas required for a modern comprehensive textbook, and in a welcome development, in line with modern practice, a number of chapters are written by experts in the areas, each with an introduction by Owen himself. There are chapters on veterinary homeopathy, homeopathic software, Miasms (by David Lilley) and the Sankaran method (Helen Beaumont and Maggie Curley), among others. David Owen himself contributes a series of thoughtful concluding chapters which cover the management of difficult problems and the 'self-maintenance' for homeopaths. All are interspersed with case histories, illustrations and points for reflection.

Dr Peter Fisher
Clinical Director
Royal London Homoeopathic Hospital
2006

ACKNOWLEDGEMENTS

'Every blade of grass has its Angel that bends over it and whispers, "Grow, grow".' The Talmud

The knowledge in this book is tiny compared to the truths of homeopathy held by the homeopathic profession as a whole. Any wisdom it offers does not solely belong to me or any other single teacher – it belongs to the total sum of the homeopathic profession and its patients, who are the reason for its existence. Those who have written different chapters and those who have both taught me and learnt with me represent the many homeopaths that have contributed to this knowledge. The bibliography at the end of each chapter introduces, cumulatively, other key texts that have been important in my learning and lay the foundation for further reading.

I am especially grateful to my colleagues and the students of the Homeopathic Professionals Teaching Group (HPTG) especially Alice, Brian, Charles, John, Peter, Andy, Lee and David who make studying and teaching such a transformative experience. One colleague who had a huge influence on my thinking and approach was Dr Lee Holland with whom I discovered more could be learnt from the difficult cases than the easy ones. It is to him, and through my memory of him to those patients which challenge me (and you), that I dedicate this book.

I would particularly like to thank Dr Jeremy Swayne who has studiously corrected earlier drafts and critically reviewed the text. Also to Patricia Ridsdale, who as an ex-student and now a colleague has encouraged and given feedback. Other inspiration came from Robin Shohet who has invited me to explore models of reflective practice and supervision and has supported me in 'finding my voice' and writing this book. I am grateful for the support of many friends, like Alan Heeks, who have reminded me of the opportunities and lessons to be learnt while writing the book, stood by me as I faced my fears and have encouraged me to share my dreams.

The challenge of writing this book would not have been possible without the patience, encouragement and love of my family. Thank you to my wife Sue, and children William, Oliver, Henry and Miranda.

PREFACE

'You must give birth to your images.
They are the future waiting to be born.
Fear not strangerness that you feel.
The future must enter into you
Long before it happens.
Just wait for the birth
The hour of clarity.' Rainer Maria Rilke

Every homeopath I know describes, at some time, entering unfamiliar terrain. This book will, I hope, be helpful to the student when navigating through such 'terrain'. To make your journey through the book easier it is designed on a spiral pattern – weaving together the philosophy, an understanding of the materia medica, the patient's case, the analytic strategies and the management issues raised. There are six sections, each with five chapters. Very approximately each year of a three-year training course on homeopathy will link with two sections. Each section will deepen and progress the ideas previously discussed.

My passion for homeopathy and the belief that it is the health care system for the future of humanity is the overwhelming reason why I decided to write this book. At times it reflects the consensus of homeopathic thinking; at others it may seem potentially outrageous to you. The principles covered here are, however, validated by my clinical experience and those of colleagues with whom I've practised and taught. These have led to a clarity and certainty of mind about the different ways that health can be viewed, described here as five different but complementary 'models of health'. This book looks at what information about our remedies and patients is needed to practice in each model. I am eager to share these with you as I have observed, over many years of teaching students and supporting and supervising practitioners, that the greatest confusion and difficulty in

practising homeopathy comes from limiting the universal principles of homeopathy.

I hope that you accept this book as an invitation to explore and journey towards your own clarity and certainty; to celebrate the diversity homeopathy offers and find a way of practising that is not only practical, inclusive and effective, but also suits the unique contribution you can bring to this healing art. This is a practice that will help those patients who wish to understand and work through their illnesses to a deeper and subtler level, leading to better health for themselves, our environment and our future. It is a way of working that is stimulating, rewarding and enjoyable for you – the future of homeopathy.

The nature of writing is that it lends itself to the expression of certain concepts and ideas better than others. I realise that, at times, it may seem as if I am making sweeping statements or being defensive about concepts that are important to me. While I am passionate about sharing these ideas with you I welcome any doubts about my interpretation of things. Learning is not easy and at times questioning different ideas and challenging assumptions and concepts will serve you better than anything you read. My belief is that if I can, in some way, share my enthusiasm, then it will help you to engage with your own inquiry and sustain you when it becomes challenging or just plain, laborious hard work.

Why you should read this book
'What lies before us and
What lies behind us
Are small matters compared
To what lies within us.
And when we bring
What is within us
Out into the world
Miracles happen.' David Thoreau

Learning homeopathy is a journey, there are no time machines, no reaching the end before leaving the beginning, no ways someone else can do the journey for you or carry you. Some of the journey is well trodden and easy to follow, some in the outer world and some in your inner world. Some of the journey is difficult, where you must make your own pathway and upon which it is easy to get lost.

The principles provide fixed and consistent markers in this sometimes unfamiliar terrain. The practice, as recorded by different practitioners, provides signposts pointing the way. At times different signposts point in different directions and you will at times feel lost and confused. This is as much a preparation for working with patients as anything else. We each have to wrestle, struggle and eventually find our own way around the world of illness that parallels and shadows the world of health. You, like me, will need to reflect, meditate and try out the different, at times contradictory or paradoxical, teachings to find your own way!

Every homeopath will also, at some point, reach a place where they feel alone and stuck. At such a moment I hope this book will remind you that you are not alone and help you to courageously move from your 'stuckness'. When you have experienced this many times you will know that these difficulties are where you find the true connection with your colleagues and from where you have the opportunity to fly above the problems and 'stuckness' to gain new perspective. My experience is that I move between uncertainty and certainty. As a homeopathic student I sought certainty but the reality of being a practitioner has made me realise that it is how I embrace and work with the uncertain that determines my personal insights and ability to see and work with patients. There will be many times in the book when I invite you to reflect on your own uncertainty. If you enter fully into this it will help you make your own map – which you will find infinitely better than anyone else's, and which will make you safer and more comfortable with the uncertain.

How you might get the most from this book

'What doesn't kill me makes me stronger'
Albert Camus

Clarifying the questions and searching for answers is essential for our development and I would not want to take this struggle away from you. If this book makes your journey more conscious (even if at times you find it more difficult) then this is, I believe, the price we pay for the privilege of studying and working as a homeopath. My belief is that we will not run out of questions to go through. In the same way as the last patient won't ever be treated, so when one set of questions is answered another will arise. Offering you the questions and answers is not just a gift but also a responsibility. For you to gain the insights that I hope you will, your perception will need to be attuned and your presence focused. One of the best ways to do this is to read this book actively, not passively. This means not assuming each subject will unfold gradually and sequentially but, at each heading, to think positively about what you already know, what you want to learn about this topic or idea, and what questions you would like to have answered about that topic. If you are attuned and focused when reading this book it will (as with the patients you see) bring insights. If you are questioning and reflective then for every insight you gain, you will discover yet another question. To help in this questioning and reflective process I cannot state too strongly the importance of being in a supportive learning environment; somewhere where you can share your successes but more importantly your failures – where you can own your fears and dream your own dreams!

In order to both broaden and deepen your training I hope you find a learning environment where your education, support and development are all addressed. It may require different colleges, courses, teachers, mentors, peer groups and supervisors at different times and for different students, to facilitate your learning. This book, indeed any book, by its nature, cannot provide all this.

There are, for example, real challenges regarding integrating homeopathy with other healthcare systems. It is influenced by the conventions of different communities that patients belong to and the beliefs and priorities that individual patients hold. Each of these cannot be covered in specific detail although the general principles are covered in the chapters which address case management. It is beyond the scope of the book to look in detail at organisational, public health or social issues related to providing a homeopathic healthcare system to a community. For this vital work to be done, the commitment of practitioners to the health of communities and populations as well as individuals is required. To work meaningfully with this requires the realisation by individual homeopaths of the importance of their own professional organisation, providing far more than examination/assessment processes and regulation. For you as a student it means that as well as an environment where you feel safe and supported it is vital for you to find a peer group and professional community.

The focus of this book is on your personal understanding of homeopathy. It does not set out to provide materia medica or to offer specific case management advice for treating patients with specific conditions. Although brief illustrative materia medica and case vignettes are used to connect the theory to the practice. It will offer you most when studied alongside other texts, when you have the opportunity for the observation of a variety of homeopathic cases and can begin to practise with careful but challenging clinical supervision.

REFLECTION POINT

- What is your learning environment like? Can you be yourself, could you have your case taken, if necessary receive treatment, share your concerns and discuss your failures, etc? What else do you need to best facilitate your learning and how will you get it?

Style

This book is written in a way that attempts to address readers' different preferences in learning. Each person will find some aspects of the book more or less useful than another. This is as it should be, and where a point is important I have made it several times – each time in a way that I hope will appeal to different readers. It does mean that some points are repeated, frequently revisited and deepened in different chapters and sections. Typically, learning consists of different stages and is approached differently by those with different learning styles (see Chapter 12). Learning a subject deeply (like treating a patient at the deepest levels) will often involve cycling through a number of stages as your knowledge of the subject (or patient) deepens. Your own preferred way of learning and consulting will be influenced by the stages and styles you feel most comfortable with, as well as how the information is presented. When paced and managed this learning cycle will naturally lead to the understanding of a subject deepening. Different readers will start in a different place and find some parts easier than others.

If you find you are distracted by something in the text then check to see if you can accurately describe the point for yourself as it may need more reflection before you can deepen your understanding. Realising your own learning style and preferences will help you assimilate and personalise the huge amount of information that studying homeopathy requires. It will also offer insight into how you relate to others – so important to understand when treating patients.

As the book progresses so the ideas may appear more challenging; they also move from historical teachings to perceptions from current practice. I am completely confident in these perceptions and their value but, being newer, they do not carry the same endorsement by other homeopathic teachers. In many cases teachers of other therapeutic modalities verify them. The homeopathic truth does not change but our interpretation and explanation does. So, for example, this book aims to extend an understanding of the principles and practice of homeopathy to include psychological concepts, e.g. observations about the therapeutic relationship including projection both onto and by practitioners, which are confirmed by the experience and observations of those using psychotherapeutic approaches to treatment.

Writing this book has provided an invaluable process for me to reflect on, and record, how I work and the principles I follow. Daily I see homeopathy revealing staggering qualities in people as they journey between illness and health and in homeopaths as they struggle to glimpse the mysteries of life. I am grateful for the opportunity to have reflected on these observations and thoughts and the privilege of being able to share them. I hope this book helps you examine both your attitudes and behaviours to yourself and others and encourages you to enquire deeply about your role as a healer and seek out those who can personally supervise your training and support your education.

I have spoken only of those models of health, approaches to treatment and methodologies to prescribing with which I am familiar. None is right, none is wrong. Other practitioners with different experiences may describe what they do, and how they work – it is for you to decide if they sit within the framework I have described. I wish you luck in developing your own style of practice to suit the situation in which you work and the patients you are likely to see. I own up to a slight sense of envy of all the excitement and opportunities that your study of homeopathy will bring to you. But I am equally enthused by the questions and opportunities that patients and students daily present.

My heartfelt desire is to engender tolerance, open-mindedness and insight amongst practitioners using homeopathy, while at the same time celebrating the difference and uniqueness that each of us has to offer. If this book helps you to clarify the principles and values you choose to work with, to find what works best for you, helps you understand those who work differently, and encourages you to extend and explore your own therapeutic 'territory' then it will achieve all that I could hope for.

Readers are invited to contact me with comments or feedback on the text; by e-mail to enquiries@thenaturalpractice.com.

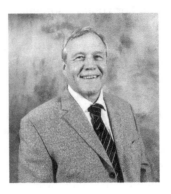

David Owen
Winchester, 2007

Section 1

Foundation

CHAPTER ONE

What is Health?

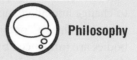 **Philosophy**

David Owen

Introduction

The laws that govern health are the cornerstones of a homeopath's knowledge. How we understand the relationship between the substance and energy of life determines the model we use to describe health. Homeopathy is the matching of a remedy to a patient based on their similarities (like treating like). Homeopaths use several different models to explain health and define illness. The model used determines the approach to treatment. For each approach to treatment there are several methods of prescribing. This chapter invites you to reflect on what you think health is before outlining five models of health.

The different relationship between homeopath and patient – where symptoms describe the interface between patients and their environment, and illness may be seen as a necessary aspect of being well – invites further reflection about homeopathic patients and the meaning of illness. How symptoms arise and communicate the patient's needs is mediated by what is termed the vitality. The natural forces that govern the vitality and the general laws of health start to describe the homeopathic laws.

Laws of Health

The science of homeopathic medicine is based on a framework of laws described by philosophers and validated over generations by observers and practitioners. The laws apply to all organisms and they follow laws that govern our environ-

ment whether we think of it in terms of objects or energy. By knowing these, it is possible to work with the great healing potential of nature and individuals.

The first law is that every action is matched by an equal and opposite reaction. When a force is directed in one direction an opposite force operates in the other direction. This law explains why every cause has an effect, why certain lifestyles produce certain symptoms and why the homeopath seeks to understand all aspects of a symptom, including those which at first may appear hidden or unconscious.

The second law is that nothing (in a closed system) is ever ultimately created or destroyed but that it just changes its form or nature. So energy will change from kinetic to potential, compounds may break into component elements, health and illness are aspects of the same thing and birth and death are considered a change in 'state'.

The third law is that change is a constant, that it is inevitable. Complex systems in time decay; simple systems in time become more complex. Organisms try to move towards or maintain a steady state, but when a steady state is approached or obtained for any length of time it inevitably becomes unstable again. The only constant is change.

The fourth law is that all observation is affected by the medium through which the perception is taking place. For example, things look different when seen through air or water, and because it takes time for us to see things, we only see them as they were and never as they are. Two people will have different views of the same things.

Lastly, the fifth law says that the same laws govern objects as govern energy. All matter has the potential to change and all change is an expression of energy, so matter has a 'potential energy within it'. Our bodies are influenced by energy, including thoughts, that we are exposed to and that we express.

REFLECTION POINT

- What do these laws tell you about health? How do these laws affect different therapeutic systems, for example the body's reaction to medicines or the remembering of thoughts from the past?

What is Health?

To stimulate your thinking about health consider the 'health' of the individual in these different situations:

Peter comes into the practice feeling completely fit and well but needing a medical for his insurance company; he has raised blood pressure and investigations lead to a diagnosis of a serious disease. Peter was obviously not healthy before he walked into the practice but he did not know this.

Lucy and James are born with identical birthmarks that will, if untreated, stay all their lives; James feels disfigured by his while Lucy feels hers is a distinguishing mark. Symptoms in different people cause different responses.

It is also important to remember health and illness have important functions in communities as well as in individuals. An individual's illness will affect their community and their community will affect them. We have a primary role to care for an individual and often a secondary role in caring for a family group or community. At times, these roles conflict:

Joan has depression and feels different from her family and community. She is an artist, and her work makes her family and community feel uncomfortable but leads to some members of her community reflecting on how they see things and brings for them greater insight. There are important questions to ponder both on the conflict that can exist between treating an individual and that

of a population, and on what benefits an illness can bring. Health is therefore not a single point of balance but a dynamic state with changing points of balance; temporary removal of some symptoms is not the same as a cure. *Joan, with depression, seeks treatment and takes antidepressants. This helps her feel less different but it alters her art and also leaves her susceptible to other illnesses.*

REFLECTION POINT

- You might like to reflect on some other situations seen in practice that inform us about what health is, and isn't. Think about the situations described below and what they tell you about health and illness.

As John gets older, his mobility reduces to a point where he finds it hard to walk to the shops unaided. He has no pain but just can't walk as far as he used to. Perception of health is related to what you expect of your body.

Julie feels 'absolutely fine' but wants to 'make sure I keep healthy'. She asks her homeopath if she would benefit from homeopathic treatment – might it make her healthier? Julie takes a remedy and feels that she has significantly more energy and an increased sense of well-being. Was she not healthy before?

David always feels at his best after a cold or cough. When is he healthy?

Jan brings her child to see you: the child is content and happy but Jan describes the child as a 'slow developer' or 'poor sleeper'. Who has the health problem?

Mike and Mary take their pet dog to their veterinary homeopath, as they want it to bark less, be friendlier to children and less protective of them. The breed is strongly territorial. Does the pet or the owners have the problem?

What is Natural Health?

People, animals, plants and micro-organisms can all be healthy without following a system of care and health. The ability to be healthy existed before any healing system was devised and natural laws alone are sufficient for healing most organisms most of the time. Symptoms are in many ways necessary for health. When you 'catch a cold', a normal and healthy response is to develop symptoms. Tiredness might lead one to have an early night; thirst, to taking extra fluids. These things will help you throw off the cold. So having symptoms is an integral part of being healthy, not an opposite.

As individuals are drawn to explore lifestyles and environments that are more varied or challenging to them, so the challenge to maintain a healthy state increases. As this happens so the individual attempts to act in a way that can help maintain or return to a healthy state. The more any treatment system takes into account each of the laws of health the more it will work with individuals' natural ability to heal themselves.

The Models of Health

This book considers five main ways of looking at illness and health. They are not exclusive and frequently are combined together to try to understand a patient's illness from several perspectives. However, each leads to particular approaches to treatment, each has strengths and weaknesses, expectations and limitations. They are represented diagrammatically in Figure 1.1.

The *pathogenic* model sees illness in terms of an external cause that can lead to a chain of causation. When the cause happens it causes the patient to 'get ill'. When the cause is treated or reversed it can enable the patient to 'get better'. The *biological* model recognises that a single cause in every living system does not always have the same effect. In non-living systems the effect of any cause is in theory predictable, for example a chemical reaction. In the biological model of health the symptoms always express the illness and represent how the healthy organism has been affected by a cause. It may therefore reflect indirectly information about causation. The symptoms represent the way an organism is attempting to re-balance itself in response to the cause. The symptoms may both be a way of overcoming the cause (diarrhoea in

food poisoning) or of repairing or minimising the damage after the cause is removed (scarring after an injury) or adjusting to the damage by modifying the environment or situation the organism is in (arthritic pain limiting mobility). In this model the absence of symptoms is an indicator of health. Throughout Sections I and II, the book focuses on what is required to use homeopathy in these first two models of health, and on how to treat on causation and presenting symptom.

The *holistic* model looks at health in a broader context than just that of the presenting illness. It sees that in more complex cases the factors that affect the health of the patient are many, and that one simple cause is unlikely to explain the illness and the illness is unlikely to be expressed through one group of symptoms. The cause and effect can simultaneously exist in many aspects of the patient and the environment – indeed at the extreme view

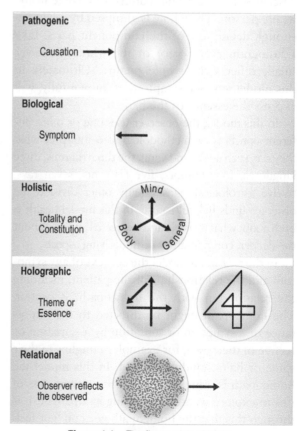

Figure 1.1 The five models of health

of this model, cause and effect are co-dependant and no one change or symptom happens in isolation. The trends and patterns in the patient both when well (constitutional state) and when ill (totality of symptoms) indicate the remedy state (see section III). In this model health is not just the absence of symptoms but also describes something of your resistance to common causations or what we call susceptibility; it also recognises that illness in some situations is necessary and even a requirement of long-term health as a way of rebalancing when the environments we are in change.

While the pathological, biological and holistic models are easily recognised in much homeopathic teaching they, like any model, have their limitations. Two other models are outlined briefly below but discussed in more detail in section VI.

The *holographic* model recognises that symptoms do not just happen in many areas of the body at the same time but that each individual symptom describes the underlying pattern of change in the whole person. The whole is glimpsed by seeing, in enough detail, any of the component parts. Like a hologram every piece of the whole, however small, reflects the whole picture. Ultimately in this model any one symptom, if known fully, will express the essence of the patient.

In this model, the observer uses one or more different concepts or methodologies to interpret what they see, such as yin and yang, the three miasms, three kingdoms, four humors, five elements, seven rays, twelve astrological signs or any other division the observer finds helpful to use. In this model health is both about what is visible and expressed and also about the deeper, compensatory or underlying aspects.

In the *relational* model the context of any symptom and the relationships of the patient, including the relationship with the homeopath, is central. The homeopath might be directed to the importance of a symptom or sensation by a sensation or feeling of their own, for example, a tingling in their spine or hairs standing on end. In this model the homeopath is using his reflections or awareness of this to explore what is happening in a patient. It is through this that the homeopath goes on 'gut feeling', on 'I feel this in my water' and I suspect this underlies most 'intuitive' prescribing. In this model health is only partially about what the patient consciously expresses and much more about what is hidden and the influence of this on the observer. The holographic and relational models in my experience offer a great deal in the management of the difficult cases. They build on and are an extension of the holistic model, and the concepts behind them are introduced gradually through this book.

Models, Approaches and Methodologies; Impression Plan and Prescription

Each model of health invites different interpretations and realisations about homeopathic remedies, cases, analyses and treatment. Although in practice these are often blended together, a thorough understanding of each in turn is a prerequisite to a rational system of care. Each of the five models of health leads to particular approaches to treatment, and each approach is served by different methodologies. Different but complementary information about the homeopathic remedies is needed to use each methodology and different aspects of the patient's case will provide the information necessary to apply each approach. These are developed and built up throughout the book but an outline of the different models, approaches and main methodologies is given in Table 1.1 with a reference to the section of this book in which they are developed in more detail.

It helps to think of the model of health as determining the overall impression of the patient, the context in which the patient's story or narrative is told (see Chapter 3). Different models often suit different types of case and this is explored in Chapter 10. Each model of health can have several different approaches to treatment and a number of prescribing methodologies. The methodology of prescribing gives the method of selecting a specific homeopathic prescription that matches the patient in a particular context. Different methodologies indicate remedies prescribed in slightly different ways and are therefore likely to have slightly different outcomes. (The idea of separating out the impression, plan and prescription in each case is developed in Chapter 8.) The different models, approaches and methodologies are often combined

Table 1.1 MODEL APPROACHES AND METHODOLOGIES			
Model of Health	**Book Section**	**Approach to Treatment**	**Methodology of Prescribing**
Pathogenic	I	Causation	Aetiological Isopathic
Biological	II	Presenting symptoms	Local Clinical Keynotes
Holistic	III	Totality Constitution	Three-legged stool Mind, body, general Morphological constitution
Holographic	IV, V, VI	Essence Thematic	Miasms Families Kingdoms Related remedies
Relational	V, VI	Reflective	Psychodynamic Emotional 'Intuitive'

in practice or emphasised in different situations but it is important to first understand each in detail.

The Pathogenic Model

In this model health is the ability to withstand causes of illness. It concerns itself with the causation of the patient's problems and is the basis of much simple and effective treatment, using many different treatment modalities including simple lifestyle changes such as avoiding acidic foods in indigestion. It also lends itself to sensible self-treatment in the home on the basis that once the cause is removed or treated recovery will follow. It is often most effective when there are single causative factors, sometimes referred to as a trigger factor. It is the level of much conventional disease treatment today, such as treating an infection by killing the infective organism.

When a patient presents with an illness, the question the enquiring physician using this model asks is 'what is the cause?'. If, despite treatment, the cause is maintained then, although treatment may give relief the illness either remains or resurfaces later as a recurrence. Not all illnesses caused by a single causative agent are superficial. Radiation exposure, asbestosis, smoking damage and nutritional deficiency can all be accommodated within the causative model, but just removing or treating the cause will not always lead to a cure as damage may have occurred over a period of time. We see that the duration and severity of the cause is central to the extent to which this model alone will heal patients.

Strictly speaking, treating on causation means treatment based on 'aetiology'. However it includes predisposing and precipitating or provoking causes. In many cases the causative association between events is less clear, such as a patient getting headaches when constipated, or very unclear, such as a patient feeling happier when constipated. In these cases the closeness in time between symptoms is important, including which symptom pre-existed the other. If the patient had never been happy before or unless they are constipated, it increases in importance. In more chronic illnesses there may be several causative factors which may or may not be connected. If a clear order of causes exists it can help to understand which was the first and which are acting more deeply.

A homeopathic treatment using causation may be chosen on the trigger event, on the factors that preceded the patient's illness, and events from which they had 'never been well since' or in combination with other approaches and methods of prescribing. The case of Alice in Case Study 1.1 illustrates this.

CASE STUDY 1.1

Alice, age 11, presented with recurrent upper respiratory tract infections. Each of these was helped to some extent by acute prescriptions but she continued to get relapses. She was brought for a consultation to see if a more deep-acting remedy might help prevent the recurrences. Taking a history the colds had started shortly after a grandparent had died. Alice had been protected from the loss of the grandparent and had not attended the funeral but neither had she had a chance to talk about her feelings. Alice was prescribed a remedy based largely on the suppressed grief but also taking into account the local symptoms. After being sad and tearful for a few days she felt much better and had a significant reduction in upper respiratory tract infections.

The Biological Model

The biological model sees health in terms of the effects of a cause. In this model health is the organism's ability to rebalance itself after a threat or cause. It is also called 'homeostasis' or 'auto-regulation'. When a patient presents with an illness, the question the enquiring physician asks in this model is 'what response has the patient had to the cause; what is the disease process that has ensued?'. It may follow (but not necessarily) that the cause is known. In the biological and patho-logical model the relationship between cause and effect is usually considered as a linear relation-ship, i.e. cause first and effect second and, at its simplest, especially in acute illness, focuses on one cause giving one effect – e.g. a fever caused by an infection. A more sophisticated biological model is one with multifactorial causes, where a number of different causative factors can predis-pose or lead to a number of effects, including a variety of symptoms. For example, poverty may be a contributing factor to poor nutrition, which may contribute to susceptibility to a particular illness.

The Holistic Model

The holistic model recognises that any single cause may, in different people, have a different effect, and any one individual can produce simi-lar symptoms from diverse causes. Susceptibility determines what causative factors the patient is sensitive to, the degree to which they respond, and what symptoms they are likely to develop, i.e. their vulnerability to particular illnesses. In the holistic model the enquiring physician investigates the 'individual susceptibility' and asks why does the patient have this particular illness with these particular symptoms and what will help them now and in the future?

In this model, whatever the pattern of cau-sation, symptoms include both the physical and psychological symptoms of an individual. These will affect the environmental preferences of the individual, what we may call 'situational' factors, as they may extend to any situation the patient chooses or 'finds' themselves in including work, relationship, cultural, etc. Taking all aspects of the situation as well as local causes and effects leads to a totality approach to treatment that incorporates local, psychological and general symptoms.

Our situations are always changing and our health in one situation does not assure us of being healthy in another. There is a quality to being healthy in the holistic model that not only addresses our ability to be in balance with the environment we are in now, but also the ability to be in balance with the situations we are likely to come across, or the changes we are likely to face. The pathological and biological models are about the individual's ability to function optimally in a set or given environment, while the holistic model provides a model to explore health as something that is sustainable.

The Holographic Model

As cases advance, particularly if they are only par-tially treated, then they get more and more com-plicated. Fewer symptoms are clearly expressed in the totality of symptoms and a holistic model becomes harder to work with. In these cases, where many symptoms become overshadowed by others and where much of the case can appear to be in shadow, an essence and thematic approach, based on the holographic model, opens the possibility of working with what would otherwise be difficult cases. The holographic model recognises that cause and effect are mutually dependent and the pattern behind the causation and expression of the illness is what points to and requires treatment.

Using this model the homeopath asks what is the order or pattern being expressed or revealed by the patient. Treatment is based on these patterns, referred to as essences and themes that are matched to the essence and themes in the homeopathic remedies (see Chapters 22 and 27) – both seeing the case and the remedies thematically go hand in hand. At times these themes relate to traits that run through groups of patients and that correlate to susceptibility, including inherited and acquired disposition. When related to the influence of a particular disease process that causes a distinctive pattern of illness, not necessarily the same as the disease itself, it is referred to as a miasm (see Chapter 17). Originally in homeopathy three miasms were described, relating to the traits set up by the illnesses of scabies, gonorrhoea and syphilis, corresponding in turn to a general pattern of deficient, excessive and disordered reactivity. Some homeopaths do not accept the theory of miasms; some do not accept the concept of essence and themes – those that do, find them a useful model for understanding more deep-seated illness and what would otherwise be confusing cases.

As a patient with deep-seated illness begins to respond to treatment, so other models and approaches may become indicated. The homeopath starts to see that returning to and maintaining health is a process that may go through several stages, often using different models of health as treatment unfolds over time.

While the pathological, biological and holistic models are relatively objective the holographic model relies on the recognition of patterns that are not a random collection of events but that have a perceived order or 'intelligence' in the observer. These patterns may be connected to the typical symptoms of a disease in the case of miasms or due

to other more abstract qualities such as a theme of rigidity (Kali salts) or performance (metals). They all, however, share an element of 'subjectivity' – that is why understanding the relationship between patient and homeopath is so important (see Chapter 23). Historically homeopaths have shied away from such interpretations but increasingly they offer opportunities to perceive cases that are difficult to treat with other approaches and that can be rigorously explored using insights on perception from modern science and the therapeutic relationship from psychotherapy.

Well-Being

The pursuit of well-being often preoccupies many patients. Many wish to feel a positive sense of well-being and to 'feel healthy'. Health, however, is not something you can be separate from or 'feel'. It is easy to find patients where health, like beauty, has become an idealised state, becoming influenced, determined and promoted by prevailing fashion, markets, culture and political norms. It is perhaps why much complementary medicine is found within the beauty sector, as an attempt to counter the dominance of the narrow objective measures of health that have more to do with fitness. Health is, however, neither fitness nor beauty.

The Relational Model

'What is crucial ... is that, according to the theory of relativity, a sharp distinction between space and time cannot be maintained ... thus, since the quantum theory implies that elements that are separated in space are generally non-causally and non-locally related projections of a higher-dimensional reality, it follows that moments separated in time are also such projections of this reality.'

David Bohm, *Wholeness and the Implicate Order*

The relational model uses the principle that the health of a patient cannot be considered as separate from those things around the patient. The patient is at all times projecting onto the surrounding people and environment and the people and environment will constantly be projecting on to the patient. This leads to an approach that

Foundation

recognises and reflects on these projections, that are not just psychological but are often most accessible in the conscious and unconscious reactions of the homeopath, leading to what are here referred to as a 'reflective' approach to treatment and psychodynamic methodologies of prescribing. Here the dynamic nature of the relationship between patient and homeopath reveals important aspects of the case (that might otherwise be hidden) and informs the treatment and prescription. It is particularly useful for understanding and working with cases that may present with a single, often overwhelming, symptom such as a tumour or where a disease is diagnosed in the absence of symptoms such as hypertension. These most hidden of homeopathic cases are sometimes called 'one-sided cases' and are often treatable when using this model at a deeper level than they might otherwise be.

The relational model requires homeopaths to reflect carefully about their physical and emotional reaction to patients and to know themselves well.

Health in the Different Models
Health as Balance

Balance can be considered in a number of ways, from returning to a previous state after being 'off balance', to returning to the same state but with the ability to resist being 'knocked off balance' again. Balance may also be a state that reflects harmony, either internal, for example, balanced emotions, or external, for example, balanced diet. It may, for some, reflect a point of development, 'I'm getting more balanced', or a positive state to attain, 'I'm looking for a better work–life balance'. For others it is something only recognised when lost. In practice a homeopath works with several different notions of balance and health within different models. In the Biological model the relevant symptoms are tightly focussed around 'the illness'. At other times a broad range of symptoms including those not immediately and directly related to the presenting illness may be considered to describe balance in the holistic model of health. While each model provides a discrete view you may already be able to see where the models can 'run into' one another.

Health Compared with Fitness

Fitness is the ability to perform optimally in a set or limited situation. For example, a sports person may perform very well in one particular sport but not in another. Fitness helps you 'fit into' a particular environment or situation. You can be fit intellectually or emotionally when you are in a particular intellectual or emotional situation, but this doesn't necessarily mean you will cope if the physical, intellectual or emotional situation changes significantly. Homeopaths see many people who work hard at their fitness, including athletes, but they often have problems dealing with things like changes in their career, ageing, or bereavements. They may be fit but they are not necessarily healthy. Many patients pursue fitness rather than health, and much of the conventional health care system is focused on being fit, getting the body to work well or in balance in a given environment.

In John's case the treatments he needs may be many, depending on his choices and the models of health that are used to understand this case. How do you understand this case through the different models of health?

CASE STUDY 1.2

John enjoyed running. It helped him cope with stress. However, he started to get pain in his right knee, which he treated with an anti-inflammatory. His knee deteriorated until he required surgery. At that time he was unable to exercise, and found he was unable to cope with the stress of his job. He was diagnosed as depressed and started on antidepressants.

Health in the holistic model is the ability and potential to maintain the integrity of the organism in a changing environment. Unfortunately, much research into health care looks at the ability of an individual to perform or operate only in a particular fixed set of circumstances over a brief time. It looks at a single outcome, or at immediate changes that give a pointer towards fitness but very little information about health. This is possibly the single biggest reason why much conventional research methodology is flawed when applied to treatments used in the holistic, holographic or relational models of health.

Fitness is something that you can train and practise for in a given environment, whereas health is more difficult to prepare for – although you can anticipate some of the likely changes that will affect you, for example as you age.

Tensions Between Different Models of Health

While no one model of health will be appropriate to interpret a patient's health needs in every setting, and while several models can be used together, they do also raise various conflicts. For example, in the holistic model a homeopath sees minor challenges to a patient's health as preparation for other more serious challenges; childhood minor acute illnesses might help a patient cope with more serious illnesses in later life. Holistically it is important for some acute illness to happen and for the patient to throw it off naturally. In the pathological and biological models, if the acute illness is treated by an approach that undermines the individual's susceptibility they may, from the holistic model, end up less healthy. In some models of health it is easier to think of health as a dynamic process rather than an absolute state. In order for the body to remain healthy it has sometimes to move out of balance. When it is out of balance it can react and come back into balance. In this way being healthy includes the ability to generate symptoms and get ill.

The Importance of Illness

The moving out of balance when a situation changes is a disturbance of the organism, a *disease*. The organism, if it responds in a healthy way, generates a reaction to the disease in order to attempt to rebalance itself. While health may be noticeable and observed by the absence of symptoms, the symptoms are vital to maintaining health. Health and illness are not so much like black and white as like shadow and light. They are like two sides of the same coin. The homeopath accepts that illness

> ### CASE STUDY 1.3
> Karen has recurrent chest infections as a child. Each is treated with antibiotics. The infections get more frequent and her resistance seems to get lower. It is suggested she goes on continuous antibiotics which she is reluctant to take. She seeks a homeopathic opinion and is supported through her next few acute infections using homeopathy. Her attacks get less frequent and, over six months, her resistance to infections improves.

has to happen, that symptoms are the body's reaction to the disease. This whole process is a healthy one and leads to an enhanced and developed resistance as Karen's case illustrates.

Balancing the Subjective and Objective Views of Health

When we combine a subjective and objective view of health we notice that the observer and what is observed are connected. To distinguish between what is inside and outside the body, the patient and their environment, is artificial. In the same way one part of the individual cannot ultimately be seen as separate from another. A holistic view recognises that the different parts of an individual are intimately connected. The holographic view recognises that when one thing changes, everything else changes – nothing changes in isolation. The relational view recognises that when there is change in what is being observed there are also changes in the observer. Monitoring and working with yourself as the observer, including your personal development, is an important part of working in these models of health.

Summary of the Five Models

No one model can accurately describe what is happening in every patient but separately or in combination, they provide insight into most situations, from the most straightforward to the most complex case presentation. In applying the different models of health, the homeopath has to hold different boundaries and to use different skills.

I frequently observe homeopaths moving over time and with experience into more individual ways of working. Blending the models and choosing the most applicable approaches and methodologies in a given situation is central to developing your optimum way of working for any given patient and clinical setting.

The five models described do not exclude others that readers will find important or even vital to how they work; other authors may name or refer to them differently. Being clear about the model used helps in determining not only the optimal treatment approach but also deciding on the strengths and weaknesses of the available methodologies and interpreting rationally the outcome of any prescription.

The student of homeopathy may find ideas in the holistic, holographic and relational models raise important questions about the 'nature of man' and the relationship of the patient to their 'global' environment and the nature of illness. The focus of this book is on the health of the patient and their physical and psychological well-being. We will touch on questions related to the health of a population but I encourage you to reflect and question each other and your teachers in relation to the spiritual nature of patients and yourself. I do not seek to answer these questions but am pleased if they are asked, as I believe they can bring you to the heart of what it is to be a homeopath.

Before moving from the models of health to the homeopathic approaches to treatment, it is helpful to focus on the homeopathic patient and how illness expresses itself – particularly what is offered by an understanding of vitality in the cause and treatment of illness.

Homeopathic Patients

'The role of the homeopath is to help patients in their pursuit of health and it requires "insight, discernment, knowledge and awareness".'

Paragraph 3 Organon, Medical Art
by Dr Samuel Hahnemann

Different patients choose to work explicitly with different approaches to treatment. Some choose simply to counter a cause, others to remove a particular effect. Some patients recognise that their health is related to things that are happening in their lives that may provide opportunities for growth and development. Still others recognise their illness in terms of their susceptibility to what has gone before, including hereditary factors. Patients with these different views will seek out different ways to be healthy and choose different treatments in different situations. Part of the challenge to a homeopath is to recognise this diversity and choose which models are optimum for each condition, situation and patient. The more open a patient is to understanding and expressing their illness and health through a particular model the easier it is to use the corresponding approach to treatment.

Reframing illness

'There is a vitality, a life force, an energy, a quickening, that is translated through you into action, and because there is only one of you in all time, this expression is unique. And if you block it, it will never exist through any other medium and will be lost.'

Martha Graham

When we think of illness as having a purpose for individuals and communities, we start to 're-frame' our thoughts about it. Rather than something to be avoided at all costs illness starts to offer opportunities, and sheds light on the relationship between our inner and outer worlds. A change to a patient's outer world, such as a change in family dynamics or diet, affects the inner world, from how they think and feel to the functioning of different organs. Many patients gain, through illness, insight into how the outer world affects the inner world. Less common is the insight into how a patient's illness and health can affect individual circumstances. If illness is an opportunity to learn, then before removing an illness it is appropriate to reflect on whether what is to be learnt has been.

A definition of health and illness I invite you to consider is that 'health is the freedom to move through the different circumstances in which you find yourself and illness is the loss of that freedom'. A healthy response to illness is to make changes to yourself and, where possible, your environment to bring them back into balance. Illness is important for keeping our environment and our bodies in balance; symptoms are what exist at the interface of the patient's inner and outer worlds. The symptoms remain necessary until the inner and outer worlds are brought into balance. Understanding that a patient's inner world and outer environment are connected allows us to tell things about a patient's inner world from the environment that they desire or fear and those they actually live in.

The Life Force and Vitality

The life force is non-material and therefore sometimes described as a 'spirit-like' force or 'dynamis' that is expressed in living organisms as vitality. In today's language we might instead talk about general well-being, resistance and immunity. If you think of a living organism like an electrical machine the life force would be the battery or generator and the vitality the electric current. If you imagine it as a spinning top, the life force might be thought of as what keeps it spinning, and the vitality as the force that throws things out to the periphery, both keep it balanced and upright.

The concept of life energy is found in many other therapeutic systems, e.g. as 'chi or Qi' in traditional Chinese medicine, as 'prana' in Hinduism and 'vis medicatrix naturae' by Aristotle. When the organism is out of balance the life force that animates the body expresses itself through the vitality. The vitality stimulates the organism to re-establish balance through the production of symptoms. At the time homeopathy was formulated in the 18th century, the idea of vitalism was common, so it was not unusual to think of all living organisms as having a vital principle that energised, co-ordinated and brought together the functions of an organism. Using this terminology allowed homeopaths historically to conceptualise on a subtler level the physical, chemical and biological changes that take place in an individual when ill.

The potential energy needed to throw off an illness is similar to the way electrical energy is needed to operate an electrical appliance. The life force can be thought of as a battery that needs charging now and then and is subject to being drained; the vitality can be thought of as the current generated when the battery charge flows. In health, life force integrates and allows the different parts to co-ordinate, including normal physiological functions.

Many patients, as Paul's case illustrates, are prepared to talk about their general feelings or general energy and this is similar to what historically might have been described as vitality. It allows the body to regulate, balance and evolve and, as such, is an intrinsic quality of life connecting the separate parts of the mind and body. Much debate that reflects on the purpose of life rather than maintenance of health takes place as to whether the vitality is intrinsically intelligent with perception and creativity (free and spirit-like) or 'blind', following patterns established in the individual that it animates (instinctive).

CASE STUDY 1.4
Paul consults with a history of recurrent minor infections; he is exhausted from overwork and a 'stressful' home life. He complains of generally feeling unwell, and when asked how he would score his 'general energy' between zero and ten, says it rarely gets above four.

Vitality

Most patients have a sense of their level of vitality and it is important for the homeopath to reflect on what it does and how it is sustained, as it is

Foundation

through the vitality that individuals are able to heal themselves. It is what allows subtle homeopathic medicines to have major effects. Changes in vitality precede illness and recovery, and indicate when there is a need for the patient to be supported or to make changes to environment or lifestyle, before remedies can act fully.

Different models of health reveal different views on whether it is the vitality or the environment that is the cause of all illness. At one extreme, in the pathological model, all cause and cure could be considered to be due to external factors, e.g. it is the bacteria that cause infection. This leads to a deterministic approach to care where patients are made ill and cured by others. At the other extreme it is the susceptibility of the patient that in the holistic model invites illness, e.g. it is the host's low resistance that lets the bacteria get established. This leads to a fatalistic approach to care where nothing can be done for or to a patient unless they do it themselves.

Integrating these different models, whether as a homeopath or any therapist, is part of the art of medicine – being able to hold a balance of seeing the inside affecting the outside and the outside affecting the inside. One way to do this is to see the vitality and the patient's circumstances and environment as directly related. On the one hand the vitality enables the body to react and change its situation when out of balance; on the other hand, the vitality is nurtured and supported (if not produced) by life experiences. When an individual gets stuck in their environment, the vitality starts to stagnate and, when the individual stops completely, it is dead. This fluctuation of the vitality can be illustrated graphically through the 'vitagram'.

The Vitagram

The vitagram schematically represents the individual's vitality over time and you will see in Chapter 3 how this links to life events as a 'time line'. It is helpful for you and your patients to appreciate that the vitality or 'general well-being' fluctuates depending on what you have been doing, e.g. a poor diet or several late nights might reduce it and alter susceptibility to illness. Normally it is

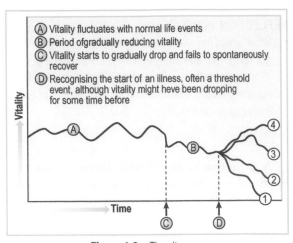

Figure 1.2   The vitagram

self-correcting and some early nights or a change in diet can improve the vitality and precede a recovery from the illness. Figure 1.2 illustrates the idea of vitality changing over time, demonstrating its gradual drop (which often is a precursor to chronic illness) and showing several common ways the vitality then changes (described below).

As the vitality drops, the individual is more susceptible to acute and recurrent acute illnesses, which is why these are often precursors of chronic illness. The four common changes to the vitality illustrated in Figure 1.2 are:

1. patients deteriorate rapidly and the vitality may drain quickly
2. the vitality may carry on draining away only slowly where they use supportive treatments
3. they temporarily stimulate their vitality but with no underlying cure they relapse
4. they may correct the imbalances of their life that have led to the low vitality or receive treatment that allows the vitality to return to its normal levels.

In order to better understand patient vitality see the reflection point below.

REFLECTION POINT
- If you are sitting in a room with someone who has a cold, what factors in you are likely to influence whether

you catch it and how does this connect to your general well-being and vitality?

- How would you score your vitality from 0 to 10, If 10 out of 10 was the highest and 0 out of 10 the lowest? What do you think improves your vitality?
- What would your 'vitagram' look like over the last 5 years? When would you think your vitality has been highest and when was it at its lowest?

The Law of Similars and Approaches to Treatment

In each model of health, the corresponding approach to treatment follows a central tenet of homeopathy, 'like treating like'. In the causation approach then using something that acts in the same direction as the cause can stimulate a healing reaction, similar to desensitising treatments for allergic illness and the stimulation of a patient's immunity by vaccination. In the symptomatic approach an acute symptom can often be appreciated as a person's way of trying to get well. For example, when a patient develops food poisoning they get diarrhoea and vomiting. This is the body's way of clearing out the food poisoning as rapidly as possible. The symptoms are the body's way of trying to return to a balanced state and the most helpful treatment works in the same direction as the symptoms. The information the body needs to rebalance itself is contained in remedies that can also cause diarrhoea and vomiting.

In the holistic model the totality approach is based on selecting a remedy that closely matches the symptom picture. It is as if the vitality produces symptoms in an effort to return the organism to a healthy state. It requires a stimulus as it has failed to resolve spontaneously. The illness is like a pendulum that has stuck. Tapping it is enough to free the gravitational pull on the pendulum to return to equilibrium. In the holographic model the pattern of symptoms expresses what the patient needs from the illness. In treatment this is met by the information available through homeopathic remedies. In the relational model the treatment approach has many similarities to 'psychodynamic' treatments that are informed by

the effect the patient has on the homeopath. The same remedies may be used in each model but are understood in different ways.

The Law of Similars is based on reliable observations that if a substance produces symptoms when taken by a healthy person, the same substance can help an ill person with a similar set of symptoms. The recording of symptoms produced when a substance is given to a healthy subject is called a proving and is explored in detail in the next chapter. Dr Samuel Hahnemann was the first to record this systematically and his life and experiments first with Cinchona bark and his thinking, as reflected in the Organon of the Medical Art, are essential study for the student of homeopathy. He observed that taking Cinchona, used at the time to treat malaria, created in a healthy person a fever similar to malaria. He successfully used Cinchona to treat fevers homeopathically and developed his thinking over six editions of the Organon.

Samuel Hahnemann (1755–1843)

Hahnemann was 35 when he conducted the experiment using Cinchona bark. At the age of 50 he published his reflections on this for the first time – 'The Medicines of Experience' – observing that medicines should be prescribed on the basis that they are similar to the disease symptoms a patient has. Medicines were chosen on the basis of the symptoms and the homeopathic remedy was known by the effect it has on healthy people (provings). In 1810 he published 'The Rational Art of Healing' – this and the second edition focus predominantly on the scientific concerns regarding the new approach to treatment. In the third, fourth and fifth editions he incorporated a more metaphysical inclination with an increasing emphasis on the doctrine of vitalism. The fourth edition introduced the theory of chronic diseases into the basic text, while in the fifth edition the dynamics of remedy preparation are discussed. The sixth edition of The Organon, written by Hahnemann in his eighties and completed the year before he died, was not published until nearly 80 years after his death and is still essential reading for all homeopathic students.

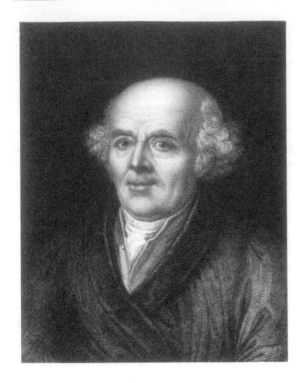

The Structure of the Sixth Edition of the Organon

There are seven main sections in the Organon and over different editions the themes of each evolved gradually. The first section is an overview of the objectives for the physician (paragraphs 1–2). The second defines homeopathy in terms of what is to be cured, what is curative in medicines and how to adapt medicines to particular patients (paragraphs 3–5). Section 3 looks at the central role that symptoms play, what the illness is and how a cure is obtained (paragraphs 6–8). In Section 4 the Law of Similars is explored – looking at how disease and medicine act dynamically and how symptoms indicate not only what treatment is needed but also, from the effects that they can produce in healthy individuals, where the curative power of the medicine lies (paragraphs 9–27).

Section 5 explores a possible mechanism of how homeopathy works in comparison with other disease treatments of the time (paragraphs 28–70). Section 6 looks at how to practise homeopathy (paragraphs 71–285) and Section 7 briefly considers the context of homeopathy in relation to other non-allopathic therapies (paragraphs 288–291) (Singer & Overbook 2004).

The idea that low doses of a similar substance could have as strong, if not stronger, effect than higher doses, and with significantly less adverse effects, he referred to as the 'minimum dose'.

The Minimum Dose

Homeopathic remedies stimulate the vital force and provide the information for the body to throw off illnesses. As the remedy is acting on a subtle level, the aim is to give the dose in an equivalent subtle form that is also the minimum effective concentration. To do this, a process of preparation known as 'potentisation' incorporating dilution and vigorous shaking (succussion) has been developed (see Chapter 20).

For some people the minimum dose has become the most characteristic feature of homeopathy, although this is incorrect. It is the process of prescribing remedies on the basis of 'like treating like' that is the most characteristic feature of homeopathy. However, Hahnemann did also observe that remedies have different effects when used in different strengths or potencies. This is reflected in the theory of hormesis, which suggests that different doses of toxins have different and at times opposite, sometimes stimulatory and sometimes inhibitory, effects (Calabrese 2001 and 2004). Different potencies often match the methodology and model of health that is being used to understand and treat a case. For example, a prescription based on causation or a single presenting symptom is more likely to require a low potency while a remedy prescribed thematically is likely to benefit from a higher potency. Of course, in many cases, more than one model and methodology may point to the same remedy.

Summary

This chapter has covered some of the core concepts of homeopathy. You may like to return to the laws of health and five models of health, both to clarify your ideas about health and illness and to help you understand the role of the homeopath in helping patients. Understanding the different views of health that patients have is an important part being a homeopath. While some methodologies will appeal to you more than others, it should be noted that some patients will only be prepared to work at certain levels and, if you are unfamiliar with the different approaches to prescribing, you will limit your effectiveness as a homeopath.

An understanding of the different models of health is also central to understanding the energetic action of the remedies and the different ways the remedy picture can be expressed and collated. Before building on this further, we look in Chapter 2 at how the information related to different remedies is expressed through provings.

References

Calabrese E J 2004 Hormesis – basic, generalizable, central to toxicology and a method to improve the risk-assessment process. Int J Occup Environ Health 10:466–467

Calabrese E J, Baldwin L A 2001 Scientific foundations. Hormesis Crit Rev Toxicol 2001 31:351–695

Singer S R, Overbook M 2004 The structure of the Organon. Homeopathy 93:151–153

Bibliography

Carlyon J 2003 Understanding homeopathy. Helios, New York

Danciger E 1987 The emergence of homeopathy. Century Hutchinson, London

Dhawle M L 1967 Principles and practice of homeopathy. Institute of Clinical Research, Mumbai

Dudgeon R 1853 Lectures on the theory and practice of homeopathy (Indian edition). B Jain, New Delhi

Gibson D M Elements of homeopathy. The British Homeopathic Association, London

Haehl R trans Wheeler M L, Grundy W H R 1922 Samuel Hahnemann: his life and work. Homeopathic Publishing Company, London, Indian edition 1995, B Jain, Delhi

Hahnemann S 1842 Organon of the medical art, 6th edn. Based on a translation by Steven Decker, edited and annotated by Wendy Brewster O'Reilly. 1995, Birdcage Books, Washington

Handley R 1990 A homeopathic love story – the story of Samuel and Melanie Hahnemann. North Atlantic Books, Berkeley

Kent J T 1900 Lectures on homeopathic philosophy. New edition 1981. North Atlantic Books, Berkeley

CHAPTER TWO

Provings

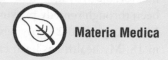

Jeremy Sherr

Introduction by David Owen

To the homeopath the remedies we use are more than just medicines. Understanding them provides a medium, through which we perceive and order the world. They provide the ideas and concepts that bring sense to a patient's story. They are not random or unnaturally 'manufactured' but represent the very world the patient lives in and are drawn from the minerals, plants and animals around us. Provings are how the information held within the remedies is revealed. The information is not secret and indeed it is expressed in many ways by the source of each remedy. However, it is the provings that rationally and minutely reveal the full picture of a remedy and as such lay the foundation to the art of case-taking and the science of case analysis. Jeremy Sherr is a leading light in the field of provings and his enthusiasm and eye for detail gives him a contemporary and relevant authority that makes his observations reliable and frequently useful in practice. To the student of homeopathy it may appear unduly technical and daunting to be talking about provings and taking part in provings at such an early stage in your study. However, before you start learning in great detail the materia medica, it is invaluable for you to understand where the information comes from. I encourage you to study Jeremy's other writings and look at some of the detailed contemporary provings that he and others have produced.

What are Homeopathic Provings?

The basic principle of homeopathy is 'like cures like'; what a medicinal substance can cause it can also cure. To ascertain what a medicine can cause, we administer it to healthy people. This experiment is called a homeopathic proving (from the German 'preufing', meaning experiment). During the proving all effects of the remedy (physical, mental and emotional) are recorded in detail. Once the experiment is over all the symptoms experienced by each volunteer are gathered into a collective record. The more comprehensive the proving, the more it represents the totality of remedy effects, which forms the basis of the materia medica. This collective totality of symptoms is used as a guide for homeopathic prescriptions. At later stages the picture is consolidated through clinical experience, and synthesised into a more concise record that may be collated with others into a materia medica.

Homeopathic remedy indications have remained effective and unchanged for the last 200 years. Beyond the scientific evaluation of medicinal effects they provide a method for homeopaths to explore and confirm their healing systems, a tool for physicians to experience their remedies and a means by which the healthy may cure the sick. They provide the most fascinating journey into nature's inner world, into our own deepest nature and our personal development.

My Experience with Provings
'The best journeys are made without ever leaving home'
Lao Tzu

I have travelled to many countries, but my most memorable voyages and greatest insights have been through remedy provings. In the last 20 years I have organised 27 provings and have participated in 18. My health has been enhanced and not damaged in any way. The personal and collective journeys into these provings have enriched, on many levels, my life and the lives of those with whom I have conducted the provings. Through them, my fellow provers and I have experienced the sting of a scorpion, the cold riches of sapphire, the opulence of jade, the cycle of salmon, the monotony of rape seed, the flight of an eagle, the enlightenment of hydrogen, the gentleness of deer, the hardness of diamond, the nurturing of olive and the rigidity of germanium. We have explored these and many other secrets from nature's treasure chest by entering into nature herself, by diving into her substances and shape shifting our beings into her mould.

In the process we have learnt, in time-honoured tradition (see Box 2.1), many things including:

- The power of the collective, experiencing the unity of a single substance influencing a large group of people providing a window into the collective consciousness of humanity (see Chapter 26).
- The need for exactness and attention to detail while organising and editing provings for publication.
- What to retain and what to discard, what is useful and what is superfluous, and how to present material in the most effective way.
- Proof of the relevance and accuracy of our experiments, as case after case has responded positively to the new remedies, based on the indications we have gathered.

The Necessity for New Provings

'Therefore, we have only to rely on the morbid phenomena which the medicines produce in the healthy body as the sole possible revelation of their in-dwelling curative power.'

S Hahnemann, *Organon, Para 21*

Provings are the pillars upon which homeopathic practice stands. Without accurate provings all prescribing indications are vague guesses at best and

---

BOX 2.1

'And further, while we were preparing the so-called old medicines we never forgot our position as explorers of the unknown world of results, of effects; never forgetting the ground-work of our healing art, we prepared from time to time new medicines also; we made a regular proving at least once a year, often twice and even three times a year. These provings were the high feasts in our church, and you cannot consider yourselves true members of it without joining in these feasts.

Proving is a most wonderful thing; the world has never known its like. We suffer, and we enjoy it; we sacrifice a little of our comfort, and gain abilities and power by it; we lose a part of a few days, and gain years of strength by it; we go to school to learn, and we increase the certainty of the healing art. At the same time, to prove drugs is of all other ways the very best, the nearest and the easiest to learn to master our materia medica. It is the way to learn; to observe the art of arts, the principal one on which all others are based.'

Constantine Hering

---

fiction at worst. The use of signatures, toxicology, clinical experience, family pictures or intellectual concepts may contribute to our understanding but they cannot approximate to the precise knowledge gained by a thorough proving.

Why More Provings?

There are billions of sick individuals, each with their own unique configuration of illness. The more precise the match between remedy and patient, the more profound the cure will be. To increase the certainty of our healing science, we need many more remedies.

A new remedy will cure a class of cases that existing remedies may only palliate. For example, many cases needing Chocolate were previously prescribed the very similar Sepia with limited success. It is likewise for Cygnus and Ignatia or Androctonus and Anacardium. To compensate for the lack of new provings, existing remedy pictures have been inaccurately expanded beyond their natural sphere of action.

Of the thousands of remedies in our materia medica, only a few hundred are well proved. Many remedy pictures are based on small and incomplete provings, toxicology, traditional herbal use or speculation. As a result they consist of common symptoms, which are of little use in prescribing, as they have too little detail to allow accurate matching to symptoms or are incomplete in areas of the body or mind, so not allowing a totality prescription.

Learning Through Provings

Taking part in provings provides great insight into the power of remedies and the various responses of our defence mechanism. It is also a practical lesson in the structure and construction of the materia medica and repertory. During the proving one gains intimate knowledge of the remedy. The remedy enters into our spirit and permeates every part of our being, just as a virus takes over a cell nucleus and directs the entire cell to its own purpose. We become the remedy and the remedy becomes us. This is the deepest level of materia medica knowledge.

Taking Part in a Proving

It is important to understand that provings can only induce symptoms which are pre-existent or latent in us. These symptoms may be from a long past or a distant future, but we are inherently capable of producing them. Thus a proving illuminates an intrinsic part of us that is yet unexplored – symptom seeds that have lain dormant within now germinate and flower.

On the simplest level, provings provide a particular stimulus to which our vital force reacts by producing symptoms. Similarly, any new experience which stimulates us to react is essentially a proving. But only the intentional uses of potencies in an experimental setting are homeopathic provings.

The difference between a proving and a crude life experience lies in the potency and force. A stimulus resulting from a crude mother tincture experience (such as vexation, vaccination, a snake bite, a movie, food poisoning or a drug) may be violent and can invoke strong or damaging symptoms. On the other hand, provings of homeopathic potencies use a dynamic force which is at once gentle and profound, and unlikely to cause any lasting damage.

Safety and Provings

'the organism of the prover becomes, by these frequent attacks on his health, all the more expert in repelling all external influences inimical to his frame and all artificial and natural morbific noxious agents, and becomes more hardened to resist everything of an injurious character, … by means of these moderate experiments on his own person with medicines. His health becomes more unalterable; he becomes more robust, as all experience shows.'
S Hahnemann, Organon, Footnote to Para 141

In all the provings I have conducted, the vast majority of provers benefited or learnt from the experience and were willing and eager to do another proving. However, it is only natural to experience apprehension before a proving. After all, one is going to experience bothersome symptoms and a change of attitude that may well be unpleasant. Provings can cause painful symptoms and may affect relationships and work.

Life is full of risks. If we take none, we will never experience new things and learn. The key is to maximise the benefits and minimise the risks. Gentle and well organised provings do precisely that. By choosing relatively healthy provers, using a minimal dose and applying close supervision while the proving lasts, the damage from provings is very small.

It is true that a small number of provers (5–10%) get stronger symptoms. Usually these symptoms do not last long, but on rare occasions I have known symptoms to continue for months. This serves to remind us that conducting a proving is no light task and should be undertaken with full care and responsibility. The safety of provers must be our main concern at all times. The proving should be discontinued if it is harmful to the subject. While there are small risks, the advantages far outweigh them. Not only does the proving create a new remedy and offer a unique learning opportunity, the stimulation of a proving actually invigorates us and increases our health and wisdom.

Types of Provings

There are many levels of proving methodology. On one hand, there is the highly organised, accurate and thorough 'full' proving. On the other, there are the casual or 'fast track' provings. Well organised and reliable provings are undertaken by a large number of people over a considerable period of time, with the purpose to fully unfold the totality of a new remedy, including physical, mental and emotional symptoms. The results are incorporated into the materia medica and repertories, making the information available for homeopathic posterity. A project such as this must naturally be undertaken with extreme care and thoroughness.

'Fast Track' Provings

The 'informal' or partial proving includes provings on oneself, a patient, or with a small study group. This is often a proving of an existing remedy. Such experiments are undertaken in order to gain direct inner experience of a remedy and are not usually intended or suitable for publication. Some provings concentrate on dreams and mental symptoms, in an endeavour to uncover the deeper meaning of the remedy. Some homeopaths conduct meditation provings, often not actually taking the remedy but just holding it. Another method is for the group to prepare a remedy by extensive trituration while paying attention to the symptoms that arise. While the advantage of fast track provings is a short cut to an inner essence, they miss many of the physical, general and long-term symptoms. Poorly prepared and conducted provings can be dangerous (and inaccurate), because they lack prover screening and long-term supervision.

By far the most frequent provings are those done by patients who inadvertently receive an inaccurate prescription, i.e. a dissimilar remedy. Such a prescription will produce proving symptoms in the sensitive patient (see Chapter 16). This is a common occurrence and a valuable source of symptoms. Unfortunately, these unintentional provings often go unnoticed or are mistaken for aggravations, random events or return of old symptoms.

Methodology of the 'Full Proving'

Creating a full proving which aims to give a comprehensive new remedy picture requires time, enthusiasm, commitment and leadership. Box 2.2 lists some of the most important factors.

BOX 2.2
The Most Important Factors in Producing a Full Proving
1. Good organisation.
2. Use provers who have studied together for a while or a group of provers who know each other. This lends a cohesion which amplifies the epidemic 'as if one person' effect.
3. Homeopaths usually make the best provers. They know what they are looking for.
4. Random provers from scattered locations produce poor provings, as do paid 'volunteers'.
5. Ensure careful and close supervision.
6. Believe what the prover tells you, however strange – it may be significant. Clinical experience will confirm or deny the symptom.
7. Hold a provers' meeting after 6–10 weeks.
8. Careful and extensive editing of the findings.
9. Attention to detail and perseverance.
10. Allow two to three months for editing and collating a proving.
11. Prepare for provers' fatigue and possible drop-out.
12. The best group size for a proving is 5–20 provers.

Relationship to Conventional Drug Trials

Some of the more conventionally minded homeopaths would like provings to emulate allopathic (Phase 2) drug trials, in a search for acceptance or total accuracy. While there are many similarities, there are also large differences.

A proving will never be 100% accurate (not that phase 2 trials are, but they strive for this impossibility). This inherent inaccuracy is a result of the many variable susceptibilities of the provers, and the huge variables of daily life. If we consider that adding an extra prover to any proving may produce a whole range of additional symptoms, while leaving out a particular prover will lose these symptoms, it becomes clear that it is impossible to have a perfect proving. The only way to resolve this would be to prove on every different type of person, but this would produce an impossible amount of information. Therefore a proving should be considered a suggestion for clinical application, rather then a final or 'complete' product.

Double Blind

While most modern provings are double blind (neither the patient nor immediate supervisor know the substance being proved), classical provings were not blinded at all, and yet they have produced very reliable results over a long period of time. Double-blind tests are supposed to compensate for bias in the observer and patient. In previous writings I suggested provings should be double-blind, but recent experience has led me to believe that it is not an essential factor in producing high quality provings.

Placebo

I and others have also suggested the use of placebo. Theoretically the placebo serves to distinguish the effects of the remedy from the effects of the proving process. According to this idea we should eliminate symptoms similar to the placebo symptoms from the proving. However it has been the repeated experience of many modern provers that the placebo produces symptoms typical of the proving. This may sound strange in conventional terms, but it is consistent with the idea of a proving being a collective infection similar to an epidemic.

This makes firm guidelines on how many provers should use placebo and how to handle symptoms from a placebo difficult to give. I tend to use placebo in 10% of provers, which serves to keep provers reflective about accuracy in the reporting of symptoms.

Choosing and Preparing the Remedy

Any substance, natural or artificial, may be used, as long as the same source is used in conjunction with this proving forever after. A substance may be selected for any reason. Often it is because of suspected medical potential, personal interest, toxicological or chemical properties. It is essential to record and verify the exact details of the original substance, such as species, gender, time when gathered, location, quantity by volume or weight, percentage and volume of alcohol, age and part of specimen, etc. In the case of a remedy made from a disease agent or tissue, precise details regarding the donor should be recorded.

In plants, one should investigate the herbal and botanical literature to discover the most potent part of the plant and the best time of gathering. It is preferable that the plant is collected from its natural environment. All substances should be as natural and free from pollution as possible. The exact mode of pharmaceutical preparation should be recorded.

The Roles in a Proving
Co-Ordinator

The co-ordinator (also called the master prover and principal investigator) is responsible for the proving – including choosing the remedy to be proved, the safety of provers, the accuracy of supervisors, and the diligence of editing and final publication. The co-ordinator oversees all the supervisors and provers, ensuring that everything is functioning properly and safely. The role includes keeping track of the dates each individual proving begins (which preferably should be around the same time so as to keep management simple) and also recording which provers are experiencing symptoms, how many doses each took, etc.

The most demanding role is the third stage of extraction, collation and editing of symptoms into the materia medica format. As the proving progresses, the co-ordinator will get to know the symptoms and develop a feel for the remedy, which will aid in the difficult process of choosing reliable symptoms.

Supervisors

'Every real medicine ... acts at all *times, under* all *circumstances, on* every *living human being, and produces in him its peculiar symptoms.'*

S Hahnemann, Organon, Para 32

Good supervision is the key to a high quality proving. Often symptoms are produced, but due to poor supervision they go unnoticed. It is the supervisor's role to identify and clarify symptoms, to separate real from random, and to encourage the prover to be diligent. The supervisor must also be alert to the prover's well-being. Consequently supervisors should have some homeopathic experience. This is a good learning opportunity for students nearing graduation. The prover's case should be taken by the supervisor prior to the proving. This is essential in order to create a baseline to compare symptoms from before and after the proving.

During the proving the supervisor takes the prover's case every day, until symptoms begin to subside and communication can be less frequent. Daily interrogation is important as provers often do not notice their symptoms or realise that they are experiencing a proving. It is often difficult to distinguish the delicate proving symptoms from daily events and life fluctuations. The prover often cannot perceive that they are changing, even when their behaviour is radically different from usual.

Provers

The prover should be in a reasonable state of dynamic health, meaning they should be able to 'bounce back' from negative situations. One should not do a proving on persons who have pathology,

serious obstacles to cure, difficult mental and emotional states and low vitality, because they lack the dynamic force to recover.

Remedy Reactions

Reactions to a proving depend mainly on the relationship between the susceptibility of the prover and the nature of the remedy proved. Other factors are potency, sensitivity, dose, repetition and timing. As the proved remedy has a random relationship to the prover, there are many possible reactions. These can be broadly divided into three main categories; the *homeopathic*, the *antipathic* (opposite) and the *allopathic* (dissimilar). It is the variety of the different effects on a large number of provers that creates a full and meaningful totality. In any proving there is a possibility that some provers will find symptoms are cured – these can be added to the proving as such. It is essential that the exact nature of the symptom prior to the cure be recorded.

In the case of antipathic action a symptom will be ameliorated first, followed by aggravation. This means that the primary action in the proving will be a sense of well-being or improvement of symptoms, followed by a worsening or aggravation of the prover's situation. In a clinical setting this would be an unfortunate result, often indicating organic pathology. However, as the prover is relatively healthy, each should be able to return to their former state once the remedy effect is over.

The third possible reaction, and the most common, is the allopathic or dissimilar reaction, which occurs when the remedy sustains no logical relationship to the prover's susceptibility. The characteristics of a dissimilar reaction are symptoms that the prover never experienced before, i.e. new symptoms. These are the most significant and reliable symptoms of a proving. Every individual will bring out a different aspect of the remedy.

Sensitivity

Some individuals are more sensitive provers than others, some are sensitive to the particular remedy and others are sensitive in general. The latter can be divided into pathologically sensitive provers, who are extremely useful provers but often difficult to cure, and healthy provers, who are very aware.

This awareness consists of a capacity to 'listen' to the gentlest changes in body and mind. Rather then pushing a proving to the extremes of suffering and pathology, provers and supervisors should become proficient at listening to these 'whispers'. Often the most important proving symptoms are brought about by one or two of the most sensitive provers, the others serving to fill out the bulk of common symptoms. Many well-known remedy keynotes and 'pictures' arise from only one or two sensitive provers. Though conventional research methodology may discount these as statistically insignificant, homeopathy considers these to be highly characteristic and extremely valuable.

Sensitive provers are also sensitive to other events taking place around them. It may be difficult to know if a prover had bad milk in their tea, or if they developed a stomach ache due to the remedy.

Seemingly Unconnected Events

During the proving particular attention should be paid to random external factors that may affect the prover, giving rise to false symptoms. These include infections, epidemics, colds, exposure to noxious influences and poisons including various forms of pollution. In addition, external physical injuries or external emotional factors such as grief, shock, fright, etc. may affect the prover, giving rise to symptoms that are unrelated to the proving. In all cases of strong external forces, or stronger dissimilar disease, it is prudent to eliminate the resulting symptoms, or even to terminate the particular proving. However one should keep an eye open for external events which re-occur in many provers, and are actually a response to the proving.

Dose

There are many diverse opinions concerning dose in provings. A study of the dose and potencies used in the history of provings reveals total inconsistency. Provings have been done with any potency from the lowest to the highest and with any dose ranging from a single dose to daily repetition over a long period of time.

As some people show symptoms easily, while others need to be pushed, I recommend a maximum of six doses over two days. If any symptom occurs, no further doses should be taken. This will generally produce a clearer proving and safeguard the prover. While symptoms are often very mild, like a delicate cobweb over one's normal consciousness, I find that at least 80% of the people developed distinct symptoms before taking all six doses, many after the first dose.

In each of my provings I have used a wide range of potencies. Occasionally after completing a proving in the lower potencies a sensitive individual can repeat the proving with a single dose of higher potency. This will produce finer and more characteristic symptoms.

Recording Proving Symptoms

The prover keeps careful notes regarding all symptoms, modalities and times using their natural language. All symptoms are identified as new, old, altered or cured. Comments and observations from friends and family are helpful; accidents and coincidences should be noted.

First Group Meeting

The group meeting is an essential part of the proving. It is also a grueling but wonderful experience. Each prover tells of their experience in detail, and supervisors comment on this. During this meeting the totality of all provers' experiences are woven together into a cohesive whole. The remedy picture is 'midwifed' into the world, and we see its face and features for the first time.

The provers' stories may well trigger awareness of many symptoms that have gone unnoticed or are attributed to 'life'. These symptoms can be extremely important, but supervisors and co-ordinators must exercise great care and discrimination when adding them. The proving meeting also serves as an important opportunity for the prover to 'discharge' the proving in a safe and supporting environment, which often feels very good to provers and allows them to come to a completion of the proving. After 6 months the provers should be contacted to check if anything else of significance has occurred.

Extraction

The prover's and supervisor's accounts are amalgamated into a single cohesive document including valid symptoms and omitting all superfluous, doubtful or irrelevant information.

Choosing Symptoms

During this stage it is essential to be precise, censorious, forgiving and sensitive simultaneously. It may be helpful to remember that many symptoms from Hahnemann's provings that seemed dubious at the time were later clinically confirmed. Extracting symptoms for a proving is a delicate and difficult task, which should be undertaken with the utmost care. With clinical experience, an annotation as to the nature of the doubt can be added.

It is also interesting to note that many of our famous keynotes, now considered leading symptoms, originated from a single occurrence in one prover. For example, the isolation of Camphor and the enlarged sensation of Platina. It is at this stage that the co-ordinators discover that good supervision constitutes 80% of the work.

Collation and Editing

The aim of this stage is to convert written diaries into materia medica format. Symptoms are scrutinised, validated or rejected, and then edited into a proving that is coherent, logical, useful and non-repetitive. The end result is more useful if it connects to how other materia medica are compiled (see Chapter 7).

During the editing careful attention should be given to retaining the original language of the prover. A delicate balance must be found between leaving in the essential and removing the superfluous. My practice during this stage is

to imagine homeopaths studying the proving in 100 years' time. They would not want too much superfluous detail, but they would want to understand the exact sensations, functions and symptoms of the prover. Cumbersome sentences and unnecessary detail should be edited for the sake of clarity. Cross references are inserted where appropriate.

Toxicological and clinical data for the substance can then be collected and added to the proving information. A pharmaceutical report and a substance report should be added. I tend to present symptoms from those who received placebo and anecdotal events in a separate section, so that the reader can decide their relevance.

Many co-ordinators strive to arrive at an essence of a remedy during this stage. To my mind it is premature to constrict the proving totality into a simple idea before having some years of experience with it. It is preferable to present the proving as a full and simple document for the unprejudiced study of the profession.

Proving symptoms also need to be added to the symptom registers, called repertories, which homeopaths use (see Chapter 9). If particular provings 'flood' the repertory with minute or repetitive symptoms it becomes imbalanced. A repertory is an index to materia medica, thus not every minor aspect of a symptom needs to be repertorised. A few years of clinical experience of the remedy can help identify the strongest and confirmed symptoms before adding them to the repertory.

Summary

Provings are a vast subject which every serious homeopath must study in detail. Some homeopaths may feel that understanding provings is irrelevant to them, but my experience is that participating in a proving is an important part of homeopathic education. Provings are the basis of homeopathy. We are fortunate to have inherited wonderful provings from our homeopathic forefathers. It is, I believe, our duty to continue this process.

Foundation

Bibliography

Hahnemann S 1842 Organon of the medical art, 6th edn. Paragraphs 105 to 145. Based on a translation by Steven Decker, edited and annotated by Wendy Brewster O'Reilly. Birdcage Books, Redmond WA. An earlier translation by Dudgeon and Boericke is also available online: www.homeopathyhome.com/reference/organon/organon.html

Kent J T 1900 Lectures on homeopathic philosophy. Ehrhart & Karl, Chicago MI. New edition 1981. North Atlantic Books, Berkeley: Lecture 28.

Sherr J 1997 The dynamics and methodology of homeopathic provings. Dynamis Books, Malvern.

For a list of modern provings and publications see *www. dynamis.edu*

CHAPTER THREE

The Homeopathic Consultation

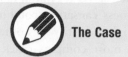 **The Case**

David Owen

'Fiction can be truer than history because it goes beyond the evidence and each of us knows from his own experience that there is something beyond the evidence.'

E M Forster, Aspects of the Novel

Introduction

We can observe the same 'truth' of the above quote in the consultation process. The written record of the consultation between doctor and patient is called the 'homeopathic case', often shortened to 'the case'. A clear case that identifies accurately 'what is wrong with the patient' leads smoothly to the case analysis where the patient and homeopath can reflect upon and explore what lies behind the patient's story, to find 'what is needed for a patient to heal'. The consultation not only records objectively symptoms and signs of the case when viewed in the pathological and biological models of health but also opens up the subjective world of the patient and explores the meaning, pattern and effect of symptoms so important in using the holistic, holographic and relational models of health.

The Homeopathic Case

This chapter focuses on the kind of case necessary for working with the pathological model of illness and identifying causation, but also identifies many core aspects to the case whatever the model or approach used. Although in some cases

causation is obvious, in others it is less so. In every case, an attempt to understand the cause will help towards knowing the 'full story' and planning the treatment, which of course may include removing a persistent causative factor, as the case of Jan illustrates.

CASE STUDY 3.1

Jan, aged 38, had a small patch of eczema in the midline below her umbilicus. This was really irritating her, having been present on and off for 12 years. She had used low strength hydrocortisone cream to treat it, and although this had helped, its effect didn't last, so she wanted to find an alternative. Around the time the eczema started, she had taken up riding horses. The eczema was occasionally better in the winter, and also when she had been away on holiday for more than a couple of weeks when she hadn't been riding. In the past, she had noticed that she reacted with a skin irritation to some jewellery. At consultation, we wondered whether her problem was due to nickel allergy, rather than a true eczema. She was advised to make sure that she wore some clothing between the nickel buckles and clasps on her jodhpurs and her skin. Since then she has had no further problem with her eczema.

At the simplest level consciously reflecting on causation often allows a patient to remove or reduce a cause of a simple problem. At the next level many patients find it an easy way to treat themselves for minor ailments. In more established illness causation combined with local symptoms might identify a homeopathic treatment. Even in more complex cases identifying causation can point towards, or away from, different remedies.

Jan in the case above remained clear of dermatitis but three years later presented with a profuse sinusitis and a non-infective irritating vaginal discharge. At this time she discussed a previous genital infection with gonorrhoea when she was aged 25 that had been treated with antibiotics. This was a deeper cause that informed a prescription based on essence. The deeper cause was connected and consistent with a pattern or what might appear as a spiral of causes that included the gonorrhoea, the skin sensitivity, sinusitis and vaginal discharge.

Understanding the patient's 'case' is intimately connected to our understanding of homeopathic philosophy and the homeopathic remedies. As we study the various remedy pictures, so we gain insights into the variety of possible causes and symptoms that can affect each of us. For example, understanding the different remedies that have anger in their picture allows us to understand how anger can be a cause and how different patients contain or express their anger. In practice there is invariably a connection between the cause and the effect. For example, Nux Vomica is a remedy that gets competitive, it will be susceptible to being irritated by the slightest sense of failure and will be hypersensitive to criticism. By studying the variety of symptom pictures described in the remedy provings it expands the homeopath's 'vocabulary' and improves the ability to hear and describe what is happening to a patient.

We can know a lot about philosophy and be aware of many remedies but if we lack the proper skills to take the patient's case, we will fail to prescribe the most appropriate remedy. Knowledge of homeopathic philosophy, awareness of the different remedy pictures and skill in taking the patient's case are all part of understanding a patient. When the homeopath's knowledge, awareness and skill are developed and in balance, a patient's treatment will often be clear.

Causation and the Models of Health

Although causation may be an indicator for treatment in its own right, it may also be part of any approach to treatment. Cause and effect are frequently described together and can be understood in relation to their interactions (like a story). Several different causes can contribute to more complex cases that can sometimes be best understood within the context of the whole patient in their historical and biographical context. A pattern of causes often reveals themes that run through a case that might be expressed in a way that brings out the fundamental pattern in the narrative. In the homeopathic relationship understanding what is projected and what this causes is key to appreciating the fundamental sensations and feelings that arise in the patient and homeopath as part of the relationship between them.

The Patient's Story

A core skill of the homeopath is to assist the patient in telling their story. At the simplest level the patient's story is 'I get these symptoms when this happens to me'. This level of association by the patient may explain the causes of many minor ailments. Some of the best known and easiest to use homeopathic remedies are used to treat simple causation in this way, as Carol's case illustrates.

CASE STUDY 3.2

Carol, a 48-year-old mother of three, fell four weeks ago while ice-skating with her children. She had rib pain that settled over 24 hours with painkillers. After a week, she started to get severe pain over the right side of her chest, where she had knocked herself. This was enough to suggest the remedy Arnica, but further confidence in the prescription was possible because she described the pain as 'an inner bruise' much worse from any pressure or touch, and she couldn't bear her children or husband coming near her in case they touched her right side. Arnica is a remedy prescribed for blunt injury where there are associated features of tenderness and aggravation from touch. Interestingly, after Arnica a bruise came up, suggesting the starting of a natural healing process.

The remedy Arnica is often referred to as a 'trauma remedy', meaning that the symptom picture that people develop after a trauma often requires the remedy Arnica. This is called the Arnica state. Matching the 'remedy state' to the 'patient's case' on the basis of similar is homeopathy.

Levels of Causation

In most straightforward cases the causes most connected to the presenting symptoms will usually point to the remedy. As cases get more complicated frequently the causes run deeper, often involving a hierarchy of causes that in confused cases can be difficult to see and might only gradually be revealed as a patient moves through a course of treatment. The most obvious association between apparent cause and effect doesn't always describe fully what is happening; contrast the previous case of Carol with Jane's apparently similar case.

It can be helpful to think of an individual organism as having features that are expressed at different depths, or within a successive number of shells like Russian dolls one inside the other (see Chapter 6). The homeopath, like a good biographer, wants to reveal what is happening at different layers in a person's life. Different layers often require different interviewing styles (see Chapter 13). The homeopath is looking for the appropriate depth of cause for the layer the patient has suffered on, as in the case of James.

CASE STUDY 3.3

Jane, age 75, presented with chest pain following a road accident. She had been driving slowly with her husband as a passenger when she hit the car ahead. The steering wheel hit her chest, and it was exactly here that she first experienced pain. Her husband's face was badly cut, which required him to stay in hospital overnight. Jane was very anxious and was prescribed tranquillisers to help her sleep. When I saw her, Arnica had not helped. Although the pain was a problem for her, much worse was her fear. Since the accident, she had not driven as she was frightened of something else happening to her husband. For her, it was the shock that required treating, and after taking the remedy Aconite, she made a speedy recovery. (Aconite is a remedy prescribed for fear, which includes the features of rapid onset after shock.)

CASE STUDY 3.4

James, 13, had always been susceptible to accidents. At these times, his parents had often given him much Arnica, with good effect. One day he presented with pain over the ribs, diagnosed as costochondritis, following a fall while skiing some time ago. Although Arnica had helped him, he still had some pain. On taking the case at a follow-up appointment, James explained that he thought he deserved the pain. At this point in the consultation his mother comforted him by putting her arm around him, covering with her hand the point where he felt most pain. His mother commented that James had been especially cuddly, needing physical affection since the birth of his younger sister. Encouraging James to talk about his feelings enabled him to talk about his jealousy towards his sister and feelings of insecurity at school that came across as shyness. The remedy Pulsatilla was chosen on the basis of his jealousy and his shyness with need and desire for affection. After this not only did his pain get better, but he also reported feeling happier and more confident in himself. Interestingly he also became less accident prone.

Foundation

There may be several different but concurrent causes such as a physical injury and an emotional shock; ordering these according to the different aspects of the case can be considered as a hierarchy of causation. In some patients the deeper causes may be painful to recall, and the symptoms themselves may be how the patient has avoided, denied or contained the causation. For example, a patient with a gastric ulcer might develop an aversion to foods that upset them, or a patient who has been bullied and is upset by conflict might seek to avoid confrontation, blame themselves for their problems and develop low self-esteem. This might attract bullies and so the hierarchy becomes a repeated pattern of causation so often observed in deep-seated cases.

In acute cases, the trigger event is often a major factor in the remedy state the individual has developed and therefore helps in choosing the prescription the patient is likely to need.

Causative factors are just as important in the psychological realm. Sometimes an initial causation can trigger a reaction that goes through several different stages. For example, after a grief, the patient may go through stages of shock, denial, sadness, anger, exhaustion, etc. A healthy group reaction would involve the patient moving through each of these over a period of time, but if the patient becomes stuck in any of them, they are likely to develop problems. By understanding the homeopathic materia medica for different grief remedies, we are able to hear the patient's story of their grief in more detail. In which state the patient gets stuck will determine which remedy they are likely to need and will be influenced not only by the nature of the causation but by their experience of previous loss, their susceptibility and the support that they have. We begin to see that it can be quite appropriate to move into a remedy state for a period of time as a way of reacting to a particular environment or situation, but it is when the patient gets stuck in this state that it becomes a problem and that a remedy is required.

Different patients have different susceptibilities to different causes. Some, if they are strong enough, will put many patients into a particular remedy state. For example, for many people, if they experience severe enough blunt injury, they will enter into the Arnica remedy state. This is important to remember, as a strong causation can, even with deep-seated symptoms, be the main indicator to the remedy. Significant illnesses can be caused by this sort of causation, for example after radiation poisoning, of course not all of them are easily reversible with homeopathic remedies. In Chapter 6 we explore how the susceptibility of the individual determines the causes that the patient is susceptible to and in Chapter 10 we explore how a population can be susceptible to, for example, an epidemic.

REFLECTION POINT
- Think of a significant life event you have experienced. How did it affect you and what did those symptoms mean to you? Has it left you more sensitive to other life-events like this? How might it have affected a different person in a different way?

Sometimes the causation of certain symptoms only becomes apparent through reflection on the case. At other times, the case becomes clear in the context of more general life events, the 'biopathography', which is orientated particularly towards a biographical or autobiographic view of the evolution of the patient's health history. When we seek to understand the case at deeper levels, and to understand recurrent or chronic disease, the evolution and change of symptoms over time is important, especially where one symptom is clearly the cause of another. In some cases, the cause can best be understood as a physical event in the patient's life; in others, it can better be seen in terms of the environment of the patient, or in psychological terms. Causation is frequently mirrored in the patient's physical and psychological state as well as the environment.

The Narrative

'Somewhere between the first year and final year of medical education, undergraduate students exchange a narrative facility for eliciting and appreciating patients' narratives for the learned experience of constructing a medical history.'

Interview skills of first-year medical students.

The story, when we record it meaningfully, is more memorable than a simple sequential record of events. Told from the patient's perspective, it becomes a 'narrative', carrying with it something of the patient's place in the world and what it means to the patient.

When relating to the patient through hearing the narrative, the homeopath begins to 'enter into' the patient's life. In the relational model of health the dynamic between the patient and homeopath is an important part of the 'living narrative' of the patient and connects with the living narrative of the homeopath. How this shapes the quality of the therapeutic relationship and the importance of monitoring our own processes when hearing a case is explored in Chapters 23 and 25. For example, when James (Case Study 3.4) talked about his pain and his mother comforted him I noticed that I felt sad. This prompted me to ask about his feelings and it alerted me to notice how his mother touched him.

Understanding and recording the patient's case as a narrative gives far more information than just documenting the symptoms. It allows us to glimpse an order and pattern behind the case that can itself lead to a prescription, or it can provide essential information to start exploring the case at deeper levels. While we want to record the events as they happen to the patient, we also want to understand the themes behind the events in the same way as we seek to understand the plot behind a story. If we record that James fell and hurt himself, it is an accurate description of what happened. It tells us the event but not much about what lies behind it. If we say that James kept falling and hurting himself, and the pain was his way of getting sympathy, then this reveals a theme and starts to reveal the narrative.

While a patient's story can be understood as a sequence of different causes and effects, and each cause might point to a different remedy, in the patient's case as a narrative a fuller description comes about when we can see the events connected to each other. The case may be better described in terms of the pattern running through it, sometimes expressed as the essence or a theme of the case.

The Language of the Case

In recording the narrative the patient's own words are important. There is a balance between using the patient's exact words to anchor the case in the patient's reality, and recording a superficial but quick summary of the case that may fail to reveal an underlying pattern or order. A good balance is to include some of the patient's phrases and dialogue verbatim, so that if you were reading a case to a colleague they would get a sense of who the patient was. Some words a patient uses can be easily summarised whereas important 'feeling' words can describe more complicated aspects of the case. For example words with emotional intensity behind them like 'sad', 'guilty', etc. can immediately connect to deeper experiences in the patient's life.

It is helpful to record any significant actions, including repetitive movements, as they can reinforce what is said and provide non-verbal clues to the case. Some young children and pets can't use words and so a fuller description of their behaviour, especially their interaction with parents or owners, can communicate aspects of their story. Some patients will respond quite differently in different company, and the observations and comments of a parent, spouse, sibling or work colleague can shed light on aspects of the patient that might not otherwise be revealed. Box 3.1 summarises some of these key points of the dynamic process of homeopathic case taking.

BOX 3.1
Key Points on the Homeopathic Case
- An important aspect of the homeopath's job is to enable the patient to tell their story fully
- Only when we have taken an accurate case can we know what is to be cured
- It is more than a simple record of events, it is more than a story with memorable themes, and it is more than a narrative grounded in the patient's experience – it is all of these together, including the patient's and homeopath's reflections

- The case allows us to see not only what is there, but also to start to see below the surface, to see the cause
- Several causes may exist as several layers
- It is helpful to have your own homeopathic case taken
- Reflect on your perception, openness, accuracy and precision in listening to and recording patients

When we talk about a patient being a certain remedy type, like a 'Pulsatilla type', we are using our knowledge of the materia medica and the language of the materia medica to sum up whole areas of a patient's case. We need to be aware of the risks involved in 'pigeon holing' a patient, or trying to extrapolate a certain behaviour into how they might act in all situations.

The Time Line

Using causation, we can usefully describe a patient's health in terms of life events and symptoms, and record the case as a 'time line' by noting when symptoms develop. Consider the time line in Ben's case (Case Study 3.5) illustrated in Figure 3.1.

In order to treat this case we can focus on the acute episode, the recurrent pattern, the trigger event, or any combination of these. Where the case is focused will depend on the patient, the homeopath and the circumstances of the consulta-

tion. For example, a parent treating Ben at home might suggest a 'right sided, sore throat' remedy for the acute picture. A homeopath, in a short consultation or over the phone, may prescribe a remedy based on the flushed and startled appearance of the patient, and the experienced homeopath, with more time, may explore the 'never well since' theme. In each scenario, the prescription is likely to be the remedy Belladonna, but the match of remedy to symptoms over the 'time line' gives the homeopath much greater confidence of a deep acting result, and the concurrence of remedy at each level informs our choice of strength (potency) of prescription.

CASE STUDY 3.5

Ben, age 9, presented with an acute fever and sore throat, worse on the right side. He flushed easily on exertion and had a startled look. He had enlarged cervical lymph glands since his tonsils were removed at age 5, and had been getting recurrent sore throats ever since a bout of scarlet fever aged 2.

It is surprising how often key events in the pathogenesis of illness are frequently not volunteered by the patient, and the information only surfaces when asking about other events. Ben's parents were surprised when they recognised that in fact he had never completely recovered from scarlet fever. The 'time line' also has a relationship with the changes in his vitality (see Chapter 1) and sheds light on how a patient might improve after the correct remedy, curing firstly the fever, then the lymphadenopathy and finally the recurrent sore throats. To the homeopath the direction of cure follows what is referred to as laws of cure (see Chapter 6).

Early causes are not always the most deep-seated and sometimes the patterns or cycle of causes are more important than just the order in which they happen. The type of causes an individual is susceptible to and the pattern or hierarchy of causes is often an important aspect of difficult cases.

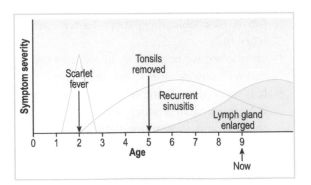

Figure 3.1 Time line used to understand Ben's symptoms

The Homeopathic Consultation

When the patient and homeopath are alert and attentive, the consultation changes in subtle ways as the therapeutic process begins.

In an ideal world every case would express all the available information. The reality is that not every patient is able, or wants, to show every aspect of themselves or their problem, no environment is equally conducive to hearing every case and not every homeopath is perceptive to all of every case. In each homeopathic consultation, especially as deeper aspects of the case are sought, the factors affecting the patient, the doctor and the consulting environment need to be considered. These three aspects of the consultation interact and as the homeopath becomes more experienced each develops a range of styles to suit different consultations.

The Consulting Room

The consulting room needs to be a place where the patient and homeopath feel at ease but focused, in 'relaxed attention', where both can feel present and receptive to each other. For the patient to relax and trust in the consultation, he must be allowed adequate time to say what needs to be said and not be worried about being overheard or interrupted.

Practically, there need to be comfortable seats and provision to record the history, as well as access to repertories and materia medica. On occasions family members will attend and although it can add something to the recall of the history it can also inhibit the patient and homeopath. In more in-depth cases, having some time alone with the patient (unless a parent is required by a child) is recommended.

Different environments will help or hinder different patients and this must be taken into account. For example Kim, a Pulsatilla child, is shy and relatively difficult to get to talk in a stuffy room with little natural light.

Some patients and homeopaths will enjoy sitting face-to-face, others prefer a more oblique sitting angle. Some are more comfortable with a desk between them, others without a desk or with the desk to one side. Some patients feel more comfortable in the middle of the room, others near a wall or in a corner. With two or three different chairs in different places in the consulting room it is surprising how much can be told about a patient and how the consultation can be helped by which they choose. One helpful exercise is to think about how the patient experiences the consultation; try sitting in the patient's chair and when studying different remedies imagine how each might feel in different environments.

Time

The time necessary to take a homeopathic case will vary depending on the homeopath and treatment approach, the patient and their complaint. Too short a consultation time is often given as the limiting factor to understanding a patient in a consultation. Whilst this is true in some cases it is possible in just a very brief amount of time to understand a great deal about patients.

It is a matter of planning the consultation so that the case can be covered in the time available; expectations need to be set appropriately for each consultation. It is important when treating complex cases to see the case building over a series of consultations and using a semi-structured record for the case can facilitate adding information to the case over several consultations.

The Patient

Some patients are much more likely to reveal their case to you than others; this in itself reflects their remedy state. Some patients are closed to all types of homeopath, such as patients needing Natrum muriaticum; others, like Phosphorous, are open to most homeopaths (see Kim and Sarah's Case Study, 3.6). Many patients can be open or closed depending on you, the environment, the type of symptoms being described and how they feel when you see them.

CASE STUDY 3.6

Kim, age 15, presents with menstrual problems. Initially she is very shy. At her second visit she is more open and talks about feelings. She responds to Pulsatilla. Sarah, age 16, has similar problems; she also is shy and remains reluctant to reveal much about her personal life. She steers the consultation away from anything personal or to do with feelings. She responds to Sepia.

When the consultation involves a third party, a parent or partner, or, in veterinary practice, an owner, it is always coloured by them. Sometimes the colour can add to the picture, e.g. the sharing of something the patient might not have noticed or been able to express; sometimes it distorts, like the behaviour of a child with a dominant and controlling parent. Many patients hide aspects of themselves if they feel ashamed or judged by others. For example, patients may deny recreational drug use or excess alcohol consumption. Certain remedy types feel a pressure to act, behave and look 'normal'; a strong need to belong and be liked might colour how they dress or what they reveal, for example about food preferences or their sexual orientation.

Factors in the Homeopath

How homeopaths interpret what is heard in a consultation will be coloured by their own state and affect what they consider relevant. For some cases and in some methodologies this is more often a problem than in others. The more insight the homeopath has into his or her own state and the more experience of working with these they have, the less problematic are the inevitable projections between homeopath and patient that accompany all relationships. It may explain why certain patients needing particular remedies are difficult to perceive accurately for some homeopaths. When supervising homeopaths, it is common for each homeopath at times to find some remedies hard to recognise and to go through

times when they see some remedies particularly frequently. These remedies often reveal much about the homeopath's condition. Ultimately the better you know yourself, the clearer your reference point and the easier it will be to gain insight into diverse and different people.

Listening Skills

One of the important skills or competences of any health practitioner is being alert, to be attentive to the patient and to themselves. It is surprising how often homeopaths having difficulties with the consultation find it difficult to pay attention to what the patient is saying. Frequently in these consultations the patient's details are hard to recall in detail. When this starts to happen it is important to re-engage with the patient. As with most skills, it is possible to develop your ability to concentrate and be attentive; the exercises in Box 3.2 will help.

At your first encounter with a patient you receive far more information than you can register consciously or record (and they also receive much information about you). By developing your attentiveness you will find it easier to invite the patient to be fully present. One of the commonest barriers to being alert to the patient is the health practitioner having strong feelings themselves and this can include being overwhelmed by feelings of vulnerability, shock, threat and even, we have to say, repulsion and attraction. When these feelings surface it is important to analyse why they are there – commonly it is because the practitioner has unmet needs or makes judgements about the patient, or professional boundaries are not in place.

Note-Taking and Record-Keeping

'He writes everything down with the very same expressions used by the patient and his relations. The physician keeps silent, allowing them to say all they have to say without interruption, unless they stray off to side issues. Only let the physician admonish them to speak slowly right at the outset so that, in writing down what is necessary, he can follow the speaker.'

S Hahnemann, Organon, 6th edition

BOX 3.2
Exercises to Help the Health Practitioner to be Alert and Attentive

- Focus on the first two minutes of a recent meeting with someone, either a patient or socially. Think about how they arrived, what was the atmosphere like when they arrived?
- What might have been influencing how they felt before you met them?
- How did you look when you first saw them?
- How did they carry themselves, where did they sit, how were they dressed?
- Describe their complexion, their breathing, and the colours they were wearing
- What other senses can you use to describe them? Did you touch them when you shook hands? What was the texture of the skin like? Was there any odour?
- If you think about them hard can you imagine, in any way, what it is like to be them? What would help you do this – can you sit like them, hold yourself like them, and are there any ways your life is like theirs?
- Can you imagine what their life is like?
- Think about this exercise and why you chose the person you did
- What people or types of people might you find this a difficult exercise to do with?
- Why are these people difficult to do this exercise with, and what does this tell you about yourself?
- If you saw them as patients how might you adjust your work to help you stay alert?

BOX 3.3
Some Practical Hints on Recording the Case

- Leave sufficient margins on both sides
- In the left margin make notations on the history and add additional objective information as it surfaces or later on in subsequent consultations. This can include the patient's expression or movements.
- In the right margin identify different themes running through the history and any speculative thoughts, including remedies, that surface and cannot be dismissed
- Place one symptom on alternate lines so that you can return later to add information about that symptom
- Make references to texts, whether repertories or materia medica, in one or other margin or in different coloured ink so they can be noted at follow-up
- Use quotes for actual phrases used by the patient that describe central features of the case or more peculiar or unusual symptoms
- Ask the patient to bring a small photograph of themselves with them at their first appointment. Having this in their file provides an instant reminder of them if you have to analyse the case away from them or when speaking on the phone to them.

There is a tension between recording what the patient says verbatim and summarising the key points, themes and observations that run through the case and also being seen to give the patient your full attention. Both are necessary and both have their place. While a straight transcript of a case may hold a full record of what was said, it won't necessarily indicate where the emphasis was

in the consultation, e.g. a patient talking about her father while making fists of her hands, or someone talking about a bereavement, and saying that it didn't affect them, while holding their throat.

The best record is one that most accurately sums up what was observed in the consultation; including what the homeopath was able to perceive even if the patient was not conscious of it. Too much writing can be at the expense of eye contact and observation, and may adversely affect the consultation. Box 3.3 suggests some practical hints on recording the case.

REFLECTION POINT

- What are you most confident about in your case taking and how have you developed that confidence? What opportunities do you have to take cases and to monitor and receive feedback on your technique? Have you considered observing yourself on video, asking a friend to give you feedback or had your case taken by a colleague?
- Do you find certain patients easier to work with than others? If so how can you modify your technique and consulting room to help these patients tell their story?
- What is important to you for creating a space where you feel comfortable and where you would feel comfortable if you were coming in as a patient?

Summary

As we explore the homeopathic consultation throughout the book we will see how the patient's story interfaces with the doctor's story and how the way we understand a case is helped and hindered by our understanding of the homeopathic remedies and the language we use. Although we separate out the philosophy, remedies, case and analysis in order to make them more manageable the practice of homeopathy intertwines each of these. Depending on the treatment approach we use we will focus on the history in different ways. When the patient has told the story, we naturally turn to ordering and prioritising the information through the process of case analysis.

Bibliography

Greenhalgh T, Hurwitz B 1998 Narrative-based medicine. BMJ Books, London

Mitchell A, Cormack M 1998 The therapeutic relationship in complementary health care. Churchill Livingstone, Edinburgh

CHAPTER FOUR

Assessing the Homeopathic Case 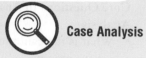 Case Analysis

David Owen

Introduction

When a close enough match of remedy to patient is made the alchemy of healing takes place.

Case analysis brings together the philosophy, the knowledge of homeopathic remedies and the case. It aims to address important questions that need to be asked before treating any patient. It includes, but is far from just, selecting an approach to treatment and applying a methodology to match a patient to a remedy on the basis of similars. Case analysis encompasses aspects of understanding why something has happened, attaching meaning, defining the patient and how they relate to their environment and to others. The ability to carry this out is a major factor in determining the competence of a homeopath.

This chapter looks at these broader issues of case analysis before exploring treatment based on causation, sometimes referred to as aetiological prescribing. Aetiological prescribing, such as Arnica for blunt injury, is a useful methodology to start prescribing for many minor ailments and is often where a homeopath starts to gain experience. However it is just one of many different methodologies covered in this book; which of these the homeopath is able to work with will determine the patients and conditions the homeopath can prescribe accurately for.

The Core Principles of Case Analysis

In many 'straightforward cases' it is possible to go straight to making a prescription and much of what is discussed below is part of an unconscious process. If when you start prescribing you take an overview of the patient's treatment and case analysis, then when you start to treat more complex cases there is a structure to return to. The structure I am inviting you to consider is a series of questions, as outlined in Box 4.1. Each represents a stage in the process of case analysis. It is helpful to answer these in every case but the more difficult the case the more important it becomes not only to finding the homeopathic remedy but also to the patient's overall management.

In practice as the case and analysis unfolds these questions represent stages of the case and analyses. The answers to each overlap and form part of the overall analyses of the case. At times, especially in straightforward cases, some of the answers are self evident, at others the clarification of one stage informs and leads onto subsequent stages. Figure 4.1 illustrates these stages as part of a cycle that in turn informs the optimum management of cases (see Chapter 15). Although you might choose to do some of the analysis at a time when the patient is not with you the consultation is not truly over until each of these stages has been completed and, where appropriate, the answers

Foundation

BOX 4.1

Core Questions to Answer as Part of Case Analysis

- What is the causation and are maintaining causes present?
- What does the case tell us about the patient's vitality?
- How 'stuck' is the case in terms of duration and depth?
- What is the conventional diagnosis or differential diagnosis of the patient?
- What is the model or models of health that give the best impression of how and why the illness has developed?
- What approaches to treatment are available in a particular case?
- According to what methodology or mix of methodologies is a remedy most reliably prescribed?
- How 'well indicated' is a remedy – including confirmatory and exclusion factors?
- What are the likely and possible outcomes?
- What general management factors must the patient and the homeopath take into account?
- Is there a clear understanding of the illness and is there an agreement with the patient about the treatment being offered and its duration?
- When is the treatment best reviewed and how will response to treatment be assessed?

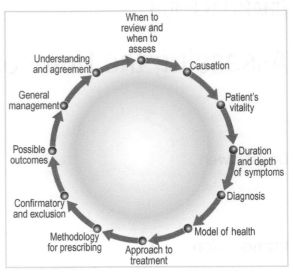

Figure 4.1   The cycle of case analysis

communicated to the patient. Failing to do these steps or communicate them is, I suspect, one of the main reasons why some homeopaths find it difficult to move from a theoretical understanding of homeopathy to practising successfully.

What is the Causation and are Maintaining Causes Present?

Identifying causal, contributing and associated factors, even when there are several different factors, is an important part of any case analysis. It is

very helpful to know what was happening to the patient when the illness started. The stronger the link between causation and illness, the more likely looking at the pathological model of health and relying on the causation approach to treatment will lead to a successful prescription. The more likely that a specific causation is to cause an illness in all patients then the more successful a treatment based on that causation is likely to be – if, of course, a treatment for that causation is known.

There is a range of causative factors, from the transient, through those that are easily changeable to others that appear fixed. They include environmental factors such as pollution and life style factors like diet. When there are fixed or maintaining causes, then the approach to treatment needs to take this into account, as in the case of James.

CASE STUDY 4.1

James presents with headaches, he drinks very little but when he drinks more water his headaches are better. He has ample opportunity to drink but just does not want to. In this case it may be appropriate to understand and possibly prescribe on the patient's lack of thirst rather than prescribe on just the head pain.

At times the illness a patient gets is a way of identifying, for the patient, what the causes are. Removing the symptoms without addressing the cause is the commonest sort of suppression and invariably leads to the illness being expressed through other symptoms. Before attempting to remove symptoms it is always appropriate to reflect on what the cause is and if it needs treating – even if this is only one factor in the eventual treatment given. For example, if we choose to give a remedy that reduces the irritating cough of a smoker without supporting the patient to stop smoking, then this may lead to a deeper illness. If instead he is given treatment that helps him deal with why he smokes, perhaps a stressful emotional environment or issue related to self-image, then the cure is likely to be at a deeper layer. For this reason reflecting on the cause is one of the foundations of effective case analysis.

Maintaining Causes

In many acute, first aid and home treatment situations the causative factors are only temporary. In more chronic illness it is not uncommon for causation to be ongoing, a 'maintaining cause'. This often needs to be dealt with as part of the curative process, as in Peter's case.

One of the tasks of case analysis is to identify specific causative factors from the past and to

---

CASE STUDY 4.2

Peter presented with headaches that were linked to stress at work. Natrum muriaticum fitted the cause and symptoms of the headache but the remedy and treatment also helped him talk about a problem that he had been 'bottling up'.

---

identify maintaining causes. For example, if we see a patient with a blister on their foot, there is little point treating the blister unless we check the patient's shoes and advise a change of footwear if that is the cause. In chronic illness poor nutritional intake and psychological stress are common maintaining causes and many patients require

basic dietary advice and emotional support. In this way the role of the homeopath, as with any health practitioner, is more than just the application of a technique and includes helping the patient become aware of possible causative factors and to find different ways to deal with or approach the causations.

What does the Case Tell us About the Patient's Vitality?

An important step in analysing any case is to gather an idea of how high or low a patient's vitality is. It will influence at what depth the case is treated and where the treatment is directed. If the vitality is low treatment might first focus on reducing the maintaining causes and building the patient up.

A basic level of fitness with good sleep pattern and a harmonious emotional environment are good indicators of reasonable vitality, as is the patient's own subjective assessment of 'general energy'. Without adequate vitality the cause may be uncertain, the symptom picture unclear, much of the holistic picture obscured and other approaches unreliable. In treating cases with low vitality it often takes a longer time to get a complete picture, as the vitality needs to increase before the case can be seen more clearly. It is usual to find that as the treatment progresses so the vitality increases. Therefore assessing change in vitality is an important part of any follow-up, as it may inform the next stage of treatment.

How 'Stuck' is the Case in Terms of Duration and Depth?

The development of a case, including its duration and how numerous and how clear its symptoms are, will help to reveal how 'stuck' it is. When a case is stuck symptoms have less clarity and change slowly, with fewer individualising symptoms. The more stuck symptoms are the more likely they are to relate to structural changes in the body and less likely they are to be symptoms of sensation (see Chapter 6 for Perspectives of depth).

When a case is stuck it is often linked to a low vitality in the patient that may be due to factors in the patient's personal circumstances, past medical history, lifestyle, environment or relationships – so-called obstacles to cure. In such cases the patient's resistance to the illness is low and recovery is slow or hindered. There are parallels between how stuck a case is and how open each patient is to making life style changes, perhaps as a consequence of how little they believe they can get better. To engage these patients and get them to see illness as more than the presenting complaint and to comply with treatments that are more than 'a pill for every ill', is part of the challenge that needs to be considered by the homeopath in the case analyses.

What is the Conventional Diagnosis or Differential Diagnosis of the Patient?

Homeopathic texts make full use of standard medical terminology, unlike some other complementary therapeutic systems such as traditional Chinese medicine. Homeopaths that are not also medical doctors sometimes find their training does not prepare them for the sound anatomical, physiological, biochemical and psychological understanding of health that the biological, pathological and holistic models of health require. A case analysis usefully includes, where possible, a medical diagnosis, but with additional information. This sometimes, misleadingly, leads to homeopaths that are doctors separating out the case into medical and homeopathic aspects that can limit the perception of the case in the relational and holographic models of health.

A diagnosis gives several benefits to the patient and homeopath. First, it gives the patient information about the different treatment options available and the ability to make informed choices. Second, it points to what the likely natural history or prognosis of the disease is going to be. It is only by having an idea of what is likely to happen with no intervention that the homeopath can accurately assess what has happened following a prescription. Third, it does, with inherent limitations, allow comparison of different treatments in different patients – although the limiting of treatment regimes to suit a diagnostic label rather than

a patient has been a significant cause of the dumbing down of medicine. Fourth, it eases communication with other health carers.

What is the Model or Models of Health that Give the Best Impression of How and Why the Illness has Developed?

Describing the 'who, what and where' of an illness is the main aim of the homeopathic case. Finding the 'how and why' is intimately connected to this and the main aim of the case analysis.

Different therapeutic systems work within different belief systems using different assumptions about health that describe different models of health. While no one model is likely to fit every patient in every situation, a collection of models of health that fundamentally share the same basic laws can, as experience has shown, work in many patients in many cultural belief systems over many generations. While some schools of homeopathic thinking often favour a particular model of health and approach to treatment, for the homeopath able to move between models of health, the opportunities exist to select a model that makes sense of a patient's illness when others do not. The varieties of models that are described in this book create the possibility of an eclectic homeopathic profession that could become a mainstream provider and maintainer of health. Which model of health to use depends on the patient and the illness, the homeopath and their preferences, and the social and cultural norms they work in.

The attraction of homeopathy as an eclectic system is that each model of health relies in part on the same philosophy, the same remedies and a connected understanding of the case. It is possible to move between and combine, cautiously, the different approaches to treatment based on what the patient and homeopath find acceptable and relevant. Sometimes it is very clear which model is most appropriate, for example, often in acute straightforward cases the biological model may suit best. In cases where there may be multiple different organs involved, a holistic model might be indicated. In others where the illness may be hidden behind one main presenting feature, the relational or thematic approach may suit. Sue's case illustrates how the agreement on what model of health to use can change.

CASE STUDY 4.3

Sue presented with twins just under 2 years old and was finding it 'hard to cope' with her hectic life. She had been used to 'being in control of my life' and to having 'protected time' for herself and her relationship with her husband. She wanted help for cramps in the calves that came on at night. She was reluctant to take conventional medicines and wondered if homeopathy might help but found it hard to talk about her feelings. Sue wanted a specific remedy for night cramps and Cuprum metallicum prescribed on the presenting symptom gave relief when taken nightly but the improvement relapsed once she stopped taking it.

At a follow-up appointment Sue discussed her feelings of heightened anxiety and panic attacks that started after the twins were born and about which she felt ashamed. It was agreed to treat her holistically and a constitutional match to Sepia was made. This helped her feel better in herself and the cramps gradually ceased.

What Approaches to Treatment are Available in a Particular Case?

In many cases the model of health, approach to treatment and methodology for prescribing each complement one another. The benefit of separating out the treatment approach is that it may include many treatment suggestions, of which a homeopathic prescription is just one. There are different homeopathic treatment approaches possible within each model of health. Deciding which treatment approach you are going to use will influence not only the methodology you follow to choose the remedy (simillimum) but will also determine other aspects of the case analysis and the treatment plan i.e. it allows treatments to be explicitly matched to a particular view of what is

taking place in the case. For example treatment might include advice on avoiding a maintaining cause, and a prescription based on a holistic view that incorporates the presenting symptoms. However in some cases it is not so straightforward. There may be clear causation but no known remedy for that causation, or there may be a sense of a clear theme or essence but no remedy the homeopath knows for this.

Planning the treatment does not require a fixed course of action as the plan may be revisited frequently, but in the same way an illness is understood in the context of how it has evolved over time, a treatment is planned in the context of how a cure is achieved through what might be thought of as a 'journey back to wellness'. In many cases the health of the patient and the disease can be perceived in a number of different ways. A plan of treatment might involve several stages of homeopathic prescribing and other treatment modalities, as well as including how to deal with obstacles to cure using lifestyle advice.

According to What Methodology or Mix of Methodologies is a Remedy Most Reliably Prescribed?

The underlying principal behind all methodologies is to find as close a match as possible between what is being treated in the patient's state and the known materia medica. The experienced homeopath is able to move between different methods of prescribing fluidly and easily, maintaining an awareness of where the different methodologies overlap and how they may be combined to lead to the best prescription. If we aim to treat patients from the most straightforward home ailment to the most complicated deep-seated pathology, there is no doubt that we are going to need a range of methodologies. Add to this the patient's preference to work in different ways with different people and we can see that no one methodology will provide the optimum prescription in every case.

In more deep-seated conditions often the best remedy is one that is indicated by several methodologies. This has led to several established 'formulas' for prescribing, such as using key symptoms and essence. Each methodology will have its own benefits and limitations – understanding these will inform the homeopath about the likely outcome of taking a remedy. If the likely outcome of each methodology is known then when several remedies are indicated the homeopath is helped in making an informed choice between them.

How 'Well Indicated' is a Remedy, Including Confirmatory or Exclusion Factors?

In any homeopathic case there can be several possible homeopathic medicines indicated. Some homeopaths talk about a single simillimum to a case, others that there are a range of similars – some closer than others (Kent 1926). Using different views of the remedy and case preferred remedies may appear more strongly or weakly indicated. While ideally the same remedy will be indicated by several different models of health, frequently this is not the case. Similarly a single methodology often points to several close remedies and how well indicated, or not, a remedy is by other methodologies may confirm or exclude a remedy. A remedy confirmed in this way is more likely to give a positive outcome. Knowing the materia medica of likely remedies is essential in recognising what features confirm a possible prescription and what features relatively contraindicate it. The most useful information about remedies that confirm or contradict a prescription is often the most unique or strongest features of a remedy, referred to as the keynotes of a remedy (see Chapter 7).

From several indicated remedies a 'best indicated remedy' that is the strongest match between the case and the remedies can be chosen.

What are the Likely and Possible Outcomes?

After identifying the best indicated remedy the likely outcomes need to be considered. It is at this point that the strength of any prescription – referred to in homeopathy as the 'potency' – and the regime for taking the remedy need to be decided. Although ultimately the patient can only get better, worse or stay the same, there are several ways these things happen. Reflecting on these before prescribing can often ease the patient's overall care and may in some cases lead to reviewing the prescription so that a better-tolerated

outcome is achieved. For example, different remedies in different strengths and taken in different regimes have different durations of action and have different likelihood of causing an aggravation (see Chapter 16). There are many patients who have given up on treatment or changed homeopath after a perfectly good prescription because the outcomes were not considered or explained – including patients who have relapsed and failed to take a repeat prescription, patients who have given up because a remedy is only acting slowly and patients who have not tolerated an aggravation. In these cases careful consideration of the remedy, the potency and the prescribing regimes, along with considering the correct information and explanation to give to the patient, are a vital part of the analysis and management.

Many patients view the effect of a homeopathic prescription as similar to conventional medicines as both frequently involve 'taking a medicine'. If you document and assess the outcomes you expect (there are several ways of 'scoring' outcomes - see pages 321 and 322) it gives you and the patient important feedback. Remember outcomes do not just have to be about frequency and severity of presenting symptoms but can also be about 'general well being', 'energy' and 'vitality'. These outcomes can often more realistically indicate progress in more deep-seated illnesses and give valuable information about choice of potency, frequency of administration and indications to change a remedy.

What General Management Factors Must the Patient and the Homeopath Take into Account?

There are several general management points that need to be considered along with the case analysis. These are the broader questions relating to a patient's treatment and include the possibilities of a remedy being antidoted, the general advice appropriate to a patient receiving homeopathic treatment and consideration of any other medicine that has been or may be required for the patient – including conventional medication or other treatments. Other general management issues include the need to document the diagnosis, advice and treatment, and to correspond with other carers to improve care, or when ethically indicated or when legally required. These and other broader management issues to be discussed later become increasingly important as the homeopath starts treating more serious illnesses.

Is There a Clear Understanding of the Illness and is There an Agreement with the Patient About Treatment and Duration of Treatment Being Offered?

Summarising the model of health, plan of any treatment and the methodologies used to prescribe, and getting agreement from the patient on this basis, as part of the analyses, is good practice. If there is no agreement or if the patient offers information that means the analysis needs to be modified then this can be taken into account and the relevant steps repeated.

This agreement includes informing the patient about the need for reviewing the treatment and that a course of treatment, in more complex cases, is likely to involve several consultations and prescriptions. While this agreement may be quite informal it should be recognised that it forms the basis of the 'contract' between patient and homeopath. If this agreement is not reached then the expectations of the patient and homeopath are likely to be different. So, for example, the patient may just wish to be rid of a troublesome symptom while the homeopath is seeing the symptom only as an alarm bell of more deep-seated illness. In later chapters the contract and its importance, in particular to the therapeutic relationship, are revisited.

When is Treatment Best Reviewed and How will Response to Treatment be Assessed?

The end of any case analysis process is clarifying what follow-up is required and setting the framework for this. It may include being explicit about expectations, so the treatment can be meaningfully reviewed. Although a full analysis does not need to take place at every consultation, steps in the process will need revisiting. The review of treatment is not only important for the patient but also for the homeopath. How a case progresses and remedies act or fail to act in a case must be moni-

BOX 4.2
Reflection on the Core Principles of Case Analysis

- Case analysis is a way of seeking 'meaning' to a case, whether in terms of external causation, an illness, susceptibility, a personal story or in relation to others. It is informed by knowledge of philosophy, the materia medica, and the case.
- The 'meaning' describes something of the journey the patient has taken with the illness and points to the journey to wellness. In anything other than the most straightforward of illnesses this is likely to be a process that 'unfolds' over time.
- Patients and their symptoms can be understood using different models of health, several of which can be used concurrently. They will determine the optimum approaches to treatment and this will indicate the most suitable methodologies to select an indicated remedy.
- Remedies are homeopathic when prescribed according to homeopathic principles applied through a homeopathic process of matching like with like.

tored in order to inform the homeopath. Even if the patient does not attend for follow-up some feedback on the treatment should be part of the agreement so that the homeopath may monitor and develop the way that it works. Before moving on you might like to reflect on how the case analysis seeks and allows communication of the meaning behind a case and treatment given.

Having looked at the broad issues involved in assessing a homeopathic case that apply to all case analyses, it is appropriate in this chapter to focus on the more specific issues that apply particularly to cases viewed within the pathological model of health and that are suitable for treatment based on causation. Before moving on you might like to reflect on how the case analysis seeks and allows communication of the meaning behind a case and treatment given.

Assessing Cases Using Causation

A cause is an event that gives an outcome. In homeopathy we observe many causative events but it is the degree of association between cause and outcome that determines how useful treating on causation is. When there is a high degree of association, we talk about causation. When there is less, we talk about causal or contributory factors and when slight, we might just notice it as an association. For example, dermatitis may have a contact sensitivity, e.g. to nickel (causation), a contributory factor like stress, or an association, worse in colder weather. In identifying the degree of causation, the symptom and cause need to be considered together – this is illustrated by Sam's case.

CASE STUDY 4.4

Sam, age 5 months, presented with discomfort during and after feeding that had been going on since starting to wean at 4 months. After eating he becomes distressed, curls up and is relieved by passing wind or from firm pressure over the abdomen (better 'from being carried over the shoulder'). On taking the history it transpired that he would occasionally have these colicky type symptoms, even when breastfed, if the mother had eaten strong tasting food such as onions or curries. Colocynthis, made from bitter cucumber, was prescribed mainly on the causation 'after eating' but also on the feature 'better from pressure'. Sam's colic settled down and his mother started introducing a range of foods that were well tolerated.

Knowing the Causation in Remedies

In Sam's case you can imagine why bitter cucumber produces proving symptoms that include colic. Interestingly there are also high levels of magnesium in this plant and remedies made from magnesium salts also work well in colic. Given the

role of magnesium in muscle contraction it is not surprising. So, although causation can point to a specific remedy it can also point to a group of remedies and while several may help, a more individual prescription is possible if the symptoms, like 'better from pressure', are taken into account.

Those factors, such as 'better from pressure', which modify symptoms are collectively known as modalities – some modalities hint at causation and the degree of association between cause and symptom. When a patient is unable to describe the detail of a symptom then causation can be particularly useful, e.g. in veterinary practice or in babies, as Victoria's case illustrates.

CASE STUDY 4.5

Victoria, Sam's twin sister, has not been bothered by colic unduly and tends to eat and breast feed in a more relaxed and less speedy fashion than Sam. However, Victoria does suffer from a worsening of her behaviour and a break out of dermatitis when teething. She becomes irritable and unpleasant towards her brother, pushes away her mother and father who try to comfort her and develops an itchy rash. Victoria had a dramatic improvement after being prescribed Chamomilla on the basis of causation from teething and it is commonly prepared as 'teething granules'.

While the symptoms are common features of teething, it would, on the basis of causation, be possible to consider Chamomilla for any onset after teething or indeed where pain and discomfort is caused in a patient and the patient is unable to rationalise the cause or see it coming to an end.

In most cases where the pathological model of health is the best to understand the case, either the illness is acute and the vitality is high (and the case unlikely to be stuck) or, in chronic illness, the link between causation and the patient's illness has been demonstrated in other patients and other models of health do not give a contradictory picture.

Treating Cases on Causation

Causation is most likely to be a useful strategy when the strength of the causative relationship is strong, e.g. if most people exposed to that causative factor would get that symptom. In later chapters we explore how to match the appropriate prescribing methodology to the depth of the case.

Dosage and Potency

Choosing the best indicated remedy is the aim of all case analyses. At the same time a choice also needs to be made on the treatment regime and dosage. Some remedies may be prescribed frequently, others as a single dose. Generally as the homeopath moves from a less confident to a more confident prescription, and as the criteria used to select the remedy match at a deeper and in a more fundamental way to the case, so a higher potency is given. As a higher potency is given it is usually repeated less frequently – this is explored in detail in Chapter 20. As a rough guide most simple and straightforward cases prescribed on causation and presenting symptoms will be treated with 'lower potencies' such as the 6 or 12 or 30 potencies. In more complex cases, prescribed for on holistic, thematic or relational grounds, a higher potency of 200, 1M or higher is often recommended. See Chapter 10 for discussion of simple and complex cases.

Acute Illness

Many first aid and trauma remedies are prescribed on a basis of causation or a combination of causation and presenting symptoms. However, it is important to note that when not all patients respond to the cause in the same way they are likely to need a remedy based more on the symptoms. Box 4.3 illustrates some causes and the corresponding remedies.

Chronic Illness

In more chronic illness the causation is less likely to cause the same symptoms in every case and so other approaches are more likely to be required – although treating on causation may provide a suitable starting place until the case becomes clearer. While understanding the aetiology will

---

BOX 4.3
Some Causes and the Corresponding Remedies

• Bruising from blunt injury	Arnica
• Cough from getting cold and wet	Aconite
• Itch from insect bite	Ledum or Apis
• Diarrhoea from food poisoning	Arsenicum Album
• Hangover from alcohol excess	Nux Vomica
• Sunburn from sun	Sol
• Hay fever from pollen	Mixed Pollen
• Insomnia from caffeine	Coffea

CASE STUDY 4.6

Philip, aged 28, presented with fatigue for 12 years. At times it improved only to relapse after exertion or upper respiratory tract infections, which he was very slow to throw off. At 16 he had glandular fever and although no-one has suggested that this was linked to his chronic fatigue, he felt that his energy had never been the same since. The glandular fever coincided with his school exams, which he was unwell for, and he struggled to progress academically afterwards. There were options to treat Philip based on the presenting symptoms of his acute flare-ups following upper respiratory tract infections or more generally on the fatigue. The decision was made, based on previous experience, to prescribe Carcinosin, a remedy that has a specific causation of glandular fever and has a reputation for helping cases that present having 'never been well since' glandular fever. One month after two doses of Carcinosin his energy was starting to improve. Gradually his well-being improved and his susceptibility to recurrent infections decreased. Three years after the initial presentation he returned with signs of fatigue that had come on following exertion during preparation for a marathon run. A further dose of Carcinosin helped him.

automatically suggest a cause – for example the use of remedies made from allergens for allergic conditions (pollen in hay fever) or remedies made from infective agents – they do not always match the case at the deepest or most appropriate layer, as Philip's case illustrates.

The link between chronic fatigue and the increased prevalence of glandular fever raises many questions. What environmental factors might affect a patient's susceptibility? Is the glandular fever the primary cause or are there other causes precipitating the glandular fever and making the patient susceptible? Why does it happen so frequently in teenage years? Why do some patients 'throw off' the glandular fever better than others? So there are many questions raised when doing a case analysis of more deep-seated conditions. In all but the most basic prescription on causation these broader management issues need to be considered.

Levels of Causation

It is possible to see cause at a number of levels. In an infection there might be factors that lead to exposure and increase the susceptibility to the infection. For example, in malaria is it the swamp, the mosquito or the malarial parasite that is causative? In many conditions a number of causes might be contributing and only those that point to remedies that can be confirmed might be considered.

In these cases the best indicated remedy is likely to match several of the causes and/or the susceptibility of the patient. For example, in post-natal depression there may be a cause from the birth, the mother's loss of independence, the surfacing of the mother's previously unresolved 'mother' issues, tiredness, hormonal imbalance, or strong emotions of fear, anger or failure about the birth. Any one of these might point to the remedy Sepia but the prescription is only likely to act deeply if it fits several of these and it will act at a deeper level if it fits the underlying susceptibility.

The concept of susceptibility is explored in more detail in Chapter 6 and throughout Section II. However, it raises an important point that

should be considered along with causation. Each patient has their own susceptibility – some will be shared with many others, such as the susceptibility to blunt injury or high-dose radiation, some will be more personal, such as sensitivity to a particular pollen. However, every patient will have certain situations where they get ill – by studying these situations we gain insight into our patients and by proving the homeopathic remedies on susceptible patients we build up our materia medica.

REFLECTION POINT

- What do you think the connection is between cause and susceptibility and provings and illness?

Summary

At the end of the case analysis the homeopath will have worked through a thought process and series of decisions about the case and its treatment. The process will, in part, depend on your level of knowledge of homeopathic principles and materia medica. Depending on the decisions you and the patient make about the treatment you will be clear on the 'context' of the treatment, including the role of other carers. As you understand more about homeopathy you will have greater choice of methodologies available to you, as well as a wider range of materia medica that will 'come alive' for you. In many cases the patient's priorities and understanding of the illness will inform the eventual methodology and prescription.

Much benefit can be obtained using homeopathy following a causative or symptomatic approach – especially in home prescribing, treatment of minor remedies, or indeed more serious and complex cases where the full picture may only become clear after preliminary treatment informed by causation. In parallel with exploring the different approaches to prescribing it is important to think about the practical considerations of prescribing including remedy strength, potency, administration, storage, availability and pharmacy. These are addressed in Chapter 20. Reflecting on these issues brings up questions relating to competence and broad issues about clinical management that are developed in the next chapter.

References

Kent J T 1926 Lesser writings. Ehrart & Karl, Chicago

Bibliography

Foubister D 1988 Tutorials on homeopathy. Beaconsfield Publishers, Beaconsfield

Jack R A F 2001 Homeopathy in general practice. Beaconsfield Publishers, Beaconsfield

Watson I 1991 A guide to the methodologies of homeopathy. Cutting Edge Publications, Kendal

CHAPTER FIVE

Introduction to Prescribing

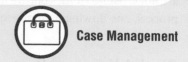 **Case Management**

David Owen

Introduction

Every treatment has its time.

This chapter explores putting the foundations and basic principles described in previous chapters into practice. Although these principles allow the most deep-seated illness to be treated homeopathically we started initially looking at more straightforward and easy prescriptions, which is where most homeopaths start their prescribing. Homeopathy means 'like cures like' (*similia similibus curentur*); essentially a patient's case is matched to a remedy picture leading to a prescription of a remedy. There are, however, different views of both patients and remedies that lead to different approaches and methodologies to find a prescription. This chapter explores the main approaches to treatment and methodologies of prescribing connected to the five models of health previously described, and goes on to look in more detail at the methodologies based on the causative approach and pathogenic view of health. In other management chapters the relevant approaches and methodologies are covered in more detail, although a brief summary to orientate the student to these different approaches is given here. It leads on to important questions about how different approaches and methodologies can be combined in practice and questions what information and competencies are needed to work at different levels of illness.

The management advice in this book is at all times intended as advisory rather than proscriptive. Homeopathy is a tool (a body of knowledge and experience) that may be used in many ways and in many settings. It can be practiced in homes, pharmacies, as part of family or general practice, in dedicated homeopathic practice, as part of a integrated practice along with other therapies and in veterinary surgeries. Consultations may be momentary or last several hours, but in every setting the practitioner develops by learning from every patient and every treatment. The more unexpected the outcome the more important the lesson, so cases that do not respond can teach as much, if not more, than those that do.

The acceptance of, and comfort and competence in using different models of health to understand and treat patients will depend not only on the homeopath's personal view but on how members of a community view their own lives and connections to others. The practice of homeopathy is more than just the prescription of a remedy. Its contribution does not just depend on how much it is used or the latest research but it expresses core beliefs and values that are important in understanding that the health of any individual is not static but always shifting – in the same way that the health of a population, community, society or culture is always changing. While throughout this book the focus is on treatment of the individual, this cannot be separated from the broader public health considerations (see Chapter 30).

When you have thoroughly assessed the homeopathic patient you have already given them much information feedback and advice that will be helpful in understanding and treating their condition. The next step is to make the homeopathic prescription and undertake to care for and treat patients. These are not separate entities but are in practice a seamless process, one flowing naturally into the other.

Straightforward Prescriptions – Minor Ailments and First Aid Situations

A straightforward prescription is one where the case is clear, the analysis is not complicated and the prescription is well indicated. Usually these are cases that do not have too many levels to them and where the layers of illness are few. In practice this often means acute illness in an otherwise well individual, with good vitality and who has not had or is not having too much other medication that might distort the presenting picture. Frequently in straightforward cases if anyone were exposed to that particular cause they would get the same symptoms. It makes sense to start one's clinical practice with such cases even though these are also often the cases that will heal spontaneously in time.

Many minor ailments and first aid situations present straightforward cases where the indicated remedy is clear and it is only necessary to prescribe superficially. The potential benefit to patients being able to treat themselves in this way is huge, for example a patient able to take a remedy quickly after trauma or at the earliest stage in a cold. The criteria that make this approach more likely to help are listed in Box 5.1.

This approach can also lend itself to a busy practice of other health care professions whether it is the use of Arnica by midwives or osteopaths or the use of one or two remedies with a clear cystitis picture in family practice. There are a small range of homeopathic remedies that can help in many different first aid and minor ailments. One of the easiest ways of working in this way is to be familiar with the causes and presenting symptoms of each and to give them when a patient presents a recognisable match. There are many homeopathic first aid kits that contain some of these remedies so they are immediately available for use. Often homeopathic patients use these to help treat problems in the

> **BOX 5.1**
> **Criteria That Make Easy Prescribing More Successful**
> - A patient with clear symptoms
> - A patient with clear causation but no ongoing causes
> - Likely remedies known well
> - A patient with high vitality
> - A patient with only minor ailments
> - An illness of short duration
> - No other treatment having been taken
> - Immediate access to the remedies so treatment can be started early

home and they are hugely preferable to treatment with the analgesics, anti-inflammatories, antipyretics, etc. that make up so much of conventional home treatments. By helping the patient to throw off minor ailments, many cases of more serious illness can be avoided and it prevents the harm caused by straightforward cases treated inappropriately with strong drugs leading to the development of more deep-seated problems. Treatment is often successful in these cases and the proportion of conditions that you will be able to treat in this way depends on the number of remedies you know.

Patients will find a number of books that can help them treat minor ailments for example in Dr Lockie's *The family guide to homeopathy* or his *Encyclopedia of Homeopathy*.

Methodologies of Prescribing Within Each Approach to Treatment

The homeopathic student will realise that many minor ailments can be helped with homeopathy, and this will avoid a patient's symptoms being suppressed and leading to more serious illness. Limiting the treatment you offer to a certain range of cases is an important way of working within your competence; it is obvious that by knowing more homeopathic remedies and understanding those you know better, you can treat more patients and gradually those with more serious illnesses. However, expanding the knowledge of remedies is, as we are already seeing, only part of a homeopath's training. Another key factor in managing patients is in understanding and being able to utilise the rich matrix of methodologies for selecting a remedy. The homeopath aims from these different methodologies to have an individualised management strategy for treating every patient. While this comes in part from experience, it is important to have a theoretical overview of the different methodologies.

Figure 5.1 gives a diagrammatic illustration of the five main approaches to treatment from the different perspectives of the 'disease', the patient and the homeopath. Where the causative approach uses the external cause of the disease, the symptomatic uses the expression of the disease directly on the patient. The totality is the overall expression of the illness through the whole patient and the constitution expresses the susceptibility. The essence approach uses the expression of the case through the interface between the patient and homeopath. The pattern of changes in the whole affects every symptom, and so the essence and themes in every part reflect the essence or themes in the whole. The relational approach uses the expression of the patient onto their world or, in the context of homeopathic treatment, onto you – the homeopath.

The causative, the symptomatic and the totality approaches are well described historically. The essence and thematic approach, based on the holographic model, and the reflective approach, based on the relational model, have more recently become major methodologies. While they can significantly improve the treatment of difficult cases, they are offered without the same historic validation that the first three approaches carry or even the same standard acceptance of the terminology. Figure 5.1 illustrates how within the paradigm of 'homeopath treating a patient suffering from a disease', the homeopath's view incorporates and is informed by the patient's state. The patient's state incorporates and is informed by the realm of the disease as an entity. As you move from the causative outwards, each approach is naturally informed by and incorporates aspects of the previous approaches.

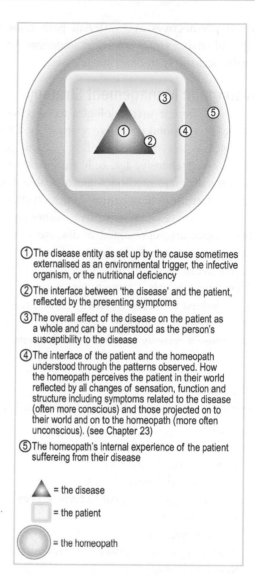

① The disease entity as set up by the cause sometimes externalised as an environmental trigger, the infective organism, or the nutritional deficiency

② The interface between 'the disease' and the patient, reflected by the presenting symptoms

③ The overall effect of the disease on the patient as a whole and can be understood as the person's susceptibility to the disease

④ The interface of the patient and the homeopath understood through the patterns observed. How the homeopath perceives the patient in their world reflected by all changes of sensation, function and structure including symptoms related to the disease (often more conscious) and those projected on to their world and on to the homeopath (more often unconscious). (see Chapter 23)

⑤ The homeopath's internal experience of the patient suffereing from their disease

▲ = the disease

☐ = the patient

◯ = the homeopath

Figure 5.1 Five main approaches to treatment from the perspectives of the 'disease' the patient and the homeopath

Subjectivity Verses Objectivity

When the homeopath moves from the pathogenic to the relational models of health, and therefore from the causative to reflective approaches, so the perspective will shift from the more objective to the more subjective (see Chapter 23). Each view has its own balance of subjectivity and objectivity and which view the homeopath finds it easiest to work with will be influenced by their own comfort and training. In practice being able to move between different perspectives and different paradigms of health will enable you to perceive, understand and prescribe accurately in many more cases.

A Systematic Management Strategy

The many different methodologies to selecting a remedy cluster around these five approaches. These methodologies are outlined in Box 5.2 but they are not a comprehensive list, only an indication of some of the different methodologies available. Each is presented in more detail either in this chapter or subsequent 'management' chapters. Although the methodologies are represented as discrete ways of matching a remedy to a patient there is a degree of overlap between them and in practice several may be used to point towards a remedy (or group of remedies) or indeed to direct you away from a remedy partially indicated by another methodology. So you might choose a remedy as it has both the aetiology

and presenting symptoms of a case or not use it if it fails to match the totality or constitution.

The analogy of trying to find someone in a crowd might help understand these different approaches. Imagine you were looking for someone in a crowd. Causation might use where they joined the crowd. Symptomatic might use where in the crowd they were last seen or where they were heading. Totality might describe what you remember of what they are wearing. Constitution might describe their general and facial appearance. Essence might describe why they are likely to be there and who they are likely to be next to. A reflective approach might use what you know of them and if you were them where you would go to in the crowd.

Given these approaches you might like to imagine you were actually looking for someone in a crowd and to think what method you might use to look for them. For example you might try to

---

BOX 5.2

Key Methodologies to Prescribing Within Five Main Approaches to Treatment

Causation
- Trigger event or aetiology
- Isopathy and tautopathy
- Nosodes and family history
- Anticipating causes, prophylaxis or preventative treatment
- Maintaining cause
- Detox, organ and drainage treatmentl
- Never well since

Presenting Symptoms
- Local or clinical prescribing
- Single main symptom
- Single keynotes
- Several keynotes in one or more areas of the case
- The complete symptom
- Epidemic remedies
- Doublet or triplet symptoms, linked symptoms
- Previous well indicated remedy
- Combination remedies
- Strange, rare and peculiar
- Confirmatory and contradictory symptoms
- Symptoms 'As if. . .'

Totality/Constitution
- All physical, mental and general symptoms
- Three-legged stool
- A mix of physical, mental and general keynotes
- Physical and psychological type
- Central disturbance

Essence
- Miasmatic
- Categories of remedies
- Remedy families and kingdoms
- Types of essence
- Related remedies (see Chapter 27)
- Herd prescribing (see Chapter 18)
- Using fundamental sensation or feelings in the patient

Reflective
- Psychodynamic using feelings generated in the homeopath by the patient (see Chapter 29)
- Intuitive

retrace their likely steps, to wait in a certain place to see if they come past you, to find one feature of clothing that stands out etc. In practice you may use several, which ones determined by the size and the intensity of the crowd, the time you have, how well you know them (representative of both the case and remedies) and your perspective (if you are taller you might find some methods easier).

Some homeopathic teachers describe and classify the methodologies differently, and while for the student homeopath this is confusing it illustrates the variety of views and methodologies available. However, to compare them and develop them for yourself, a model in which to think of them, such as the one in Box 5.2, is important. It is hoped that the homeopath inquiring scientifically into these methodologies will remain aware that one methodology is not isolated from any other, they are not an exclusive list and that the art of homeopathy requires a palette of methodologies that different homeopaths will mix in different ways to suit different patients.

REFLECTION POINT

- Reflect on what the different words used to name each methodology mean to you in the light of what has been covered in this section so far. How might each tell you something different about a patient and their health?

Which is Most Homeopathic?

In every case there are different assumptions that are made to allow us to observe patients, identify their illness and suggest treatments.

It is valid to use homeopathy in any of these ways but each has its own strengths and limitations. Throughout this book I try to refer consistently to these approaches and methodologies with the aim of helping you develop a familiarity with a range of approaches and methodologies while appreciating that what homeopathy can offer is bigger than any one. In some patients, the best remedy may be indicated by more than one approach or methodology. In other patients several different remedies may be indicated by one methodology and a choice made between them.

Each methodology invites you to look at your patient's and your own world in a slightly different way. There is therefore a process of personal development for the homeopath who wishes to become competent in a wide range of approaches. A preference by groups of homeopaths for some of these different approaches and methodologies rather than others accounts for the different schools of thought within homeopathy.

An important practical consideration is that each of the different methodologies differs in the information used to select the homeopathic remedy. They each have a slightly different emphasis on what is the most relevant part of the case history, and they look at slightly different information in the materia medica. They lend themselves to different practice settings, and prescriptions often used in different potency and with different intervals of repetition of dose. They each bring slightly different expectations and are likely to give different outcomes. While not wanting to restrict the homeopath's choice of approach or methodology some student homeopaths might find it easier to develop and build their approaches to treatment and methodologies for prescribing by stages.

Treating Causation

Understanding causation can point to many interventions in addition to the other homeopathic methodologies. An overwhelming infection will point to the need to control the infective organism. Onset after a physical trauma such as a whiplash injury might point to a manipulative treatment of the spine, or orthopaedic intervention. In addition, life style changes might be indicated to remove maintaining causes. Remembering to consider other treatments reminds the homeopath of the importance of the context of general health care and maintenance in which you work, not just as a prescribing technician. You might like to reflect on the broader management that is indicated in Anne's case (Case Study 5.1).

Trigger Events

Many remedies are renowned for their trigger events or causative factors, and working with this model it is always worth asking when studying the

CASE STUDY 5.1

Anne, age 27, has a cough that keeps recurring. She uses regular cough linctus that helps her sleep. She has an underlying asthmatic element that is aggravated by dust mite and animal dander. Anne is helped by isopathic treatment of her dust mite sensitivity by using a homeopathic preparation of her known allergens. She fails to make a further improvement from homeopathic treatment based on other approaches. She eventually finds another home for her pets, takes steps to minimise inhalant allergens and her cough stops.

CASE STUDY 5.2

Jill (28), a hairdresser, presented with dermatitis of the hands aggravated by her work. After several unsuccessful prescriptions using different methodologies, the skin improved temporarily using the remedy Castor Equi, made from the rudimentary thumbnail of the horse. Following this Jill obtained more significant benefit with a remedy prepared from a mix of different human hairs. If she repeated this monthly she was able to carry on cutting hair.

homeopathic remedies, 'what factors are likely to cause illness in patients needing this remedy?'. Often in more complex cases a mix of causes might be present. In others the causation is summed up as the patient being 'never well since' something happened. How confidently this methodology points to the best remedy, like any other, depends on the depth of the case and the extent other methodologies confirm the remedy.

Isopathy and Tautopathy

One method of treatment on the basis of causation is to focus on the use of medicines derived from pathogenic agents of the disease or from a product of the disease process, e.g. allergens, infective organisms, infected tissue or discharges. This is collectively known as isopathy and is one of the easiest ways of prescribing. Homeopaths differ in whether the selection of medicines on the principle of identical (as isopathy is sometimes referred to), rather than similar criteria make it less 'homeopathic'. There are many cases where it can ease symptoms or help a clearer picture emerge even if it does not cure. But in more deep-seated cases the benefits will often be limited in scope and duration.

Examples of isopathic treatment include the treatment of shoe leather, chlorine or nickel sensitivity with remedies made from leather, chlorine or nickel respectively. Jill's case illustrates

a simple prescription that helped in a case that did not initially improve with more complicated methodologies.

Tautopathy is a type of isopathy where the causative agent is a conventional drug, where the adverse effects point to their range of action and they can be helpful when prepared homeopathically in treating iatrogenic disease or in reducing adverse effects. For example, a potency of a vaccine can help 'unlock' a case of vaccine damage. In more complex cases a previous or concurrent prescription of a conventional drug can prevent a case responding to a deeper-acting remedy. In these cases a tautopathic prescription of the drug in potency can make a significant difference to the case and allow another methodology to be used, allowing a deeper remedy to be seen clearly or to act more fully. We will return to how drugs can act as an 'obstacle to cure' in Chapter 15.

Another situation where this methodology can help is in patients seeking assistance in reducing conventional medication, for example in the withdrawal of benzodiazepines, where careful tautopathic doses can reduce the severity and duration of withdrawal effects. Isopathic medicines can also be used for the reduction of recreational drugs, e.g. nicotine, amphetamines and hallucinogenic drugs – although these conditions should only be treated when a more general appreciation of homeopathy has been gained so that reactions to prescriptions can be fully understood. If the conventional or recreational drug is still being taken the benefits are unlikely to be significant or long lasting. Some remedies used isopathically have been proved and a fuller picture of their materia medica is known, which allows them to be selected according to other methodologies in addition to causation, as the case of Lydia illustrates.

CASE STUDY 5.3

Lydia, who is 35, presented with palpitations that had been present for 3 years. She had been fully investigated and had no organic heart disease, although she was getting occasional runs of atrial fibrillation and at times her pulse would be quite high. She had been treated conventionally with digitalis but it was increasingly failing to control this adequately and she wanted to explore homeopathic treatment before going down further conventional treatment routes. One of the aggravating factors for the palpitations was coffee and she had avoided this in her diet. She gave a history that prior to the palpitations she had sleep problems, which also had been aggravated by coffee. Coffea might have been prescribed on an isopathic basis but in this case it also fitted because in the materia medica of coffee there is an unusual extreme sensitiveness and susceptibility to nervous agitation. As a confirmatory she disliked tight clothing.

Interestingly, after getting a substantial improvement in her palpitations after Coffea she was able to reduce her digitalis, although she did relapse on two occasions after taking strong coffee.

Other examples of isopathy include prescribing allergens like pollen in hay fever, infective agents or disease discharges in infections, and healthy and diseased tissues in disease of specific organs and tissue.

Nosodes and Family History

Homeopathic medicines derived from diseased tissue including micro-organisms, diseased animal tissue or diseased plants are called nosodes. They may be used isopathically and are particularly useful when there is a history of the particular illness in the individual, or in the family or society, as these may all indicate a particular susceptibility to an illness. For example, a patient who has been unwell since influenza may benefit from a remedy prepared from the influenza virus. The susceptibility of an individual due to an illness from the past is considered as a trait or taint. Groups of patients often share certain taints, e.g. many patients appear to have a susceptibility related to a past history or family history of tuberculosis. These taints are referred to as 'miasms' – an important concept in understanding more chronic illness and helpful in managing otherwise confused cases (see Chapters 15, 17, 22).

In many remedies made from disease agents and drugs there are provings that frequently correspond in some ways with the disease picture and side effects but with the sort of enhanced detail only possible from a detailed proving. Some homeopaths use the disease picture and adverse effects of certain drugs as a way into the materia medica of these substances.

Anticipating Causes, Prophylaxis or Preventative Treatment

In some cases it is possible to anticipate likely causative factors, e.g. childbirth, surgery, exposure to infection (such as a sibling's chicken pox), or susceptibility to travel sickness. It is possible to use homeopathic treatments prior to the (causative) event in the hope of stimulating the vitality, so that it is already 'keyed up' or 'keyed in' to respond to the causative factor. Many patients find using remedies this way helpful to reduce the likelihood of illness and to reduce the severity of any symptoms that develop. Preventative treatment raises important questions about how accurately the effect of any event can be predicted and to what extent and at what level remedies can act to prevent illness. This is explored in Chapter 6 when health and illness are considered in terms of the presence and absence of information. It is important to remember that effects are also capable of being causes in their own right and that cause and effect are not always best understood as a linear or one-way reaction. For example, the Bach flower remedies recognise the feelings the patient has as both an effect of something that has happened to them and also a cause of other things that are happening.

Bach Flower Remedies

Bach flower remedies are prescribed on the basis of key emotions, and it is interesting to look at how they were developed using the feeling faculties of the homeopath. Dr Edward Bach, when feeling particular, strong emotions, was drawn to certain plants and substances. He found that by using medicines made from those plants, those emotions were alleviated. This led to the development of his range of flower essences. These are very useful when you are starting to enquire about the patient's emotional state and wanting to support the patient emotionally, but not yet able to match a remedy at a deeper level.

Maintaining Causes

The presence of maintaining causes is, as you would expect, a common cause of relapse or of limited response to a prescription based on those causes. A cause may still be present or ongoing such as an allergy where the allergen is still present or an infective organism is present. In practice there is often a hierarchy of causes and this may only become clear over a course of treatment. Identifying maintaining causes that the patient cannot throw off is one indication that a deeper causation exists.

Detox, Organ and Drainage Treatment

Detoxification treatment is based either on seeing toxicity as causation, or on recognising that certain organs are actively engaged in detoxification and need support and/or stimulation during treatment. For example, lead and other heavy metals or environmental pollutants, at levels much lower than are thought to be toxic in the normal population, may be toxic in susceptible patients. Homeopathic medicines made from toxins such as these appear to help by assisting elimination of the toxins or by reducing susceptibility. Supportive treatment for organs

that are involved in a disease process or involved in detoxification uses remedies based on the affinity that some homeopathic remedies have for particular organs (organotrophic remedies), e.g. Chelidonium and Nux Vomica have an affinity for the liver.

Sometimes there may be a disordered organ due to a previous illness, family susceptibility, particular illness or environmental poison, to mention just a few causes. It is unlikely that a remedy selected this way will match at a very individual or deep level but it may be a methodology to help see a clearer case, relieve a patient's suffering or to support other treatment approaches. Sometimes these may be isopathically prescribed, e.g. a homeopathic preparation of thyroid gland may help normalise symptoms in patients with thyroid problems when used alongside other treatments. Many herbal remedies are known by their action on different organs and some of the homeopathic remedies made from these herbs have affinities with these organs. This organ-based methodology is useful not only in patients with an unclear deeper picture but also those with a low vitality when organ support and drainage can be an important initial stage of treatment while the vitality builds or a deeper picture emerges. Sometimes this is refered to as clearing the case.

Toxins may include metabolic products sometimes referred to as homotoxins and some remedies, or combinations of remedies (antihomotoxins) are prescribed on the basis of reversing this or as an antidote (A O'Byrne 2003).

Treating Symptoms

This approach (see also Chapter 9) identifies homeopathic remedies in terms of the presenting symptoms, e.g. prescribing Ipecac for nausea.

A combination of the location and presenting symptom gives many conventional diagnoses e.g. tonsillitis – 'itis' meaning an inflammation of the tonsils. Prescribing based on a single main symptom or diagnosis is sometimes referred to as local prescribing. It becomes more unique and individual the more the symptom 'sums up' the patient in a unique and individual way. The stranger and more peculiar the symptom to the disease or to the patient, or both, the more likely the remedy will match the patient's needs.

At the next level several symptoms may be taken into account, to see which remedies fit each of the symptoms. When two or more symptoms are linked together in the same illness or at the same time they are referred to as concomitant. Depending on the association of the symptoms, how fully they describe the case and how unique they are, they can indicate a very individual remedy. Throughout Section II the symptomatic approach is revisited.

In cases with many different symptoms and layers of illness it can be helpful to identify the central or most unique aspect of the case, sometimes referred to as the 'central disturbance'. Prescribing on the central disturbance is more likely to give a remedy that matches the most central and deepest aspects of the patient's case.

REFLECTION POINT

- Before considering other approaches to treatment and their methodologies reflect on the strengths and weaknesses of using causation and symptomatic approaches. What sort of cases would they work well on and when might they not be indicated?

Treating Using the Totality and Constitution

Each individual is influenced by many different experiences, both physical and psychological, and the complete clinical picture encompassing all symptoms, signs and investigations is the totality. The totality approach (see also Chapter 14) is sometimes described as like a 'three-legged stool' combining local, mental and general symptoms – and like a stool all three legs are needed to make a stable and reliable base from which to prescribe.

As homeopaths, working holistically, we see all our patients having psychological changes due to their somatic condition and somatic changes due to their psychological state. In a 'world without gaps', when one thing changes all aspects change. While the totality is the complete clinical symptom picture when a patient is ill, the constitution is an expression of the sum susceptibility of the patient. Together they

make up the 'two sides' of the whole and they are explored in much greater detail in Section III. The complete totality would encompass every symptom, however minute, and the exact constitutional would cover everything to which the patient is susceptible. In practice these methodologies can only approximate to an individual and may point to different remedies.

The constitutional methodology is described by Watson (1991) as taking the whole person into account as far as is possible, and treating the person simultaneously on all levels – physical, mental and emotional. The expression 'treat the person not the disease' is central to this methodology. The correlation between the constitution and a person's resilience to illness leads some homeopaths to promote the prescription of a constitutional remedy as a way of preventing illness. The constitutional approach embraces several different methodologies that are connected in that they see aspects of the 'nonpathological features' of the patient reliably indicating remedies that either reflect the susceptibility to certain situations or the totality an ill patient is likely to develop. It includes the constitution described on physical features like body shape, hair colour and morphological type, such as phosphoric, carbonic and fluoric types. It also encompasses the constitution described in terms of the psychological character, including emotional type, which became the dominant methodology for many homeopaths in the latter part of the 20th century and is sometimes referred to as the Kentian method after James Tyler Kent. The materia medica studied or used to match to the constitution is sometimes referred to as the constitutional picture of a remedy, and the patient as fitting a constitutional type.

'Ten years of practice will be a revelation to you, so that you will understand people and their minds. You will almost know what they are thinking, and will often take in a patient's constitution at first glance.'

James Tyler Kent, Lesser Writings

Treating Using Essence and Theme

Running through constitutional and totality 'pictures' and 'types' are different themes used both to compare remedies and to prescribe on more thematic and essence criteria. The essence and thematic approach (see also Chapters 22, 29) selects a treatment on the patterns of symptoms, signs, and behaviour of the individual and matches them to the essence and thematic pattern of the remedy. This description often allows a more 'joined-up' description of the patient where each symptom is connected to other symptoms and forms an overall pattern to the case. While some patterns are clear 'for all to see', for others the patterns are not so clear and like some Impressionist paintings different observers may see and interpret the case and picture differently.

The essence methodology focuses on matching a single central pattern that expresses itself throughout the patient's case and remedy picture. It was described and used in many cases that would have been difficult to treat using other methodologies by George Vitoulkas. The emergence of this methodology has coincided with, and some would say enabled, an understanding of illness with increased awareness of how a single pattern or gestalt can run through a patient's psychological and physical state. Frequently in chronic illness this pattern can be expressed or noticed as linked to a core emotional state.

The thematic methodology, which has developed from using essence, observes that in many patients and remedies a single theme fails to adequately express or explain all the symptoms. By observing several patterns or themes running through patients and remedies, we can more often accurately match patients and remedies. There are some themes that run through a number of remedies and this has led to a significant development in the studying of homeopathic remedies based on grouping remedies together. Often the same or similar themes run through groups of remedies that are connected in other ways, including by biological families, chemical composition, location of remedy source, etc. For example, remedies with high levels of carbon in their source material share qualities of trepidation, anxiety and fear; they are often pessimistic and have negative attitudes. It is helpful to

be aware of this in the early stages of studying homeopathy so that themes, when they exist, can be noted when studying 'related remedies' or differential diagnosis.

There are also themes that run through groups of patients connected by, for example, appearance, family, race, etc. This can be an important pointer when prescribing for young children on themes that run through the parents or in veterinary prescribing, where there may be themes running through species, herds of animals or even between owner and pet.

Some themes can be very specific and indicate a single or small group of remedies or patients. Others can be more general and represent large groups of remedies or patients. For example, the many Natrum muriaticum (common salt) qualities such as reserved sensitivity that runs through many, but by no means all, English patients.

There are many different ways of seeing and expressing the patterns within groups of patients and remedies. One of the best-known looks at links related to the historically common illness of scabies (psora) and the deep-seated illnesses of syphilis (syphilitic) and gonorrhoea (sycosis). These patterns of illnesses set up themes that are inherited and are referred to homeopathically as miasms, the 'traits' referred to earlier, and lead to a miasmatic approach to prescribing. While these three miasms have a long history in guiding homeopathic prescribing, the recognition of other miasms or themes, due to previous, inherited or cultural illness can shed light on otherwise difficult cases (see Chapter 22).

The understanding of remedies in groups also allows the homeopath to begin to look at the relationship between remedies above and beyond those that have been historically noted and to think of what remedies might complement, follow well or be closely linked to remedies in the same group or family.

The Reflective Approach to Prescribing

Changes in ourselves, including our emotional state, reflect what is happening around us.

Likewise, what you become aware of in yourself in a relationship is a guide to what is happening in the other person and to the treatment required. For example, noticing the desire to comfort a typical 'Pulsatilla' child and using this to influence a prescription is an example of this 'reflective' approach. In fact this is a factor in all 'relationships'. This can be an important guide to the treatment required and by making it conscious it can inform the homeopathic process.

While the reflective approach to prescribing (see also Chapters 23, 29) is not historically described as a core homeopathic methodology it does, in experienced homeopaths, contribute to the choice of remedy. Perhaps more importantly, when not understood, it can lead to difficulties recognising certain remedy types or bias in prescribing certain remedies. The relationship between patient and homeopath influences (in the author's experience of supervising other homeopaths) much prescribing, whether consciously or unconsciously, constructively or destructively. Using a reflective approach underlies the description of different remedy pictures as if they are people, where a collection of symptoms and signs reflects a pattern that is described as if it has a personality, a history, a future, a life – so-called 'living materia medica'.

The psychodynamic methodology is greatly informed by the psychotherapeutic concepts of projection (transference and counter-transference) explained more fully in Chapter 23. The potential to understand this has been facilitated greatly by the description of emotional intelligence. Emotional intelligence refers to the capacity for recognising and working with our own feelings and those of others. In a medical context emotional intelligence gives insight into patients from observing their emotional state and the effect *of* their emotional state on us and informs the advice and treatment given. It is distinct from but complementary to academic intelligence focusing on analytical and cognitive capacity and measured by IQ (Gardener 1983, Salovey & Mayer 1990). The emotional and academic intelligences are sometimes colloquially described as 'left brain' and 'right brain', reflecting different brain wave activity and different areas of the brain associated with each intelligence (Springer & Deutsch 1981). The relational model, reflective approach and psychodynamic methodology are explored in more detail in Section VI, where the techniques that seek to use small and subtle changes including emotional changes in the observer to help give insight into what is happening in a patient are explored further.

Different Approaches in Practice

Different homeopaths will use different approaches to prescribing in different cases. All the approaches can help the homeopath to prescribe a similar remedy based on 'like treating like'. Some approaches will be better suited than others to finding the closest match (the simillimum). Each homeopath is likely to develop personal preferences of these different methodologies and over time and in different situations these preferences will change.

Different methodology might well point to different remedies. By matching the methodology used to prescribe to the depth of the case, some guidance is possible as to which method might be most useful in what sort of case. An informed decision can be made between remedies indicated by each methodology and the likely prognosis for each can be predicted. Distinguishing between remedies selected on a particular methodology or combination of methodologies helps in predicting the outcome and progress of any treatment. Recording the approach and methodology used in making a prescription will also help at follow-up in assessing a treatment.

Self-Healing

Each individual has huge capacity to adjust to threats and changes to their environment and situation with imperceptible or minor symptoms. Many are recognisable as the body 'telling us something', e.g. tiredness, particular food desires, a twinge in the leg, a mild sore throat.

Foundation

The homeopath should always remember that most patients with most illnesses get better on their own. If the self-healing process is unfolding without hindrance then at best we may make just a slight improvement in the speed of recovery and at worst we may slow, prevent, or manifest a new deeper illness. Giving no prescription is always an option. It is not the same as giving no treatment, as reaching this decision will have already included elements of a therapeutic consultation and identifying obstacles to cure. Not prescribing is important if a disturbance is resolving rapidly as there may be no clear case to prescribe on or a previous remedy may be acting.

Straightforward Cases

Having looked at the range of different methodologies and approaches available to the homeopath, it is appropriate to concentrate first on what are generally the easiest conditions to prescribe for. These are generally the conditions where there is a clear and single causation – what we will call a straightforward case – and those conditions where there is a clear symptom picture of recent and relatively quick onset, typically an acute illness, what we often call a simple case. These will, if the vitality of the patient is good and the trigger not overwhelming or persistent, respond well to treatment. In many cases the methodologies will be on causation and/or main symptoms but a totality or other methodology may be used if the remedy suits the patient.

The example of some of the local remedies used in treating acute sore throats is given in Box 5.3; there are many others but it gives the sort of information that can distinguish them. While sore throats are often amenable to local treatment some may indicate a more deep-seated condition, particularly if they are recurrent or persistent. Certain remedy pictures are more tuned for these chronic presentations. The selection of potency and frequency of administration of remedies is covered in Chapter 20. For those new to homeopathy and while developing your knowledge and skills

BOX 5.3
Treatment of Sore Throats
- Aconite for a sore throat started after being in a cold wind or after a shock. Especially if burning, redness, smarting, dryness, tingling in the throat and if it hurts to swallow water.
- Baryta carbonica for recurrent cases of sore throat following exposure to cold and chill, and better for drinking. The tonsils are frequently large, especially the right tonsil. Suited to timid children. Offensive foot sweat. Better swallowing fluids.
- Belladonna often has a viral type fever with a dry and burning sore throat. The tonsils are often inflamed and bright red with a red, hot face and skin. Worse talking and any touch but with little or no thirst.
- Gelsemium has a sore throat that develops several days after exposure to warm moist relaxing weather, they are very shivery but with little thirst.
- Lachesis for a similar burning pain in the throat worse from swallowing liquids but due to over use of the voice with pain worse on the left side. The throat appears more blue or purple colour than red and is characteristically much worse for any constriction around throat.

I advise you start by prescribing for straightforward and simple cases the 12c or 30c strengths of remedies. In the most acute situations these may be needed every half hour (or more) and as symptoms improve the interval between repetitions can be increased. As a general rule, repeat a remedy as often as is needed but stop when no further improvement is obtained. Be warned that it is very easy to get diverted into hunting for a perfect potency, with each text and school suggesting different potencies, rather than concentrate on the most important task of finding the closest remedy match possible.

In many straightforward cases the symptoms a patient gets are acute because the causative factors happen suddenly, or certainly reach a threshold suddenly. The causative factors may be physical (trauma) or emotional (shock) but tend to be quite large and the situational and environmental change that precipitates the illness is often the most apparent factor leading to the remedy. The importance of understanding the cause is that if a number of different individuals experience the same cause then many of them are likely to get the same illness and need the same remedy. If the strongest stimuli present an individual with a situation they are just not prepared for and do not have the information to cope with they will get 'ill'. Untreated it is likely to take some time for an individual to re-balance and take on board the information they need to cope with that situation – homeopathic treatment can greatly speed up this process.

The strength of the cause and individual susceptibility will determine the extent and degree to which this is true. In some individuals there might be a predisposition to particular causes so one patient might find a specific food upsets them but not others. In others there may be a cause that affects most individuals, e.g. a strongly toxic substance in the environment. In others a patient might only be sensitive in certain situations such as being sensitive to an allergen only when they are stressed or at a certain threshold of exposure.

Summary

At the end of Section I you have examined the basic principles and laws of homeopathy, how the information of materia medica is derived from provings, and looked at the homeopathic case as a way of understanding the patient and the illness. In Chapter 4 we explored the broadest principles behind analysing cases homeopathically and the important questions upon which we need to reflect. In this chapter the different approaches to treatment and methodologies for prescribing have been covered to create an overview of the homeopathic approaches and this lays the foundation for managing homeopathic patients. Prescribing on causation and presenting symptoms can offer a great deal in the treatment of acute illnesses but a solid foundation of the principles will also prepare you for exploring the methodologies and approaches necessary to tackle more deep-seated cases and more chronic illness. In the next section we look at factors which affect prescribing in simple cases and introduce the idea of complex cases and their management.

References

Gardener H 1983 Frames of mind. Basic Books, New York

Salovey P, Mayer J 1990 Emotional intelligence. Imagination, Cognition and Personality 9:185–211

Springer S, Deutsch G 1981 Left brain, right brain. W H Freeman, San Francisco

Watson I 1991 A guide to the methodologies of homeopathy. Cutting Edge Publications, Kendal

Bibliography

Bellavite P, Signorini A 1995 Homeopathy: a frontier in medical science. North Atlantic Books, Berkeley

Blackie M G 1976 The patient not the cure. MacDonald and Jane's, London

Cameron D M 1951 Low potency prescribing. Br Homeopath J 41(2):77–92

Lockie A H 1989 The family guide to homeopathy. Elm Tree Books, London

Lockie A H 2000 Encyclopedia of homeopathy. Dorling Kindersley, London

O'Bryne A 2003 The symphonic architecture of antihomotoxic medicine. Explore 12:3

Roberts H A 1936 The principles and art of cure by homeopathy, a modern textbook. Homeopathic Publishing Company, London

Vithoulkas G 1980 The science of homeopathy. Grove Press, New York

Section II

Causation and the Presenting Symptoms

CHAPTER SIX

The Symptom, Susceptibility and Hierarchy

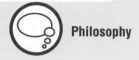 Philosophy

David Owen

Introduction

Symptoms occur when a patient is not in harmonious balance with their environment. The environment includes any relationships, their life situation or circumstances and their life style, as well as the 'ecological environment'. All these together contribute to the patient's 'environment'. This chapter explores the way the patient and environment relate. The interface between the patient and environment reflects in its broadest sense the symptoms a patient has.

Section I looked at symptoms arising from a cause in the environment. In this section symptoms are explored through the susceptibility of the patient as this determines what causes they are susceptible to. The relative significance, value and importance of each symptom is important to understanding the susceptibility of cases with several symptoms. Homeopathically symptoms are compared and ordered by looking at the breadth of systems affected, the depth and severity of symptoms, and how one symptom relates to another. Being clear about the order or hierarchy of symptoms is important to understanding more complex cases and interpreting the reaction to treatment. It helps the homeopath plan an appropriate treatment and predict the response to treatment.

Understanding the range of possible responses to treatment enables the homeopath to assess how curative any treatment may be. Particular patterns of response are found to be so reliable as an indicator of a good outcome that they have become known as the homeopathic 'laws of cure'. These laws of cure, like many other aspects of homeopathy, have developed over many years of careful observation.

While the approach and response to treatment is influenced by the disease a patient has, the homeopath is more interested in the patient who has the disease. For this reason it is helpful to speak less about how acute or chronic an illness is but rather how simple or complex a case is. While acute illness is often present in straightforward and simple cases and chronic illness in more complex cases, this is not always so. A complex case may present with an apparent acute illness or symptom that is in fact simply the 'tip of the iceberg' as far as the case is concerned. A simple case may present with a longstanding chronic symptom but when the cause is removed or a local remedy given the symptom goes completely.

Symptoms in the Different Models of Health

- The pathological model sees the illness happening to the patient, the symptoms being predominately useful as pointers to causation (although in practice this is often combined with the biological model).
- The biological model sees the illness as the effect or reaction within the patient in terms of symptoms that the patient describes and signs that can be observed. (Hereafter, both signs and symptoms will be referred to as

'symptoms', unless the distinction needs to be made explicit.) Symptoms can either be directly related to the illness in which case they are called 'local symptoms', or incidental to it, i.e. non-local. In physical illnesses non-local symptoms are often the mental and emotional symptoms, or those relating to the physical environment called general symptoms. In the symptomatic approach to treatment it is usually the local symptoms that are identified and on which treatment is based.

- In the holistic model the local physical symptoms, the mental symptoms and the general symptoms give the case.
- In the holographic model the qualities that run through several symptoms or the pattern expressed through the symptom are most important.
- In the relational model it is the deepest most fundamental sensation and feeling that underlies the symptoms and how this affects others that is used to select a prescription.

Illnesses in the Different Models of Health

Different models of health provide the homeopath with a spectrum of views of patients that can 'make sense of' a wide range of illnesses. The pathogenic model perceives the world of disease through aetiological agents (infections, toxicity), the biological model perceives the world of disease through effects (organ, disease process/inflammation). In the totality model the disease is seen in the context of the world of the patient (mind, body, general). In the holographic model the disease is seen in the context of a pattern or theme running through the disease and patient (overactive, underactive etc) and in the relational model in terms of the effect of the individual on their situation, including their effect on the homeopath.

Table 6.1 suggests some of the trends that run across the different models of health, although these are not hard and fast and many cases can be helpfully perceived through several models or views of health. Identifying these provides part of the information for assessing the type of case that best describes a patient (see Chapter 10) and on which management decisions are made. For example many prescribers will use a different remedy potency depending on their view of the case (see Chapter 20).

In the pathological model the illness is caused by something that disturbs the equilibrium of the patient and is to be overcome. In the biological model the illness is a change in the patient

Table 6.1 THE FIVE MODELS OF HEALTH AND SOME TRENDS RUNNING ACROSS THEM

Models of Health	Focus On	Perspective of the Homeopath	Localisation of the seat of illness	Suitable for cases that are: (see Chapter 10)	Potency (see Chapters 15 & 20)
Relational	The Therapeutic Relationship	More Subjective	More internal to the patient	More hidden	Higher e.g. 10M
Holographic	The Pattern or Sensation behind the Symptoms			More confused	e.g. 1M
Holistic	The Patient's Totality and Susceptibility			Complex	e.g. 200c
Biological	The Illness and Presenting Symptom			Simple	e.g. 30c
Pathogenic	The Illness and Its Cause	More Objective	More external in the patient's environment or situation	Straightforward	Lower, e.g. 12c or 6c

expressed as symptoms that are the reaction of the individual to the cause (influenced by the patient's susceptibility). The homeopath seeks to find a remedy through an approach that takes account of several significant symptoms. In practice the pathological and biological models are understood through the dynamic between patient and the situation they are in. Both often see illness as a threshold event where patients often believe that the onset of an illness is sudden. In many cases however, when a careful and comprehensive history has been taken it may become clear that the illness has been developing for some time.

REFLECTION POINT

- Any 'model' will only be accurate to a certain extent and different ways of understanding illnesses and patients will each provide different strengths and weaknesses. What do you think the strengths and weaknesses of the five models of health presented are?

Table 6.2 gives a suggested comparison of the models presented so far and two other complementary ways that you might like to study further, e.g. five-element theory provides one way of seeing patterns that run through cases and remedies (see Chapter 21 page 279) and is used extensively in traditional acupuncture (Maciocia 1989). There is no reason why you should use any particular number of different models or stages and you may seek to connect and merge a number of different systems,

e.g. aspects of Sankaran's levels, and how they may connect to the models of health (Sankaran 2004).

The Cause Behind the Cause

When we assess a patient in the biological model, we endeavour to understand the symptoms. Causation will not suffice if it does not explain such questions as:

- why has this happened now?
- why has it caused these particular symptoms?
- why, even when the cause is removed, have things not improved?

For example, in many 'infections' it is not a complete or accurate account of the disorder to blame only the infective organism, we need also to understand the terrain that allows the infection to thrive. When trying to understand the way the illness has developed we must ask how or why a patient's health was originally disturbed to become susceptible to infection now.

REFLECTION POINT

- Remembering that healing is something that happens within patients rather than something the practitioner does to or for them, you might like to reflect on the purpose of illness and the qualities of healing. What are the implications of the different views each model of health offers on the homeopath's role in the healing process and understanding of what a cure is?

Using Different Models and Approaches

When it is difficult to see one remedy that links the causes and the different symptoms together some homeopaths respond by treating each group of symptoms separately. This can lead to a rather piecemeal approach to treatment. Another option is to look at the patient from another perspective such as the holistic model of health, where one remedy may cover a greater proportion of the case. Each model sees illness and health in a different way and if one model of health leads to only a partial

Table 6.2 COMPARISON OF MODELS OF HEALTH WITH FIVE ELEMENT THEORY AND SANKARAN'S LEVELS		
Models of Health	**Five Element Theory**	**Sankaran's Levels**
Relational	Ether	Energy
Holographic	Fire	Sensation
Holistic	Air	Delusion/emotion
Biological	Water	Fact
Pathogenic	Earth	Name

understanding of the case another model may provide a better understanding – and several together an even better understanding. In the holistic model, every aspect of the patient is important and the susceptibility of the patient and the hierarchy of the different symptoms become central to understanding the case. The holistic model invites a view where illness and health are not opposites but aspects of the same whole (see Chapter 11). In later sections of the book the holographic and relational models of health invite you to reframe your concept of illness, where health and illness are informed by the relationship to the observer and illness can be seen as a necessary part of being healthy, both for an individual and a population (see Chapter 26).

These evolving principles and perspectives provide both a rich and wide interpretation of illness and reflect the uncertainty and art of clinical practice. The model of health used to best understand the case will most often determine the approach to treatment and point to the methodology to select the remedy. Any homeopathic remedy can be prescribed according to any approach as long as the relevant homeopathic picture of the remedy is available. In practice some remedies are better known in some approaches and methodologies than others. To help unravel this it is necessary to examine the symptom and its depth or hierarchy in relation to the patient's susceptibility.

Susceptibility

'If a man were in perfect health, he would not be susceptible. Whatever man is susceptible to, such he is, and such is his quality.'

John Tyler Kent

'By susceptibility we mean the general quality or capability of the living organism of receiving impressions, the power to react to stimuli. Susceptibility is one of the fundamental attributes of life, upon it depends all functioning, all vital processes, physiological and pathological. Digestion, assimilation, nutrition, repair, secretion, excretion, metabolism and catabolism as well as all disease processes arising from infection or contagion depending on the power of the organism to react to specific stimuli.'

Stewart Close, The genius of homeopathy

Symptoms are produced by the individual in response to the situation they are in. Those symptoms bear a relationship to the patient's situation, including the causative factors. In response to certain strong causative factors most individuals will get symptoms. In response to other causes, whether an individual gets any symptoms or what those symptoms will be is determined by susceptibility. In this way both the cause of any symptom and the symptoms themselves reflect the patient's susceptibility. If a student in a class of 20 has an infection then if very virulent all the other students might catch it, if less virulent only those with susceptibility will get it. Each student who catches it might get slightly different symptoms – how these symptoms differ point to each individual's susceptibility. While several of the students might respond to the same remedy the more unusual the symptoms the more it points to a unique susceptibility and the more likely a remedy will be needed to suit that individual's susceptibility.

As the causes and symptoms become more complicated the more the homeopath aims to build a deeper picture of the patient. This is achieved by understanding both the cause and effect from the perspective of the patient's susceptibility. The susceptibility of each of us shapes our tolerance to different environments, our resistance to different illnesses and our sensitivity to particular remedies. By determining our response to different stimuli and challenges in our environment, our susceptibility colours every aspect of our nature and behaviour.

In more complex cases different symptoms each reflect the patient's susceptibility; this is taken into account in the holistic model of health and is why susceptibility plays such a central role in understanding cases holistically (see Section III). Deciding which symptoms are more central to the case helps us to know how strongly they should be considered and is done by deciding on their place in the 'hierarchy of symptoms'. The most central symptom often points to the 'centre of the case' and is sometimes referred to as the 'deepest disturbance'.

Hierarchy of Symptoms and Perspectives of Depth: Penetration, Levels, Breadth, Layers and Intensity

If susceptibility and symptomatology express a patient's unique individuality, then hierarchy provides the structure through which it is expressed and the perspective through which it is seen. Each model of health has a slightly different way of perceiving the depth of symptoms (Table 6.3). I suggest when talking about causation or aetiology it is helpful to think about how deep a cause 'penetrates'. Thinking about localised symptoms it helps to identify the 'level' of the symptom, sometimes on an axis of peripheral to most central. In the totality or the constitution each feature or symptom is viewed in the context of 'breadth and continuity' with other features and symptoms through the whole picture.

Thematically, symptoms can be understood as connected to a series of layers, overlapping and overlaying each other. In an essence approach then those symptoms with themes that run through other symptoms are linked together – if there were several themes each could be thought of as a layer that might each cover part of the whole or that might be understood as one intertwined with another. We might talk about a Phosphorous 'layer' or the Tubercular 'layer'; both these remedies might be partially indicated in the same case (see Chapters 26, 27). In the relational model it is the 'intensity' of the feeling, sensation and relationship that indicates its importance. So the strength of feeling and how unusual the feeling is both influence how important it is.

Each model of health allows perception of the patient and the illness at different depths and the information from one may give more useful and deeper information than information from another. It is not the case that causation always gives more superficial information than a theme or relational insight. Table 6.4 illustrates the sorts of perception possible in each model.

In taking and analysing the case the homeopath often combines several different approaches and therefore systems of ordering the symptoms. The same feature or symptom might be interpreted differently in each model and according to the approach used. It may help to think of these perspectives as different axes or different ways of viewing or 'focusing' on the case (Swayne 1998) – these are considered in more detail in each relevant section. Approaches based on 'cause and effect' mirror much of the conventional practice of weighting the importance of aetiology and presentation of clinical symptoms. Many homeopathic students,

Table 6.3 WAYS OF EXPRESSING DEPTH IN RELATION TO THE FIVE MODELS OF HEALTH

Modes of Health	Perception
Relational	Intensity of relationship
Holographic	Layer of theme
Holistic	Breadth of constitution/totality
Biological	Level of symptom
Pathogenic	Penetration of cause

Table 6.4 THE SORTS OF PERCEPTION POSSIBLE IN EACH MODEL

Penetration of Cause	Level of Symptom	Breadth of Constitution/Totality	Layer of Theme	Intensity of Relationship
A coffee kept me awake	I'm restless	I like to be on the go	I digest things quickly	Friends say I'm 'wired'
I'm tired as I didn't sleep well	I'm weak and lethargic	I always want to be busy	My digestion and bowels are rushed'	I make others 'buzz'
I've not slept well since we moved	I fall asleep at work	My body and mind are always sluggish	Everything in my body works too fast and my mind speeds all over the place	The patient's homeopath is exhausted by the consultation

who are aware of the conventional model of disease classification, find biological and pathogenic models of health an easier place to identify the hierarchy of symptoms, so initially find it easier to either prescribe homeopathically in these models or prefer remedies indicated more strongly by these approaches.

Each of these different perspectives of symptoms can be considered in terms of their clarity, duration, uniqueness and influence on the patient (and homeopath). A causation may be more important the longer it has been going on. A local symptom will often be most important the stronger it is and the more it restricts a person's life. In a totality or constitutional approach the more unique or unexpected the symptom the more it might reflect the patient's individual state and so point to a remedy with the best indications. This is why symptoms that are strange, rare and peculiar (SRP) are so important at giving person-specific 'keynotes'.

REFLECTION POINT

- Sam's case illustrates some of these different perspectives. You might try to decide which fits which approach to treatment and how the perspectives compare.

CASE STUDY 6.1

Sam, 12 years old, was prone to recurrent upper respiratory tract infections which he had had since pneumonia when 3 years old. Sometimes he got ear infections, helped with Belladonna, sometimes sore throats, which improved with Ferrum Phos. Despite local treatment, symptoms kept recurring. He was worse in the cold air and craved cold drinks, especially cold milk and iced water. He liked a lot of attention and sympathy when ill and wanted to be held or stroked by his mother. He always had a fear of the dark and a dislike of loud noises and this theme of 'sensitivity' seemed to underlie his need for sympathy. He made the homeopath feel that they wanted to reassure him.

As a local approach to treatment had failed to cure Sam a totality approach was taken. In this approach the symptoms related to Sam's behaviour and personality were important, as were those relating to temperature and food, especially the more unusual ones. He had themes of the remedies Pulsatilla and Phosphorous. The feeling in the homeopath also revealed aspects of the case. Sam was prescribed the remedy Phosphorous on a balance of information from different approaches. After three doses of the 200c Sam's recurrent acute problems stopped and his mother reported that he generally seemed to have 'more energy' and was less 'clingy'.

Given the importance of the distinction between the different models I recommend you clarify for yourself – if necessary revisiting the tables above – what you understand when we talk about depth, level, hierarchy, breadth, layers and intensity of symptoms.

Combining Different Models and Approaches

As the case of Sam illustrates, in practice as you learn about and become experienced in different models and approaches they will often point to the same remedy and reinforce the confidence of any prescription. In more difficult cases you may have to choose between remedies partially indicated; the clearer you can be on the different approaches and the perspective each gives, the easier it will be to manage these cases. While attempting to clarify these different approaches it is possible that you will be tempted to over simplify or unrealistically separate out the information available in each model. In practice each model influences the others and how symptoms are perceived.

Aetiology has to be interpreted in terms of its symptoms, its influence on the totality and constitution. It will bring forward some themes and be interpreted in light of the relationship between you and the patient. Each local symptom is in balance with its cause, is related to the totality, will be part of a theme and create a certain response in you. Each theme has a cause, an effect and has its own complete picture and effect on you. Each reflection is caused by something, produces and notices particular symptoms, colours the totality and relates to a theme.

Laws of Cure

'In all diseases, especially acute cases, the patient's emotional state and entire behaviour are the surest and most likely of the signs showing a small beginning of amelioration or aggravation. Where there is the slightest beginning of improvement the patient will demonstrate a greater degree of comfort, increasing composure, freedom of spirit, increased courage, a kind of returning naturalness ... This can be easily seen if one observes with exact attentiveness but it cannot be easily described in words.'

S Hahnemann, Organon, Paragraph 253

Whichever model of health is used, the first indication of change in the direction of cure, i.e. the first indication that a true healing process has begun, will be an improvement in vitality and general well-being. Changes in symptoms may accompany this, or follow on from it as the vitality of the patient improves.

When we recognise that illness comes about in relation to natural laws that incorporate the hierarchical relationships of symptoms that have been described, then it should be apparent that reversal of illness or 'cure' will also follow a similar order. Understanding this allows us to judge if a treatment has effectively stimulated the healing process before having to wait until the cure is complete. Hering first referred to this in 1867 in his book 'An analytic therapeutic of the mind, volume 2' but it was not until 1910 that Kent first talked about direction of cure (in the reverse order to which symptoms appeared) and in 1911 that Kent wrote about Hering's Law (Saine 2000).

Hering's Law

Constantine Hering noted that cure proceeds in reverse order of appearance of the symptoms, from the most important organs to the least important organs, from within outwards (i.e. most central organs first), and from above down. In other words, essentially improvement follows a rever-

sal of duration and depth. When treating a single severe symptom there may well be other aspects of the case to treat once the most severe symptom is controlled. In these cases we see a cure proceeding with an overall improvement in how a patient feels as they move from more severe (life threatening) to less severe symptoms.

Understanding the laws of cure will tell you when a remedy has acted, when it is continuing to act and the direction of the action. It also indicates whether and when a change of prescription (potency or remedy) is needed.

By understanding the journey an individual has to go through to get well, we can start to understand and note where an individual is on that journey from the symptoms they are experiencing in response to the treatment. Fundamentally the journey into illness is cured by a journey out of illness, i.e. retracing your steps, when the symptoms disappear in the reverse order to which they appeared. It can be thought of as a centrifugal force 'throwing' the illness out. This clearing of symptoms may involve several healing reactions; the main two to be distinguished are aggravations and healing crises (see Chapter 10).

REFLECTION POINT

Before moving on, take a few minutes to answer the following questions:

- What is the scope for an individual to self-heal and do they always have the information needed to adjust to the circumstances they find themselves in?
- If, in response to an illness, an individual becomes healthier, can we expect as life goes on that individuals will become more and more healthy?
- If suffering acute illnesses in childhood helps develop resistance to difficult situations in later life, is it healthy to have an absence of illnesses as a child?
- Are there only three possibilities when you suffer an illness?
  1. You gather the information to cope with the situation you are in
  2. You modify the situation you are in (or your circumstances)
  3. You succumb
- Can you have more than one illness at a time?

The Patient, the Environment and the Symptom

By considering an illness in terms of the relationship between the patient and their situation, the homeopath understands the importance of each in developing a subtler understanding of illness. The interplay between an individual's susceptibility, their environment and the symptoms generated by their vitality can be illustrated by thinking of the analogy of a boat, what it is designed for, the different conditions affecting it and the way it is crewed (Fig 6.1).

An individual's journey through life might be compared to a voyage in a small boat where the boat represents the individual. The sea and weather conditions represent the environment or situation the boat is in. The crew that can alter course or 'man the pumps' represent the vitality. The vitality, like the crew seen from a distance, will not be apparent, rather they are noticed by changes in the behaviour of the boat equivalent to symptoms.

REFLECTION POINT

- Boats, like human beings, all have much in common with each other, although their ability to respond to changing conditions varies. There is no single or optimum environment for all boats. Much depends on the configuration of the hull, the specific design of the vessel, where it is taken or the tasks it is used for. Different designs (patients) give different performance (susceptibility). There is no one perfect design, rather an optimum design for different situations and conditions. How a boat performs in certain conditions might represent its health, which varies from 'plain sailing', going where you want to without a problem, to 'making heavy weather', to being 'submerged', 'awash' or even 'swamped and sinking'.

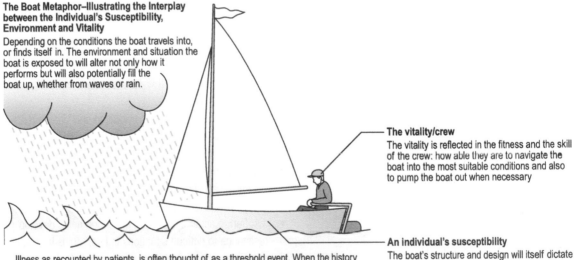

The Boat Metaphor–Illustrating the Interplay between the Individual's Susceptibility, Environment and Vitality

Depending on the conditions the boat travels into, or finds itself in. The environment and situation the boat is exposed to will alter not only how it performs but will also potentially fill the boat up, whether from waves or rain.

The vitality/crew
The vitality is reflected in the fitness and the skill of the crew: how able they are to navigate the boat into the most suitable conditions and also to pump the boat out when necessary

An individual's susceptibility
The boat's structure and design will itself dictate the situations and conditions in which it sails most favourably, and the situations and conditions in which it struggles. This is equivalent to the individual's constitutional susceptibility. To some extent it will determine where the boat can safely go, although modifications to it and careful crewing can extend the range of the environments it can move into.

Illness as recounted by patients, is often thought of as a threshold event. When the history is carefully taken, the boat can often be seen to be leaking, taking on water or not performing optimally for some time before suddenly sinking. In the same way, although patients may think an illness starts at a certain point in time, often the history will reveal there has been a gradual onset, sometimes going on for many years before the patient first reports they have become ill. By understanding the environment, susceptibility and the vitality, one can paint a dynamic picture of the health of the individual. As the situation gets more hostile, so the integrity of the boat and the skill of the crew become increasingly important to maintaining health. Different boats, like different people, perform at their best in different environments.

Figure 6.1   The boat metaphor of the interplay between an individual's susceptibility, their environment and the symptoms generated by their vitality

The Environment

Different individuals find different environments challenging to them. The environments that the patient is exposed to will be determined in part by choices they make; when considering a patient's environment it is important to assess not only the physical but also emotional and intellectual state. Factors such as stress, anxiety and fear often have a significant impact on well-being.

The Individual

The characteristics we share in common determine both the families and species we belong to and our core susceptibilities. All individuals are susceptible to certain environments. Some are specific and peculiar to the individual, while others may be common to the species, family or culture we belong to. In nature when groups of organisms share basic characteristics, those characteristics categorise that group's preferences for and optimal situations where they flourish.

Different individuals' susceptibility may vary from the trivial to the seriously life threatening; the effect will also depend on the degree of environmental exposure. For example, some patients might be very sensitive to slight increases in exposure to sunlight, while all patients will be sensitive to excessive exposure to sunlight. The more unusual the susceptibility or greater the sensitivity the more it tells us about the individual.

The Vitality

A patient's vitality is revealed by the way the individual adapts to the environment, and how particular organs and systems function in particular environments. These adaptations are taking place all the time, and include slight changes in the healthy functioning of organs, such as a shift in preferences for food or temperature, or a mental or emotional reaction that might, for example, lead to particular dreams. Often these changes are only noticed when something 'goes wrong'; when symptoms develop, they become the way that we interpret the energetic state or vitality of the individual, although to the trained clinician these changes can often be detected even before a patient notices them.

Another way of describing vitality is in terms of a patient's resistance to getting ill. In this respect it is similar to the conventional idea of immunity. If the vitality is low then we are less able to cope with a change to our environment, as the case of Samantha illustrates.

CASE STUDY 6.2

Samantha, age 23, suffered from eczema as an infant and sporadically through childhood and adolescence, which responded to a reduction of dairy products. She consulted in her early twenties with a recurrence of the eczema and premenstrual syndrome that aggravated her skin. When her vitality was challenged by premenstrual symptoms she become less able to cope with dairy products and her symptoms deteriorated. The homeopathic remedy Aethusa was prescribed on her local symptoms and dairy sensitivity. It produced an initial aggravation of the skin, but this settled when she avoided dairy products. Once the aggravation settled, her premenstrual symptoms had improved, the eczema improved and she was better able to tolerate dairy products.

REFLECTION POINT

- Reflect on the triad of the environment, the individual and the vitality and how these three factors affect how an illness is experienced. How does the classification of illnesses as immune, acquired or inherited depend on which of the three the attention is focused on?
- In Samantha's case which aspects correlate to the environment, the susceptibility and the vitality?

The Symptom

The symptom is how the organism's self-regulating mechanisms respond to environmental challenges. In provings, susceptible individuals produce symptoms when they are 'challenged' by the remedy. The symptoms that develop, including any changes they seek to make to their situation and the environments they seek out or avoid, describe the remedy state. The case of Peter illustrates the importance, in unravelling more complex cases, of understanding the relationship between symptoms, environment and susceptibility.

CASE STUDY 6.3

Peter presented with constipation and haemorrhoids. He liked drinking coffee and eating spicy food that gave him an initial 'buzz,' but later aggravated him, causing increased irritability and restlessness. He noticed that when he became irritable and restless he craved more spicy food and coffee. Peter also reported a contrary reaction to alcohol; having initially avoided it, he discovered it was a useful means of 'slowing down.' Nux Vomica relieved the constipation and haemorrhoids and he discovered, after the remedy, it was easier to avoid the foods and drink that aggravate his symptoms.

REFLECTION POINT
- The question posed is which comes first – the susceptibility of the individual to the diet or the diet causing the susceptibility?

As a general rule, to operate effectively as a homeopath it is important to be aware of the environmental factors affecting the patient and, where appropriate, to support a patient in removing these causative factors. When an appropriate remedy is prescribed an individual is better able to tolerate the situation and is often enabled in making environmental modifications that may appear to happen spontaneously, such as preferring healthier foods, sleeping better or dreaming more.

Treating Symptoms

The body is far more than just a collection of its parts. A damaged car would not repair itself but the body often can. This is a distinguishing feature of living organisms and depends on the dynamic relationship between the susceptibility, the environment and the vitality. When patients become ill, they frequently recover their health and discover a new way of being healthy without 'treatment'. When this natural process requires assistance the homeopath provides treatment to facilitate these changes.

However, there exists a tension in treating symptoms. On the one hand symptoms are how illness expresses itself and therefore the aim of cure is their removal. On the other hand symptoms occur due to causes and susceptibility and if these are not modified by treatment then symptoms recur or new symptoms come about. In simple cases with minor or temporary causation prescribing solely on the presenting symptoms may be adequate to throw off the symptoms and give a cure. In more complex cases an approach that takes into account the many aspects of a patient's life style and susceptibility needs to be considered; in such cases thinking of illness and treatment in terms of pieces of information can be helpful (Wheeler 1948).

Remedies as Information

When ill, patients often make spontaneous changes to their life style or situation. Animals are drawn to helpful herbs, children ask for a cuddle or patients make simple diet changes or sleep more. Illness often leads the patient to make the changes necessary for healing. These qualitative changes can be thought of as providing something required for healing and this can be thought of as a type of information. For example, in simple iron deficiency anaemia treatment might consist of material doses of iron or, as is often the situation in mild cases, something that helps the digestion, absorption or utilisation of iron may be adequate. Some herbs increase absorption of certain nutrients, as might the prescription of homeopathic iron; see the case of Sandy in Case Study 6.4. In this way the remedies might be thought of as providing information for a natural process to function better and for the patient to move to a healthier state than before – although this information, or some would say 'energetic' view, does not preclude there being other models for how homeopathic remedies act.

> ## CASE STUDY 6.4
>
> Sandy, a woman of 35, presented with exhaustion. She had always suffered from heavy periods but during the past 7 years they had become heavier and there was no evidence of uterine pathology. Her haemoglobin count was 10.6. She was diagnosed with iron deficiency anaemia and prescribed iron supplementation. The iron made her constipated, so she stopped it. Despite high levels of dietary iron and supplementation her iron stores still registered as low. When she presented homeopathically she said, 'I bruise easily' and she also had a peculiar symptom of being sensitive to noises. She felt an immediate improvement in her energy on Ferrum Phos 12c once a day and after a month of treatment her haemoglobin had marginally improved. After 3 months the haemoglobin was 11.8 and after 6 months it was 12.4. Her heavy periods decreased and after a year she stopped taking the remedies regularly and needed only a short course after a heavy bleed or when she felt tired.

> ## CASE STUDY 6.5
>
> Maxine, age 5, suffered from recurrent ear infections that responded temporarily to homeopathic Belladonna but then recurred. A more comprehensive case history was taken indicating treatment with Calcium carbonicum. Her mother reported that Maxine was more energetic following treatment, was more 'alert' and was sleeping better and less anxious. Maxine had 'given up' milk after taking the remedy and had started to stand up to her brother more. After two subsequent minor ear infections she remained clear of ear infections.

Discovery Versus Recovery

Each individual develops certain symptoms in response to their particular environment, depending on susceptibility. Getting better, so that they no longer 'need' these symptoms, requires a change in the environment or their susceptibility, or both. In practice the three elements of the triad of the patient, the symptoms and the situation each change dynamically and a healthy state is one that is evolving as each aspect of the triad changes. It is a process of discovery, not just recovery. While the homeopath may provide support in this process it ultimately requires a change by the patient. Maxine's case shows this even in an acute illness.

Perhaps the giving up milk and standing up to her brother was just because she was feeling better.

Equally, perhaps they represented important shifts in her situation. The more deep-seated the illness the more the treatment is likely to alter the state of the patient and to lead to a change in situation and the environment they choose to live in. They may change their temperature or food preference or change how they relate to other people; in some cases it is prudent to warn patients of these possibilities.

Working with Life Style Treatments

When a lifestyle cause is obvious and removable, one approach to treatment is to encourage the patient to make simple life style changes, e.g. change of diet or reduction of stress. Indeed if causes are not removed and symptoms treated alone the illness is likely to express itself in some other way or treatment may be unsuccessful due to a 'maintaining cause'. Homeopaths recognise the need to work with life style factors alongside the correct prescription in order to obtain and maintain health. The homeopathic case informs the homeopath about diets, rest, exercise, relationships, etc. and a homeopathic prescription can facilitate what might otherwise be difficult life style changes. For this reason a homeopath is more than someone who prescribes homeopathically – they are also aware of and supportive of other treatments and advice that facilitate this healing process.

Working with Other Treatment Modalities

In some cases a symptom can be in its own right a cause for another symptom. Treatment, in practice, often requires working with a variety of different interventions and may involve bringing together several different strands of treatment to plan a programme that takes several aspects of a patient's situation and susceptibility into account. John's case is an example.

CASE STUDY 6.6

John, aged 28, had a history of eczema since childhood and asthma starting in his early teens. The asthma responded only partially to a well-indicated homeopathic remedy. He had a mildly kyphotic spine and poor posture. John had a course of osteopathic treatment that 'made him feel taller' and after this the same homeopathic remedy became more effective and the asthma started to improve.

Many types of treatment can be utilised to clarify a case and help in its overall treatment. This book concentrates on the homeopathic interventions but other approaches and their effect on the case and response to treatment need to be considered as increasingly complex cases are treated. If remedies are thought of as information then they might be likened to a blueprint or an architect's plan of a building. In order to construct or repair a 'building', in addition to the plan, physical building materials are required. The absence of the right material and support such as adequate diet, rest, and relaxation (including emotional) accompanying the correct remedy is a common cause for a well-indicated remedy failing to act.

REFLECTION POINT

- If information is required for health how might this relate to psychological, energetic, chemical or genetic information? How is treating a patient by modifying their situation or environment different from treating their susceptibility? How does this affect their 'resistance' to other illnesses?

Summary

In many minor ailments and acute cases prescribing on the presenting symptoms with or without causation gives a well-indicated remedy. Treating more complex conditions requires identifying the deeper symptoms and understanding the hierarchy. In later sections we will revisit the foundations set in this chapter including maintaining factors, obstacles to cure, low vitality and aggravations.

We have introduced two important concepts, one of health as an interplay between the patient's susceptibility, vitality and situation (or environment), and a second of understanding health in terms of information as well as gross material factors. These concepts will inform the subtle examination of the materia medica and the homeopathic case in this section and allow you to develop a structure for approaching more complex cases in subsequent sections. They are not always easy concepts and they may require further reflection in order to put them into practice.

This chapter invites you to start to 're-frame' health in energetic terms, with illness a way of adapting to changing circumstances and environment. Disease process provides an opportunity for the organism to respond to a stimulus and acquire knowledge and resistance to illness that allows the individual to explore many different evolving and changing life situations. While patients with simple illness can often do this themselves over time, it can be greatly speeded up using a homeopathic approach. Simple cases when the natural healing process is not facilitated or is blocked by drug treatments (even mild analgesics, anti-inflammatories, antibiotics and antihistamines, for example) are a major cause of more complex cases. For this reason being able to treat acute conditions and simple cases homeopathically and isopathically – whether in the home or by the homeopath, the family doctor, the nurse or the pharmacist – is important in preventing more serious and increasingly complex disease.

References

Maciocia G 1989 The foundations of Chinese medicine. Churchill Livingstone, Edinburgh

Saine A 2000 The method, lectures on pure classical homeopathy II. Lutra Services, Eindhoven

Sankaran R 2004 The sensation in homeopathy. Homeopathic Medical Publishers, Mumbai

Swayne J 1998 Homeopathic method, implications for clinical practice and medical science. Churchill Livingstone, Edinburgh

Wheeler C 1948 An introduction to the principles and practice of homeopathy, 3rd edn. William Heinemann, London

Bibliography

Close S 1924 The genius of homeopathy. Lectures and essays on homeopathic philosophy. Boericke and Tafel, Philadelphia. Indian edition 1959; Haren & Brother, Calcutta. Also available online: www.homeoint.org/books4/close/index.htm

Clover A 1989 Homeopathy reconsidered, a new look at Hahnemann's Organon. Victor Gollancz, London

Gaier H 1991 Encyclopaedic dictionary of homeopathy. Thorsons, London

Hahnemann S 1896 trans Tafel L 1896 The chronic diseases, their specific nature and their homoeopathic treatment, 2 vols. Boericke & Tafel, Philadelphia. Reprinted 1998 Homeopathic Book Service, Sittingbourne

Hahnemann S trans Dudgeon RE 1852 The lesser writings of Samuel Hahnemann. W Headland, London. Indian edition 1995 B Jain, New Delhi

Johnston L 1991 Everyday miracles: homeopathy in action. Christine Kent Agency, Van Nuys, CA

Shine M 2004 What about the potency? Food for Thought Publishing, London

Vithoulkas G 1979 Homoeopathy: medicine of the new man. Thorsons, Wellingborough

Vithoulkas G 1980 The science of homeopathy. Grove Press, New York

Vithoulkas G 1991 A new model of health and disease. North Atlantic Books, Berkeley

CHAPTER SEVEN

The Materia Medica

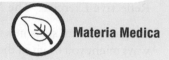 **Materia Medica**

David Owen

'What we had repeatedly found confirmed by cures, day after day, week after week, and year after year, is what we took as our basis, as true gain in the new science; these were what we called the characteristics of the drug.'

C. Hering

Introduction

The materia medica is how we know the unique qualities and characteristics of each remedy, what it can cure. Homeopaths must know this information or how to find it so that they can match the appropriate remedy to the case. The homeopath gathers this information especially, but not only, from provings (see Chapter 2). Many homeopaths see that the information about each remedy is also expressed in other ways, including toxicological and clinical effects but also through such things as the appearance of the source material, where the source material is found, cultural relevance of the source material, etc. The information about a remedy is recorded in the materia medica, but these vary greatly in what sources of information are included, the level of detail and how they are laid out.

Different materia medicas suit different approaches to treatment and methodologies. For example, those that best suit first aid and acute prescribing are often brief and focus on causation and presenting symptoms and are not the same as those that fit essence or thematic prescribing. One way to think of the different materia medicas is like different maps that might describe or portray the same place but in different ways. In the same way as a map identifies key features we explore key symptoms or 'keynotes' of the remedies.

The remedies represent a huge amount of different information and it is helpful when embarking on learning it and deciding how to reference it to explore your own preferred style of learning. It is worthwhile spending a little time thinking about and comparing different materia medicas so that you can, over time, build your own personal materia medica in a way that suits you and that can be expanded as you broaden the range of approaches and methodologies you wish to use.

Levels of Detail in the Materia Medica

Ultimately, all materia medicas are a collection of symptoms. The detail and the way they are collated determine both their size and how applicable they are to finding remedies according to different methodologies. Each has different priorities and includes remedy details to suit some situations more than others. Choosing the most appropriate level at which to study each remedy is influenced by many factors. These include the patients and diseases likely to be treated, the homeopath's preferred approach to treatment and learning style, and the practice environment in which the remedies are likely to be used. Likewise the materia

BOX 7.1
Reflective Exercise: 'The Maze'

Imagine you are stuck in a maze. In what different ways might you be given the directions you need to get out? In a straightforward maze you might start with trial and error and in many cases this might 'get you out' – equivalent we could say to self-healing. As the maze gets more complicated then you might need to think about it in different ways and use different approaches to find your way out.

At the causative level you might just retrace your steps and, if not too far in, follow the daylight or draught. At the presenting symptom level there may be one key junction at which to choose the right direction, or a series of junctions – followed one junction at a time with separate 'local' directions for each junction. The totality model would seek to form an overview of the maze, a map of it, and to use this overview to navigate out. It may be possible to recognise a pattern behind the map that would equate to an essence or theme, e.g. to always turn left, or mostly to turn in the direction that makes you go furthest. It might be valid to try to understand the design or designer of the mazes and how they are 'relating' to you. If it is to tease you it may always take the least likely direct direction, if it is to relax you it may take you the easiest route when offered a choice.

Each of these methods can, of course, be combined in practice– as can the homeopathic models and approaches, but the information and interpretation of the information that each uses is different.

medica you know and the texts you have available will influence how you are able to analyse the case. This is one reason why those who carry out provings and compile the materia medicas are at the centre of homeopathic development. The exercise in Box 7.1 provides an opportunity to reflect on the different levels of information that might be found about remedies and how they correlate with the five models of health using the metaphor of a maze.

Selecting the Materia Medica According to Approach

The information needed to use each of the five main approaches to treatment covered in this book is slightly different.

Causation

When there is clear causation it is helpful to see this in the case and in the materia medica. The modalities often hint at causation even if it is not clearly stated as such, e.g. a condition reliably and frequently aggravated by wet weather may be caused by it. In some remedies the source material may point to the cause directly, e.g. the remedy Radium Bromide, made from radioactive radium, can in potency help patients with radiation damage and is sometimes given to patients receiving radiotherapy.

Presenting Symptoms

In many simple cases the presenting symptoms point to a likely remedy. The stronger the symptom in the patient and the more notable the symptom in the remedy the more likely a remedy matched on this basis is to work. In addition it can help greatly to understand related aspects of the symptom such as things that make them better or worse, other symptoms, the nature of any pain, etc. – what we refer to as the complete symptom. Communicating both the strength and the connections between different symptoms is an important aspect of the materia medicas and is done through different methods of 'weighting' different symptoms and building what is referred to as a 'symptom picture'. Table 7.1 looks at the information about the remedies most useful for each approach, both in the case and in the materia medica.

Table 7.1 FEATURES OF MATERIA MEDICAS LINKED TO EACH APPROACH

Model of Health	Main Information	Linked to	Example of Remedy
Causation	Causative factors	Features that make symptoms better or worse, called amelioration (>) and aggravation (<)	Aconite after exposure to cold wind
Presenting symptom	Main symptoms and keynote symptoms including some 'strange, rare and peculiar' symptoms	The complete symptom including the typical clinical presentation, location and modality	Night cramps helped by Cuprum metallicum (copper)
Totality	Symptoms related to the patient's mind (mentals), body (physical) and environment (generals). It may be laid out in the words of the provers or systematised into mentals, parts of the body and generals	Stronger more unusual and unique symptoms. The intensity of symptoms is illustrated by scoring them, using italics, bold type or underlining.	Remedies that we know and use widely in chronic and acute cases and for disease of many types are sometimes referred to as 'polychrests', e.g. sulphur
Essence	The pattern behind symptoms, describing the themes or trends in remedies. Often describing a group or family of remedies and what they have in common particularly in relation to the sensation or feeling behind the symptoms.	Groups of symptoms that share similar qualities or shared patterns of symptoms. Several different themes can run through the symptoms of a case	Graphite showing qualities of carbon remedies, also of mineral remedies
Relational	Not frequently described in the materia medica but the feelings that emerge in a remedy state and sometimes those generated when thinking about or working with patients needing a remedy	How these remedies make the homeopath or those around the patient feel. Different homeopaths might feel differently but if they are in a 'steady state' their feelings can reliably point to the remedy	Feeling like the Pulsatilla patient needs a hug

Totality

As cases become more complex they are likely to need a remedy prescribed on a diverse symptom picture, which in turn needs a much more detailed materia medica to describe them. When using the totality approach symptoms from the mind, body and general symptoms are included. Remedies known to have a clear totality picture and that are frequently indicated using this approach are sometimes known as 'polycrests'. Sometimes remedies less well known or used are called 'small remedies', although when studied more fully or in different situations they may indeed have a broad range of action. In different cultures and over time the frequently used remedies change. In practice many materia medicas are cumulative in that those describing the totality include causation and the presenting symptoms.

Essence and Theme

Essences and themes in different remedies frequently relate to patterns that run through several remedies, particularly those whose source materials share some features, such as a group of remedies that come from the sea or a group of remedies belonging to a particular botanical family (family materia medica) – each showing some common and some slightly different symptoms.

Relational

In the relational model the dynamic between the patient and homeopath is often something developed by experience in the profession as a whole; the individual homeopath can draw upon this common insight to point to the remedy, e.g. the feeling of wanting to comfort or 'hug' a child needing the remedy Pulsatilla. This is sometimes described as 'situational' materia medica. It also includes any personal but reliable experience the homeopath has and how different remedies can make them react and feel.

Depth Versus Breadth on Learning Materia Medica

The remedies are the tools of the homeopath's trade – the more that are known the greater the range of tasks that can be undertaken. But the tools are only useful when combined with the craft of the operator. For most homeopaths it is a practical matter of learning a range of remedies in sufficient depth to suit the methodologies favoured, supported by knowing how to access more information about the remedies when needed. This is followed by gradually extending both the range of remedies and the details about each, often learning through new provings, the experience of other homeopaths, and through their own cases.

In simple cases, a few well-known remedies (and importantly having them available when you see the patient) may be all that is needed. In complex cases where a greater sense of individualisation in matching the remedy is needed a greater breadth of remedies is likely to be required. Ultimately a good homeopath will have both a breadth and depth of remedy knowledge. They build their knowledge of the remedies from a variety of descriptions of the remedies as well as from clinical experience.

Sources of Information

There are thousands of proved remedies available to the homeopath and this number is growing steadily. In addition there are any number of remedies that may be used on other indications. About 70% of the remedies that have been 'proved' are plants. Most other remedies are from animal products or minerals. A few are known as 'imponderables' and made from such things as electricity, radiation, sunlight and magnetism.

In compiling the materia medicas there are many different sources of information about the remedies. Not all remedies and certainly not all materia medicas make use of information from each of these but a variety of sources help to build a complete and memorable remedy picture. The provings are central to this but other sources also provide important information (Box 7.2). It is possible to think of information about each remedy corresponding to the different approaches to treatment and models of health, giving a picture built up with several different, but often complementary pieces of information – as Figure 7.1 illustrates for the remedy Belladonna. The name comes from bella = beautiful and donna = woman, and it was used as eye drops to dilate the pupils, itself a type of proving. It contains atropine, which has well known pharmacological effects and is a rapidly acting poison (also called deadly nightshade). Sometimes characteristics are linked to the botanical solanacea family to which it belongs. Sometimes it is related to the remedy calcium carbonate, to which it is described as the 'acute' – meaning that in many acute illnesses and simple cases responding well to Belladonna the underlying picture can be Calcarea carbonica.

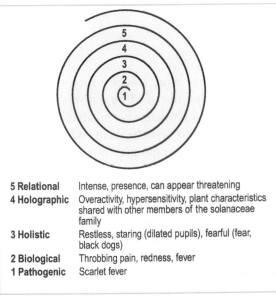

5 Relational	Intense, presence, can appear threatening
4 Holographic	Overactivity, hypersensitivity, plant characteristics shared with other members of the solanaceae family
3 Holistic	Restless, staring (dilated pupils), fearful (fear, black dogs)
2 Biological	Throbbing pain, redness, fever
1 Pathogenic	Scarlet fever

Figure 7.1 Different levels of materia medica information correlated by model of health to the remedy Belladonna

BOX 7.2
Sources of Information About Remedies

Main Sources
- Provings e.g. China Officianalis
- Toxicology e.g. Lachesis, venom of the bush-master snake
- Recorded clinical use e.g. Euphrasia (eyebright)

Subsidiary Sources
- Appearance or behaviour of the source e.g. Silica in sand and glass
- Environment of the source e.g. Arnica growing on mountains, also called fall-herb
- Disease patterns e.g. nosodes
- Historical, including herbal usage of the remedy e.g. Caulophyllum known as squaw root from its use in childbirth.
- Traditional/cultural usage e.g. Anhalonium
- Pharmacological including adverse effects e.g. Lithium Carbonicum
- Connections with biological families
- Mythological e.g. Aurum from the use of gold

- Symbolic including shape and colour of source (Doctrine of Signatures)
- Case history pointing to an affinity with a substance e.g. nickel allergy
- Personal or cultural use of a remedy e.g. Coffea or Cannabis indica use etc
- Emotional and intuitive insights such as in the Bach flower remedies

Other Systems
Other systems use other criteria to determine how a remedy acts e.g. the Biochemical tissue salts and Bach flower remedies. As these are not prescribed on provings they are not always considered homeopathic, although they act as 'energetic' remedies. Biochemical tissue salts use a range of 12 inorganic salts prepared similarly to homeopathic remedies. Bach flower remedies are a range of energetic remedies prescribed on the dominant emotional state of the patient.

Sometimes other sources of information, in addition to the provings, are particularly significant in the adoption of a remedy. Any substance can, when prescribed on the basis of like treating like, be considered a homeopathic remedy, but the accurate matching possible when a comprehensive remedy picture is used allows both deeper-acting and more confident prescriptions to be made. This chapter considers provings, toxicology and clinical use, although the other sources are referred to elsewhere and not only provide useful detail but can serve as an aide-memoire to key points of the materia medica.

Provings

Provings present a wealth of information about the reactions that take place when individuals are exposed to remedies; how these are conducted has been covered in Chapter 2. Reliability of proving symptom is influenced by the objectivity of the symptom, repeatability in differ-

ent provers, and the rigour and protocol of the proving. How the symptoms are collated and arranged determines how easy it is to find this information. Some original records of provings give complete detail about the reaction of each prover in a descriptive style. Others combine similar symptoms from different provers, while some systematise the proving under mind, part of the body and general headings. As a way of systematising the materia medica this structure has gradually evolved, often requiring a trade-off between ease of use and completeness.

Toxicology

There are many accounts in literature and in folk-lore of the effects of poisoning on the human organism. From the early days of homeopathy accounts of poisonings have helped in developing the materia medica and are the source of many symptoms in the early materia medicas. One of the earliest recorded poisonings was of Socrates with Conium maculata; it gives a description of the ascending paralysis that can respond to this remedy. Knowledge of toxicology has also influenced what substances are selected for proving as it points to substances that have a significant effect. The toxicology of Belladonna from a medical herbal of 1834 gives an account of the poisoning of a group of soldiers:

'... *dryness and burning heat of the throat and mouth, vertigo, dimness and confusion of sight; dilation and immobility of the pupil; delirium, coma, an eruption resembling that in Scarletina, and occasionally strangury ... The greater number were delirious, but the delirium was gay; a great number also lost their voice, and others spoke confusedly; there was also much motion of the hands and fingers; several were blind for some time; and in all, the pupils were dilated.*'

Clinical Experience

Some homeopathic remedies are chosen in specific conditions as much on their clinical reputation as on their provings e.g. Chamomilla, Ferrum Phosphoricum and Euphrasia (Eyebright). This can sometimes be adequate for treatment of acute conditions at a symptomatic level although provings reveal a more complete picture, allowing a more accurate and confident match. Mostly this clinical information limits the use of the remedy to local or clinical methodologies. It is sometimes possible to see remedies favoured by certain groups of homeopaths. For example, in an international study on treating upper respiratory tract infections in the UK, Ferrum Phosphoricum was well used as it has a 'clinical reputation', but in the USA it was much less used.

When new symptoms emerge as a patient is being treated with a particular remedy it is possible they are related to that remedy. In a way this is like making a proving on a sick person and although frowned on in principle, because the patient's sickness will alter the remedy reaction, in practice many early provings were done on patients.

Clinical experience offers a way of updating information about remedies when provings were completed some time ago or in different cultures. For example when Arsenicum Album was proved

photography was not common but a feature of patients responding to Arsenicum Album is that they frequently become less anxious about their photograph being taken. Extrapolating from this, a fear of having a photograph taken may point towards the remedy Arsenicum Album. We can be more confident about this because it is consistent with the concern about appearance and control that we observe in Arsenicum Album.

REFLECTION POINT

- If remedies provide information that helps a patient move to a new balanced state, why should this information produce these symptoms in provings? And to what extent might this same information be expressed in the appearance of the remedy, where it is found and any effects, myths, beliefs that are associated with it?

Symptoms In The Materia Medica

Symptoms, including signs, are the language of the case (see Chapter 8), disease (see Chapter 6) and the remedy. As every substance has in theory the potential to challenge someone who has the susceptibility to that substance, every substance could be a remedy. A remedy may provoke as a proving anything from a single subtle symptom to a comprehensive symptom picture. Weighting, or evaluating the strength of each symptom indicates the relative importance and reliability of that symptom. Different materia medicas indicate this by using different typefaces (capitals, bold, italic, underlined, etc), or using numbers (+2, + 3 or in 'aversions' −2, −3, etc.), or by labelling symptoms in some way e.g. as keynotes. (Similar ways to indicate the importance of symptoms in talking about or recording a case are also used.)

Keynotes

Certain symptoms and causations are observed as reliable indicators for certain remedies; these often relate to key features of the remedy called the keynotes. These are reliable symptoms observed in provings and may also be observed in toxicology or clinical practice. They are sometimes claimed to describe symptoms of a remedy uniquely and in local prescribing may be matched to the characteristic symptoms of the individual's expression of the disease process. Examples of keynotes are the irritability and sensitivity to pain in Chamomilla and the fearfulness in Aconite.

Importance of Keynotes

Keynotes may be used as relative inclusion (confirmatory) and exclusion (eliminatory) checks before prescribing. For example, a keynote of Sulphur is that it is untidy and it would be unusual (but not impossible) to prescribe Sulphur in a very precise, tidy and fastidious case; a keynote of Argentum Nitricum is a desire for sweets and it would be unlikely to be prescribed in a case that did not have a desire for sweets. An exclusion symptom relatively eliminates from consideration those remedies that do not have that symptom (see Chapter 9).

Keynotes are often summaries of something observed in many provers and represent an abbreviation of often more complex symptoms. In clinically-based materia medicas using keynotes allows them to be shorter, making it easier to find your way around them, to make comparisons and to memorise. Keynotes of presenting symptoms are sometimes called 'guiding symptoms'. Personal keynotes may also be symptoms that you reliably observe in patients. For example, I am confident that many Staphisagria patients talk with a fixed lower jaw as if they are talking through their teeth. Arsenicum Album patients often have not only an aversion to being photographed but also an aversion (or desire) for red foods like tomatoes and beetroot.

Strange, Rare and Peculiar

Keynotes, like other symptoms, become more important the *stronger* they are, in the remedy or the patient, e.g. 'I must eat something sweet every half hour'. However they also become more important the more *striking* they are in a particular case or remedy picture. So in a remedy that is generally worse from heat but has a headache better from heat, the headache better from heat is more distinctive. These things make the keynote more individual to the patient and remedy – and therefore more important. They may be more individualising because they are strange, rare or peculiar. Strange in that they are paradoxical in a particular situation, rare in that they occur infrequently. Or they may be peculiar in that they would not be expected in a particular situation. A symptom may stand out due to its own uniqueness or because of the things that modify (modalities) the symptom's expression.

Modalities

Modalities are factors that modify the behaviour or degree of intensity of a symptom or sign. They may be a normal physiological function, an emotional state, an activity or environmental factor. They include palliative measures the patient may use to minimise the symptoms, such as rubbing or scratching a rash, or holding a painful part of the body.

Modalities (see also Chapter 8, p. 101) can be strong or weak and are scored in the same way as symptoms. If a modality is especially strong, strange, rare, peculiar, or fits several symptoms it can be considered a keynote. For example, a patient whose joint symptoms are aggravated from movement but who also generally hates moving about when feeling ill, describe the modalities of the remedy Bryonia, where 'worse (<) from movement' is a keynote.

Appearance

Some physical features of patients indicate certain remedies, e.g. a 'saddle nose' may be a feature of patients fitting Syphilinum, and red hair may be a feature of Phosphorous patients. Information about the appearance of patients is most likely to be based on the appearance of individuals that clinical experience shows responds well to that substance, or types of patient susceptible to poisoning by it, or to those most likely to exhibit strong proving symptoms to it. Sometimes the appearance of the patient can change during a proving, e.g. during a proving of Sepia a sallow complexion may develop.

Different Materia Medicas

Materia medicas vary in layout, number of remedies, amount and sources of information, and from brief outline descriptions to verbatim reports of provers. Some, such as Hughes, concentrate on local cause and symptoms. Others, like Hering, used much clinical information and verification. Some, such as Kent, draw out a picture of mental and general symptoms that directly lead to thinking of remedies as a totality. Some of the most significant materia medicas historically are listed in Box 7.3 and to put these and the development of homeopathy in context some world events are included (Figure 7.2). Many of these early materia medicas share some of the same sources of information; some repeat content but use different layouts. It is interesting to compare this historical record and the wealth of relevant information collected over this time with the relative transience of much of currently conventional medicine that has its origin in the apothecaries and barbershops of the 19th century. At the time Hahnemann was developing his ideas on homeopathy, most illnesses were thought to be due to an excess of blood or impurities in the blood. Healing required blood-taking and blood purification using emetics, purgatives, agents causing salivation, perspiration, urination, drawing plasters, etc.

Only after 1980 do the remedy descriptions really begin to draw out the essence and themes in the remedy pictures. Vithoulkas was one of the

---

BOX 7.3
The Most Significant Materia Medicas

Materia Medica Pura, S Hahnemann
In the materia medica pura are some original provings before potentised remedies were used.

Chronic Diseases, S Hahnemann
Includes theory of chronic disease and a list of provings of 23 new medicines as well as several already published. Hahnemann no longer offers the name of provers as they were probably drawn (contrary to his own rules) from his patients with chronic diseases, and it includes apparently inert substances like Silicea, Natrum muriaticum and Lycopodium. Provings used the 30c potency and the distrust of these provings together with hostility to his new theories resulted in a split in the homeopathic camp. All the remedies were later proved in Vienna and generally substantiated.

Allen's Encyclopaedia of Pure Materia Medica
A large collection of provings, all with references – some dangerously toxic and using high dilutions. High potency provings tie up with clinically useful symptoms e.g. the uterine prolapse sensation in Sepia which was a minor symptom in 'Chronic diseases' got into bold type in Allen as a result of a single proving of the 200th potency which emphasised it. Both Hughes and Hering were major contributors to Allen's work.

Hering's Guiding Symptoms of our Materia Medica
Less interested in the provings and 'old school' symptoms than in those symptoms which had been shown in the light of clinical experience to be useful. Free of annotations with one symptom per line making it easy to read, and with markings indicating the most well verified symptoms. Used by Kent in grading of symptoms for his repertory (see Chapter 9).

Hughes' Cyclopaedia of Drug Pathogenesy
Hughes had co-operated with Allen's Encyclopaedia but did not agree with high potency provings and provings made on patients. It contains toxic and material drug proving symptoms from healthy provers and gives detailed information on causation and presenting symptoms. It gave rise to a number of the clinically orientated guides based on 'local prescribing'.

Kent's Lectures on Materia Medica
Descriptions of individual remedies assumed an easy narrative style. Talk about 'the Sepia patient' or 'Pulsatilla patient' was the beginning of the idea of constitutional prescribing.

Clarke's Dictionary
Eclectic and practical, and each remedy starts off with an interesting account of cured cases and includes a list of common conditions.

Boericke's Materia Medica
A succinct summary of the materia medica with useful preamble and well chosen italics for emphasis, a good desktop guide.

Boger's Synoptic Key of the Materia Medica
A combined repertory and materia medica organised along lines promoted by Boenninghausen emphasising modalities, localities and sensations.

Tyler's Drug Pictures
A chatty and readable materia medica using frequent quotations from other materia medicas.

Vithoulkas's Essences
A thematic interpretation of the materia medica using imagination, feeling and a considerable knowledge to bring to life and reinterpret the remedies through a modern and memorable psychological picture.

Sankaran's Situational Materia Medica
Reflects the adaptive way an organism responds to a real or imagined situation. Explores the fears and delusions behind each remedy state. Symptoms centre around a particular type of reality distortion, e.g. the remedy Tarantula has dancing and desire for music in its provings. Perhaps explained by the organism trying to attract attention due to a basic delusion of unrequited love i.e. trying to attract the attention of the loved one.

Scholten's Homeopathy and Minerals
Certain characteristics being associated with different anions and cations e.g. calcium and Muriaticum elements, combining to form a composite picture. He relates characteristics to the element's place in the periodic table.

first to describe comprehensive patterns that run through a remedy that he named 'essences'. These patterns have developed alongside materia medicas looking at groups of remedies based on similar clinical pictures, such as Borland's children's types, and sometimes on the source material of the remedy, such as Scholten's use of the periodic table. Materia medicas with constitutional, thematic and relational information are less common than those with causation, presenting or totality symptoms. Constitution is reflected by situational preferences including the environment sought out (reflected in generals) and relationships moved into and away from (reflecting psychological preferences). Sometimes referred to as 'situational materia medica'.

Themes are reflected in the feeling world both of physical sensations and emotional feeling. The sensation (that runs through a theme) or feelings that runs through a case or remedy is represented in emotional or thematic materia medica.

Relationally it is important to know not only how a patient needing a particular remedy makes you feel but also what it is like to be that remedy yourself and how do you relate to those aspects of the remedy that are in you? This is sometimes called living materia medica.

Different tools are needed for different jobs. The ideal materia medica needed for each separate prescribing methodology varies, and the homeopath developing a range of prescribing methodologies will benefit from using several different materia medicas. Box 7.3 shows how the structure of the materia medicas has evolved and also offers insight on how the different approaches to treatment (and, less explicitly, the models of health) have developed.

Causation and the
Presenting Symptoms

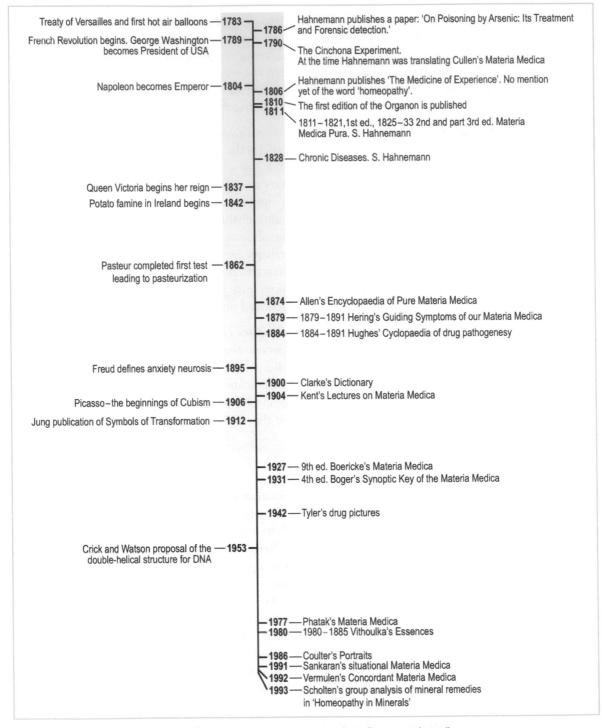

Treaty of Versailles and first hot air balloons — **1783**

Hahnemann publishes a paper: 'On Poisoning by Arsenic: Its Treatment and Forensic detection.' — **1786**

French Revolution begins. George Washington — **1789**
becomes President of USA

1790 — The Cinchona Experiment.
At the time Hahnemann was translating Cullen's Materia Medica

Napoleon becomes Emperor — **1804**

1806 — Hahnemann publishes 'The Medicine of Experience'. No mention yet of the word 'homeopathy'.

1810 — The first edition of the Organon is published

1811 — 1811–1821,1st ed., 1825–33 2nd and part 3rd ed. Materia Medica Pura. S. Hahnemann

1828 — Chronic Diseases. S. Hahnemann

Queen Victoria begins her reign — **1837**

Potato famine in Ireland begins — **1842**

Pasteur completed first test — **1862**
leading to pasteurization

1874 — Allen's Encyclopaedia of Pure Materia Medica

1879 — 1879–1891 Hering's Guiding Symptoms of our Materia Medica

1884 — 1884–1891 Hughes' Cyclopaedia of drug pathogenesy

Freud defines anxiety neurosis — **1895**

1900 — Clarke's Dictionary

Picasso – the beginnings of Cubism — **1906**

1904 — Kent's Lectures on Materia Medica

Jung publication of Symbols of Transformation — **1912**

1927 — 9th ed. Boericke's Materia Medica

1931 — 4th ed. Boger's Synoptic Key of the Materia Medica

1942 — Tyler's drug pictures

Crick and Watson proposal of the — **1953**
double-helical structure for DNA

1977 — Phatak's Materia Medica

1980 — 1980–1885 Vithoulka's Essences

1986 — Coulter's Portraits

1991 — Sankaran's situational Materia Medica

1992 — Vermulen's Concordant Materia Medica

1993 — Scholten's group analysis of mineral remedies in 'Homeopathy in Minerals'

Figure 7.2   Time line of the development of significant materia medicas

Layout of the Materia Medica

The aim of a materia medica is to communicate as effectively as possible, in an orderly and systematic way, the use of remedies in different situations. Since the time of Kent, in most detailed materia medicas the symptoms from different sources are often collated according to anatomical location, as in the Boericke materia medica (Box 7.4).

Choosing a Materia Medica

Different homeopaths favour different texts and while initially you are likely to be influenced by those that teach you, over time homeopaths often select different texts that suit their way of working.

BOX 7.4

Example of Layout of a Materia Medica

Based on Boericke

Name and source

Introduction, including pointers on usage and
generals

Mind

Head

Eyes

Ears

Nose

Mouth

Throat

Stomach

Abdomen

Rectum

Urine

Kidney

Genitalia

Respiratory

Back

Extremities

Sleep

Fever

Skin

Modalities: what makes symptoms better (>)
and worse (<)

Relationship to other remedies, follows
well, etc.

Information on dosage, frequency and duration

Given the diversity of texts easily available there is no reason why a homeopath should not have a range of texts available in books or electronically to enable a variety of approaches to suit different patients. Many homeopaths will start with a keynote text for ease of use, supported by a more 'totality orientated' text with access to the individual provings when the remedy picture is unclear. The bullet points below cover some of the things to think about in selecting a text and some of the limitations of some materia medicas. Does it:

- detail likely causation and common primary symptoms?
- give a totality picture? (in practice some materia medicas are more 'diseases centred'; others are more 'person centred')
- collate information from a range of provers?
- integrate clinical observations and toxicological information?
- detail aspects of the constitutional type?
- give information on essence and theme?
- point to how these remedy types behave and interact with others and in a consultation?
- suit your way of working and is it easy to use? (there is often a trade-off between ease of use and comprehensiveness)

Limitations

- Many were compiled from information from provers of previous generations where the language of expression of symptoms is very different from that used currently.
- Given the amount of information and the numbers of individuals collecting and collating it, errors naturally occur. Proving symptoms may be recorded incorrectly, inaccuracies may be copied, unreliable sources used. For example, in their proving of Aethusa (Fool's Parsley) Hartlaub and Trinks got the symptoms mixed up with those of Conium (Hemlock). From there the error was copied and handed down to numerous materia medicas and eventually corrected in Allen's Encyclopaedia.
- The possibility for error increases when symptoms are abbreviated, or symptoms from one prover are combined with another. If footnotes

or references of each prover for every symptom are used the text becomes unwieldy.

Comparing the Different Materia Medicas

The descriptions below are edited extractions from the mind section of the remedy Silica in four materia medicas and one repertory. A repertory is a systematic list of symptoms of a homeopathic medicine, usually from several sources, indicating the degree of association or strength of the symptom (see Chapter 9). Using extractions from a repertory, the relevant rubrics that contain the remedy at a particular level of association, strength or uniqueness, or a combination of these things can be constructed.

These five sources illustrate something of the variety of layouts, including how symptoms are abbreviated and weighted in different texts. The weighting in the first uses plain type, italics and capitals to represent increasing degrees of strength or association. The second and third use plain type and bold for the same purpose. In the third, keynotes are put in double brackets << >>. The fourth is not weighted.

REFLECTION POINT

- Different practitioners prefer different materia medicas – what qualities are most important to you and why? From the example below, what features of materia medicas and repertories might you find helpful to your study of the remedies and what make it harder?

BOX 7.5

Extracts of Mental Symptoms for the Remedy Picture of Silica (Sil) from 5 different sources

Vermulens 1992
Faint-hearted, anxious. Nervous and excitable. *Sensitive* to all impressions. Brain fag of businessmen, lawyers, preachers and students. Obstinate, headstrong children. Fixed ideas; thinks only of *pins*, fears them, searches for and counts them. Yielding. Sensitive weeping mood. Cries when kindly spoken to. Sullen. Loss of self-confidence; dreads failure, but unfounded. Starts from slight noise. *Confusion worse < conversation.* Forgetfulness better > after eating. *Prostration of mind after writing. Remorse about trifles.* Indisposed to talk loud. *Unconsciousness after taking cold water.* ANXIETY DURING MENSES. Clairvoyance. CONSCIENTIOUS ABOUT TRIFLES. CONSOLATION aggravates. *Intolerant of contradiction; Dullness in children.* Dullness from damp air; after dreams. *Fear of literary work. Homesickness.* Inconstancy. *Irresolution.* INTERNAL RESTLESSNESS. *Restlessness while sitting; on waking. Sensitive to voices. Starting when touched.* TIMIDITY ABOUT APPEARING IN PUBLIC. Undertakes nothing lest he fail.

Boericke 1927
Yielding, FAINT-HEARTED, ANXIOUS. Nervous and excitable. SENSITIVE to all impressions. Brain-fag. Obstinate, headstrong children. Abstracted. Fixed ideas; thinks only of PINS, fears them, searches and counts them.

Morrison 1993
<<Yielding, refined, delicate patients.>> Quiet and self-contained. THE PATIENT WILL ADMIT TO HAVING CONVICTIONS WHICH HE DOES NOT ARGUE, even seeming to acquiesce to another's viewpoint though internally keeping his own view. <<Anxious conscientiousness over small details.>>

<<Anxiety from noise.>> Anxious and depressed.

<<Stage-fright.>> Performance anxiety. Test phobia.

Mental dullness. Dreads or is aggravated by mental exertion.

Weak memory. Mental deterioration. Dementia.

Fear of pointed objects or pins.

<<Obstinate>> children who 'weep when reprimanded'.

Shy children who will not answer the prescriber directly but instead whisper to the mother who must relay the information.

Psychic capacity; clairvoyant.

Fixed ideas.

Tyler 1942

Silica, they say, lacks grit – needs sand. And doses of Silica stimulate mightily these weaklings who are going under, to put up a fight, mental and physical

You look up, as poor little Silica is dragged reluctantly in. He is listless; not interested; not frightened.

You see a pale, sickly, suffering face; and you realise at once that there is something deeply wrong there;

He doesn't get on, he doesn't thrive. He doesn't learn; he doesn't even play. He is irritable and grumpy. He is always at the bottom of everything, and his teacher can't make no think of him; she writes, see! – 'he shrinks from effort, from the least responsibility, and is utterly lacking in self-confidence and self-assertion.' Doesn't seem to have no 'go' in him. He doesn't seem to be able to think! He can't fix his mind. He can't read or write. And yet he's always worried to death over little things he's done wrong. That's it: he's so odd, and so unlike the others.

He gets violent attacks of headache, she says, and complains that the back of his head is cold. That's where the pain is, but it goes all over his head. He says his head will burst. He wants it tied up tight. He wants it warm. Warm and tight, that's what his head has got to be – when he gets one of his attacks.

And a funny thing she has noticed, he's always ill with the new moon!

Look at his nails – rough and yellow; and feeling as if he had got a splinter in his finger. Or gets red, swollen finger that throbs and feels like a felon. Or look at that finger, how it is swollen, and the bone feels big. He wakes crying, and says his hands have gone to sleep...'

Repertory Extraction from Kent 1877

Below is the result of a search of the mind section of Kent's repertory for Silica where it occurs in second (italic) or third level (bold) with no other remedy sharing the symptom with the same or higher grade. No entries for silica at the first (lowest) level are shown. It therefore only shows the stronger symptoms that Silica may have but it also shows some of the remedies that share the symptoms of Silica. It gives an interesting view of the strongest and/or most particular symptoms, as well as an idea of other closely related remedies, for example Phosphorous (phos) is in three of these rubrics and it is known to be closely homeopathically related to Silica.

Mind; ANXIETY; fright, after (read as anxiety coming on after a fright): acon., gels., lyc., merc., nat-m., op., rob., *sil.*

Mind; ANXIETY; menses; during: acon., *bell.*, calc., canth., cimic., cina, coff., con., ign., inul., kali-i., merc., *nat-m.*, nit-ac., nux-v., phos., *plat.*, sec., **Sil.**, stann., sulph., zinc.

Mind; ANXIETY; noise, from: agar., alum., *aur.*, bar-c., caps., *caust.*, chel., nat-c., petr., puls., **Sil.**

Mind; CONFUSION; conversation agg.: *sil.*

Mind; DELUSIONS; images, phantoms, sees; sees, all over: merc., *sil.*

Mind; DELUSIONS; needles, sees: merc., *sil.*

Mind; DULLNESS; writing, while: acon., arg-n., cann-s., chin-s., glon., mag-c., nux-m., rhus-t., *sil.*

Mind; FEAR; work, dread of; literary, of: nux-v., *sil.*, sulph.

Mind; PROSTRATION of mind; reading, from: aur., *sil.*

Mind; PROSTRATION of mind; writing, after: *sil.*

Mind; REMORSE; trifles, about: *sil.*

Mind; RESTLESSNESS; waking, on: am-c., ambr., bell., canth., cedr., chin., cina, dulc., hyper., ph-ac., phos., sep., *sil.*, squil., stann., tarax.

Mind; UNCONSCIOUSNESS; cold; after taking: *sil.*

Mind; WEEPING; afternoon: carb-v., cast., cop., dig., phos., *sil.*, tarent.

Computer Materia Medicas

Several computer programmes hold details of a number of different material medicas. It is possible to both scroll through computer screens to look at different pages of material medica and to search for key words, phrases or combinations of words. They are frequently combined with a computerised repertory (see Chapters 9, 19). Some patients and homeopaths feel there is a subtle change of the relationship between the homeopath and patient when a computer is used rather than books. Others recognise the potential of having all the literature in one source and not needing to swap between different books.

Dynamic Materia Medica

In most materia medicas each remedy is portrayed essentially through a list of symptoms. As a result it is easy when studying the remedies to construct a fairly fixed picture of the remedies. In practice a more fluid picture is helpful in grasping the full expression of the remedy – a remedy picture developing over time and according to the changing life situation of the patient. If we don't understand how a case develops over time (see Chapter 3) we can find it hard to make sense of seemingly contrary information. For example, Phosphorous starts off with huge levels of sensitivity and is emotionally open, but then becomes emotionally exhausted, when the sensitivity focuses internally through worry and anxiety.

Once we understand these contrary, sometimes opposite and paradoxical symptoms, they add a new dimension to the understanding of a remedy picture and how it can unfold. A comprehensive remedy description will indicate something of how a remedy picture is in its various stages; a comparison with other remedies might point to how one remedy state can move to another. For example, the exhausted and 'burnt out' Phosphorous case may move to the remedy picture of Phosphoric acid, which can have fatigue and marked mental then physical debility. In this way it can be helpful to think of the remedies as having a life cycle.

The Life Cycle of Remedies

Nux Vomica as a remedy state has a clear relationship with stimulants, e.g. caffeine and spicy foods. At one stage it craves these stimulants and will invariably use them excessively. Over time patients needing this remedy frequently become upset and averse to these foods, simply because they aggravate their symptoms. The symptoms on show will depend to some extent where that remedy is in its life cycle.

Causticum provides another example of 'a life cycle' of a remedy. It starts out with a high level of emotional sensitivity to those who are suffering and will be drawn to helping those who are in pain or suffering. However, later on in the life history of the Causticum patient, when they may have given a great deal to others, they will start to 'break down,' and their symptoms and the underlining pattern may become more brittle and rigid. They may then enter a state when they actually withdraw from and avoid those in need as a way of protecting themselves from their own sensitivity. A single, one-dimensional description of any one remedy may express contrary symptoms that different patients express at different times in the remedy life cycle. Understanding the pattern that unfolds, through the different stages of a remedy's manifestation, is often a start to recognising the themes and essence in the remedy. For example in Aurum metallicum, made from gold, there are frequently issues related to golden objects, self esteem (the golden child), money, etc. (Gutman 1937).

In this way the remedy is more than just a collection of symptoms; rather it has a character that may be compared to characters in a film or book. In the same way that every patient has a story that unfolds over time, so too does every remedy. As you develop a comprehensive picture of the remedy through the materia medicas, and from seeing it in patients, so you start to become aware of how the remedy picture unfolds over time in different environments. Matching how the remedy unfolds to how the case unfolds over time is one example of thematic prescribing.

Evolving Materia Medica

Given the dynamic relationship between the remedy states produced in patients and the environments we live in, it is not surprising that as our environment changes and as the illnesses people get change so we see new materia medica becoming more prominent. For example, in a society that starts to abuse more recreational drugs including cannabis and hallucinogenic substances it is not surprising that we see the remedies of Cannabis Indica and Agaricus (from a toadstool that contains muscarin) becoming more often indicated. As we see more patients suffering from allergies, then those substances to which patients have increased sensitivity are likely to become more important remedies. Interestingly, these changes do not seem to manifest just on those who have used cannabis and hallucinogenic substances or who have allergies but, albeit to a lesser extent, in a whole population.

As homeopaths, when we look for homeopathic remedies we need to stay alert to the environment our patients are in. The range or 'palette' of remedies we might need is informed by the environment in which we live. Historically, herbalists have always used plants that grow in similar environments or climatic conditions to the environment a patient has lived in. Of course, with increased globalisation the ability of patients to travel both geographically and emotionally from culture to culture has changed. So individuals are faced with increasing diversity of environments. As each environment can present a different challenge to a differently susceptible patient, it is consistent that as the variety of environments we meet increases so the number of remedies to provide the best information to cope with that challenge also increases. Therefore the homeopath in cultures that are cosmopolitan and changing fast is likely to need to be aware of a wide range of remedies and alert to new challenges and remedies to treat these.

Summary

The materia medicas are an essential tool that include information about medicines expressed at different levels of detail and in different formats, and lend themselves to different ways of working. It is important to explore different materia medicas in order both to discover remedies that are new to you and to deepen your knowledge of the remedies you already know. Taking part in provings, and recording your own experience of remedies and clinical practice will consolidate your own knowledge of remedies and extend the knowledge of the remedies available to the homeopathic profession. Although not the easiest to use, access to original records of provings of remedies is helpful in making judgements about the reliability of information, and to reveal detail of information about the context in which any one prover generated proving symptoms.

References

Boericke W, Boericke O 1927 Pocket manual of homeopathic materia medica. Boericke and Runyon, Philadelphia

Gutman W 1937 Homeopathy: fundamentals of its philosophy, the essence of its remedies. Homeopathic Medical Publishers, Bombay

Kent J T 1899 Repertory of the homeopathic materia medica. Examiner Printing House, Lancaster PA. Last edition 1957. Ehrhart and Karl, Chicago. Reprinted 1986 Homeopathic Book Services, Sittingbourne

Morrison R 1993 The desktop guide to keynote and confirmatory symptoms. Hahnemann Clinic Publishing, Grass Valley, CA

Tyler M L 1942 Homeopathic drug pictures. Homoeopathic Publishing Company, London

Vermulens F 1994 Concordant materia medica. Merjlin, Haarlem

Bibliography

Gibson D 1987 Studies of homeopathic remedies. Edited for publication by Harling M and Kaplan B. Beaconsfield Publishers, Beaconsfield

Tyler M, Weir J Repertorising. British Homoeopathic Association, London

Causation and the Presenting Symptoms

CHAPTER EIGHT

Taking the Case

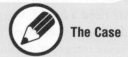 **The Case**

David Owen

Introduction

As homeopaths we look for hints, gestures, half-remembered characteristics, as if we are trying to recognise friends at a masquerade.

This chapter looks at the homeopathic case from the starting point of the presenting symptom but goes on to see that every symptom and modality is important in shaping the overall case and that there is a continuum from prescribing on a local or presenting symptom to evolving a case to prescribe on many (often seemingly) unrelated symptoms as a totality. The aim, in practice, is for the case-taking to be a seamless process, often appearing as a relaxed and informal conversation but needing to be a comprehensive, fluid and reflective exchange between the homeopath and the patient. To achieve this, the homeopath needs an appreciation of all areas of a case that might be relevant and experience of taking and recording a case. The presenting symptom is a good place to begin. Although to an observer and patient the process may appear passive, in every case the homeopath is actively seeking to recognise information so that when interpreted through one or more models of health, the meaning of a patient's situation and illness is clear. There are a number of different styles and skills involved in case-taking that a homeopath will need to develop in order to meet the needs of the patients that they are likely to see. This chapter starts to explore those styles and skills.

In practice the symptom picture will have evolved over time but most cases, and therefore most case-taking, will share the same start, the presenting symptoms and first impressions.

Making a Start

The first few minutes of the consultation establish much about how the rest of the consultation and even subsequent consultations will go. It is interesting how often even the most complicated cases will start by saying something like, 'I just wonder if you have anything for my arthritis'. It is only later you find out that it is one of many problems that have perhaps gone on for decades. In any case-taking initial impressions are important. The first perception you have of the patient is unique and often things can be glimpsed in the first few moments of a consultation that are otherwise difficult to see. For example how a child is playing in the waiting room, where someone is sitting, how eager or happy they are to meet you, who they are with, their expression, how they hold themselves, how are they dressed etc. It is worth remembering that the patient is also assessing you from the outset. What you and your practice do and how you come across will influence the tone of the consultation, e.g. if before the first meeting you can provide information explaining how you work it may help to relax the patient.

Type of the Case Related to Model of Health

The type of history you choose to take will be influenced strongly by the models of health you

Causation and the
Presenting Symptoms

choose to work with. In situations where you work on causation, local or clinical prescribing you may only need a brief history that may not, in the first aid setting, even need recording in any detail. If you are integrating homeopathy into a busy family or general medical practice you may have serious time limitations. Generally as you move through the models of health the focus of the case widens from the local illness to the broadest considerations and the detail required increases, as does the time to take the case.

As cases get more complex, patients present several different illnesses each with presenting symptoms. Starting by establishing each different complaint, possibly numbering the different symptoms, can help keep track of them and make sure that modalities are identified and recorded for each. Different symptoms may naturally link together, and some order or pattern may emerge. Sometimes this may only become clear over several consultations. An indication as to which is the most deep-seated disorder can sometimes be established by asking the patient what order the symptoms appeared in, or which symptom troubles them the most, or which one they would most like to be without (see Hierarchy in Chapter 6).

Another way to record this is as a mind map, particularly useful for those who use a very visual style

of learning and to reveal connections and themes running through a case. Figure 8.1 illustrates this based on a case presented later in this chapter.

In cases when there is a very complicated or confused picture or where the history cannot be obtained clearly in this manner, another approach that can be helpful is to suggest the patient talks through their life from birth through childhood, up to today. It describes a 'time line' but with several strands that may each represent different problems, leading to the question: 'And what brings you to consult with me now?'.

As we move through the different models, so a broader, less structured or standardised consultation may take place. The homeopath may invite the patient to 'tell me everything about yourself' or may find and explore how the patient's state is expressing itself in the consultation, including how the patient and homeopath relate.

In practice of course these are not discrete and different styles, but just as one model of health will rarely be used alone, elements of each are often combined, leading to a range of case-taking techniques. Different groups of patients may each require special experience for example in the case of children (Shepherd 1938, Herscu 1991, Wynne-Simmons 1993) or in veterinary practice (see Chapter 18). In this chapter the focus will be

Figure 8.1 Mind map of Sharon's case.

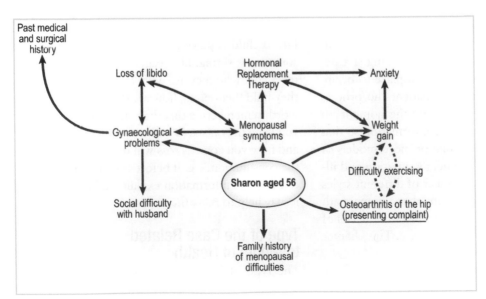

on the biological model, starting with the presenting symptoms but extending to other connected symptoms.

Overview of the Case

'A human being is part of the whole, called by us the Universe, a part limited in time and space. He experiences himself, his thoughts and feelings as something separated from the rest – a kind of optical delusion of his consciousness. This delusion is a kind of prison for us, restricting us to our personal desires and to affection for a few persons nearest us. Our task must be to free ourselves from this prison by widening our circle of compassion to embrace all living creatures and the whole of nature in its beauty.'

Albert Einstein

Initially while you are gaining experience, it is helpful to have a basic structure in mind for a consultation. In practice having explored the main presenting symptom the case will often flow onto another related area of the case and all the areas mentioned in Box 8.1 can be covered in the style of a semi-structured interview. Box 8.1 gives a checklist of the main areas of the case that the homeopath may need to enquire about. Each area may reveal vital information about the presenting symptom, may provide vital confirmatory or exclusion symptoms and contribute to the totality. The psychological, general, family and social areas of the case are covered in Chapter 13.

A central essence or theme or relational aspect of the case may emerge in any of these areas and because the presenting symptom is frequently discussed or handled in a certain way, it is often first most noticeable or hinted at in areas of the case away from the presenting symptoms or by unconscious movements of the patient's hands or body or by a change in the observer, such as the prickle in the hairs of the neck of the homeopath, the curiosity about one phrase or word, an emotional reaction from a nervous giggle to the eyes watering etc. The practitioner must never allow the structure of case-taking to pre-empt the spontaneous flow of the patient's story, sometimes in quite unexpected directions.

> **BOX 8.1**
> **Outline of the Homeopathic Case**
> - *Presenting symptom*: the complete symptom including the causation, time, location, sensation, intensity, modalities and treatment history
> - *Other main symptoms*: may be more than one, include treatments given
> - *Past history*: illness, treatments, accidents, operations
> - *Review of systems*: bowels, urinary, stomach, respiratory, skin, allergies, headache, fits or faints, genitourinary, gastrointestinal, respiratory, neurological, cardiovascular, ear, nose, and throat (ENT), the senses musculoskeletal, skin etc
> - *Significant life events*
> - *Mental*: psychological[*]
> - *General*: environmental and dietary history[*]
> - *Treatment history*
> - *Family history*: illnesses in both sides of the family; add parents and grandparents[*]
> - *Social history*: deepening the case, marital, economic status, career etc., social habits, smoking alcohol, drugs, exercise[*]
> - *Examining the patient*
> - *Making a diagnosis*: including the homeopathic diagnosis

[*]Covered in Chapter 13.

The abbreviated case of Sharon shows how a case might unfold; in another patient with similar symptoms or to another homeopath it might unfold differently. Remember that all cases given in this text are abbreviated to show only the most relevant information for the point being illustrated and a great deal more information is taken and recorded in the full case.

Figure 8.1 shows one way of understanding how the different areas of Sharon's case connect and how a remedy that acts deeper than just symptomatically might fit this pattern. In Sharon's case Calcarea carbonicum fitted not just her presenting symptoms but it was confirmed by her appearance, food and general symptoms. She felt better

CASE STUDY 8.1

Sharon, aged 56, attended for help with osteoarthritis of the hip. She had over 5 years put on 5 stone in weight and wanted help losing weight; she found exercise difficult. The weight gain came on after starting on hormone replacement therapy (HRT) for menopausal hot flushes but Sharon is unhappy with her relationship with her husband and comfort eats. Sharon described the weight gain, then the hot flushes and the alternatives to HRT she had tried and that she had recently stopped. Other treatments and investigations Sharon had had, including thyroid function, were discussed. She went on to talk about her past gynaecological history and other past history, including a review of other systems. After prompting she shared details of her mother's menopause and other family history. She was anxious about having the same problems as her mother and this lead to her discussing her fears and anxiety. Steering the consultation back to her hot flushes the consultation explored her general temperature preferences and other environmental factors – this led to a review of the effect of her symptoms on her daily life. Sharon spoke about the effect on her libido and her disrupted sleep pattern and how this affected her marriage. At this point she spoke about her deep worries about the future and her children.

following treatment and her symptoms improved gradually.

The Importance of the Beginning of the Case

You only get to begin once.

It is a well recognised feature of medical consultations that patients will sometimes reveal crucial information, even their real reason for attending, as they are about to leave the room. Equally, the first things the patient observes and communicates are often things of significance to the whole case and set the tone of the consultation. While the centre of the case may be unclear or unconscious at this stage, much of its importance is revealed by discussing those areas of the patient's life which are most greatly restricted by their illness – what they can't do, what they want to change, how the symptoms affect them. Helping the patient to be at ease and to talk about symptoms will set the tone and pace of the consultation and will be of help later in completing the symptom picture. How the first consultation begins will influence the rest of that consultation and also all subsequent consultations.

Rapport

It is surprisingly easy in the attempt to gather information about the symptoms to forget the importance and priority of establishing rapport and developing an understanding of the patient – 'in chasing a prescription the patient can be lost'. Always reflect on why the patient has the illness and what needs to happen for them to be well.

Hearing the Symptoms

While a symptom may at its most straightforward be expressed as a single observation, the homeopath is often concerned with the detail that makes this symptom unique. Its character, the type of pain, the colour of discharges, location – e.g. which side, which particular finger and the pattern of symptoms – i.e. how often it comes, what makes it better and worse and what it alternates with. All this information helps complete the symptom. The description of a symptom may also include its causative factor, and so we see the symptomatic approach incorporating the causative.

The Complete Symptom

A complete symptom can, because it is particularly individualising, point to a clear and well indicated prescription. The complete symptom gives information about causation, location, sensation (such as the type and radiation of pain in a painful condition), and modalities including timings of the symptom, and also intensity. The intensity of symptoms or those features that modify symptoms can be indicated by using capitals, underlining or scoring the symptom in the same way as in the materia medica (see Chapter 7). So a strong burning pain may be BURNING PAIN, *burning pain* or burning pain (2). By convention most symptoms are scored between 1 and 3. The complete symptom also includes extensions and concomitants and is described in more detail in Chapter 9 (p. 111)

Modalities

Modalities are things that change the symptom. They are influenced not only by changes in the environment but also by co-existing clinical conditions, the patient's emotional state, activities and behaviour. They also point to aggravating factors that may be an extension of the causative factors. Remember they are indicated by < for aggravation and > for amelioration, and the intensity can be indicated as << strong aggravation (equivalent to '2' or single underlining or *italic*) or <<< very strong aggravation (equivalent to '3' or double underlining or **bold**), as in Jonathan's case.

CASE STUDY 8.2

Jonathan, aged 42, presented with a reactive arthritis following a throat infection. The joint pains were <<wet, < cold and >> from warmth > rubbing the painful joint and < at first then >> from gentle movement. He responded to Rhus tox with gradual improvement of his joint pain.

In some cases a modality can be shared by several different symptoms, e.g. joint pain better for stretching and sore throat better for yawning (a type of stretch). If this is the case the importance of the modality is increased. If the modality appears in symptoms of different body systems, e.g. cough worse for talking or moving and diarrhoea better for lying still, then it is again increased and some would then consider it a general symptom and all

remedies that are generally < movement might be considered. These characteristic modalities become increasingly important as the homeopath moves from analysing cases based on causation, through local prescribing on presenting symptoms to cases analysed on totality, essence or thematic prescribing.

Sometimes language fails to describe the exact symptom or quality of symptom. There are many different types of pain or grief and our ability to hear, communicate and cross reference the exact symptom is limited by this. In other cases there is the language but exactly what each means may not be clear, e.g. fever may be considered hectic (consuming and high) or insidious, relapsing, remitting; pain may be sticking, gnawing, biting, etc.

There may be modalities that run counter to the general symptoms – the more unusual a modality the more it tells us about the individual's unique susceptibility. For example, contradictory modalities like burning better by warm applications, exhaustion with obsessive tidiness, breathlessness better lying flat, or unusual sensation as if head will fly off.

Presenting Symptoms

Most straightforward and simple cases have one main presenting symptom. There are three aspects of any presenting symptom that need to be taken into account – the situation in which the patient became ill, the symptom itself and how the presenting symptom relates to any other symptoms that emerge as a more complete history is taken. The more all three aspects are covered by a prescription the better the chance of recovery. If we return to the principle that no one symptom alters in isolation then associated symptoms will inform us about each other, although they may not be directly causative or predisposing, e.g. 'my head aches when I am constipated', where the constipation may or may not be a predisposing or provoking factor. The closer the association the more important this link, e.g. 'I always get constipated when I've a headache'. Although at first it appears there is a clear distinction between causation and a modality, in practice there is a gradation from a clear 'A causes B' through different degrees to 'A is associated to B', on to the opposite extreme that 'A and B are not associated and have no connection'. Establishing where A and B lie in relation to each other is part of case-taking.

Other Main Symptoms

Some patients particularly used to working with causation or local approaches may not always notice or volunteer symptoms in areas other than their main presenting complaint.

As cases get more complex so they may appear to have more seemingly unconnected presenting symptoms. In taking the case there may be modalities that are common to several. For example, several symptoms may be worse in the morning, or be relieved by the application of heat. These common modalities are likely to be linked to the patient's susceptibility. They may include symptoms that describe the individual's mental, general or physical state.

CASE STUDY 8.3

Joan, aged 52, presented with a sore throat made worse from swallowing liquids. When the importance of other symptoms is explained she reveals that she suffers from extreme jealousy and is suspicious of her husband. When Joan is especially jealous her sore throat is often worse. After taking the remedy Lachesis, she feels her jealousy recede and feels better in herself. Joan comments that the sore throats she has been getting were only a 'small part of my general problems'.

While patients often want to talk mainly about the presenting symptom, because they are most worried by them, when the importance of other symptoms is explained the case can often proceed into these other areas, as happened with Joan. Often if the presenting complaint is physical then psychological symptoms can be under-reported.

Past Medical History

The presenting symptoms are in many cases only the 'tip of the iceberg'. While the tip is what you see there are frequently significant factors in other areas of the case. Asking when the patient was last completely well often allows them to see their illness in a historic context and make links to other events. One reason for some cases to be more difficult to treat is because large parts of the case are apparently invisible (see Hidden cases in Section VI). Many patients present their past history of illnesses in a way that is unrelated to their main complaint. To the homeopath the past history frequently points to the susceptibility and what lies behind and below the current problems. An unresolved illness or one where symptoms have simply been suppressed through allopathic treatment is not uncommonly a cause for present illnesses. This is why understanding symptoms and causation in terms of levels is so important, as Joy's case illustrates.

CASE STUDY 8.4

Joy, aged 36, had a 20-year history of irritable bowel syndrome (IBS) – especially diarrhoea and urgency when needing the toilet. In the consultation she was anxious and fidgety and she said this had been bad since her IBS. She gives in her history that at age 16 she suffered from food poisoning that was treated with drugs to stop her diarrhoea. The symptoms of IBS started soon after the food poisoning and the remedy picture of Arsenicum Album was indicated on the symptoms of the original food poisoning, as well as modalities of the IBS and keynote symptoms of anxiety, coldness of the extremities and craving for lemon juice. Arsenicum Album helped her symptoms and at follow-up Joy commented she felt more relaxed and was sleeping better.

It is interesting that Joy had become more anxious since having the IBS and it is common that changes to a person's physical well-being influence their psychological well-being and vice-versa.

That is why we seek to understand our patients and remedies as both physical and psychological entities and why cases other than the most simple often benefit most from an approach that is closer to the totality than local approach.

Review of Systems

When a patient is keen to talk about a particular complaint or group of complaints they may neglect to mention other aspects of their health that may provide valuable information to the homeopath. One of the best ways of quickly reviewing those other aspects is to ask about the different organ systems – digestive, respiratory, circulatory, musculoskeletal, etc. Another way of reviewing the systems is to ask if the patient has had any problems with any other part of the body, running from top to bottom, e.g. any headache, neck ache, arm problems, chest problems, stomach problems, pelvic problems etc. Even quite minor problems in the past might be significant to the homeopath.

Significant Life Events

Given what we now know of the holistic nature of health, the significance of a particular life event as a possible causative factor or influence on susceptibility would appear obvious. I frequently explain the relevance of significant life events in terms of how we know moving house or experiencing bereavement can affect health, even causing measurable changes in the immune system, and that even apparently minor events can be relevant homeopathically. I ask them to list significant events, the effects they have had on them and the ages when they happened. Patients are usually good at recalling significant life events although it helps some patients to think about this before they attend, as they may ask family members to remind them of events that they might otherwise not remember or, if they happened as a child, they are unaware of.

Treatment History

Treatment history will often come up during discussions of past or present problems. It is surprising how many patients take medication for conditions they forget to mention. It is vital to understand this aspect of the case as not only does it frequently alter the characteristics and modalities of the patient's presenting symptoms, but also it is a major factor in causing new symptoms (see Suppression in Chapter 11). Treatments include not only conventional drugs and surgery, but also psychological interventions like counselling, and any complementary medical treatments. It is helpful to ask patients to bring with them any medication that they are taking or to list any treatment they have had in the past. The longer the symptoms have gone on, the more important it is to go further back in the treatment history. For chronic illness, information about vaccinations, birth history, early infant traumas, etc. are all relevant, as Paul's case illustrates.

CASE STUDY 8.5
Paul, aged 38, presented with many allergic symptoms for which he had over the years been prescribed much medication. It was difficult for Paul to see any link between symptoms and trigger factors after all this time, especially since his symptoms had been modified by so much treatment. Through exploring Paul's treatment history and symptom time-line it suggested his allergies started shortly after a smallpox vaccination aged 8 and being taken abroad. This pointed to a remedy Thuja, that was confirmed by keynotes and which helped his allergy.

If a patient has had previous treatment by a different homeopath it is worth noting, particularly detailing any reactions to former treatments given. This leads on to making contact with previous and inter-current carers to request treatment details. It may also be the place to discuss with the patient issues relating to their shared care with other health carers.

Mental Symptoms, General Symptoms, Family History, Social History

These are covered in Chapter 13 as they are often considered more important in the totality of a case; however, a patient may present for help due to symptoms in any of these areas.

Examining the Patient

Taking a homeopathic case history and examining the patient are complementary to understanding the individual and the case – either without the other is flawed. The relevant examination of the patient in relation to the presenting pathology can be vital in reaching a diagnosis, as well as revealing important information about presenting symptoms. For example, if a patient has a rash, how and where exactly does it appear? Any signs observed are enquired about in the same way as symptoms in order to give a complete picture – what are the modalities, causation, locality, etc.

Observing the patient also reveals much about their physical constitution (body shape, hair texture and colour), their generals (how many clothes do they wear, where do they sit) and mentals (how expressive they are, their appearance and their style of dress). It is surprising how much information can be gained simply from shaking hands with a patient, whether it is the moist 'soggy' handshake of a 'Calcarea carbonicum patient', or the light, tentative 'cold' handshake of the 'Arsenicum Album patient'.

An accurate and complete record of the consultation should also include a contemporary note of the patient's movements and mannerisms during the consultation. Even subtle movements and mannerisms give clues to important aspects of the case and indicate where the case might need to be expanded. A patient may appear to be holding back something by covering their mouth, or touch their body when emotionally moved by something or be trying to communicate something when they make certain movements – pointing or making a fist might be obvious but small movements are just as important. As we move into the holistic perspective every movement, sign and physical characteristic may encapsulate and transmit key points of the consultation.

Above and beyond this information, physical contact with the patient as part of a relevant examination engenders trust and a deepening of the therapeutic relationship, which is important both for the patient and the doctor. Frequently new and sometimes important information surfaces during or after an examination.

Investigations

If there are indications then the examination may be extended to include necessary investigations. They tell us not just about the conventional diagnosis and severity of illness and response to treatment but can also point to homeopathic remedies. With more sensitive interpretation of test results it is possible to get pointers to many remedies, e.g. the low normal thyroid function of Sepia, the slow clotting time of Phosphorous, and the low normal iron and haemoglobin of Ferrum salts.

Making a Diagnosis

The diagnostic label we give to a patient's illness is an attempt to simplify and codify the reaction of the 'vital force'; to label how the patient's vitality and environment reach a point of balance.

Making a diagnosis is important but the homeopath wants more than just a disease label. 'Jimmy has a sore throat' tells us something of his presenting symptom and 'Jimmy has a virus' may tell us about causation, but neither gives much information about his susceptibility or how to distinguish between the many local remedies that might help patients with sore throat. More information is needed to make an accurate and useful assessment and homeopathic diagnosis. Has Jimmy got enlarged tonsils? Has he over-used his voice? Was he exposed to a very cold wind before he felt ill? Where exactly is he feeling the pain? What is the pain like? Has he stopped eating or drinking? Does he have recurring sore throats? These are all important qualifications of the diagnosis.

Often homeopathically a diagnosis is a description to include conventional disease terminology. Rather than a label, it becomes an abbreviation of the patient's story, a summary or an overall impression of the patient and their symptoms.

Impression – Plan – Prescription

It is helpful at the end of the consultation to clearly document what your impression of the consultation has been, the plan of how you have agreed to manage the case, and any methodology used and prescription advised. The impression leads on to a plan of treatment and management issues such as liaison with other health carers, advice on concurrent medication, how treatment might progress and possible reactions to treatment. This leads on to recording specific prescription advice given and the need, or not, for feedback and follow-up. As more complex cases are managed the usefulness of separating out each of these steps increases.

Discussing the impression with the patient shares the meaning we have constructed from the case and helps patients gain insight from their experience of the illness. It also allows any inaccuracies made by the homeopath to be checked and is likely to improve compliance of any advice given. Explaining the plan to the patient promotes understanding of what the patient can expect from homeopathic treatment and importantly, as often is the case in more deep-seated illness, when treatment needs to be seen as just a step in the process of cure. This is an important step in clarifying and reviewing the agreement between the patient and homeopath about the treatment process. This in turn affects the rapport and empathy between homeopath and patient and will in difficult cases prepare the ground for seeing a deeper case at the next appointment.

REFLECTION POINT

Consider some of the tensions that exist in taking a case and reflect on how you will respond to these in your own practice:

- The patient prioritises what they feel are the worst symptoms but what makes a symptom more or less important to the homeopath?
- So much happens spontaneously and unconsciously – how can this be made more conscious without interrupting the spontaneity?
- In a consultation, how much detail should be recorded and how can this be done without interfering in taking the case?
- It is not uncommon during a case for some remedies to suggest themselves, how can the potential to bias the case towards or away from these remedies be managed?
- There are many benefits to disclosing treatment plans and prescription details to patients. Are there times when this may not be the beat course of action? If so, when and why?

The Case and Seeking Agreement to Work a Certain Way

There are certain styles and skills to case-taking and the successful homeopath will develop a number of these to suit different patients at different times. No one set of skills or particular style will suit every situation – what is strength in one situation can be a weakness in others. The trainee homeopath is well advised to explore different styles and different skills to develop a range of approaches to case-taking. Two of the best ways to develop this are by observing others at work and to experience having your own case taken. Once there is an awareness of the variety of styles and skills available and what they each reveal, then experience and practice will allow the homeopath to personalise the case-taking for each case. It is always worth reflecting on what makes a homeopath successful at identifying symptoms, particularly ones that the patient might be reluctant to show, or even be unconscious of. Some of the different styles are covered in this book and the contrast between 'taking the case' in this chapter and 'receiving the case' in Chapter 13 is intentional.

Identifying the most appropriate model of health, approach to treatment and method of prescribing in each case at a particular time develops alongside taking the case. The homeopath may adopt many, sometimes very different, styles of case-taking to suit different patients. Case-taking can seem like a hunter 'hunting down' the symptoms and the

BOX 8.2
Reflections on the Homeopath as a Hunter

- How does being familiar with the location that you are working in help you detect subtle changes of atmosphere or symptoms?
- Be prepared to wait with patience to allow the symptom to present itself.
- How might you create opportunities for the symptom to reveal itself, particularly the deeper, more hidden symptoms which are frequently more characteristic?
- Might the right sort of bait, or provocation, entice the symptoms to the surface? The bait might include pauses, invitation, explanations, mimics, challenge or provocation.
- How might modelling back to the patient the behaviour of a parent, a partner or even themselves allow patients to get in touch with or recreate a symptom, e.g. unresolved feelings? (If this isn't done consciously the homeopath may unconsciously be subject to these projects anyway.)
- When is the time to gently challenge a symptom that is partly revealed? Challenging it might simply be naming it or an attempt to understand it.
- The one that got away – there will always be symptoms that are just out of reach; sometimes there will just be a sense that there is something more to the case and it may not be until follow-up or sometime later that the symptom will surface and be seen clearly.

exercise in Box 8.2 compares some of the skills of a hunter to a homeopath working this way.

The Invitation and the Pause

The homeopath creates a space for the remedy to reveal itself.

For the case to emerge – especially the more embarrassing, unconscious or psychological symptoms – it is important to be able to create a safe space for taking the case. Psychological space is created through the pause or measured silence, that to be safe needs the patient (and homeopath) to be comfortable. In this space the deeper aspects of a case often unfold and small observations about words, movements and behaviour reveal a great deal.

Using open-ended questions helps patients to feel invited to reveal symptoms. For example asking 'can you share with me some of the things that have made you happiest and saddest?', then sensitively asking for clarification or more detail is very different from closed questions that have their place but reveal much less, e.g. 'that must have made you happy?'

Classify the Symptoms

'Each individual symptom must be considered. Every symptom must be examined to see what relation it sustains to and what position it fills in the totality in order that we may know its value, whether it is a common symptom, a particular symptom, or whether peculiarly a characteristic symptom.'

James Tyler Kent

Once symptoms are revealed and explored completely then it is possible to order them not only by weighting but also by their relationship to other symptoms. This can be in terms of chronological appearance, hierarchy, sphere of action (mental, general or local), how strange or rare or peculiar. Sometimes it is only while trying to classify or weigh a symptom that it becomes clear that the symptom is far from complete, at other times the importance of other symptoms surfaces, as Mary's case illustrates (Case Study 8.6).

The Case as a Journey

By seeing how an individual operates in different environments a homeopath observes the individual's susceptibility. The fears and anticipations that an individual has will reflect the fear and anticipation of the circumstances they might find themselves in. Their delusions, dreams, imaginations and hopes will reflect the environments they

CASE STUDY 8.6

Mary describes herself as full of fears. Taking the case, it becomes clear that she is most fearful of illness but only after describing all her symptoms does the one she is most fearful of, heart attack, surface. When we explore what symptoms are related to this fear she describes small points of pain over the chest that she thinks her father, who died from heart disease, had. On examination, pressing the costal cartilage, which she describes as being 'stabbed in the heart,' reproduces her chest pain. She is reluctant to talk about her relationship with her parents. She responds to Kali carbonicum, a remedy that includes fear of heart disease and well-circumscribed pains. After the treatment Mary had less pain and fear and was able to talk about unresolved issues regarding her relationship with her father.

are drawn to or away from. During the homeopathic consultation, by exploring these things we ask a patient to journey into those different circumstances. We explore how the symptoms are linked with those different environments.

Deepening the Case

Often the illnesses a patient gets reflect, and are influenced by, their journey through different environments and life situations made over some time. During a course of homeopathic treatment, and particularly in patients who use homeopathy over a long period of time, patients often move from thinking about their health in terms of what has been done to them by external causes, to thinking of their health in terms of optimum well-being and as an internal process which provides an opportunity to learn, change and grow. Helping patients to navigate through this transformative process is for some people more important than getting rid of the symptoms. The homeopath requires a mental agility to not only apply the right approach at the right time but also the skill to clarify the optimum approach at each stage. As difficult cases open up so the approach to prescribing deepens, then as

the patient improves and the case becomes more straightforward so the approach to treatment can become more straightforward.

The Use of Questionnaires

Questionnaires can facilitate consultations but they can also make them less spontaneous. They facilitate by allowing a large amount of data to be prepared by the patient beforehand and by orientating the patient to the areas of importance to the homeopath. For example, a question about significant life events can make patients begin to see the relevance of life events.

Jane presented with anxiety symptoms that she thought were menopausal. After listing life events a correlation between the anxiety and her children leaving home was clear.

On the down side, when patients talk about things that they have already recorded in their questionnaire, they can be more difficult to weight and their connection to other aspects of the case may be less clear. For example, symptoms may be 'glossed over' or patients may come emotionally prepared, so the normal pointers that something is particularly significant may be filtered out. Some of the strengths and weaknesses are listed in Box 8.3.

In addition to being given in advance, questionnaires can also be used as a 'work-book' or checklist during a consultation – useful when starting in practice or developing new approaches to treatment that each offer a slightly new approach to case-taking. Questionnaires may be useful at different times in your career, initially when you need a checklist to ensure you have covered all possible areas of case-taking. Later on they may enable you to focus on the areas of the case that you consider most relevant while just quickly checking over areas not dealt with in the consultation. They can, when designed by you, help complement your style of working and as such will evolve as you evolve. I would caution against using someone else's standard questionnaire other than as a checklist at the very beginning of your practice, rather you should design and modify your own – for this reason a model questionnaire is not offered.

BOX 8.3
Strengths and Weaknesses of Questionnaires

Strengths

Saves time at the appointment, especially in detailing basic information such as address and date of birth. Enables the patient to reflect on their health before the appointment and also to find out and write down chronological events, current medication and past medication, significant events in the past, details of family history. It may also allow them time to complete a life style questionnaire over a period of time, when they can observe their life style, e.g. a dietary history over one week. It may allow patients to ask family members and friends for feedback on how they come across, aspects of their temperament or details about the family history. It also allows broad questions to be asked about past medical history; which may not always be covered in the consultation if other things take greater priority. It may reveal the patient's style of writing and handwriting and can be combined with the 'consent to treat' form.

Weaknesses

It may interfere with spontaneity and may be considered intrusive by the patient. It may take time for the patient to complete, which they might be reluctant to give. It may make patients feel that things other than on the questionnaire are not relevant, so they might be less prepared to explore them. It may make patients feel the consultation is more recipe-like than necessary. It allows patients to list their different symptoms with no clear priority hierarchy.

REFLECTION POINT

- Do you agree or disagree that the consultation is far more than just 'finding the remedy'? What do you consider your own strengths and weakness in case-taking to be? To what extent are cause and effect inter-related, so that the disease is observed as not just having a simple cause followed by an effect, but rather that cause and effect can be related to and help understand each other? Having thought about taking the homeopathic case and studying Box 8.3, do you think a questionnaire for patients will be helpful; if so what would you include in it?

Summary

Enthusiasm for case-taking and exploring cases in their entirety is central to the homeopath's qualities. Mastering the ability of case-taking is essential to becoming a good homeopath and leads quickly on to how to order the information that is revealed from the case. The next chapter looks at how, in case analysis, we start to sift though the information generated by the case and how we can use this information to give meaning to the treatment we are able to offer.

References

Herscu P 1991 The homeopathic treatment of children. North Atlantic Books, Berkeley

Shepherd D 1938 The magic of the minimum dose. Homoeopathic Publishing Company, London

Wynne-Simmons A 1993 The children's toy box. British Homeopathic Association, Luton

Bibliography

Foubister D 1963 The significance of past history in homeopathic prescribing. Br Homeopath J April 52(2):81–91

Leckridge B 1997 Homeopathy in primary care. Churchill Livingstone, New York

Roberts H A 1937 Sensations as if, a repertory of subjective symptoms. Boericke & Tafel, Philadelphia PA. Indian edition. 2002. B Jain, New Delhi

CHAPTER NINE

Local Prescribing and Repertorisation

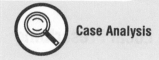

Case Analysis

David Owen

'To be a genuine practitioner of the medical art, a physician must:

Clearly realise what is to be cured in diseases, that is, in each single case of disease (discernment of the disease, indicator),

Clearly realise what is curative in medicines, that is, in each particular medicine (knowledge of medicinal powers),

Be aware of how to adapt what is curative in medicine to what he has discerned to be undoubtedly diseased in the patient, according to clear principles. In this way, recovery must result.

Adapting what is curative in medicine to what is diseased in patients requires that the physician be able to:

Adapt the most appropriate medicine according to its mode of action to the case before him...'

S Hahnemann, Organon, Para 3

Introduction

Having identified what is wrong, where possible what is causing what is wrong, or at least what was going on when things went wrong, it naturally follows to ask what needs to happen to help the patient back to a new state of balance, to plan a course of treatment.

The realities of practice are that there is often a spectrum of information between the purely local symptoms, aspects of the totality, the patterns running through the case and the interaction with the patient, on which to base a prescription. A broad range of factors can consciously and unconsciously influence the final selection of the remedy. While a broad understanding of the local symptoms within the totality will emerge as this chapter proceeds it is helpful to start by focusing on the analysis of cases on the presenting symptom. The skills and knowledge learnt in using each model, approach and methodology overlap with and inform the study of the others. There is no absolute reason why the homeopath should develop prescribing in the order suggested through this book, although it may be wise to gain experience in managing cases from the simplest to most complex. An appreciation of each approach will help the homeopath maximise their treatment strategies for different cases. This chapter also starts to develop the importance of matching of the model, approach and methodology to the level of complexity of the case and the idea that in any one case several methodologies may each point to a remedy. When it is the same remedy, our confidence in the prescription increases; when it is not the same remedy strategies that require an understanding of the strengths and weaknesses of each methodology help select an optimum prescription.

While the analysis of any case has to address the key questions identified in Chapter 4, many of these take place as the case is taken – the analysis chapters of this book will now look predominantly at the question of finding the indicated homeopathic remedies. Focus in this chapter is particularly on the approach to treatment based on the local symptoms and the methodologies for matching the local but complete symptom to the remedy, a method frequently suited to treatment of localised and acute conditions.

Local Prescribing

Treating on presenting symptoms (local prescribing) is often incorporated with causation approaches and is often a starting point for homeopaths treating simple or straightforward cases with acute illness. The aim is to identify a remedy that circumscribes the case, that covers all the main features and, if possible, to cover both causation and presenting symptoms.

There are several reasons why treating on causation alone may not be indicated or successful. In some acute illness there is no strong, clearly indicated precipitating or causative factor. In others there may be lots of different causes – when there is no clearly indicated remedy from the cause or where a prescription based on causation fails to act fully. In these cases the homeopath wanting to look more widely for a remedy may first consider the presenting symptoms.

Some homeopaths are critical of local prescribing, believing it fails to act deeply enough, perpetuating a lengthy and (I believe) wasteful schism in homeopathy. When a local prescription has acted, an individual is not only freed of their acute symptom but they frequently feel generally better and happier as well. They are less likely to get a recurrence and from the evidence of families who have used homeopathy in the home over many years it appears their general resistance to chronic disease is improved. As such local prescribing seems a completely valid and appropriate use of homeopathy for simple or straightforward cases (in Chapter 10 the different types of case are described). Not only can the use of local remedies and first-aid remedies in the home and by health carers greatly help to reduce acute suffering, but they can also do a great deal for the health of the population by reducing the amount of symptoms being masked by conventional drugs and reducing iatrogenic disease.

In some more deep-seated cases only an acute or local picture may be manifest, or the homeopath may choose just to focus on the local symptoms.

In these cases local treatment may be just the start of a process of gradually deepening understanding and treatment. Indeed, this process of gradually treating at deep levels is what much chronic disease treatment is all about.

Different Methodologies of Local Prescribing

Box 9.1 lists the main local methodologies. Each has different advantages and disadvantages. Each may be, and often is, combined with another (and with other approaches) to improve reliability. Establishing for a particular patient in a particular context the most important symptoms and how they are related is the beginning of any case analysis.

Single Main Symptom

Choosing a remedy on the single presenting symptom or sign is sometimes referred to as 'clinical' prescribing. It is quick but often many remedies share the same symptoms.

Single Keynotes

The main presenting symptom is not always the most useful. A hierarchically significant symptom – including 'strange, rare, peculiar' – in the case matching a significant symptom in a remedy may be a strong pointer to a remedy match. This is where

BOX 9.1
Methodologies of Local Prescribing
- Single main symptom
- Single keynotes
- Several keynotes in one or more areas of the case
- The complete symptom
- Confirmatory and eliminatory symptoms
- Epidemic remedies
- Doublet or triplet symptoms and linked symptoms
- Previous well indicated remedy
- Combination remedies
- Strange, rare and peculiar

the weighting of symptoms and knowledge of the keynotes in the materia medica is very useful. So for example the patient with cold extremities who finds relief when they are in cold environments would be peculiar and link with keynotes in just a few remedies.

Several Keynotes in One or More Areas of the Case

The more unique, stronger and representative of the case keynotes are, the more likely they lead to a good prescription. Identifying the weighting and hierarchy of keynotes again makes case analysis much easier.

Remember, if you are finding it difficult to weight a symptom in order to compare its value to other symptoms, then it is worth considering its intensity, its uniqueness, its depth and duration. Consider how strongly the symptom is affecting the patient, how much it is limiting normal function, how 'strange, rare or peculiar' a symptom is, whether it is a quality that affects several symptoms or been present for a long time, and how deep or central it is, i.e. does it affect a vital organ like the heart or kidneys?

The greater the number of symptoms, the more important it is to have a hierarchy. Not seeing an order to the symptoms can blind the homeopath to the most relevant symptom.

The Complete Symptom

The complete symptom looks at all aspects of the symptom that the patient presents, to include causation, location, sensation, modalities and concomitants and extensions. This is illustrated in Figure 9.1 as symptoms being like a cube, having six faces. The location is the part of the body or personality most affected and may include an idea of how narrowly focused a symptom is, e.g. whether a pain is felt at a specific point or more generally. The modalities are those things that modify the symptom and often provide the characteristic that makes the symptom more individual. The sensation is what best describes how the symptom feels to the patient and it is possible in several apparently diverse symptoms to find a

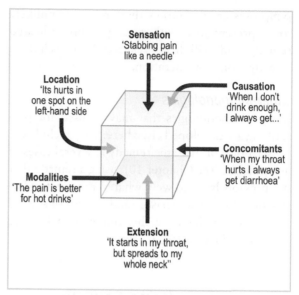

Figure 9.1 The complete symptom

similar sensation. Sensation may connect to other aspects of the case, including thoughts and feelings. Concomitants or extensions (where anatomically a symptom moves or extends to) are how one symptom relates to symptoms in other parts of the body, and so also starts to point towards a wider totality. Two or three related or concomitant symptoms are sometimes referred to as doublet or triplet symptoms.

Confirmatory and Eliminatory Symptoms

Inclusion symptoms are often other presenting symptoms, but can also be other aspects of the patient such as mental and general symptoms, that confirm or reinforce the indication of a particular remedy. The more aspects of the case the remedy fits, the more confident the homeopath can be with the prescription.

For example, in a case of food poisoning when the remedy Arsenicum Album is indicated on the basis of the causation, it may also be indicated by the presenting symptoms of diarrhoea and/or vomiting. Restlessness, anxiety and chilliness are the confirmatory symptoms that significantly increase the confidence with which a prescription could be made. Likewise eliminatory symptoms are symptoms that are highly unlikely to be present in an otherwise possibly indicated remedy and will lead 'relatively' to exclude a remedy from consideration.

Other Methodologies

Other methodologies that may be used for prescribing are developed elsewhere. They include the prescription of the same remedy in several cases of an epidemic (see Chapter 10), using a remedy that has previously acted well, whatever the methodology on which it was based, and the use of several remedies combined together that may each cover aspects of the case (see Chapter 26).

Case Analysis Using Causation and Local Symptoms

The aim of each methodology is to match the case to a remedy or 'shortlist' of likely remedies, the shortlist being sometimes referred to as the 'differential diagnosis'. Once several remedies close to the case emerge they may be compared from their materia medica pictures. As the symptoms become more numerous and complicated it becomes more difficult to identify and remember which particular symptoms relate to which particular remedy.

While for simplicity's sake prescribing on causation as opposed to local symptoms has been separated out, in practice both are very much connected. A remedy that is covered by both is much more likely to act than one covered by only one of them. Local treatment based on symptoms alone is most useful when it is only possible to see the case at the level of symptoms expressed locally and there is no obvious maintaining cause. The patient's life style and circumstances and their susceptibility will still, of course, have an effect but these are not always visible or amenable to treatment.

Matching the Case to the Remedy

Given the desire to match the patient's case with a homeopathic remedy, it makes sense to develop a way of presenting and learning the remedies that

allows them to be compared with the symptoms that emerge in the homeopathic case and with other remedies. When prescribing on causation there may be just one or two remedies to distinguish between. When prescribing on presenting symptoms there may be several. Books with lists of remedies for different conditions can be useful in prescribing for common or well recognised causes and presenting symptoms, and the modalities can indicate the relative closeness of different remedies to the picture the patient is presenting. Here, too, confirmatory symptoms can be helpful. In more obscure symptoms remembering where to find them in the materia medica can be difficult, and an index of symptoms with the remedies that have each symptom is helpful – this is a repertory.

It makes sense always to use the easiest but also the most efficient and accurate method to match the remedy to the case. In more simple cases a step-by-step method like a flow diagram may work best. In more complicated cases, matching several different symptoms in the case and remedy by a process of comparison (like comparing two pictures – one the patient, one the remedy – to see if they are similar enough), may need to take place. When using comparison, different skills are required and different interpretations are possible. It is possible for different homeopaths to come up with different remedies because they have seen the priorities of the case or information about the remedies differently.

Step-by-Step (Flow Diagram) Case Analysis

At its simplest, a remedy and case can be matched through a process of comparing a shortlist of possible medicines to the case – as in first-aid type prescribing. For acute illness there may be several steps in making the match and these can be thought of as 'flow diagrams' that allow several possible remedies to be compared (Figure 9.2). From the questions asked about the symptoms, remedies can be confirmed or eliminated. It relies heavily on keynote information in the case and in the materia medica of the possible remedies. This flow diagram or decision-tree

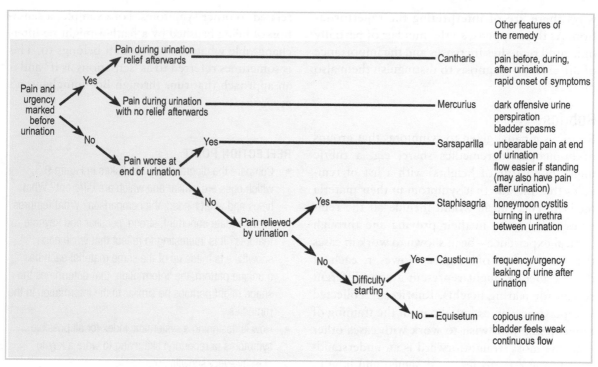

Figure 9.2 Flow diagram of common symptoms in cystitis (with thanks to Dr A Gove)

approach lends itself to cases where there is a fairly clear diagnosis or symptom picture, with not too many symptoms or modalities. When we approach materia medica in this clinical way we are able to make comparisons between different remedies, for example in urinary infection between Cantharis and Sarsaparilla, to see which is best suited to any simple case. For many health practitioners this flow diagram approach to selecting a prescription is one of the easiest ways to start prescribing, and is a good way to start integrating local homeopathic prescribing with other treatment approaches.

Comparison or Picture Matching Method

When patients present a variety of symptoms the overall collection of the symptoms may be thought of as resembling a picture. This picture can then be matched to the symptom picture of the remedy, and the analytic process is similar to the puzzle of comparing different sketches or cartoons to spot the differences and to find the

two pictures (patient and remedy) that are most alike.

One way to systematise this approach is by trying to match each of the important or characteristic symptoms of the case to the important or characteristic symptoms of the remedy. This can be helped by using a repertory that consists of symptoms, each of which has attached to it a list of remedies that have that symptom in their materia medica. Each symptom and its collection of remedies is called a 'rubric'. Within each rubric there may be sub-rubrics of that symptom but with different modalities and therefore more detailed elaborations of the main rubric. There may be several levels of rubric, sub-rubric, sub-sub-rubric, etc. – studying them will give an idea of the different symptoms and modalities a remedy picture has.

Remedies can be compared in cases with several symptoms on the frequency with which the remedy occurs in the different rubrics. As the approach to treatment broadens from the local towards the totality so more information is included in the analysis, the greater the individual's susceptibility is represented, and the more

Causation and the
Presenting Symptoms

ways there are of interpreting the repertorisation. As this happens, so the number of partially indicated remedies increases and the importance of differential diagnosis to distinguish them also increases.

Rubrics

Rubric is a name given to symptoms that groups of homeopathic remedies share, e.g. a rubric might be 'a fear of heights' with a list of remedies that include that symptom in their materia medica. This rubric would include all the remedies that have – in their proving and through clinical experience – been shown to work in cases that have a fear of heights. However, each of those remedies might represent a very different reason for fearing heights. Rubrics are collected in repertories; an essential part of the training of homeopaths who wish to work with cases other than the most straightforward is an understanding of how repertories are designed and how to use them. They are an invaluable tool for searching for the information about different remedies and discovering those remedies that fit particular symptoms.

As one expects, in the compiling of repertories, at each removal from the actual language that the prover uses to describe their experience of a remedy proving, there is potential for error. While rubrics and repertory are an essential aid to matching cases there is no replacement for comparing the actual language of the original provers with the language that patients use to describe their symptoms. Although many repertories are large, they do not include every symptom – especially not the complete symptom. As such, finding a rubric for a particular symptom is difficult and learning to use a repertory is an important part of the homeopath's training. The homeopath needs to be not only a detective but also a translator, matching the symptom expressed by the patient to a symptom or rubric that has been translated from a proving. Some homeopaths feel that the quality of the complete symptom, e.g. as reflected by the modality and sensation, can be analysed using the same modalities and sensations, even if

related to other symptoms. For example, a sensation of being brushed by a feather might be interchangeable whatever symptom it belongs to. This is sometimes referred to as 'sensations as if' and is an approach that runs through Boenninghausen's repertory.

REFLECTION POINT

- Compare the diagrams of snowflakes in Figure 9.3, which ones are similar and which are different? What helps and what hinders the comparison? What features might equate important, strong, peculiar and keynote features? It is interesting to reflect that while each snowflake is made up of the same material each has a unique pattern, the 'information' that determines the shape might perhaps be similar to the information in the remedies.

- How is designing a systematic index for all possible symptoms (a repertory) like trying to write a key to classify every snowflake?

- What might the fact that every snowflake appears different but is made from identical material say about the 'information' that determines the shape of a snowflake?

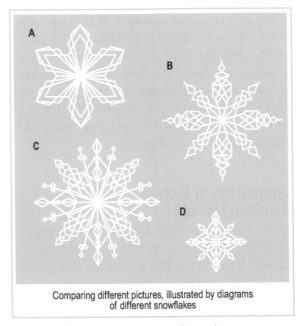

Comparing different pictures, illustrated by diagrams
of different snowflakes

Figure 9.3   Comparing different pictures

Differential Diagnosis

An exercise that helps us in differential diagnosis is to examine the different character of remedies sharing particular symptoms. For example, when we consider remedies that have an element of fastidiousness we want to understand why they might be fastidious and how they show this trait, so that they can be distinguished from other fastidious remedies. Difficulties arise in any analysis strategy when patients fall between different remedies. In these cases we must often take another look at the case to see if there are other symptoms we have overlooked, to consider remedy pictures other than those so far considered and to look at other analysis strategies.

Related Remedies

We also find that some remedies are related to one another – sometimes because they often appear together in the same differential diagnosis, sometimes because they may be an acute or chronic complement to one another, and sometimes because one may frequently be observed to follow another well in a treatment strategy. These relationships may point to groups of remedies that might need to be considered in a case favouring one remedy over another. They may appear in the materia medica or in a separate 'relationship' repertory and are discussed further in Chapter 27.

Repertorisation

'A tool for finding the best indicated remedy'

The word repertory comes from the Latin *reperire* (to find). The repertory lists the remedies relating to each symptom, like an index, and is the reverse of the materia medica (which lists the symptoms of each remedy). Through the repertory homeopathic remedies can be selected, compared and contrasted using different methodologies.

As the materia medica grows in both the number of drugs and the symptoms and features of those drugs, so the repertory grows. Most of the repertories we use today have drawn their information from preceding repertories, adding remedies and rubrics (symptoms) from past and present provings and clinical experience, and making corrections, alterations and modifications. No repertory is ever complete and some repertories contain information that is not in another.

Great care has to be taken in compiling repertories to make sure the information is accurate. Even so, there can be considerable difficulties in turning a symptom from the materia medica into a form that is appropriate to the repertory. This is a limitation that has to be borne in mind when using the repertory. Some repertories have tried to preserve the language of the patient and prover (Knerr, Allen) and as a result have many more rubrics than others.

The Structure of the Repertory

Most of the repertories are divided into chapters, each covering a bodily system. The divisions vary quite a bit from repertory to repertory and you have to get used to the structure of each one; an example of the structure of Kent's repertory is given in Box 9.2. Some, like Clarke's and Phatak's, have no chapters and are strictly alphabetical. Kent's repertory and those based on it include information about the laterality of symptoms (e.g. right or left) and the time of incidence of symptoms (e.g. morning, afternoon), before the alphabetical list of modalities, which is followed by the extension of symptom to other parts.

The order of rubrics throughout deals with the general before the particular. For example in 'extremities', pain is taken in general first (i.e. those things that affect all the extremities), then it moves to joints and bones, then to particular parts of the arms and legs. Then it repeats the whole process with each different type of pain going alphabetically from aching to tearing.

In extremities the parts are listed from above downwards, so shoulder is listed first, going down to fingers, then from nates (buttocks) and hip down to toes. Other sections, such as the abdomen or head, list the parts alphabetically, e.g. hypogastrium before umbilicus. Generalities are also in alphabetical order except for time, which starts the chapter (laterality is under 'side'). Box 9.3 illustrates some sub-headings found in Kent's repertory.

BOX 9.2

The Framework of Kent's Repertory

- Mind, i.e. mental symptoms
- Vertigo, head, eye, vision, ear, hearing, i.e. special senses
- Nose (including smell), face
- Mouth (including taste), teeth, throat, i.e. all alimentary system
- External throat, stomach including desires and aversions to different foods and thirst
- Abdomen, rectum, stool
- Bladder, kidneys, prostate, i.e. urogenital system
- Urethra, urine, genitalia (male)
- Female genitalia including menses, leucorrhoea
- Larynx and trachea including voice
- Respiration, cough, expectoration
- Chest including heart symptoms and breast
- Back, extremities, i.e. locomotor system
- Sleep including dreams
- Chill, fever, perspiration
- Skin
- Generalities including food aggravations.

The Grading of Remedies

Most repertories include a useful introductory chapter on layout and how remedies have been weighted, including the number of gradations and how they are indicated. The grade a remedy is given in a rubric is not, as it is in a case, an indication of the intensity of the symptom it produces, but represents how frequently and easily the symptom is produced.

In Kent's repertory **bold** remedies brought out the symptom in 'all or a majority' of the provers, each confirmed by reproving and having been extensively verified clinically. Second grade (*italics*) remedies brought out the symptom in 'a few' provers, confirmed by reproving and occasionally verified clinically. Third grade (ordinary type) remedies brought out the symptom 'now and then' in provers. These had not,

BOX 9.3

Sub-headings of Kent's Repertory Using as An Example The Headings Under Which a 'Pain in the Head' Might Be Looked Up

Sides
Time
Modifications
Extending
Parts of the head
  Sides
  Time
  Modification
  Extending
Kind of pain
  Sides
  Time
  Modification
  Extending
  Parts of the head
    Sides
    Time
    Modification
    Extending

at the time the repertory was published been confirmed by reproving 'but stand out pretty strong' or have been verified clinically. In this grade are also included those remedies that did not cause the symptom in provers but have cured the symptom in patients.

The Evolution of the Repertory

There have been hundreds of repertories published, often sharing some common source material. Relatively few of these are still in common use today. Box 9.4 gives details concerning some of the most well-known and used paper repertories; computer repertories are covered in Chapter 19.

Card Repertories

Repertorisation by hand is a slow process. In an effort to reduce the time and effort of writing down rubrics and remedies for repertorisation, punched card repertories started to be developed

BOX 9.4
Different Repertories

Manual of homoeopathic medicine – G H G Jahr

Translated in 1836 by Constantine Hering and the other members of the faculty of the North American Academy of the Homoeopathic Healing Art in Allentown, Pennsylvania. Used two levels of gradation (roman and italic). Jahr started work on this for Hahnemann while he was still a medical student in the 1810s.

Boenninghausen's therapeutic pocketbook – T F Allen

First published in 1846. This was Boenninghausen's small concise pocket book of his major work, the 'Repertory of the antipsoric remedies' published in 1833. It has many very large rubrics because symptoms were divided into characteristics that are not limited to a single symptom, but run through the remedy picture, e.g. 'burning' is a characteristic sensation running through many symptoms in the remedy Arsenicum Album. It sees five levels of gradation and gave rise to the so-called 'Boenninghausen method', the precursor of essence and thematic prescribing.

Encyclopedia of pure materia medica – T F Allen

First published in 1879. It has only 75 remedies, compared to Kent's 654, but almost twice as many rubrics.

Repertory to the more characteristic symptoms of the materia medica – Constantine Lippe

First published 1880. Based on the repertory found at the end of Jahr's 'Manual of Homoeopathic Medicine'.

Repertory of Hering's guiding symptoms – Calvin Knerr

First published 1896; derived from Hering's 10-volume materia medica – contains guiding symptoms by his student Knerr. The rubrics are more exact and longer than most other repertories, making it ideal for seeing if a remedy covers exactly a patient's symptom. It has nearly three times as many rubrics as Kent's repertory but a third of the number of remedies. Uses five levels of gradation.

Repertory of the characteristic symptoms, clinical and pathogenic, of the homoeopathic materia medica – Edmund Lee

First published 1889. An enlargement of Lippe's repertory.

Repertory of the homoeopathic materia medica – J T Kent

First published in sections starting with the 'Mind' in 1897. First complete edition published in 1899. Subsequent editions: 2nd 1908, 3rd 1924, 4th 1935, 6th 1957. It was based on the repertories of Lippe and Lee. Used by many homeopaths for much of the 20th century. Uses three levels of gradation (roman, italic and bold).

Clinical repertory – J H Clark

First published 1904. This repertory is actually five repertories in one book. Only the clinical repertory is relatively complete but it illustrates how different methodologies suit information presented in different ways.

1. Clinical repertory – has an extensive range of pathological rubrics
2. Repertory of causation
3. Repertory of temperaments, dispositions, constitutions and states – this is where you find 'scrawny women, foxy persons and worn out business and professional men'
4. Repertory of clinical relationships
5. Repertory of natural relationships

Materia medica with repertory – Boericke

Ninth edition published 1927. Compared to Kent it has 394 more remedies, only about an eighth of the number of rubrics, but very many clinical and pathological rubrics not in Kent. It is a useful 'pocket guide'.

Boenninghausen's characteristics and repertory – C M Boger

First published in its present form in 1936. It was based on Boenninghausen's repertory and enlarged with additions and new rubrics. Stressing modalities for local symptoms as applicable to the whole person followed by concomitant symptoms (i.e. attendant symptoms), then sensations and then the location of the symptoms.

Sensations as if – H A Roberts

First published 1937. A repertory of sensations.

Dictionary of sensations as if – Ward

A repertory of sensations. Two volumes.

A concise repertory of homoeopathic medicines – S R Phatak

First published 1963. Designed by Dr Phatak to be a very compact and handy repertory; based on Boger's 'Synoptic key'. Arranged like a dictionary in one complete alphabetical list without division into chapters of body systems so a useful first repertory for simple cases.

Synthetic repertory – H Barthel & W Klunker

First published in 1974. The three volumes are drawn from sixteen sources and it is one of very few repertories to give the source of every entry. It has 40% more remedies than Kent and uses four levels of gradation.

The final general repertory – Pierre Schmidt

Published 1980 to correct and extend Kent's repertory

Synthesis – editor Frederik Schroyens and the complete repertory – Van Zandvoort

Both Synthesis and the Complete are comprehensive repertories that are based on Kent's structure but with many additional rubrics and remedies. Because they are so large they can be difficult to use in the early stages of studying the repertory, but they are recommended for the repertorisation of the totality. They include information about where additions to the repertory come from and form the basis of the main repertory programmes used in the computer repertories, although many repertories are available in the computer repertory programmes (see Chapter 19).

from 1888 but were very limited by the number of cards needed; one for each rubric. But they did ease the conceptual transition to computer repertories. An example is W J Guernsey's Boenninghausen Slips, produced in 1888 with 2500 cards.

Computer Repertories

The computer has revolutionised the homeopathic repertory and access to the materia medica. Some of the advantages are given in Box 9.5 but this is covered in more detail in Chapter 19. Some programs are also able to search the materia medicas and journals to create rubrics that can be used as part of any analyses. The flexibility of analysis strategies and options to extract information about symptoms using for example phrases, expressions or words that the patient uses is able to generate quite individualised rubrics.

How to Repertorise

When looking for the best remedy homeopaths are trying to find a remedy that covers the most important features of the patient. The repertory has two ways of helping this, as a simple and straightforward index to the materia medica and as a method for systematically processing the symptoms and rubrics in what is called 'repertorisation'. This technique indicates how well a particular remedy is represented in the rubrics selected, allowing comparisons between remedies and levels of confidence in a prescription to be formulated.

The Use of the Repertory

In repertorisation the symptoms can be weighted and are matched to rubrics in the repertory. In all cases the hierarchy of symptoms points to the grad-

BOX 9.5
Some Advantages of Computerised Repertories

- It is usually far quicker to refer to a computer repertory than the book
- Repertorisation is dramatically quicker – almost instantaneous – and as a result can be done during the consultation
- Additions and modifications to the repertory can be made very easily
- Production and distribution of repertory upgrades on disk are far cheaper and quicker
- It may allow the user to add personal rubrics and remedies
- Every remedy in every rubric can be tagged giving its source/author
- It enables rapid searches for information: (a) key words, (b) synonyms of key words and (c) remedies
- Rubrics from the same repertory or different repertories can be combined to give a more complete rubric
- A range of different analysis strategies or combination of strategies can be used with the ability to change from one to the other instantly; with different strategies the analysis can compensate for different features of either a) the case or b) the strengths/ weaknesses of the repertory.
- Graphical display of the analysis makes interpretation a great deal easier

ing and weighting. Homeopaths using different models of health see the hierarchy of symptoms differently and to some extent the layout of repertory reflects the priority of the compiler. The remedies in the rubrics and the strength or grade required are identified. Then, most simply, repertorisation adds up how many times each remedy occurs in the selected rubrics, taking into account the grading of the remedy in the rubric, and the weighting of the symptom to achieve a numerical score.

There are different ways of scoring each remedy; the most common is to add the grading for each remedy in all the rubrics with the grades scored as ordinary type = 1, italics = 2, bold = 3, (and those repertories with bold italics = 4). By taking a selection of rubrics and sub-rubrics that represent the case and scoring the remedies in these it is possible to generate a numerical score for each remedy.

In theory the simillimum should be the remedy that covers the greatest number of the selected rubrics to the highest degree. However, if the numerical result is to be correct there are several presuppositions that need to be fulfilled. These are discussed in more detail in Chapter 14, page 181. The result is that repertorisation is only a guide to the possible correct remedies even if the repertory contains the rubrics required to find the simillimum and the remedy that is the simillimum.

Analysis Strategies

There are a number of different analysis strategies possible with repertorisation. In local prescribing the grades of the remedy in each rubric are added together to give a total or 'rubric score' that is used to indicate the most likely remedy match. These use the principle of inclusion and exclusion presented earlier, where the remedy with symptoms found in the case will increase the likely inclusion of that remedy while remedies without a symptom can be relatively excluded. How strong or central the symptom is and how clearly the remedy does or does not have that symptom will give the strength of the inclusion or exclusion. This is similar to using a strong or key symptom as an 'eliminatory' rubric, where to aid analysis only those remedies in one or two key rubrics are considered as possibilities, while others are effectively eliminated.

Other strategies are covered in Chapter 14 but they include looking at small remedies, emphasising rare remedies that have few symptoms in the repertory. In small rubrics, the smaller the numbers of remedies in a rubric, the more the remedies in that rubric are emphasised – equivalent to 'strange, rare and peculiar' symptoms. Prominence emphasises remedies that are unusually strong in a rubric, – basically keynotes. Finally, it is possible to bring out family groupings of remedies that are indicated.

Using the Repertory in the Consulting Room

Some homeopaths are always dipping into the repertory throughout the interview. Others, especially when focusing on the case, repertorise at the end. Some hear the patient mention an unusual symptom and seek it in the repertory, others hear it and want to know what's behind it; both are relevant. In the repertory the remedies shown guide which confirmatory and eliminatory questions to ask. Of course sensitivity is needed when browsing in the repertory with the patient present but sometimes the pause allows the patient to share something useful they might not otherwise. As cases get more complex, so deciding the priority of what to repertorise increases. Flicking through the repertory searching for rubrics can help to both focus on and free-associate around the case, leading sometimes to the sudden exciting discovery.

REFLECTION POINT

- Try using several repertories to analyse a simple case using local symptoms. What makes one repertory easier to use than another, and what are the limitations of each?
- When looking up symptoms why is it important to distinguish between a local modality and a general symptom, e.g. 'worse during menses' may be found under 'menses' in 'generalities' or under many other symptoms that are worse at the time of menses? Do not look in 'female genitalia, menses' as it deals with the particular types of menses and lists other modalities affecting the periods.
- What are the strengths and weaknesses of the imaginative use of the repertory when the patient's state is seen indirectly or symbolically through the rubric?
- What influences the order in which you set about searching the repertory? Do you naturally find yourself thinking of some rubrics as more important than others? How does this relate to any grading of symptoms? How might you use confirmatory and eliminatory rubrics?

- Consider how one symptom might be looked up in a repertory in different ways. For example, how might hypochondriasis be expressed differently by different patients or looked up differently in the repertory (anxiety pains, fear death, thoughts of disease)?
- Finally, reflect on how the repertory might help you learn the picture of a particular remedy. You might look up features of the remedy being studied to see how prominent the remedy is in the rubric and what other remedies are present, especially those that are of the same or higher grade.

When analysing by hand many homeopaths start by choosing rubrics of a 'middle' size. For example, in a tonsillitis case – *Throat, pain, swallowing, on*: contains about 120 remedies that are too many to work with easily and it is a very common symptom. Alternatively if you take *Throat, pain, warm room amel.*, then the only remedy listed is Magnesia carbonicum. Even if this is a strong peculiar symptom it is not useful on initial repertorisation because the right remedy, unless it is Magnesia carbonicum, might be excluded at the start in such a small rubric. Rubrics like *Throat, pain, extending to the ear*, which has about 30 remedies, and *Throat, pain, warm drinks, amel.*, which has 12, are much more manageable. At the end of the analysis the large rubric can be brought in to support or oppose the choice of likely remedies.

Summary

In Chapters 1 to 9 the homeopath will, along with teaching from other sources, have developed skills and knowledge to enable the treatment of many self-limiting diseases and some more serious diseases. The same principles are used and extended in dealing with more deep-seated cases but a thorough grasp of the idea of the importance of identifying the symptoms in detail and matching the symptoms to the materia medica through repertorisation is the centre of totality prescribing, where much homeopathic prescribing takes place. In parallel with looking at different methodologies the perceptive homeopathic student will start to notice how cases might unfold over a period of time. The more local methodologies may well fit illnesses in their early stages but later more deep-seated approaches may be required.

Acknowledgements

Dr Lee Holland and Dr Charles Forsyth

Bibliography

Barthel H, Klunker W 1973 Synthetic repertory, vol 1: Psychic symptoms. Haug, Heidelberg

Barthel H, Klunker W 1973 Synthetic repertory, vol 2: General symptoms. Haug, Heidelberg

Boenninghausen C 1891 Boenninghausen's therapeutic pocket book, 2nd edn. Translated by T F Allen. Hahnemann Publishing House, Philadelphia

Boericke W, Boericke O 1927 Pocket manual of homeopathic materia medica. Boericke and Runyon, New York

Boyd H 1981 Introduction to homeopathic medicine. Beaconsfield Press, Beaconsfield

Clarke J H 1904 Clinical repertory to the dictionary of materia medica. Homeopathic Publishing Co, London

Henriques N 1998 Crossroads to cure, the homeopath's guide to the second prescription. Totality Press, St Helena

Kent J T 1877 Repertory of the homeopathic materia medica. Ehrhart and Karl, Chicago

Kent J T 1990 The development and formation of the repertory. The Homeopath 10:3.

Kent J T, Schmidt P, Chand D H 1980 Kent's final general repertory of the homeopathic materia medica. National Homeopathic Pharmacy, New Delhi

Phatak S R A 2004 Concise repertory of homeopathic medicines. B Jain, New Delhi

Rastogi D P 1990 Boenninghausen's repertory. The Homeopath 10:3

Roberts H A 1937 Sensations as if, a repertory of subjective symptoms. Boericke & Tafel, Philadelphia. Indian edition 2002. B Jain, New Delhi

Saine A 1990 The story of Kent's repertory. The Homeopath 10:3

Schroyens F (ed) 1993 Synthesis – repertorium homeopathicum syntheticum. Homoeopathic Book Publishers, London

Tyler M, Weir J 1912 Repertorising. Homeopathic World 47(4): 149–170

Tyler M, Weir J 1912 Repertorising (contd). Homeopathic World 47(7): 296–301

Tyler M, Weir J 1983 Repertorising. Br Homeopath J 72(4):195–208

CHAPTER TEN

Managing Different Types of Cases

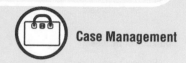 **Case Management**

David Owen

Introduction

When treatment strategy is based primarily on the presenting clinical features of the illness, categorising illness as acute or chronic provides important information about prognosis. Of more importance for person-centred medicine is to put the patient who has the illness at the centre of the case. This allows and requires a subtle but important change of focus that acknowledges both the disease process and the whole state of the individual who is presenting it. This we collectively refer to as the homeopathic case. The case allows us to discern the most appropriate model of health and approach to treatment for that individual and the methodologies and management strategies that are most likely to help. Homeopathic cases can be categorised using a spectrum that extends from the straightforward and simple through the complex to the difficult – this should not be confused with what some homeopaths refer to as simple prescribing (single remedy) or complex prescribing (using mixtures of remedies; see Chapter 30).

While acute illness is often part of a simple case and chronic illness part of a complex or difficult case this is not always so. Difficult cases are divided into those that are relatively confused and those that are relatively masked or hidden. In this chapter we explore these different categories of cases and the implications for their management. In the same way as acute illness may develop into chronic illness, so simple cases may become complex and complex cases may become

more difficult. While not all simple cases are simple to treat, they will have a clear picture and often a clearly indicated remedy. In managing more complex and difficult cases it is important to understand how they have often evolved from simple cases and how as treatment progresses they become simple again. Behind every difficult case is a complex case, and behind every complex case is a simple case.

Before looking at the management of complex cases there is much still to understand about what is to be cured, the types of cases and the management of the simple case.

The Homeopathic Continuum

Establishing where on the spectrum a particular case lies is an important aspect of homeopathic diagnosis. The type of case will often be a major factor in determining the predominant model of health and approach to treatment. The type of case will influence the style and focus of the consultation, the treatment options and expectations, and the knowledge and resources the homeopath may need to call upon. Figure 10.1 describes five categories of case; each might best be understood through a different model or mix of methods of health as previously described. The symptom picture of the different cases is illustrated graphically as a 'wave form' where the two axes might be thought of as intensity and location of the symptoms. In this way each case can be represented as

Causation and the
Presenting Symptoms

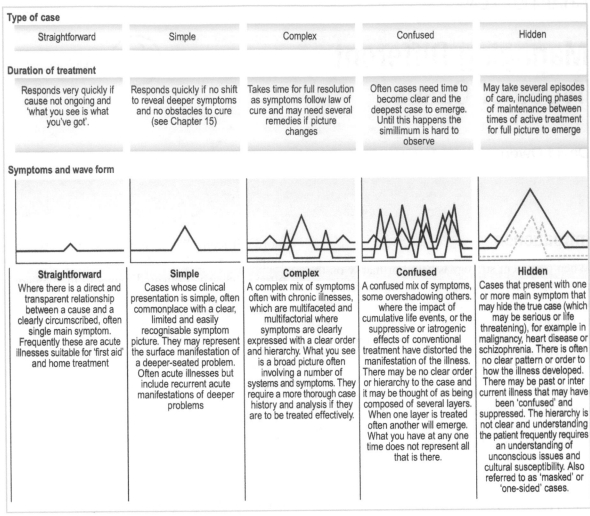

Type of case				
Straightforward	Simple	Complex	Confused	Hidden
Duration of treatment				
Responds very quickly if cause not ongoing and 'what you see is what you've got'.	Responds quickly if no shift to reveal deeper symptoms and no obstacles to cure (see Chapter 15)	Takes time for full resolution as symptoms follow law of cure and may need several remedies if picture changes	Often cases need time to become clear and the deepest case to emerge. Until this happens the simillimum is hard to observe	May take several episodes of care, including phases of maintenance between times of active treatment for full picture to emerge
Symptoms and wave form				
Straightforward	**Simple**	**Complex**	**Confused**	**Hidden**
Where there is a direct and transparent relationship between a cause and a clearly circumscribed, often single main symptom. Frequently these are acute illnesses suitable for 'first aid' and home treatment	Cases whose clinical presentation is simple, often commonplace with a clear, limited and easily recognisable symptom picture. They may represent the surface manifestation of a deeper-seated problem. Often acute illnesses but include recurrent acute manifestations of deeper problems	A complex mix of symptoms often with chronic illnesses, which are multifaceted and multifactorial where symptoms are clearly expressed with a clear order and hierarchy. What you see is a broad picture often involving a number of systems and symptoms. They require a more thorough case history and analysis if they are to be treated effectively.	A confused mix of symptoms, some overshadowing others, where the impact of cumulative life events, or the suppressive or iatrogenic effects of conventional treatment have distorted the manifestation of the illness. There may be no clear order or hierarchy to the case and it may be thought of as being composed of several layers. When one layer is treated often another will emerge. What you have at any one time does not represent all that is there.	Cases that present with one or more main symptom that may hide the true case (which may be serious or life threatening), for example in malignancy, heart disease or schizophrenia. There is often no clear pattern or order to how the illness developed. There may be past or inter current illness that may have been 'confused' and suppressed. The hierarchy is not clear and understanding the patient frequently requires an understanding of unconscious issues and cultural susceptibility. Also referred to as 'masked' or 'one-sided' cases.

Figure 10.1   Types of case illustrated as a 'wave' and correlated to models of health and approach to treatment

REFLECTION POINT

- In what ways do each type of case lend themselves to being understood in each of the five models of health and approaches to treatment?
- Thinking of the case as a wave form or shape (as in Fig. 10. 1) how might what you see be influenced by the time you have available, the case taking skills you have and the case the patient is prepared to reveal? How would what you perceive influence the treatment you offer?

an individual picture based on the symptom 'frequency', similar to each individual sound having its unique 'sound wave'.

As cases become more complex so more symptoms are seen and overlap. In confused cases one symptom can overshadow and distort what is seen of another. In hidden cases a single symptom might completely mask other aspects of the case. Finding a remedy simillimum involves finding the remedy pattern (from provings) and matching it to the symptom picture. If you imagine each symptom as a triangle then in a simple case one main presenting symptom with all its modalities represents a single triangle that can be matched to a remedy. Confused cases have a number of symptoms that each may partially disguise others, like several triangles overlying each other. A similar remedy can be chosen on a few of the key symptoms (keynote prescribing) or on the overall pattern if recognised (thematic prescribing).

In confused cases, aspects of the symptoms are missing from the picture and the theme may resemble more the silhouette of the compound shape – as the case is treated so more detail becomes clear. In a hidden case a single (or sometimes several) main, often serious, symptom presents like a huge triangle; the symptoms behind it are effectively masked from normal view. Additional aspects of the individual and the case will be expressed and perceived in the context of the homeopathic relationship (see Chapter 23). In simple cases matching the symptom to what is seen now is adequate but as cases become more complex, the symptoms that are overshadowed also need to be considered. In confused and hidden cases it may require several treatments before the overshadowed and masked symptoms are revealed – finding the simillimum is more like matching a three-dimensional model than a simple two-dimensional 'wave pattern'!

Naming these different types of case is to some extent artificial in that any homeopathic case may start at any point along this continuum, and then move as the case deteriorates or resolves. How the case is perceived is both a function of how it is presented and how the homeopath chooses to see it. You may see the same case in several different ways, influenced by such things as the time available, your experience and the aim of the treatment. Each way of seeing the case brings its own emphasis to the case, materia medica, and analyses and different management expectations.

Straightforward Cases

In the most straightforward cases the cause usually has a predictable clinical effect and therefore the susceptibility of many people to that cause is the same. Self-healing will often occur once the cause is removed, e.g. many minor ailments such as a blister from tight shoes, not sleeping due to noise, a sore throat from over use of the voice, a soft tissue injury, sunburn, etc. Treatment here is often based on avoiding or removing the cause and assisting the person's general well-being to aid recovery – homeopathic treatment is selected on the causa-

tion. If the cause is strong, persistent or recurrent the case is unlikely to remain straightforward.

Simple Cases

In simple cases a cause triggers an understandable and often predictable symptom picture. Often this focuses around a single group of symptoms, which is why it is sometimes thought of and referred to as 'local' (not to be confused with local treatment when used to refer to applications or injections applied locally/topically to a particular site). In simple illness the same cause may present slightly differently depending on the individual patient's susceptibility; one local picture may be due to several different causes. Most acute diseases can be thought of as having a single trigger and are either straightforward or simple. There is a simple or straightforward relationship between the cause and a clear symptom picture. If the patient is otherwise well 'what you see is what the patient has got'. Patients show a quick response to correct treatment and the remedies that are indicated are remedies that act quickly, often derived from sources that have a quick and dramatic effect on people such as poisons. Remember there is a link between the speed of onset, the 'clarity' of symptoms and the speed of response as they all reflect the patient's vitality.

As simple cases get more complicated, and the illnesses more chronic, so the relationship between cause and effect is more complex and the case picture and approach to treatment changes. For example, headaches due to a hangover are straightforward, those due to stress might be simple or complex, while migraine might be complex or confused. A headache as the sole presenting symptom of a brain tumour would be a hidden case. If a case presents with more than one acute illness it may be a more complex case but if treated as a simple case then it is what has changed the most or most recently that indicates the acute cause that is nearest the surface and requires treatment first.

Understanding the type of case helps interpret many aspects of the case and helps in clarifying the management and expectations of treatment. Table 10.1 shows some of the variables that distinguish simpler cases from more complex ones and the general implications for their management.

Table 10.1 COMPARING SIMPLE AND COMPLEX CASES

Aspect of the Case and Treatment	Simple	Complex
Causation	Single	Multiple
Onset	Rapid	Slow
Illness	Acute	Chronic
Focus of the case	On the illness	On the person
Symptoms	Often one main one	Several
Symptom focus	More external/superficial	More internal/deeper
Time to take the case	Shorter	Longer
Treatment	Easy	Difficult
Response to treatment	Fast	More gradual
Style of case	Taken	Received
Use of potency	Low to mid	Mid to high

Complex Cases

The distinction between acute and chronic illnesses is not black and white; nor is it between simple and complex cases. Many factors affect where a case lies on this spectrum including the cause, previous illnesses and treatment, hereditary predisposition and the ability of the patient to remove causative factors and/or move to a healthier situation. Over time simple cases inevitably either get better or become more complex, and it is frequently possible to see how a complex case has evolved from a relatively simple onset. This is one reason why it is so important to let simple illness heal properly, especially in children, so as to prevent cases becoming more complex. Likewise, complex cases either move to more simple cases as their cure proceeds or become more complex and eventually confused.

In a simple case it is often quite obvious how the symptoms help the patient deal with the illness – a pain may ensure a joint is rested, tiredness may indicate a need for rest, etc. In this way the symptom can be thought of as an interface between the patient and the environment. In complex cases it is often harder to see a direct link between the symptoms and the case but part of understanding the case is making this clear – the symptoms are how patients protect themselves or what, at one level, they need to have to survive their situation or environment.

Symptoms as an Interface Between Patient and Whole Life Experience

We may consider the development of symptoms as the organism's way of rebalancing itself, and illnesses a necessary way of adjusting to change or challenge in circumstances. In this way the body 'gives off' symptoms like a centripetal force acting in the direction of the law of cure, that is to say from within outwards. The symptoms themselves, whether commonplace (such as discharge, sweating, fever and heat) or more various, are ways for the body to 'clear itself out'.

It is not uncommon for patients to feel better after an acute illness because they have literally cleared their system out in this way. Sometimes the body just needs an opportunity to throw things out, e.g. the headache that accompanies any moderate fast or excess alcohol consumption is a sign of the body throwing off metabolic toxins. It is therefore not surprising that this curative process of developing acute symptoms often follows a prescription of homeopathic remedy that stimulates self-healing. This healing reaction is an important part of the process of cure. Seeing symptoms as an expression of an inner energy restoring equilibrium (in physiological terms, homeostasis), also allows us to conceive symptoms as an interface.

Figure 10.2(a) illustrates symptoms patients develop as an interface or boundary between them and their situation. The three perspectives relate to how the symptom is seen from outside, how it can be seen from above and how it can be understood from a cross-sectional perspective. Different symptoms provide different sorts

of boundaries where the presenting symptoms can be imagined as 'the front line' or 'outer defences'. In the analogy of a castle the patient's inner nature or final defence might be likened to a castle's keep. In more complex cases there can be many symptoms and they can overlie each other giving separate levels in a similar way that walls surround a castle's keep. The interface between patient and situation, like a wall, appears quite different when seen from the outside and from above.

In simpler cases the presenting symptom is likely to stand out, to be obvious. More complex cases, as illustrated in Figure 10.2(b), may have several symptoms – the more deep-seated ones being more central and important, representing, so to speak, the more desperate attempts of the

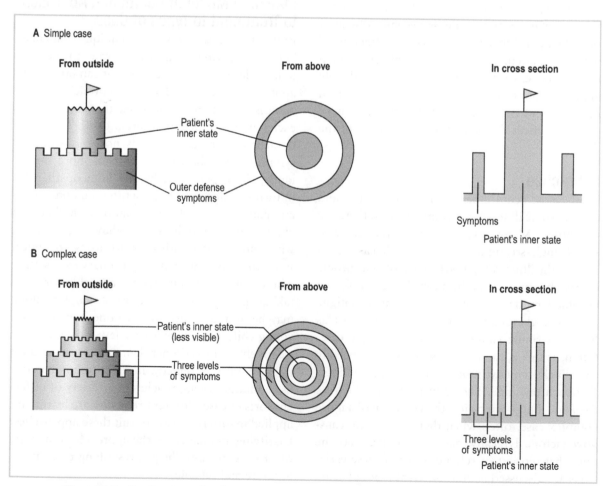

Figure 10.2   Symptoms as an interface between the patient and the situation: (a) simple case (b) complex case

organism to defend itself. So the inner might be considered higher than the outer defences, like the increasingly high walls around a castle. What is perceived will be influenced by where you are looking from and how well you can see through the symptoms. In complex cases the inner walls will not be completely visible from outside and it is necessary to see through or treat the outer levels or walls to see the deeper aspect of the case clearly, a process sometimes described (forgive the mixed metaphors) as 'like peeling an onion'.

Confused and Hidden Cases

In confused or hidden cases the deeper symptoms may be invisible behind the outer presenting symptom (see Fig 26.1). When several causative and contributory factors and levels of symptoms exist the picture becomes progressively confused until the true nature of the illness becomes obscured or hidden, and 'what you see is just a fraction of what the patient has got'. In completely hidden or masked cases there may be no immediately apparent connection between the outer symptom or 'wall' and the inner symptoms that are more likely to reflect the patient and real nature of the illness.

In Practice

While most acute illnesses are simpler cases and most chronic illnesses are complex cases, there are exceptions. Many cases that have 'never been well since' single strong triggers are simple cases even though the illness might be thought of as a chronic disease because of its duration. For example the chronic lymphadenopathy, sore throats or fatigue following glandular fever can be thought of as having a single cause and hence a simple case. Often, if this is the case, it will respond speedily to a single remedy; more akin to an acute illness than a chronic one. The opposite can also be true. An acute illness can be just the visible tip of a more complex case, often when there are several causative factors. Typically these acute ailments are the ones that reoccur or relapse; some of these variations are discussed later as different types of acute

illness. They may represent just the acute phase of a chronic illness – after the acute phase clears, the deeper picture begins to be seen. In the glandular fever example, for instance, an underlying chronic susceptibility may be revealed when a full family history is taken or as treatment unfolds.

Not only is there a gradation between cases of different degrees of complexity, but also the complexion of a case may change both as it is treated and as more or different information is revealed. Initially as more of a case is revealed the picture may deepen; then, as treatment progresses and the symptoms unfold, the case may revert to a simpler picture. Cases may need several different approaches to treatment over time; understanding this progression is central to working with difficult cases.

Matching Model of Health and Approach to Treatment to Types of Case

Each type of case offers its own unique challenges, but by classifying them in some way it is possible to learn lessons from one case that can inform our approach to another. No one approach to treatment is in itself better or worse than another, but each will be optimal in different cases. The development of the case depends not only on what symptoms are shown, but perhaps more importantly, those perceived by the homeopath. This in turn will depend on the setting the homeopath and patient are working in, and their implicit and explicit choice as to how they will work, including what models of health they are using to understand the problem. In a busy primary care setting where only a few minutes are available for case-taking, attention to the outer-most symptom alone may be all that is possible. To one homeopath a young child may present very few indications for treatment, but to another their emotional reaction might point to a remedy. In practice homeopaths use a mixture of approaches in a variety of different sorts of case; different remedies are learnt and applied in different ways to suit these approaches. Clarifying and matching the approach to the type of case significantly helps prescribing to be more accurate and reliable.

As cases get more difficult and there is more to be done for the patient to be well again, then treatment takes longer. We must be aware of the risks of both a too intrusive and a too superficial approach to treatment. As in psychotherapy, an approach that addresses deep issues in the circumstances or psyche that the patient is not ready or adequately supported to address may do harm. If a case is treated too superficially the response may be minor and/or short lived, leaving the real problem unresolved. Sometimes no remedy fits the patient's case in the model being used. In these cases another model may point to a different approach to treatment and a better indicated prescription. Learning homeopathic materia medica is a matter not only of knowing more remedies but also of building up the detail of each remedy picture according to each model of health.

REFLECTION POINT

- Think of some cases you have seen. How would you categorise these cases (simple, complex etc) and how might you draw both the symptom time line (see Fig 3.1) and represent the symptom intensity/frequency (Fig 10.1)? What is the implication if just one symptom in a complex picture is removed?

- Imagine a symptom or set of symptoms like a set of clothes or a protective barrier around you. How might the clothes you choose be determined by the situation you are in and how might it both protect you and how, if you are unable to remove them even in different situations, might this hinder, inconvenience or restrict you?

- Reflect on how a remedy might be learnt differently according to the type of cases it will be used to treat and the model of health or approach to treatment it is used for. For example, the remedy Staphisagria has causation from grief, cystitis symptoms, a full mental and physical picture, themes of suppressed anger and sensitivity to criticism and strong feelings of frustration and injustice.

Types of Simple Cases and Acute Illnesses

There are several types of simple case that each reveal aspects important in the management of acute illness, and that inform our understanding of how simple cases may become chronic.

Epidemics

Epidemics affect a number of people in a similar way; they are caused by a particular aetiology combined with a shared susceptibility. The infective organism, if there is one, is only part of this. Those who contract the epidemic disease share a common susceptibility that may point to a deeper cultural susceptibility. When epidemics start to 'die out' often it says as much about the population's susceptibility as the eradication of or specific resistance to the 'infective organism'.

Epidemics need not always be a serious illness. For example, Molluscum contagiosum is a commonplace epidemic condition in school children, and while it will usually resolve untreated in time, it is often disturbing and can become infected and temporarily disfiguring. This epidemic illness tells us something about the susceptibility of the affected children and their underlying susceptibility to veruccas and warts which, together with Molluscum, are caused by viruses that create small benign tumours. The epidemics in a community tell the homeopath about the susceptibility of the population as well as the individual. In this case it reflects a tendency to tissue overgrowth.

Knowing who else has suffered the illness, how it manifested in them and what treatment helped can point to the best treatment for others, known as the 'genus epidemicus'. Often a small group of remedies will help many patients in the same epidemic, and in so doing inform the homeopath about the susceptibility of a population.

Contagious Illnesses

Contagious diseases are similar to epidemics and are due to exposure to a particularly virulent agent spread by close proximity or contact. Their immediate cause appears as an organism that is prevalent in groups of people living close together, transmitted, by definition, by direct or close contact. There is likely to be shared or community susceptibility. The disease is often thought of as a spreading infection or infestation, but can also be seen as having a different dynamic. Just as a specific cause can be blamed for hysteria or shared grieving that passes quickly between members of a community (where it could be argued that it is the emotional susceptibility of the community that is responsible), so we can attribute contagion both to an infective agent and to collective susceptibility.

This concept of group or community susceptibility is the domain of public health, addressing, for example, communal problems of hygiene, poverty or nutrition. The role of homeopathy in helping to understand susceptibility has much to offer an understanding of a healthy environment, and could do much to inform a 'holistic' public health agenda (see Chapter 30). It is vital for the homeopath wishing to understand susceptibility to be aware not only of the illnesses that an individual patient suffers from but of the illnesses that exist in the environment and the community within which the patient lives. A common example of contagion is head lice in school children – the condition itself is not that serious, but what it tells us about a population and its susceptibility is important.

Endemics

These are illnesses or cases where the environment the individual lives in is such that causative factors are likely to occur, e.g. malaria in areas of the tropics. Changes focusing on the environment are an important part of its prevention and treatment. The concept of endemic illness may also help us to understand other illness such as joint aches and pains in low-lying areas, or respiratory problems in urban areas with high levels of pollution. The illness can inform you about the patient's situation and reaction to the environment, and can be prevented or treated by changes to the environment. If environmental changes are not made, but become a maintaining or reoccurring cause, then even if the symptoms are treated appropriately the case may deepen and become more complex, and

others in the population will suffer the same illness. As specific epidemic, endemic and contagious illness become less prevalent it can appear to be only as a result of successful treatment (or vaccination) where as in fact there are as many factors that will determine the susceptibility and resistance of a population as there are for an individual.

Acute Mental Illness

In acute mental illness the same rules and indications apply as for acute physical symptoms, and treatment requires the same approach. In the same way as an apparently simple predominantly physical case may reveal a deeper underlying psychological susceptibility, so a simple mental case may have a deeper, underlying physical susceptibility. If these deeper causes are not dealt with the condition will either not respond or relapse. For example, a patient with anxiety may be well matched to an anxiety remedy, but if the anxiety is secondary to physical causes such as the use of cannabis, overconsumption of coffee, poor sleep, or occupational stress, then these causes need to be dealt with.

Recurrent or Relapsing Acute Illness

When the patient continues to get the same acute illness, it is as if, despite seeming to resolve, the body never completely throws it off. Treatment may have failed to stimulate the individual's resistance but just, for example, eradicated an infection that then returns. This is a common occurrence in the conventional treatment of recurring infections treated with antibiotics, e.g. in ear infections or cystitis. In a patient with recurrent ear infections, swollen adenoids, increased mucus production or sensitivity to dairy products may need to be taken into account. A patient with recurrent cystitis may need to increase fluid intake or make an alteration in life style.

From the homeopathic point of view there are several, possibly interconnected reasons for this. There may be a maintaining cause, even a very simple one such as headache after eating a particular food, or earache from continued exposure to the cold. There may be blocks or obstacles to recovery (see 'Obstacle to cure' in Chapter 15) such as a patient using strong eucalyptus oil that antidotes the remedy. Or the case may be expressing a deeper disturbance and the patient's susceptibility is not being fully taken into account.

Recurring Similar Acute

In some patients there is an acquired or familial susceptibility that means similar illnesses reoccur. This deeply programmed susceptibility may be thought of as a taint or miasm (see Chapters 14, 17). For example, early birth trauma can cause a deeper susceptibility to acute illness or being accident prone, where the patient seems to keep returning to an 'acute' situation without the ability to break this pattern. There are many different triggers for this state – sometimes referred to as the 'acute miasm'. When the underlying susceptibility is treated the patient's susceptibility to acute disease is reduced.

Situational Acute

Another cause of difficulty that may need to be addressed in complex cases is a tendency for the same or a similar causation to be revisited by the patient time after time, as if drawn to a situation in which they get ill. This repeats itself until the patient has resolved whatever it is that needs to be addressed. It may mean avoiding certain foods, alcohol, emotionally damaging or abusive relationships or certain physical environments, such as cold sores activated by excessive sun. When the recurring pattern is recognised, the illness can be seen as a 'shot across the bows' – a stimulus to make changes to the patient's life situation or environment, or an opportunity for growth and development.

Acute or Chronic

A more deep-seated illness may underlie a sporadic acute picture. For example, hay fever may only temporarily respond to local treatment if there is a deeper allergic susceptibility. Even when the remedy is correct, if the susceptibility is high a remedy may need to be used in high potency or a deep acting remedy found (see Chapter 20). For example, after an injury a patient benefited from Arnica, but it failed to hold and the patient would get Arnica symptoms from the slightest knock.

This patient was susceptible to Arnica at a deep level and found it hard to move out of the Arnica state, almost appearing drawn to minor injuries (accident prone). In this case the past history revealed the patient had an earlier head injury and required a closely related remedy (Natrum sulphuricum). After this they were much better and less easily put into the Arnica state. The recurrent acute illnesses that a patient gets tell a great deal about susceptibility; one of the important questions in taking a homeopathic case is 'what sort of minor ailments are you prone to?'.

Partially Expressed Acute

When the individual fails to express the acute picture clearly in response to an acute cause, then it may be indicative of a more serious disturbance, and/or a low vitality that can itself be a sign of deeper susceptibility. In these cases a more complex picture frequently emerges.

Masked Acute

A patient who presents saying 'I never normally get ill' may just be in a state of denial. Some patients do need to be encouraged to 'listen to' their symptoms and see illness not as a weakness but (the ability to have symptoms and resolve them) as a sign of a dynamic healthy state. If they really are not getting any acute illnesses, then they may have too low a vitality or be easily suppressing their acute illnesses – either way it is not a very healthy state. In a healthy state people are likely to generate acute symptoms quickly and easily when challenged or their environment is changed. Looking deeper into such cases may reveal an underlying susceptibility; if their vitality is low patients may require more general life style advice to 'build' them up before the case becomes clear.

Relationship of Acute to Chronic Illness

Everyone encounters situations in which they are susceptible to acute illness. If these are not expressed and a curative process followed then a chronic condition is more likely. As a case becomes chronic and deepens the patient develops more internalised symptoms. Correct treatment of straightforward and simple cases is one of the best preventions of more deep-seated illness. Often overlooked when assessing the benefits of homeopathic treatment, this would only really be seen with long-term studies, as the case of Pamela illustrates.

CASE STUDY 10.1

Pamela is 48 and has been susceptible to recurrent chest infections each winter since childhood. She finds the damp environment difficult to cope with. When she gets acute chest infections she seems to go downhill in herself, her catarrh gets worse, she gets short of breath and requires treatment for asthma. On antibiotics she will often throw off the acute illness but in recent years it has taken longer to respond and she has needed a repeat of antibiotics several times a year; she has also been started on inhaled steroids for her asthma. Pamela is starting to get breathless with catarrhal symptoms throughout the year. She presents to her homeopath in an acute phase and wants to try an alternative to the antibiotics. She is wheezy with a peak flow of 310 and is on a steroid and a salbutamol inhaler. She has bronchitis and is coughing up thick, white phlegm but does not have a fever.

Antimonium tartrate (alongside her inhalers) is prescribed on local symptoms and is carefully monitored – over 12 hours her acute chest symptoms improve. After this she describes feeling a bit more energetic. Pamela finds using the Antimonium tartrate controls her chest flare-ups and they get less frequent. She is advised to avoid damp environments due to suspected mould sensitivity. After 18 months her peak flow is consistently 420 and she reports gradually reducing and then stopping her asthma medication.

In chronic disease some patients experience acute exacerbations. The acute symptom may be a diagnostic pointer to the deeper chronic illness, and treating the exacerbation or acute flare-up may be enough to give a deeper response. If the acute flare-up is in response to homeopathic treatment, sometimes no further treatment is requried.

Management of Simple Cases

There are four ways in which a medication may act. You are likely to be managing patients who are using, or have used, several medications in sequence or together and it is therefore increasingly important, as you manage more complex cases, to understand how the different remedy actions might affect the case and picture presented:

1. The *homeopathic*, where the remedy creates a symptom picture similar to the effects of the illness that it is treating.
2. The *isopathic*, where the pathogenic or aetiological agent responsible for the illness itself is used to treat it; e.g. potencies of infective organisms (see 'Nosodes' in Chapters 5, 18).
3. The *allopathic* approach, where the drug has an action that bears no direct relationship to the symptoms of the illness – 'Neither similar nor opposite but quite heterogeneous to the symptoms of the disease' (S Hahnemann, Organon, para 22).
4. The *antipathic* (also called palliative) method, in which the action of the drug is in direct opposition to the effects of the illness; e.g. the use of codeine to cause constipation and 'counter' diarrhoea.

The homeopath sees the presence of acute illness not only as part of the process of prevention and recovery from chronic illness but also as an important part of developing a strong and healthy ability to resist disease in later life. Although it is understandable to want to avoid the discomfort of an acute illness it does the organism no favour in developing its overall resistance if all acute illness is avoided or symptoms are suppressed. This is one reason why the homeopath is concerned about the over-use of vaccination, allopathic or antipathic treatments.

When an illness is not expressed or resolved the underlying susceptibility of the patient changes. Section III explores the way in which suppression of simple cases leaves a pattern of increased susceptibility that contributes to the development of complex cases.

Partial Treatment

Treating only part of the presenting symptom picture may, if the vitality is high and the illness not too deep-seated, be enough to stimulate complete self-healing. Otherwise it may lead to partial relief but not complete resolution. An illness that is only partially cured is more likely to reoccur after variable periods of dormancy or express itself through other symptoms. This is why when treating even simple cases it is best to persevere until symptoms have completely resolved. When there is ongoing exposure to a causative factor there is a risk of recurrent symptoms. The patient who wants to stay well but is unable to remove the causation will need occasional review appointments, because if the condition relapses repeatedly and is not treated effectively there will, over time, be a drop in vitality and an increase in susceptibility. It is frequently the case that the carefully attuned homeopath will detect these things at an earlier stage than the patient, like the alert mechanic who recognises that a car needs tuning. Treatment at this level is much easier and speedier than when the case has been left and becomes more deep-seated.

An inaccurate local prescription that matches only a small part of the case may alter only select aspects of the presenting symptomatology. This type of partial treatment (and conventional palliative treatments) can lead to a more complex and, in time, distorted or confused picture. If the vitality is low or the local symptoms are only part of a deeper picture, prolonged treatment of just some symptoms may make the case more confused. For this reason some homeopaths warn against all local prescribing, saying that it is important to always prescribe on the deepest aspects of the case – unfortunately this denies many patients treatment that can significantly boost their health. Certainly caution about dose, repetition and care-

ful monitoring – even of local prescribing – is advisable.

Be Aware of Any Other Treatment the Patient is On

Some patients may respond quickly and deeply to treatment based only on the presenting problem. In these cases it is important that the prescriber is aware of other problems that may not have been part of the local or presenting problem, and of how these may be affected by the response to the treatment of the more circumscribed problem, as Jean's case illustrates.

CASE STUDY 10.2

Jean, age 37 and a mother of two, presented with premenstrual tension (PMT) and received a local prescription of Sepia 30 to take once a day for 5 doses around mid-cycle. After two months she presented to another homeopath with an improvement of her PMT but a deteriorating sleep pattern and anxiety. She complained that although her PMT was better she now felt worse. Jean had been on thyroxine (thyroid supplementation) for 9 years, since the birth of her second child. On testing her thyroid level, she was found to be hyperthyroid. The Sepia had evidently stimulated a far-reaching improvement in Jean's whole health status. Stopping her thyroxine rapidly improved her symptoms.

Monitoring other treatments is important as the homeopathic remedy can change the patient's physiological state and alter the reaction to other treatments. Care should be taken when the patient is on conventional medication as the picture may be confused and may change suddenly; or a change in the level of conventional treatment may be indicated in response to physiological changes induced by the remedy. For example, in a case prescribed homeopathic Lithium carbonica while on allopathic doses of lithium (prescribed for mania) the patient's serum lithium levels increased and conventional dosage needed to be reduced. Unmonitored, lithium toxicity might have resulted.

Remember – Acute Pictures Change

Many acute diseases present different stages that can shift back and forward over time. This may require a review of the case each time the symptoms shift, if the case is not improving. For example, in a patient with pneumonia, several stages may be gone through, each possibly needing a different remedy. A patient might respond to one remedy in any stage if that remedy fits them deeply, equally the patient may need a different remedy in each phase. Even where there is no change in the conventional diagnosis, the symptom picture may change, and a change of remedy required.

When to Prescribe Deeper

If an individual produces unusual symptoms in response to a common trigger then the symptoms tell us more about the patient than the cause, hence the importance of 'strange, rare and peculiar' symptoms. These cases benefit from repertorisation to find which remedies have these individual symptoms.

In simple cases strong symptoms are likely to have been expressed by many provers of the relevant remedy. Hence these symptoms are often keynotes of the remedy, and reliably found in the materia medica and repertories. These keynotes express specific information in the patient and the remedy; matching them is like matching a key to a lock – once unlocked, and with the missing information provided by the remedy, healing can take place. Sometimes the keynote symptoms are characteristic for a disease leading to what are considered disease-specific treatments. For example, the symptom picture of scarlet fever presents very close to the materia medica picture of Belladonna, and homeopaths since Hahnemann have considered it 'specific' to that disease.

Signs of Change

Remedy reactions are covered in detail in Chapter 16 but it is useful here to reflect briefly on what

might indicate favourable and unfavourable reactions to local treatment. Change is important either if the symptoms have altered for better or worse, or if there is a change in the patient's general well-being or 'energy'. The possible changes are summarised below.

- *Favourable*
  - Symptoms improve with no new symptoms
  - A temporary aggravation of symptoms
  - General increase in energy
  - Improvement of normal physiological functions, including better sleep, more regular menstrual cycle, etc.
  - A return of previous symptoms according to laws of cure
  - Proving symptoms of the remedy given
  - An improved disposition of the patient
- *Unfavourable*
  - Symptoms worse but not following laws of cure or proving symptoms
  - A prolonged aggravation of symptoms
  - Increased discomfort
  - No change after a reasonable time
  - Lower energy
  - Disruption of normal physiological functions including poor sleep, disrupted menstrual cycle, etc.

Interpreting the Changes

The time it takes for a remedy to act is variable depending on the remedy, the dosage, the patient and the illness. In some cases, especially those that develop rapidly, a response may be felt within moments, in others with deep-seated illness it may take weeks. A useful rule of thumb is to allow a tenth of the time the patient has felt ill for recovery to take place, although early signs of change may be noticed well before this. As deeper, more difficult, cases are treated so they take longer and several remedies are likely to be needed.

If the remedy has not acted, four possibilities need to be considered: the wrong remedy was given, the remedy was antidoted, there was a block to prevent cure (obstacle to cure), or the remedy was not taken correctly. (Very occasionally it may be due to the wrong potency being given but in most cases the right remedy in any potency will give some effect – see Chapter 16.)

Levels of Competence

Finding at least one remedy for which there are indications is rarely a problem in homeopathy, and yet it is this aspect that new homeopaths spend most time addressing. What is much more challenging is choosing the best indicated remedy to suit what the homeopath and the patient are trying to achieve. If the homeopath is clear about the different models of health, and how they govern and shape the individual's health, then the management of cases becomes more straightforward even though more complex cases may need to progress through several prescriptions.

The science of homeopathy is about matching the remedy to specific criteria. The art of homeopathy is in understanding which models of health it is appropriate to work with in which patient, about seeking agreement with the patient, gathering the information to work successfully at that depth, and knowing how to progress during a course of treatment. The more deep-seated and complex the illness being treated, the more important the balance of science and art becomes.

As the homeopath becomes more competent, through study and experience, each is able to work successfully with more deep-seated and complex cases. Having support with difficult cases is one of the homeopath's biggest opportunities – learning from such examples is central to developing competence.

In many of the great historical homeopathic books there are discussions of using remedies in serious situations such as acute shortness of breath, fits, coma, bleeding, shock, mania. These cases need to be considered and managed within the context of other therapeutic systems available. The homeopathic treatment may not be used alone or indeed be the priority. The competent homeopath knows this and can advise patients within a framework of care that will include other treatment approaches and other health carers.

Many experienced homeopaths realise the need for integrating different treatment approaches and

will work closely with other health professionals. It is essential to be sure that your level of competence is appropriate to the work that you choose to do, and to bear in mind what other systems of health care are available that might help a patient, and what other areas of knowledge may need to be involved. Simple cases like cystitis, acute ear infections and dysmenorrhoea may be part of more deep-seated illness, and clarifying the patient's expectations, and how the homeopath and patient are to work together, is the foundation of the therapeutic relationship.

Introduction to the Therapeutic Relationship (See Chapter 23)

The agreement between the patient and the homeopath as to what will take place during the treatment process is an important part of case management. It allows an understanding of where each party is coming from and what each would like to see happen. A clear agreement allows the exploration of symptoms in more depth than would otherwise be possible, or even proper. Often this understanding evolves over the course of a consultation, and is reviewed during a course of treatment. For example, the initial agreement in an acute illness might become an agreement to help prevent further acute illnesses. In simple and acute cases the agreement is often 'obvious' – get rid of this problem or deal with that symptom. Even in these situations it can be important to clarify your role as the homeopath. It may simply be a matter of re-framing the patient's implicit wish, e.g. 'I will help you throw off this problem or symptom,' or 'I believe it is important that you understand why you have this symptom and that we treat it *and* your susceptibility'. Difficulties with contracting are at the centre of many cases that are perceived as being difficult but need not be so.

REFLECTION POINT

- Reflect on the difference between homeopathic and conventional drug treatment. How are they different and how are they similar in the treatment of acute illness? What advice would you give to a patient choosing between these two approaches?

- In a patient receiving homeopathic treatment for an acute illness why is it important to review the patient and what are the different possible reactions?
- Why is no remedy in itself homeopathic but only acts homeopathically? What advice would you give a patient who wants to treat the minor ailments of their family homeopathically?

Summary

The foundations of homeopathic thinking laid in the first two sections of this textbook will prepare the homeopathic student to treat minor ailments, first aid problems and some more serious illness where a local symptomatic approach is indicated. These foundations will prepare the homeopath for thinking about, assessing and prescribing for more deep-seated cases.

Homeopathy can help patients with a variety of diseases, whether in the home, as an adjunct to other therapeutic disciplines or as an approach to deep-seated chronic disease. Those using homeopathy at this deeper level are advised to understand the different emphasis on 'the case' rather than 'the illness' that homeopathy makes. By separating cases, as this section has done, the homeopath is preparing the way to understand and treat complex cases and to use strategies that can help in more difficult cases that are frequently confused, hidden or have aspects of each. At this early stage of practice you need to remember that you rarely work in isolation. What other treatments or advice the patient has received or is following are important to 'factor in' to patient care. The homeopath works alongside the patient's natural ability to provide healing – when the patient fails to recover there are a number of reasons.

The homeopathic case reflects the susceptibility and sensitivity of the patient including the symptoms. Further, it raises the question of how the health of the individual interfaces with the health of the community. Subsequent sections look at the holistic, holographic and relational models of health that build on the patient- and case-centred view of health as opposed to the illness- and disease-centred approach that is so much a part of current Western medical systems.

By examining some of the management issues in treating patients with more straightforward and simple cases the student has been introduced to issues that will be met again when treating more deep-seated illness. It is likely that the student preparing for this challenge will be gaining experience of cases within their competence – realising the importance of the case as far more than just a record of the presenting symptoms and preparing to blend together a number of different treatment strategies. Remember that when the management of cases does not go as planned or as you expected, a learning opportunity exists and it is how you use these opportunities that will determine the development of your knowledge and practice as much as any theoretical learning. Starting to sit in with experienced homeopaths and develop experience of taking and managing cases, under close supervision, is an important part of your training.

Section III

Totality and Constitution

CHAPTER ELEVEN

Holism and Understanding Complex Cases

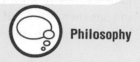

Philosophy

David Owen

'It is the theory which decides what we can observe'
Albert Einstein

'Theory, like mist on glass, obscures facts'
Charlie Chan

Introduction

A holistic model of health, taking an overview of the patient including their mind, body and spirit*, their circumstances and life situation, is central in evolving a curative approach to chronic disease and complex cases. The holistic view uses the totality and the constitution to find a remedy that suits a patient, rather than just the disease. This is a major shift (sometimes referred to as a paradigm shift) from the conventional model of how illness is viewed and treatment approached and if

---

*NOTE

Spirit is used to represent the non-material aspects of an individual – when the material aspects include the physical, intellectual, emotional and instinctual 'bodies'. The spirit means so many different things to different people that no one definition or belief serves all patients. However, for most patients the view or description of their spiritual nature allows their story to include aspects of their nature and 'purpose' that might not otherwise be articulated, and so are important aspects of the whole person. It is helpful for the homeopath to be aware that patients will hold many different beliefs that influence both their perception of normality, what is right and wrong, and their 'place' in their world.

you have practiced in this conventional model for some time the paragraphs below on 'Symptoms, susceptibility and suppression' may need several readings to be clear. A homeopath applying the holistic model no longer sees one part of a patient as disconnected from another part or from the life situation they are in. It provides an opportunity to explore the intimate connections between the psychological and physical, and the personal and environmental aspects of health.

A holistic model and totality approach allows treatment of patients with symptoms that are serious, deep-seated, long-standing and manifold. It means essentially that regardless of how many different symptom complexes and apparent illness patterns or levels of disease a patient may have (in however many different systems or areas of the body and mind), from a holistic model, a patient only ever has one fundamental disturbance to be cured. The constitutional approach recognises that even those features that are not symptoms of the illness are part of the individual's case and may guide treatment. For those whose predominant training has been in the currently dominant Western model of cause-and-effect then grasping this model may at first be difficult.

My personal belief is that the material bodies 'reflect' and parallel the spiritual. It is the material bodies that get 'dis-eased' and that are in the remit of the homeopath to work with. Your personal beliefs will both inform and colour your perception of the situations patients find themselves in. As such the more conscious you are of what 'spirit' means to you, the more aware you may be of what patients believe spirit is. The more secure you are in your own belief and values the less they need to be projected onto others.

Symptoms, Susceptibility and Suppression

In acute illnesses and simple cases, a cause leads to an effect or symptom. The effect itself can be a cause for other symptoms that can lead to a complex case. Unfortunately chronic illness and complex cases can rarely be understood solely in terms of symptoms and susceptibility. The picture is invariably changed in some way by the reaction of the patient or those around them. When this is not in a curative direction it gives rise to suppression and palliation.

Susceptibility and suppression are the keys to understanding complex cases and are expressed in cases through the hierarchy of symptoms and the presence of disease at different depths (see Chapter 6, page 71). A characteristic of the hierarchy of symptoms is that symptoms express themselves in a certain order. When a symptom is suppressed it will express itself at a deeper level – the second part of this chapter explores suppression, its distortion of the totality and veiling of the constitution, and the importance of grasping this to understand cases as they become more complex.

Looking at how susceptibility and suppression are dynamically linked starts to reveal why some symptoms are more central and others more peripheral. Whether symptoms are expressed in the realm of sensation, function or structure can be an important indicator to the depth and breadth of the symptom and therefore not only to the susceptibility and suppression but also to the likely response to treatment. The effect of suppression (from medication, hereditary and cultural factors) on the symptoms and susceptibility lays the foundations of most complex cases. When symptoms are suppressed from view they distort or mask the case, giving rise to confused and hidden cases. Throughout this section you are both

invited to explore and develop a holistic view to help you practice using totality and constitution while at the same time recognising their limitations in dealing with confused and hidden cases.

The Totality and the Constitution

In acute illnesses and simple cases it is usually possible to understand them either in terms of causation (A) or a linear cause and effect relationship (A causes B). The link between cause and effect is frequently transparent. In chronic illnesses and complex cases the homeopath wishes to understand the interplay between the symptoms and the patient's susceptibility (why B is sensitive to cause A). As cases get increasingly difficult we see that suppression actually alters the susceptibility of an individual (that treatment C contributes to B being sensitive to A). In practice symptoms, susceptibility and suppression each influence and 'shape' the case.

Each of these aspects has to be taken into account in interpreting the case and planning the management. Within this wider perspective, the totality of symptoms and the constitution of the patient (which reveals the underlying pattern of susceptibility), provide probably the two most commonly used homeopathic treatment strategies in chronic illness. A constitutional picture of a patient does not necessarily include the clinical symptoms and a prescription based on the totality does not necessarily take into account the constitutional picture (Swayne 1998)

The Totality

The totality includes all the symptoms of the illness, including all features of the case that have come about since the patient was healthy. Symptoms may be considered as physical, mental or general and may be a normal part of the disease, such as joint pain in a patient suffering from arthritis, or be more unusual, such as a craving for a particular food or skin rash in the same patient. While to perceive every aspect of every minute change due to an illness and its effects is the idealised goal, the reality is that those which are hierarchically most important will tell us most about the illness and the patient's response to it (see Chapter 6). In the totality it is the breadth of the picture combined with the most unique and peculiar features that describe the case. It is usually because the perceived totality is incomplete or the hierarchy unclear that in some cases the totality is unable to reveal what is required to be treated – these are the confused and hidden cases. It is often only over a period of treatment that in a confused case a clear totality, reflecting the hierarchy of the case, becomes apparent.

The Constitution

The constitutional pattern of a patient is described by a picture painted by broad brush strokes but often including some unique or personalising feaures. It may be most easily identified in different people by anything from just one or two key features to an intricate pattern of comprehensive and connected characteristics. This will depend on what their constitution is, how strongly it is expressed and how clearly it is seen. The patient's constitution, characteristics and reactions when well determine both susceptibility and, conversely, resilience and resistance to illness. We therefore refer sometimes to strong and weak constitutions. There is much confusion over how different homeopaths use the term 'constitution'. I recommend that both the constitution and the totality are always considered together and that it is remembered they are two sides of the same coin – but that at any one time one may be more visible or helpful in finding a remedy than the other.

The holistic case and our ability to articulate ideas and concepts about it are determined by our ability to describe a patient's totality and constitution. In this way both the totality and constitution describe essential aspects of the case, and either or both may be used as a valid approach to treatment when viewing the patient holistically. While it is important for the homeopath to try separating these two aspects out, in practice they are closely related. When thinking of a deeper case as having several layers it can be thought of as like several coins stacked on top of one another. What is a symptom at one level may

be part of the constitution on another level as Alice's case illustrates.

The constitution determines:
- the likely reaction of individuals to any situation they find themselves in, including the situations that may provoke illness
- the symptoms by which they are likely to express that reaction
- the remedies that they are likely to need.

The constitutional characteristics of a remedy are built up from those of patients who respond most sensitively and strongly to the remedy together with the observed characteristics of individuals most sensitive to the experimental proving of a remedy. The constitutional picture of a patient or a remedy is based on the picture that the individual presents when 'healthy' – the 'healthy state' being that prior to the onset of illness, or prior to the effects of a proving or in between episodes of illness. Aspects of the constitution will stay the same over several episodes of illness. When symptoms are very different or suppression strong there are likely to be subtle changes in the constitution. In this way constitutions may 'evolve' and change depending on the circumstances and illnesses the patients experience.

In some schools of homeopathy, however, the concept of 'constitution' is used to refer predominantly to the physical type and appearance of a patient; to avoid confusion it may help to refer to these as 'morphological constitutions' (see Chapter 12).

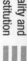

Totality and Constitution

REFLECTION POINT

- Think about a complex case you have seen. Identify those features of the case that relate to symptoms, susceptibility and suppression. Consider how different cases with the same 'disease diagnosis' might have different symptoms, susceptibility and suppression. How may the case be understood as made up of symptoms of different 'depth' and how is it informed both by the totality and the constitution?

The Paradigm Shift or Shift in Models of Health

The totality model of health is significantly different from the models of health so far described. It raises important questions about how the component parts of an individual are each less than the whole, how cause and effect are connected to each other and the situation in which the cause and effect happen. It also raises important questions about the appropriate tools to investigate and experimentally validate it (see Chapter 24). Each different model of health is only partially explained or understood by natural progression from other models of health. Moving between each model (paradigm) of health requires a shift in assumptions, values and interpretation of observations.

Each model provides you with the opportunity to explore different ways of understanding and viewing health. No one model will be optimal in every setting. However, the shift to a holistic model from the models based on a linear relationship between cause and effect provides a challenge and opportunity to the homeopath to see things differently. The cause and effect models are served by conventional medical language; the holistic model builds on this to include the interface between the mind and body, the individual and the situation. In the holistic model an illness has as much to do with the patient's susceptibility and events and experiences leading up to the illness as trying to establish an immediate cause and identify a single disease process.

The holistic model invites an appreciation of the interconnectedness of all aspects of a person (molecules, cells, tissues, thoughts, etc.) and all aspects of the patient's environment. It suggests a common thread running through the mind, body and environment to explain and allow for order, context and relationship (Bellavite & Signorini 1995).

Remedies as qualities and information

One way of understanding this common thread is as a quality or in terms of 'information' and that an individual may be thought of as being healthy when they have the qualities or information that are necessary to function in a balanced way that does not require or generate symptoms in the situation they are in.

When the situation patients are in changes so the information they need to be healthy also changes. If the individual already contains the information required for the new situation then each will adapt to it without the need for symptoms. In this way the homeopathic remedies may be thought of as providing the information a patient needs to cope with the situation. This may explain the well-observed phenomenon that having one illness seems to make some patients more resistant to others. For example, a study of 6000 children showed hay fever to be 14% less common in those contracting measles than in those not infected (Lewis & Britton 1998).

Revisiting Causation

In the holistic model causation is broader than a single aetiology. There can be a number of different causations and contributory factors in any case and during treatment different factors become apparent. Instead of cause it can be helpful to think of factors that influence susceptibility or trigger events. The case of Gupta illustrates how a complex case presenting with a clear symptom picture can be considered to have causes in several different areas of life. Different therapists, carers, advisors and friends would suggest treatment depending on where they saw the problem. A holistic approach attempts to understand a patient's narrative from as broad a perspective as possible, and Figure 11.1 suggests some of the different areas where causation might be considered in Gupta's case.

- Reflect on different cases that might present with symptoms of a gastric ulcer and consider the different dimensions in Figure 11.1 that may play a part in these cases. How do different treatments link to these different possible causes and how might these causes relate to each other? Causation might be sought and contribute to the case in any and many of the different aspects of the patient listed in Figure 11.1 – where each practitioner will see the cause and focus treatment will be influenced by their perspective. In Gupta's case how might a counsellor, a gastroenterologist, a surgeon, a dietician, a friend or a priest have seen the case differently?

CASE STUDY 11.2

Gupta presented wanting help with a gastric ulcer because she was not tolerating conventional treatment well. It was based on blocking production of histamine at the cellular level. She had received treatment for an infection in the stomach with triple antibiotic therapy, which had given short-term relief. Neither of these approaches would have been available 20 years ago. Common treatments then were based at a tissue level, cutting the vagal nerve and reducing the nerve supply to the stomach, or at an organ level, by removing part of the stomach.

Gupta eats much spicy food and might have been treated by dietary modification. She also had a stressful life with a young family and demanding job. The stress was partly social in that she was in an arranged marriage that she felt unhappy in but didn't feel able to talk to her husband about. Her extended family was helpful with her children but she felt would be very unsupportive of her criticising her husband. She spoke about cultural differences between her work life as a shop assistant and home life, and the confusion about her identity this presented. When talking with some friends they suggested this was her 'Karma' and had to be accepted as it was, while others suggested she should not be expected to put up with things as they were. She decided to see a homeopath.

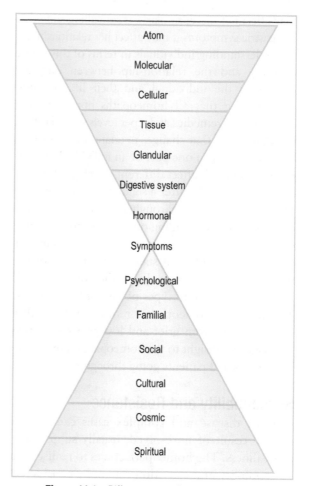

Figure 11.1 Different ways of viewing causation

In many cases the deeper symptoms are assumed to approximate to the cause, and the true primary cause may well be disguised as the case becomes more confused and hidden. It can help to remember that the deepest causes in a case can be thought of not only as a reaction to something in the environment but as subtle, energetic and information changes and that in potency, homeopathic remedies provide subtle energetic and information qualities that can help a case on several levels or in several areas of the body at the same time. So in the case of Gupta it is possible that the right remedy can be found from viewing the case in one of several different ways but when this right remedy is given it may correct the disturbance in other levels. So if something was to shift in Gupta's relationship, it may affect her ulcer; similarly, if something shifted in her gastric symptoms it may affect her relationship.

Understanding individuals in terms of this subtle anatomy and the relationship between different aspects of the individual and their life situation is something that all homeopaths hoping to use homeopathic remedies at deeper levels should reflect on. Remember that changes in anatomy, physiology or functionality in one part of an individual or their environment will affect different people in different ways. For example, after a sudden bereavement five people might each go through a similar grieving process. However, depending on the susceptibility each of those five patients may experience problems (or get stuck) in a different state. Other aspects of the totality and constitution do, in the holistic model, reveal many different types of susceptibility to loss. The different homeopathic remedy pictures that have ailments from grief and loss give substantive language and insight to the homeopath on the grieving process and patients going through it.

Susceptibility and Resistance

Chronic disease and complex cases can be the natural result of unresolved, usually suppressed, acute illness. The homeopath comes to realise that susceptibility and causation cannot be considered separately. It is necessary to 'blend together' the aetiological factors and the susceptibility to see the complex case. Which chronic illness a person develops will be influenced by individual susceptibility – including acute illnesses in the past and the reaction to them. It is therefore important to note the acute precursors of any chronic disease.

All individuals have a resistance to some things and a susceptibility to others. It is a question of working out a profile of susceptibility and resistance for each patient. This is true not only of individuals but also within all social and cultural groups. For this reason knowing the susceptibility and resistance of the patient's family, colleagues, culture, race, etc. are important. When one disease becomes less common in any group, the homeopath reflects on what has become more common. The strengths and resistance of patients can helpfully point to the best remedy match as much as the weaknesses and susceptibility.

Vitality and 'The Constitution'

As a disease progresses it can be seen to be moving deeper and deeper into a person, in what we can term a centripetal direction. The life force, through the vitality, might be considered to resist this progression by throwing symptoms out towards the extremities, centrifugally. What happens on the outside reveals what is being expressed from the inside. When the life force and vitality are low the centrifugal force is less, and symptoms less clearly expressed (Roy 1999).

Given sufficient vitality, then any illness expressed in an unobstructed way would give acute symptoms. These would express themselves on the most superficial or peripheral aspects of the individual. This is why many homeopaths claim that in the evolution of all complex cases, if the individual could develop an acute illness the chronic disease need not manifest. It is due to susceptibility to certain causes and obstruction of the expression of symptoms that complex cases with chronic diseases come about.

REFLECTION POINT

- What do you think keeps an individual's vitality high? A healthy person often appears more flexible and adjusts well to change. One of the first signs of patients improving is often they will be more creative and more active, and will make life style changes. If the vitality is fed and nurtured by moving between different life situations, then both the cause of illness and the maintenance of health rely on the interaction between the individual and the changing situations. What are the implications on your role as a 'healer' when health and illness are so closely related?

Depth of Disease

This book has already introduced the reader to the importance of understanding cases, of looking at symptoms in terms of layers, levels and hierarchy. As we move into considering more complex cases the homeopath must consider two further measures that reflect the depth of a disease – one is the difference between hereditary or acquired

Totality and Constitution

influences, the other the difference in a symptom or illness depending on the whether it is expressed through the qualities of structure, function or sensation. Often the more structural or hereditary a disease the deeper it runs and in these cases there are often several levels of symptoms and different layers of remedies running through the case.

Hereditary and Acquired

Homeopaths differ in the relative importance they attribute to situational (environmental) factors and susceptibility in complex cases. The resultant schism has been a recurrent tension between different schools of homeopathy; this mirrors the difference between those who see acquired factors and those who view hereditary factors as most central to a case. One school focuses on susceptibility. As Kent expresses it:

'...*it is not from external things that man becomes sick, not from bacteria nor environment, but from causes within himself ... measles and smallpox are not on the outside. Man is protected on the outside; he is attacked from the inside when there is susceptibility.*'

This susceptibility is expressed in the holistic model as the 'constitution'.

Other schools focus on the external or acquired causation of disease and the immediate symptoms produced. These may be the local symptoms or the totality of what is changed. In managing increasingly complex disease both these ways of understanding illness, represented by the constitution and the totality, are valid and need not be mutually exclusive. (It is interesting that despite the validity of both a constitutional and totality approach to prescribing holistically that one or other is frequently claimed to be more holistic or more 'classical' than the other.) Circumstances including hereditary predisposition and acquired influences are intimately related with our holistic understanding of the evolution of the patient's state. Unravelling this narrative is important in making sense of the more complex case and becomes central in clarifying and unmasking the confused and hidden cases discussed in later sections.

Structure, Function or Sensation

Symptoms can express themselves in qualitatively different ways. They may manifest on a level of structure, function or sensation – it is common to see chronic illness developing first in sensation, then in disturbance of function, before moving into structural damage at a tissue or organ level. During curative treatment this order is reversed. Sensation changes include feeling sick, numb, hot, pain, etc. Functional changes affect the working of a bodily system, e.g. diarrhoea, sweating, restricted movement, etc. The body might restrict function in order to reduce an unpleasant sensation, such as not walking with an inflamed knee joint. Structural changes include bone and joint degeneration, skin lesions, tumours, infarction, etc. (see Chapter 15).

A patient will often get symptoms moving through each of these overlapping phases. For example, a patient with a chronic sore throat may have thirst and burning pain (sensation), dryness and difficulty swallowing (function) and swelling (structure). The relationship between these three

Totality and Constitution

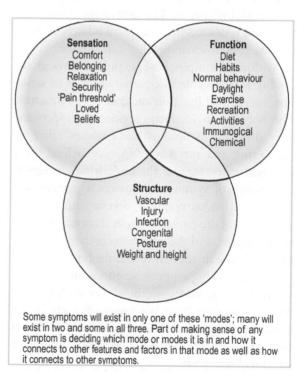

Some symptoms will exist in only one of these 'modes'; many will exist in two and some in all three. Part of making sense of any symptom is deciding which mode or modes it is in and how it connects to other features and factors in that mode as well as how it connects to other symptoms.

Figure 11.2 Three modes of symptom expression, with some of the factors influencing the quality of symptom expression

tells us about the severity of an illness, the prognosis, and the likely response to treatment. Figure 11.2 illustrates these three modes of symptom expression, with some of the processes that need to be taken into account when understanding symptoms in each one. You might reflect on how these three realms encompass the different causes given in Figure 11.1. Usually disorders of structure are reflected in a disturbance or limitation of function and disorders of function are mirrored in the realm of sensation. It is not a coincidence that structure relates to the body, function to the inter-action with environment (generals), and sensation to the mind and nervous system.

Many symptoms of sensation, such as pain, may relate to a physical part of the body but have qualities of 'feeling'. General symptoms, such as feeling hot or cold, describe how a patient functions in or reacts to the environment; physical symptoms, such as swelling, usually relate to a disorder of structure. The homeopath is interested in how different symptoms or syndromes express a common (sometimes referred to as fundamental) sensation, function or structural disturbance. The greater the disturbance the more restricted the individual is likely to be to the diversity of situations they can tolerate.

Within all complex cases expressed through the totality it is possible to observe qualities of sensation, qualities of function and qualities of structure. The homeopath is always seeking to understand how different symptoms and qualities relate to each other and the whole. In approaching more confused cases, sensing the underlying changes in the quality of symptoms provides a pattern that connects what may appear diverse and contrary symptoms of the patient's physical appearance and temperament, and the environment they choose to live in. Those drugs that mimic the body's normal functions have big suppressive effects on functional symptoms, e.g. corticosteroids. Those drugs that distort sensation have big suppressive effects on sensation symptoms. Those treatments that distort structure (surgery) have a big effect on suppressing structural symptoms.

REFLECTION POINT

- Sandra's case illustrates some of the different factors that influence a complex case. Try to identify the different levels of symptom – which are totality factors and which are constitutional factors? How do inherited and acquired factors influence it and can the features be distinguished on qualities of structure, function or sensation? How might her symptoms be affecting her vitality?

CASE STUDY 11.3

Sandra, a 28-year-old single lady, had been having premenstrual pelvic pain for 7 years. She had an operation for termination of pregnancy when she was 20 that she still feels very guilty about although she knew it would have been 'a mistake to carry on with the pregnancy'. Since the operation and signing the consent form for it she had found it increasingly difficult to sign her name on cheques and forms, and this increasingly interfered with her life. Lately she has had weakness and some wasting of the muscles in her right hand. She is right-handed. The pelvic pain had started six months after the termination of pregnancy and had been a problem premenstrually since. At age 25 Sandra started to get a swelling in the left lower abdomen, diagnosed as a large ovarian cyst. Endometriosis was also present. She was angry about the termination and did not want further surgery. Her mother suffered from painful periods and had treatment for breast cancer when Sandra was 15 years old. Sandra was treated with homeopathic Staphisagria and the pelvic pain gradually improved. After expressing her anger about the termination she described feeling stuck and a great sense of having to do 'the right thing'. After homeopathic Carcinosin she was able to accept her mixed feelings about the termination. Gradually her difficulty signing her name improved, and after 3 years of treatment her cysts and endometriosis had completely resolved.

Totality and Constitution

Suppression

Suppression is the 'treatment of a symptom or condition so that it is relieved but is not resolved. It may remain dormant, or become manifest in some other, possibly more serious or deep-seated disorder' (Swayne 2000). In simple cases the exact cause or how the patient comes into contact with the cause largely determines the symptom picture. In complex cases the symptoms that manifest and the situations to which they are sensitive are determined by the patient's constitution and susceptibility. These in turn are largely influenced by hereditary factors and suppression. Figure 11.3 illustrates how simple cases are moved towards complex cases (and on towards confused and hidden cases) by suppression.

If treatment is not to be suppressive it needs not to transitorily improve the symptoms at the price of the individual's susceptibility by sacrificing the flow of the vitality. The understanding of the dynamic between vitality, susceptibility, constitution and suppression might be helped by reflecting on the analogy of a river and the terrain it runs through.

If you think of the vitality as a river flowing through an individual's landscape, then certain features in the landscape (constitution) may inhibit or enhance its natural flow. The resulting course of the river will make it susceptible, in

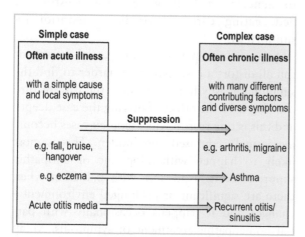

Figure 11.3 Simple cases are moved towards complex cases by suppression

different places at different times, to flooding or drought. If the river's course is artificially blocked or diverted (suppression) this will lead to a build up on one side of the blockage and a deficiency on the other (symptoms). Exactly where the blocks are likely to take place depends on the terrain or constitution (susceptibility), as well as the nature of the obstacle. A block in one place often leads the river ultimately to follow a new route, leading in turn to new excesses and deficiencies. In other words, what is suppressed in one place eventually expresses itself in another. Ultimately if it is not possible for the river (vitality) to flow, then the landscape becomes barren.

Both disease symptoms and suppression symptoms are due to disruption of the dynamic balance of the organism's susceptibility and its situation. As such, symptoms from suppression can be considered and treated in the same way as other symptoms. Suppression often takes place in response to the expression of symptoms – therefore suppression is often the internalisation or driving inside of a symptom.

Common Causes of Suppression

Suppression may be from medication, over-the-counter treatment and/or recreational drugs. There may also be emotional and cultural causes, as well as those from a secondary illness. The suppressive effect is to confuse or divert the expression of an illness through an action that either bears no direct relationship to the symptoms (allopathic) or indirect opposition to the symptoms (antipathic) (see Chapter 10, p. 132).

Suppression as a block to a natural expression or flow can be compared to putting a lid on a saucepan of boiling milk, without turning down the heat. When this starts to boil over again, further suppression puts more lids on until a virtual pressure cooker is present. It is a common reason why an occasional acute illness and simple case becomes more chronic and increasingly complex, e.g. analgesic-induced headaches.

As symptoms affect more central and vital organs so the amount of suppression needed to stop symptoms surfacing increases and the amount of force to keep suppressing symptoms increases. If suppression is likened to holding down a balloon or ball under water then the deeper the water the greater the force required to hold it down. Suppression often demands a great deal of force, especially to suppress more deep-seated symptoms – this leads to, and is a major cause of, blocked and depleted vitality, which in turn leads to failure to express a clear picture and an increasingly confused or hidden picture of the case. In order of magnitude, suppression of a structural symptom (e.g. by surgery) will be greater than the suppression of functional symptoms (e.g. anti-diarrhoea agents and anti-pyrexials), which in turn is greater than the suppression of symptoms of sensation (e.g. by pain killers or indigestion remedies). There are many causes of suppression but allopathic and antipathic treatments are a major factor in developing increasingly complex, confused and hidden cases.

Not all conventional drugs are equally suppressive. The degree of suppression depends on the extent to which they disturb the body's natural reaction to a stimulus and how long they have been given for. Any suppression may lead to the emergence of new symptoms; it is these that are often the adverse effects of the medication. This should be distinguished from those factors that can, despite a correct remedy, prevent a patient from improving. These are considered 'obstacles to cure' (discussed more fully in Chapter 15) and include a maintaining or persistent causative factor.

Palliation, Suppression and Partial Cure

Palliation and suppression are the lessening of symptoms without cure. A useful distinction between suppression due to medication, either antipathic or allopathic, and palliation due to modification of the environment and the patient's circumstances can be made. Historically in homeopathy, palliation has sometimes been used to describe the antipathic suppression of symptoms. Both suppression by medication and palliation by modifying the environment need in the homeopath's mind to be distinguished from

using homeopathic remedies or other natural remedies that only fit part of the case. This partial treatment may or may not help reveal the deeper underlying symptoms, but it is quantitatively and qualitatively significantly different from suppression and palliation.

An ill patient may reasonably seek to modify the situation to cope with that illness – indeed illness can be a major reason for seeking change. It might be a change of job, diet or life style, e.g. a hangover might encourage someone to give up drinking alcohol. You may also seek out an environment that helps you to cope with your symptoms, e.g. moving to a house with no stairs if you have mobility problems. This may give the appearance of being free of symptoms.

In cases where palliation is strong the patient may not even be conscious of actively choosing a certain environment to avoid symptoms. What palliates a particular symptom is essentially removal of what causes a symptom. Unfortunately palliation of more superficial symptoms is a way of coping with a disease but isn't a curative process and frequently leads to other aspects of the disease becoming manifest. It may be an important part of managing an illness both while the patient is pursuing a curative approach (avoiding allergens while the underlying susceptibility is being treated) or to give time for the vitality to build up sufficiently to generate a healing response (resting in bed, eating carefully or being emotionally supported).

Suppression, palliation or partial treatment can all distort a case making it harder to find the simillimum. Anything that alters the case picture can also have the effect of driving the case deeper and this is one reason why complex cases become increasingly confused and hidden. This is most likely to happen with allopathic or antipathic suppression. It is possible with palliation when there are significant or prolonged environmental changes and it happens occasionally with partial homeopathic treatment of symptoms. Many homeopathic students are overly cautious of suppression due to partial treatment of symptoms but in my experience this is minimal compared with the suppression that takes place from the use of antipathic and allopathic medication. Cautious modification to the environment and treatment of local symptoms can actually support an individual over a difficult period of problematic symptoms and allow them in time to present a clearer case, amenable for treatment at a deeper level. A certain amount of palliation and local homeopathic treatment does in practice often help reveal a deeper case that isn't visible initially. Where I would advise caution in the partial treatment of symptoms even homeopathically, is if new deeper symptoms are developing, if repeat dosages or high potencies are needed or if improvement is not following the laws of cure (see page 73). In these cases it is possible to confuse or mask a case. Exposure to culturally accepted suppressants like coffee, nicotine and other recreational drugs can also play their part in suppressing and confusing the remedy picture. Although palliation can provide a necessary temporary environment for healing to take place, it does, if prolonged, set up an environment where the individual's vitality and self-healing can be stifled. If the underlying health issues are not addressed, then as the disease progresses, many patients increasingly palliate their symptoms by successively withdrawing from their physical and psychological environment. So, for example, a patient with food sensitivity who doesn't deal with the underlying susceptibility but instead simply avoids or excludes a particular food group will find that over time they increasingly need to avoid other food groups and become 'more sensitive'. In a patient with chronic fatigue, if the underlying susceptibility is not dealt with, then they may increasingly have to palliate their environment using bed-rest, special diets and particular psychological attitudes and environments in order to cope.

Cultural Palliation and Suppression

As different environments suit the expression of different symptoms, then it follows in any culture that certain symptoms or illnesses are more common and others less. In every culture different behaviours and actions are designed to protect from certain symptoms – each of these can have a suppressive or palliative effect, e.g. the fluoridation of water, the use of preservatives in foods, culturally-accepted recreational drugs and the containing of emotions such as the bottling of grief or control of anger. It is often cultural palliation that prevents expression of minor but irritating symptoms until ('as if by magic') a deeper often confused or hidden case emerges.

Suppression and Vaccination

Vaccinations are given before symptoms are manifest in an individual and therefore are best understood not as suppression of an individual but rather as a form of cultural suppression and palliation. One reason why they are so controversial is that the aims of treatment or whom the 'contract' for treatment is with are not always made clear. There are, of course, different priorities when thinking of treating a population or an individual (see Chapter 30).

Many patients report adverse effects and some complex cases seem to track back to vaccination. If you wish to understand the principles at stake I invite you to return to the idea that health relies on having the right information to cope with a particular threat and that a cause can be considered a challenge that the individual is unable to accommodate without the need to generate symptoms (see Chapter 6). Vaccination might provide the information for some individuals to cope with a challenge they may be exposed to, while at the same time in some individuals (and there may be an overlap between both groups) the vaccination may cause symptoms. If the situations that any one individual can accommodate are determined by susceptibility, then a question arises as to whether an individual can ultimately have complete health and no susceptibility. If this was the case they could operate in any situation – this is patently not true. It therefore seems likely that every individual's susceptibility is finite. In this case gaining new resistance to a situation could, if the limit to an individual's susceptibility has been reached, lead to the loss of some other resistance as 'the price' of new resistance. Adding resistance to one thing may leave the individual susceptible to another that the patient was not previously susceptible to.

An individual or population may well make an informed choice to protect against particular illnesses but it is always important to consider the possibility that the choice the individual is weighing up is an increased resistance to a serious but rare illness against the increased susceptibility to a less serious but more common illness.

Palliation and Suppression Affecting the Totality and Constitution

The totality of the individual is gathered from the expression of all the symptoms in the organism. The totality will be influenced by palliation, suppression and local or partial symptom treatment. This in turn will change aspects of the individual's susceptibility and constitution. These changes themselves may be thought of as layers or stages in the case and need unravelling and taking into account during a course of treatment.

Every symptom needs to be understood in context of the possible effects of palliation and suppression. Hence the importance of understanding what treatment a patient has already received and possible adverse and side effects of such treatment. As the treatment progresses stage by stage, so the case changes to reflect the unveiling of these influences. The journey into illness follows a course and direction which can be discerned by careful study; the journey into well-being follows a reversal of this process. Hence the more suppression and palliation in the evolution of an illness, the longer treatment is likely to take.

REFLECTION POINT
- Think about a patient you have seen with a chronic disease – what can you imagine about the 'flow' of energy in this case, where is it blocked and stuck? Where might there be excess and where deficiency? Both are always present, although one may be more apparent than the other.

Types of Chronic Disease and Complex Cases

For many patients their first experience of homeopathy is when they have a chronic disease. Although in some of these cases, the symptom picture will be clear, in others there will be a certain amount of suppression. This often makes these complex cases more difficult to treat and the patient may need some explanation about how we approach chronic diseases. It is helpful to recognise different types of chronic disease and complex cases each requiring a slightly different strategy to their management.

Pseudo Chronic

When chronic illness is caused predominantly by environmental and life style factors it is referred to as pseudo chronic. This includes illness caused by mechanical causes such as repeated injury, or injury that fails to have an acute resolution, and more superficial illnesses due to poor diet, toxicity, extreme weather, pollution, stressful lives, stimulants, recreational drugs, etc. A cure may be obtained by removal of causation.

Confused and Hidden Cases

In more complex cases, where the whole picture cannot be seen and the constitution or totality are not clear, the case may appear confused and hidden. In confused cases the totality is not clear and the pattern or themes that run through the symptoms or the narrative of the case may be more clearly perceived and reveal more about the individual and the nature of the illness than the 'distorted' totality. Ultimately in hidden or masked cases just one symptom or sign may be all that is obvious (see one-sided cases, Section VI).

Incurable Cases

Incurable cases are those cases where the vitality is too low or the disease too advanced for a cure to be obtained. Often the illness will have been present for some time before curative treatment is sought. In others the suppression and palliation is such that the journey back to health is not possible by a reversal of the disease process, e.g. treating patients after surgical removal of glands or fusion of joints. In these cases relief of symptoms may be all that is possible.

Palliative Care and Local Treatment

Troublesome symptom complexes, even though they do not reflect the deepest aspects of the case, may be treated, e.g. nausea after chemotherapy, the anxiety of the terminally ill. The patient may be made as comfortable as possible by modifying their situation – including special diets, emotional support etc. In terminal care careful support and palliative management may allow a gradual drawing in of the life force or vitality. This compares favourably to the sudden and, at times, brutal spiralling downwards of the vitality when using increasing doses of suppressive drugs.

REFLECTION POINT

- Which is the healthier person – one who performs optimally in most environments seeking out challenge, or a person who seeks out the environment in which they do best? Some patients will seem to be 'drawn to' situations where they become ill. It is as if the susceptibility determines the situations the patient seeks out. Why do you think this might happen and what does it say about an individual's unconscious attempt to be healed?

Summary

In this chapter we have moved fundamentally from illness being something that happens due to events outside of us to something that through an understanding of totality and constitution is seen to connect us to our world, patients to their world and therefore patients and us. While there is initially a simple interplay between a patient's symptoms and susceptibility, it is unfortunately almost immediately confused in many patients by suppression and palliation. 'Homeopathic patients' who understand this and who minimise suppression and palliation are often surprisingly healthy, throwing off illness remarkably speedily and when they require a homeopathic remedy responding

deeply. Working with these homeopathic patients is dramatically different from working with those who, often from an early age, have been subject to 'much dosing' with the favourite allopathic or fashionable antipathic drugs of their day.

Given the prevalence of cultural and medicinal suppression and the nature of most patients' life styles, a holistic approach must have an understanding of suppression and palliation right at the centre of an understanding of patients' susceptibility and symptoms. It is the suppression and palliation of this generation and our ancestors that causes so many complex cases and chronic diseases to present as confused and hidden. It is only by recognising the relationship between symptom, susceptibility and suppression and reconciling these contradictory and somewhat discordant themes that we can begin to reverse this trend.

The homeopath requires not only an understanding of the patient's illness but also the context in which each subject presents, both in terms of other previous and concurrent interventions and the cultural and social influences each is subject to. To hold this dual focus requires a level of personal knowledge, insight and development that can make the homeopath's training arduous, all-encompassing and, at times, lonely. We explore in later chapters how sitting with the discomfort this can bring is as much part of the homeopath's training as learning materia medica and analysing cases.

We have developed the philosophy that allows us to work with and treat complex cases; looking at how causation, susceptibility, suppression and palliation tie in with the vital force and the symptomatology; explaining how suppression causes the case to deepen. We have revisited the importance of the holistic approach taking into account mind and body, including the emotional sphere of an individual. And we have talked about symptoms in relation to sensation and function and structure and the inter-relation of these. These concepts, when mastered and with some experience gained in putting them into practice, allow the homeopath to explore more confused and masked cases. They are important in choosing and working with totality and constitution and prepare the homeopath to work with thematic and relational approaches. Increasing our understanding of the hierarchy of suffering and disorder within the individual allows us to work deeply at the core of the problem.

Finally in this chapter we looked briefly at the types of chronic disease and types of complex case the homeopath will need to manage. We introduced the idea that symptoms themselves are both an expression of something about individuals, their situations, their response to the challenge of illness and also an expression of what may have been suppressed, and the important part that may play in the evolution of the illness. All this allows us to start to make meaningful comments and observations about the different types of therapeutic intervention available to the homeopath at different times.

References

Bellavite P, Signorini A 1995 Homeopathy: a frontier in medical science. North Atlantic Books, Berkeley

Lewis S A, Britton J R 1998 Measles infection, measles vaccination and the effect of birth order in the aetiology of hay fever. Clin Exp Allergy 28(12):1493–1500

Roy M 1999 The principles of homeopathic philosophy. Churchill Livingstone, Edinburgh

Swayne J 1998 Constitution. Br Homoeopathic J 87: 141–144

Swayne J 2000 International dictionary of homeopathy. Churchill Livingstone, Edinburgh

Bibliography

Allen J 1910 The chronic miasms: vol 1 Psora and pseudo-psora, vol 2 Sycosis. Chicago

Blackie M 1986 Classical homeopathy. Beaconsfield Press, Beaconsfield

Bodman F 1990 Insights into homeopathy. Beaconsfield Press, Beaconsfield

Chappell P 2005 The second simillimum. Homeolinks Publishers, Netherlands

Cusins P J 2001 Holistics. CandleFlame Books, Orkney

Dossey L 1982 Space time and medicine. Shambala, Boulder

Sankaran R 1991 The spirit of homeopathy. Homoeopathic Medical Publishers, Bombay

Twentyman R L 1989 Science and the art of healing. Floris Books, Edinburgh

Whitmont E 1980 Psyche and substance. North Atlantic Books, Berkeley

Totality and Constitution

CHAPTER TWELVE

Dynamic Materia Medica

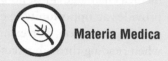 **Materia Medica**

David Owen

'Myth, legend, poetic imagery all represent a proving in one way.'

Ralph Twentyman

Introduction

In the previous chapter we saw that the totality of symptoms and the constitutional picture of each remedy provide two important aspects of each remedy picture. By considering both of these the homeopath is helped to understand both the case and the remedies themselves in a much more detailed and subtle way than on the presenting symptoms and keynote symptoms alone. A more complete understanding of remedy pictures involves seeing the remedies as dynamic pictures representing a spectrum of states, with aspects to it that evolve over time or in response to different situations. A remedy may have quite a different presentation early on in cases, when in different relationships or depending on life style.

Different homeopaths will perceive remedies and learn about them in different ways. Not only does developing a detailed picture allow matching at the level of the totality and constitution but also it brings broader understanding of the variety of different ways a patient might react to different circumstances. This richness of materia medica gives language to the different expressions of the case in different patients, and allows the homeopath to conceptualise and compare one case to another and develop a rational approach to the holistic treatment of each patient.

Studying in increasing detail a growing number of homeopathic remedies can appear a daunting task. The homeopath will find it helpful to develop a range of approaches to studying to help understand and remember the many aspects of these remedies. Remedy pictures are not random but have clear coherent patterns and wherever possible it can help to observe order in them expressed as trends and themes. Observing these patterns prepares the homeopath for connecting and extending the materia medica through the consideration of 'related remedies'.

Seeing how remedies have trends of symptoms in common or share constitutional features allows comparison between them, so that they are seen not in isolation but in a context and in relationship with and to each other. This is a prerequisite for deepening the use of related remedies within a treatment strategy.

Remedy pictures represent a range of different possible reactions, some of which are opposite and paradoxical, in response to different situations. Knowing something of these paradoxes reveals not only what symptoms and themes the remedy might show in different situations but also some of the most important and central points to be explored in the case. In this chapter we explore the idea of patterns of symptoms and constitutional features that run through the remedies. At a meta level the pattern (and therefore remedy) can be thought of as an expression of 'information' and we can consider these patterns in terms of them running along different axes, between different poles.

Learning the detail of each remedy's materia medica challenges most homeopathic students and provides an opportunity to explore the limitations of our perception. For example, it is often easier when reading through a remedy picture to see and recall certain aspects of its materia medica. This same, unconsciously selective, view and recall of patients is a major handicap to seeing the true totality or constitutional picture. It is through the personal development that goes with developing a more dynamic way of studying that our clinical work, as well as our knowledge of the materia medica, can become broader and deeper, more rounded and comprehensive.

REFLECTION POINT

- What remedies do you find it difficult to study or remember and why do you think this is? What aspects of your own psychology might make learning particular remedies easy or hard? If there are remedies you find it easy or hard to study in depth, how might this influence your prescribing?

Totality and Constitutional Materia Medica

'To treat a patient you have to find out what is wrong with them, to the homeopath the materia medica is part of the language needed to hear the case as much as it is part of any cure.'

The pattern or information running through a remedy will express itself in the slightest detail of the materia medica, whether elicited through proving, clinical observation or toxicology. The remedy also has a material and physical effect but by including the quality of the remedy as information it reflects the sense that the remedy enables and facilitates a healing process rather than itself being the healing process. Every remedy expresses itself in mental, emotional and physical features, and through changes of sensation, function and structure. It has intense features, peculiar features and reliable keynote

features that are reflected through weighting of symptoms in the materia medica and in the rubrics of the repertory. A remedy (and its information quality) also expresses itself through features of the source material itself – how it occurs in nature, the sorts of people that are drawn to or are sensitive to it, its social, cultural and mythological connections. These two sources of knowledge, like the totality and constitution, frequently complement each other and work holistically to inform a complete understanding of the remedy.

The better known the remedy the more this richness of materia medica applies. In some remedies the known totality is incomplete, perhaps because only a few provings have been done or there is a lack of up-to-date information. In others, especially little used remedies or those whose source material has little apparent significance to the treatment population, the constitution may be poorly defined.

Can the Complete Picture Ever Be Fully Expressed?

In the same way as every patient has aspects of themselves that are manifest at a certain time and aspects that are hidden or unconscious, it is helpful to think of remedies as having aspects that are revealed or hidden at different times and in different situations. When studying a complete remedy picture the homeopath seeks to know all aspects and to understand how the hidden side may become manifest over time. Thus different aspects of the remedy may be seen in different patients or over a period of time and features in the patient can seem to alter between being symptoms or constitution – as Gill's case illustrates in Case Study 12.1.

The more we understand the remedies as a story, and realise that the stories have parts which are shown and parts which are hidden, the more we are able to perceive the completeness of the materia medica. This is one reason why remedies can have opposite symptoms, e.g. the usually gentle Pulsatilla can show intense sibling jealousy. Indeed, remedies frequently have opposing symptoms within

CASE STUDY 12.1

Gill presented in her teens with hay fever. She was highly sensitive, energetic, focused and intuitive. She was tall and thin, bruised easily and had a reddish tinge to her hair; she responded well to Phosphorous.

In her late 20s she had several episodes of drug-induced psychosis and presented aged 28 as 'burnt out' and 'scatter brained', getting bruised from the slightest contact and having become anorexic. She worked as a clairvoyant but complained of nightmares. Gill was helped greatly by Phosphorous but complained that she had become less clairvoyant. Over time she ate better and put on weight, her hair colour changed and she became less of a typical 'phosphorous constitution'.

their picture at different times in the same patient or in different patients. These markedly contradictory characteristics of the same remedy are sometimes described as the remedy's 'polarity'. As you develop a rounded picture of a remedy state not only can the remedy appear to have its own 'life cycle' with different symptoms manifest at different times but also it can consist of axes of symptoms, where the axes might run between opposite symptoms.

Many of the remedies have a side that is best known but sometimes the presence of symptoms that would normally be hidden, which might include 'strange, rare and peculiar' symptoms, are a strong confirmation of a remedy.

The Constitution

'The Constitutional Remedy is a picture of the sum total of the strengths and weaknesses of the person mentally emotionally and physically.'

Margery Blackie

The constitution is the sum of the constituent parts – while it is not the presenting symptoms or 'clinical picture' it does connect to this. In practice 'the constitution' reflects a susceptibility to certain causes and symptoms, and both the constituent characteristics and particular susceptibilities are described together. So, for example, a Phosphorous constitution includes a susceptibility to bruise easily as well as a 'phosphorescent' personality that is sensitive to atmospheres. They may be features that are within the normal range or become symptoms. Subjects who most often prove a remedy, and patients who respond to the same remedy, often share similar features – the most distinctive of these features, if not symptoms, make up the constitutional picture. Identifying common characteristics of patients in this leads onto the 'typing' of patients into different 'constitutional' categories. It introduces the idea that different patients and remedies share certain features and belong to constitutional groups that may share common themes (see Chapters 21, 22).

Constitution Types

The four humours described by Galen are a historic example of this. He described the nervous, bilious, sanguine and phlegmatic types – and each has some shared susceptibility. Unfortunately the potential richness for medicine in developing these has been neglected in many developed cultures in favour of the understanding of disease in terms of external causation – particularly infection.

Morphological Constitutions

Some constitutions are described predominately on body shape and are sometimes referred to as the 'bio-typology' or 'morphological' constitution. These types in turn connect to the susceptibility of patients or proneness to certain illness. The morphological constitution is most often described as the physical appearance (Box 12.1) but is also reflected in many structural components of the organism. An important lesson for the homeopath is that it is valid to gather information on a physical constitution from the appearance of muscles, nails and hair or even at the organ, tissue and cellular level. Using morphological types is helpful to complement the totality – and is especially useful in children and veterinary practice (see Chapter 18). One of the implications of seeing morphology linked to the constitutional type is that it makes the constitutional type appear fixed. In my experience, constitutions do change but not in an unpredicted or disconnected way; rather they evolve and unfold.

Historically, Eduard von Grauvogl described the three constitutions of endomorphic, mesomorphic and ectomorphic appearance (referred to as oxygenoid, hydronoid and carbo-nitrogenoid type functions), linked to 'morbid constitutional type' (Clarke 1999), and later developed in relation to the fluoric, carbonic and phosphoric groups of remedies (Vannier 1998).

There is a correlation between different elements and their relationship to the different typology, e.g. the different effects of carbon, fluoride and phosphorus on tissues correlate with the different types and, in turn, to remedies containing these elements (Vijnovsky 2000).

REFLECTION POINT

- Which of these best describe you? Can you think of friends that fit the others?
- What illnesses do you suspect each type might be particularly susceptible to?

Matching an Individual's Constitution to a Remedy's Constitutional Picture

An individual's constitution includes morphological appearance, colouring, complexion, and personality, as well as susceptibility to certain symptoms. Any classification of remedies on constitution aims to blend features and characteristics and to build a picture that can be of practical use. If the picture is complete, the homeopath may feel confident using it when the totality is unclear; if it is unclear, you may require confirmation from causation or aspects of the totality, including 'strange, rare and peculiar' (SRP) symptoms and keynotes. Learning a constitutional picture to the many homeopathic remedies is something that often comes with experience as few texts clearly describe these pictures.

BOX 12.1
Main Morphological Features of Physical Constitution (According to Vannier)

Fluoric

Slack skin and ligaments with a gangly demeanour. They have joints at wide angles, prominent dilated veins, poor dentition, irregular dental lines and an asymmetric face. Their movements are jerky and they may have a lumpy muscular or skeletal structure. The hands and feet may look overdeveloped to their limbs and bodies and they may appear slightly asymmetric.

Phosphoric

Often tall and thin, sometimes to the point of waif-like type. They seem at times ethereal and poorly grounded, moving in a 'floaty' or drifting type of way. They typically bruise easily and are hypersensitive to their environment. Their limbs may look over-developed to their body.

Carbonic

Short, rounded and sometimes move as if having to overcome a great deal of inertia. They may have narrow angle joints and be short and round. The skin can be engorged with sclerotic veins and arteries. Their limbs may look underdeveloped in relation to their body and head.

A typical constitutional picture of the remedy Pulsatilla is described in the case of Jeni, in practice it is combined and complemented with some symptoms – together revealing more than either alone. Although brief, it reflects susceptibility of structure, function and sensation. The totality and constitution often 'fit together' like hand and glove.

The Psychology of the Materia Medica

Working holistically we need to know and match the psychological picture of the remedies as well as their physical and general characteristics. The

CASE STUDY 12.2

Jeni, age 6 years, has blonde hair and blue eyes. She is jealous of her younger sister. Her parents describe her as gentle, yielding, and wanting many hugs; she cries easily. Jeni feels better in open air and sleeps with the window open. She 'must have' natural daylight and is prone to feeling flat on 'grey days'. Her favourite colour is purple, she is self-conscious about what she wears and timid when she goes out.

Her digestion problems are aggravated by heat and fatty food and she is thirst-less when ill. Her indigestion symptoms move around the body. She gets catarrh easily and after antibiotics for an ear infection had thrush with a thick bland discharge.

psychological profiles of different remedies reveal subtle but important distinctions between otherwise closely related remedies. The ability to discriminate between them in this way is likely to develop in parallel with our psychological understanding of patients and ourselves. While this is also true for our ability to discriminate between other aspects of different remedies and patients, it is in the psychological sphere that the most sensitive and discerning comparisons are to be made – often with the greatest value in differential diagnosis.

Polychrests

'There are a few medicines the majority of whose symptoms are of the commonest and most frequent occurrence of human diseases, hence very often found in efficacious homeopathic employment, they are called polychrests'
    S Hahnemann, Materia medica pura, 2nd edn

Remedies where there are symptoms in many areas of the body and that have recognisable constitutional features are, not surprisingly, those that are used in a wide spectrum of acute and chronic disease. They are frequently prescribed and are collectively called polychrests. Different

homeopaths sometimes identify slightly different remedies as polychrests – the value of this label is chiefly to teach the student those remedies that are used frequently and about which more should be known in the early stages of practice. They are well proven and well used, and because the features of those who respond most strongly can be confidently observed they often have the clearest constitutional pictures and will be the first remedies you are likely to get experience of. However, the practical usefulness of polychrests does not absolve the developing homeopath from the need to build a wide repertoire of remedies that can be used holistically on totality and constitution. Frequently a case can appear difficult just because it does not fit a major polychrest!

For polychrests in particular the remedy name has become synonymous with a 'constitutional typology' and a clear set of symptom keynotes. So we speak about the Phosphorous type, Pulsatilla type, Sulphur type etc. Homeopaths often learn remedies by gradually building up the picture in layers that frequently correspond to the different models of health and approaches to treatment. So, for example, the causation and common presenting symptoms might be learnt first, followed by keynotes, SRPs, totality and constitution. Only after this are the patterns, themes and relational aspects of the remedy drawn out.

While this suits those who wish to build their materia medica knowledge one piece at a time, for others, immersing themselves in learning a remedy in all its aspects includes thinking of a patient needing a remedy and how they might view themselves and others (including the homeopath) and how people (including the homeopath) might relate and feel towards them (see Chapters 21, 22, 27). Developing an understanding of how different remedies relate to others in a group or family has been a major step forward in broadening the range of remedies available to the homeopath. When a remedy is learnt well it is possible to understand other remedies in part by how they relate and compare to them (see 'Related Remedies', Chapter 27, p. 374).

Totality and
Constitution

III

Caricature

In some remedies there are just a few well known constitutional features and symptom keynotes, in others there may be several particularly strong features, where the unusual or strongest features are emphasised. The main features might be considered as drawing something of a cartoon or caricature of the remedy, At times there can be huge amounts of information about the patient and remedy that can be overwhelming and obscure the simillimum, at other times there may be minimal information. In both situations it can help to match the patient to a caricature of a remedy. Sometimes it is easier initially to learn a caricature or outline of a remedy, and look up or gradually add other information from the materia medica.

Remedies and Their Source

The caricature often links in some way to the origin, source, mythology or practical use of a remedy. The link between the non-material qualities of remedies on the material world invites reflection on possible mechanisms of action of subtle remedies, perhaps similar to the relationship seen between Jungian archetypes and symbols (see Chapters 21, 27).

As homeopaths working holistically we recognise a world full of connections where each part is informed and understood by exploring its connections within the whole. Homeopathic remedy pictures can provide a way that allows apparently diverse aspects of a case to cluster, essentially allowing order and meaning to radiate through a case. It is perhaps understandable that a remedy picture may include connections with the source of the remedy. Box 12.2 lists some more obvious examples.

Related Remedies

Sometimes the concept of a particular constitutional attribute, e.g. 'a sensitive constitution', is used to describe a collection of remedy types that share that attribute. Or it may be used to describe remedies that share some common characteristic of the source material, e.g. 'a plant constitution' or a 'phosphoric' type. The practical importance

---

BOX 12.2

Examples of Connections and Symbolism Between Remedy Source and Patient

- A patient needing a bird remedy (e.g. a remedy made from dove feathers) may dream of birds or flying, or feel 'disconnected to the earth' or even have a fear of birds
- A patient who may respond to a particular plant remedy may like that plant, or like the flowers from the plants within the same botanical family
- A Pulsatilla patient might be attracted to light purple, the colour of the Pulsatilla flower, or a Sepia patient may dress in deep purple, similar to the colour of sepia ink.

---

of this is that when a constitutional remedy is not clearly indicated or fails to act fully, this kind of shared attribute may point to a related remedy (see Chapters 22, 27).

There is no doubt that getting to know one remedy well, and then exploring its relationship to other remedies, is a useful way of building a materia medica picture. One of the first times this was done was by Douglas Borland (1938) who established groups of remedies in children linked together into five groups, using a pragmatic and eclectic method mixing psychological themes (depression and 'nervy'), sphere of action (skin affinity) and related remedies (Calcaria-like).

REFLECTION POINT

- The snake is symbolically used to express many different characteristics, including in relation to healing. Having read the materia medica of one or two remedies made from snake venom, reflect on the positive and negative qualities you see in yourself that relate to 'the snake'. How do the positive and negative qualities mirror each other? How can qualities in remedies be recognised in people that they are not the simillimum of?

Deepening the Materia Medica

'We remember 20% of what we read, 30% of what we hear, 40% of what we see, 50% of what we say and 60% of what we do, and 90% of what we see, hear, say and do.'

C Rose (1985)

Knowing and understanding the homeopathic remedies provides different challenges depending on the model of health through which a patient is perceived. Different homeopaths make different remedies a priority and prefer different ways of learning about them. The homeopath learning materia medica by memorising keynotes is likely to work using keynotes; the homeopath learning remedies by understanding themes and essences is more likely to include themes and essences in prescribing strategies. Some of the theory and practice about developing a learning style provides development opportunities, allowing you to understand how you can see cases from different angles, and facilitate the learning of materia medica.

Figure 12.1 illustrates one model of learning styles based on work by Peter Honey and Alan Mumford (1992) but informed by the work of David Kolb and using the ideas of four polar states in the nature of man (see Chapter 14). These in turn are informed by four key psychological functions described by C G Jung. The dif-

ferent quadrants describe each learning style – see Box 12.3 – although we each have qualities from several quadrants, most have a preference. There is, of course, no right (or best) one but each helps understand the remedies or aspects of remedies in slightly different ways.

BOX 12.3

Activists

Activists like to be involved, are open-minded and enthusiastic about new ideas, but get bored easily. They tend to act first and reflect afterwards, enjoy groups and like to be noticed. They learn best when involved and like problem-solving. They learn less well when listening passively or when reading, writing or thinking on their own.

Reflectors

Reflectors like to stand back and think carefully before reaching conclusions. They observe and listen to others, learning best when they can review what has happened and think about what they have learned in a relaxed way. They learn less well when having to lead or role-play with no time to prepare.

Theorists

Theorists adapt observations into logical theories and approach problems step-by-step. They can be detached and perfectionist. They learn well when in complex situations, using their skills and knowledge in structured ways with a clear purpose. They do not like having to participate in emotional and feeling situations, especially if they are not sure of the basic principles.

Pragmatists

Pragmatists like to try things out. They are practical and 'down to earth'. They learn best when they see the application or see it in practice. They like to try it out and appreciate feedback. They don't like it if there is no obvious or immediate benefit or if there are no practical guidelines.

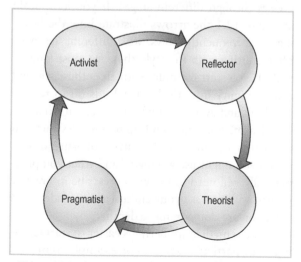

Figure 12.1 Learning styles (after Honey & Mumford 1992)

The challenge for each student is how to make best use of their strengths while avoiding having 'blind spots' to remedies or aspects of remedies. Although learning can be separated out into stages, in practice all these activities are happening simultaneously and different subjects might be learnt in different ways. Given the volume of new materia medica learning that most homeopaths undertake, and the different qualities and information about each remedy it is helpful to reflect on and see if you can develop your style of learning.

Homeopaths will not only be more likely to use accurately the remedies they know but also will use the approaches to treatment that reflect the qualities of their learning style. For example, those who prefer a more practical learning style may prefer learning causes and presenting symptoms that are observed or taught in a practical setting. They may then favour working with the pathological and biological models of health. What works best for each individual will be influenced by what they are learning, their preferred approach to studying materia medica and the likely setting they will work in. It is only by consciously developing outside your natural strengths that you will grasp the full breadth of the diverse materia medica and the full range of different models of health in which homeopathic principles may be applied.

Sometimes the student homeopath may feel there is a daunting amount of information to learn. There are, however, many different situations and activities in which you can learn, some of which are given in Box 12.4. Individuals with different learning styles will favour some and struggle with other learning activities.

Learning

Different learning activities can be understood as favouring different types of 'intelligence' or different aspects of the personality. They include linguistic, logical, visual, musical, physical, social or emotional intelligences – each of which might give a different perspective to a remedy picture.

BOX 12.4
Examples of Learning Activities
- Reading materia medica
- Putting what you have read into a mind map, a poem or a cartoon
- Writing index cards for each remedy
- Studying the repertory
- Reading case studies
- Lectures
- Observing others in practice
- Brain-storming
- Questions and answers
- Role-play
- Being tested
- Supervised practice
- Discussing what you have read with someone else
- Listening to a tape of someone's experience
- Attending a lecture, small group work, working in pairs, working alone
- Taking notes, making mind maps, using mnemonics
- Taking cases and supervised clinical experience

The Learning Cycle

Learning in depth often follows a cycle and progresses through different stages. If you look again at Figure 12.1 the arrows illustrate how the learning cycle frequently flows, with different 'learners' often starting with the style they are most familiar with. If you start naturally with an enthusiastic and active enquiry into a subject it leads on to reflecting about and even imagining things about what you have learnt. This can then lead to a more structured evaluation or theoretical analysis of situations in which you might use a remedy, and what you pragmatically will need to know to prescribe it. Practice in turn will increase your enthusiasm to understand what you are doing in more depth.

Some remedies are perhaps easier to start learning with particular styles. For example, remedies where structure and order are required, such as many mineral remedies, may benefit from a very structured approach (see 'Use of the periodic table', Chapter 22). Some homeopaths attribute the qualities of structure, relationship and sensation to remedies of mineral, animal and plant origin respectively. A more sensitive, artistic teacher may best colour in the different shades that exist between closely related plant remedies, and a relationship-focused author might breathe life into animal remedies.

One way of reframing the learning of the materia medica is to change it from being a necessary task to being an opportunity for growth. There are a huge number of different remedy pictures available for the homeopath to study, each offering insight into oneself and one's world, and each bringing with it an opportunity not only to develop a remedy picture but also to develop insight into how different patients see and experience their world.

Some students will have gushing and enthusiastic styles and need encouragement to explore the more reflective, logical and practical areas of the remedies, patients and their own case. The imaginative style may suffer from seeing too many possible ways of proceeding and be reluctant to pay attention to the practical aspects of case management. The very practical student may be over influenced by their last similar case or the latest study. The logical student may reflect on things so much that they analyse things to paralysis, wanting certainty before moving forward. Understanding your style and how it shapes your approach to both the materia medica and cases is an important part of training.

Making the Materia Medica Your Own

As you get to know the remedies better they move from a simple description of a static state and become a narrative with a beginning, a middle and end. They represent a process that unfolds over time, depending on the environment and stimuli that the remedy, as expressed in the patient, is exposed to. The remedies start to take on a life of their own and become characters. If your learning style is too restricted you are likely to have blind spots for some aspects of remedies, and some remedies you will find hard to 'see' at all.

A purely theoretical knowledge of the materia medica is always going to be limited. As the remedies are used and understood they become like members of a family with an emotional and situational picture. The interaction of the patient with their surroundings is central to understanding the importance of themes that run through both patients and remedies (see 'Thematic approaches to materia medica', Chapter 27). The way certain remedy patterns, and their manifestation in certain patients, impact upon the psyche of the homeopath is a major influence on how a homeopath experiences their patients and perceives the remedies. It is at the heart of the relational model of health (see 'The relational approach', Chapter 26 and 'Relational approaches to living materia medica', Chapter 27).

REFLECTION POINT

- Looking at Figure 12.1 and Box 12.3, and Box 12.4 reflect on your preferred learning style and activities. What strengths and weaknesses do these present to your learning of materia medica and how might it also influence your case-taking? Think about how in a group of students each might prefer a subject to be taught in a different way. What is your preference and how do you respond if the teacher tends to teach in a different style? Would one or several styles be best in developing an all-round and, one might say, 'holistic' view of a remedy being studied?

Summary

This chapter develops the understanding of homeopathic remedies in terms of totality and constitution. It allows for an approach to the treatment of an individual based on susceptibility and symptoms and sets us up to explore suppressed cases in subsequent chapters.

The information expressed about major remedies not only enables a prescription on the simillimum but also helps the homeopath in conceptualising, pursuing and ordering a 'whole person' narrative. Studying remedies as living and dynamic expressions of human experience not only broadens the tools at the homeopath's disposal but also fundamentally extends and deepens your perception and comprehension of patients.

Finally, we discussed how your understanding of remedies and approach to learning them is affected by your own personal style. To broaden your understanding of remedies you will need to reflect on your personal learning style and develop those qualities you may currently find hardest. If you do not do this then you are likely to find 'blind spots' that will continue to make some cases more difficult than they need to be.

Broadening the understanding of materia medica to different remedies in different situations leads naturally on to receiving a different case from the one that is required for local prescribing. It also leads into discussions of more complex case analyses and management. These are developed in subsequent chapters in this section. The self-reflection and deepening of the understanding of materia medica to look at what might be called 'living' or 'emotional' materia medica lays the foundations for working in the holographic and relational models of health.

References

Borland D M 1938 Children's types no. 1. Homoeopathy May 7(5):143–150

Borland D M 1938 Children's types no. 2. Homoeopathy Jun 7(6):173–181

Clarke J H 1927 Constitutional medicine. Homoeopathic Publishing Company, London. Indian edition 1999. Jain Publishing Co, New Delhi

Honey P, Mumford A 1992 The manual of learning styles. Honey Publications, Maidenhead

Rose C 1985 Accelerated learning. Accelerated Learning Systems, Aylesbury

Vannier L trans Clement M 1998 Homeopathy human medicine. Homeopathic Publishing Company, London

Vijnovsky R 2000 Tratado de Homeopatia. Editorial Paidotribo, Barcelona

Bibliography

Campbell A 1981 Concepts of constitution in homeopathy. Br Homeopath J 70(4):183–188

Foubister D 1969 Constitutional types. Br Homeopath J 58(2):77–81

Gutman W 1978 Homeopathy: the fundamentals of its philosophy, the essence of its remedies. Homoeopathic Medical Publishers, Bombay

Kolb D 1983 Experience as the source of learning and development, experimental learning. Prentice Hall, New Jersey

Leary B 1983 Constitutions again. Br Homeopath J 72(4):214–216

Rose C, Goll L 1992 Accelerate your learning. Accelerated Learning Systems, Aylesbury

Twentyman R 1989 Science and the art of healing. Floris Books, Edinburgh

Totality and Constitution

CHAPTER THIRTEEN

Receiving the Case

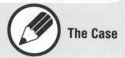

The Case

David Owen

Introduction

When in consultation with a patient the universe shrinks and your senses extend to encompass the patient in a dynamic interaction, allowing you to perceive the patient at a deeper level. Your world becomes your consulting room and when you truly see the case in its entirety the past stands still and the room disappears as you dance the homeopathic dance.

In this chapter we look at how we perceive the totality and the constitution to build a comprehensive picture of the whole person. The holistic model recognises that what is happening inside the patient is reflected in what is happening outside and vice versa. This chapter explores how patients, including their unconscious, can be observed through their connection to their environment and in their relationships with others, including to the homeopath (see Chapter 23). The case may develop, like treatment, over a number of consultations and can be thought of as a gradual but continuous process rather than a series of distinct and separate stages. How the case unfolds is intimately connected to the explicit and implicit agreement between the homeopath and patient (see Chapter 25). This agreement clarifies what information is important for the patient and helps make the consultation a safe place for the patient's story to be told.

The title of this chapter, 'Receiving the case', is intentionally distinguished from the title of Chapter 8, 'Taking the case'. It may at first appear too 'passive' a description, as there is certain information that is needed and much that builds naturally on aspects of 'case-taking' covered previously. Combining these styles presents challenges to the homeopath. How do you draw on both the more structured and directive style previously covered and the more facilitative and contemplative style suited to allowing the totality and constitution to emerge? In practice aspects of the case lend themselves to each and you guide the patient both by the explicit agenda you (and they) hold and also by the excitement and passivity that you (and they) use to direct the consultation.

The first part of this chapter reflects the passive style of receiving the case while the second part tackles some of the difficulties and compromises the homeopath will face in developing a personal style. Some of the techniques that allow the homeopath to see aspects of a case that might otherwise be unseen are discussed in the knowledge that, as other models of health are explored and the homeopath's understanding of the materia medica deepens and broadens, each is likely to develop a more individual approach to consulting that will shift between different styles and models as circumstances require.

The Art of Receiving the Case

Taking the case is about taking what the patient consciously offers or the homeopath deliberately elicits of the case history. Receiving the case is about being receptive to all aspects of the case, including many that the patient may disregard or be unconscious of.

Receiving the case is a natural step on from taking the case. Both can happen synchronously but to receive the case it is necessary to be attuned to what you might receive – for this reason experience is important. To gain this experience a homeopath can allow distinct phases in the consultation to 'hear what is there but might not be being said'. Sometimes this is at times of silence, at others by returning to important but incomplete areas of the case-taking and observing different details of the consultation, such as the exact words being used, how the patient sits and moves and how you respond to what is being said.

It is often the deepest symptoms that are hardest to see; they may be the ones the patient has become most used to, are most structural or have been suppressed or palliated. Some symptoms will only reveal themselves in later consultations after rapport has been deepened and the context of the case and patient's life situation understood. For the homeopath to be able to make as much of the case conscious as possible, perception of the constitution and totality requires all of our senses and depends upon you seeing the potential relevance of everything that takes place during the consultation.

If the patient is not in a balanced state then 'holistically' every aspect of the patient will express this in one way or another; when the remedy state is suppressed key features may be more difficult to observe but they will express themselves at some level – although this may be unconscious to the patient or indeed unconscious to the physician. Remember – everything that happens is relevant!

As a general rule allowing the patient to narrate their story with as little interruption as possible allows what is important to surface. However, there are ways of supporting the patient, particularly inviting them to explore areas that might be painful.

The pace of the consultation can 'speed up' and seem to skip over difficulties. At other times it can slow down and seem to stop at an aspect of the case that is 'stuck'. Noticing the change in pace may be enough to focus your attention on an important point. You can influence the case in many ways and we will look at some of these later in the chapter. For example, with an anxious patient who is rushing their history, you may well invite them to slow down by asking them to slow their breathing or doing a simple relaxation exercise with them before continuing with the case. Indeed, just by slowing your own breathing you may slow the patient down, or synchronising your breathing with theirs you can increase rapport.

Presence

'The patient complains of the process of his ailments. The patient's relations tell us what he has complained of, his behaviour and what they have perceived about him. The physician sees, hears and notices through the remaining senses what is altered or unusual about the patient.'

S Hahnemann, Para 84,
Organon of the Medical Art, 6th edn

By being in the 'here and now' the homeopath opens up their senses to 'hearing' the case and experiencing the case, not just with the ears but with all the senses. This attitude in itself models for the patient and invites the patient to adopt a more present and open attitude. In practice there are aspects of the history and times in the consultation when it is easier for patients to show more of themselves and for the homeopath to be more fully present. Being present is not about overwhelming the patient but being attuned to and noticing what the patient is presenting, making 'present' the patient physically, intellectually and emotionally (Box 13.1).

Observation

When symptoms are not easily expressed, e.g. in children, animals and those who have difficulty expressing themselves, then it is even more important to use every faculty of observation. Physically a symptom may be expressed through the individual's posture and movement, and this may affect your own. For example, when a Kali bichromicum

BOX 13.1

Reflection Exercises

Reflect on the different roles the homeopath might be asked to play – this may include doctor, healer, facilitator, friend and witness, or even confessor. What other roles might there be? List them and think about what appeals to you or perhaps challenges or disturbs you about each role. Which are your strengths and what are the potential pitfalls that you might face in each role?

Focus on the first few minutes of a recent consultation or social encounter. List everything you can remember about it. Now close your eyes and imagine describing the encounter to someone who has never met the person before – how exactly they were dressed, their complexion, their breathing, the colours of their clothes, their hair, shoes, make-up or jewellery. Can you use other senses – was there a smell, what was touching them like, what exactly did you hear? How did they meet you, where and how did they stand or sit, how did they move and how did they speak? Try sitting or standing like them. Who do they remind you of, and what do you have in common and what is different from that person?

Now look again at the list from the first part, how accurately does it describe them compared with the second part?

patient presents with their rigid posture I naturally find that I am sitting up a bit straighter (indeed this is quite frequent with many of the Kali salts). Their mental state may be expressed through their relationships to others; e.g. the relationship between child and parents, or pet and owner. General symptoms can be observed by seeing how the individual interacts with the physical environment. For example, their clothing, where they sit, etc. might indicate symptoms related to temperature. The precise words a patient uses are important not just for what they communicate directly but also what else is communicated. The repeated use of a word,

especially ones that are otherwise 'out of place', words that are used on a continuum from one pole to another on a particular axis, (such as words on a spectrum between success and failure may indicate issues about self-esteem) and the use of words that can have more than one meaning all indicate that something important is surfacing.

With this in mind we will return to consider aspects of the case that were not covered in Chapter 8. Although the styles of taking and receiving the case may appear opposite or exclusive, in practice both are needed and run in parallel. There is the need to gain focused and specific information, through a sort of magnifying lens, and to receive the broadest and subtlest of information, through a sort of wide-angle lens. It is as if the homeopath needs the eyes both of the hawk (depth) and of the hare (breadth). I describe the two as discrete but they are just separate styles and skills that, as you become more experienced, you move between and hold together to perceive most clearly each case. It is frequently in the realm of the patient's life situation, the mental and social aspects away from the minutiae of the presenting symptom that the broader issues reveal how the many aspects of the case tie in.

General Symptoms

General symptoms relate to the patient's reaction to their situation, particularly those physical environments in which the patient generally feels better or worse (temperature, rain etc.), food preferences (indicated by a +) and aversions (indicated by a −), and appearance or body shape. Also sometimes included as 'generals' are other features that indicate how the patient might interact with their situation or environment, including how they choose to modify or influence this. Some of these factors may be psychological or behavioural, e.g. how they dress, their mannerisms, gestures and behaviour during the consultation, areas of the body touched as they speak, where they look, the tone of voice and sounds they make, their handshake and where they live.

General symptoms also include aspects of body function such as perspiration (where, when and odour), menstruation and sleep. Finally under 'generals' the subjective sense of energy that the patient has may be noted. The patient might be asked to score their general energy out of ten. This frequently seems to equate to how the homeopath would 'score' the patient's vitality. It is both an indication of cases that may need support for their vitality before a clear case can be expressed and a change in it may indicate the first signs of a remedy acting.

General features are often a good indicator of the habitual constitutional state of the patient as well as contributing to the totality of symptoms when they are ill. Significant change in them, for example a cold person becoming hot, can be a strong indication that the remedy state is changing, either in the course of the illness or in response to treatment. Matching strong general symptoms in the case and in the remedy picture provides reliable confirmatory symptoms. Like modalities it can help to invite a patient to indicate where on the axis between two extremes their symptoms lie, e.g. where do they lie in body temperature between very hot or very cold?

Mental Symptoms

Every patient has an effect on you – you might as well use the feeling you get as a clue.

These include a patient's psychological symptoms and also pre-morbid features reflecting their psychological 'constitution' or predisposition, such as how they view themselves, and their fears, hopes, delusions and dreams. How a patient walks in, how at ease they are, their expression and how they respond to you will give you much information not only about their mind symptoms but about how to take and receive the case. In babies much information may have to come from the parents and understanding the different expressions the baby has (perhaps asking the parent to mimic it or describe when it happens). As mental symptoms emerge they inform the whole case-taking and receiving, they always run in parallel to the rest of the case – although you might choose a time to focus on the psychological picture and to 'check' you are noticing the mental state of the patient. It

is useful to have some questions that you can ask to broaden this out if the patient needs encouragement to talk about themselves. Some that I find helpful are 'how do friends (or family) describe you?', 'what are your goals and aims in life?', 'how does your illness affect you?', 'what are the best (or worst) things that have happened to you?' and 'how would you like to be different and what might you do if you were well?'.

Like other symptoms, the strength and uniqueness of mind symptoms are important in deciding how central to the case they are. Remember that some symptoms can appear disguised when they are understated or whispered – modesty or a sense of what is permissible may shape what the patient says. Paradoxically the partially expressed symptoms or 'what is not said' can reflect more important aspects of the case. It can be particularly helpful to note phrases that are mentioned out of place or those attributed to other people, such as 'John always says…'. As you might expect from what you have read so far patients may well spontaneously deny things that are in fact central to their case – 'I'm not at all afraid' or 'I've no reason to dislike…' may mean the exact opposite. To explore this you can sometimes invite the patient to imagine what it would be like 'if you were afraid' or 'if you did have a reason to dislike'.

In cases with much suppression of physical symptoms, the mental symptoms may be less disguised and give a clearer pointer to a patient's case, hence their importance. In psychological illness, however, when psychotropic drugs, anti-anxiety drugs, antidepressants, recreational drugs, etc. suppress or distort mental symptoms, the physicals and generals are more reliable.

Emotions

Frequently, strong feelings in the patient, e.g. sadness, anger or anxiety, are important parts of the case. Subtle modalities to these feelings may be noticed or teased out when patients talk about the different circumstances in which they arise. Patients can be invited and encouraged to re-experience and 'sit with' these feelings in the consultation. Often a strong feeling can be triggered when talking about the past (key life events), social situations (relationships to others) or family history (childhood, parents, etc), and if this happens before a patient really feels ready to talk about them, or you feel ready to receive them a decision has to be made whether to explore them at this stage in the history or to return to them later. With experience it is possible to move backwards and forwards between taking the case and receiving the case, between creating the structure for the case and allowing the case to just flow. Sufficient trust and rapport will need to be established to allow patients to sit with these feelings in the consultation, which is perhaps why some homeopaths only feel the consultation is 'really starting' when some emotion – whether laughter, tears or anger – has surfaced.

Some patients prepare themselves before the consultation to only show what emotions they think it is permissible to show. In understanding the complex case it is particularly useful if the patient experiences the feeling in the consultation, rather than dispassionately describing a feeling that is experienced elsewhere. In this way the homeopath creates something of the different situations the patient has been in or is avoiding and invites the patient, in the consultation, to journey into this and explore how this feels. Importantly, the patient is both made to feel safe to do this and is witnessed in this. So you might ask a patient to imagine what a situation feels like, what they would like to say to someone or how they might react if something happened. It is surprising how often some initially unspoken thought or feeling reveals itself in this way and how often this gives clues to the deeper aspects of a case. In many initially confused cases clarity appears when this is revealed. Even when there are strong common feelings such as anger or sadness there are invariably deeper feelings that relate to situations the patient is seeking to avoid (fears and anxieties) or is in some way seeking out (delusions, fancies and sometimes dreams).

Fears and Delusions

Really hearing means understanding a patient's construct of their world, what their reality is in terms of their anxieties, fears, hopes, dreams and delusions; how they enact this in their behaviour, beliefs and symptoms.

Fears are often reflected in what the patient imagines might happen, as if by trying to avoid something they are almost drawn to it – the deeper the fear the stronger the denial. It is reflected in the consultation by what the patient fears might happen but feels unsafe to name. It is often these issues that surface when specifically exploring the therapeutic agreement (see Chapter 25).

Delusions, on the other hand, often represent what the patient secretly desires including how they see themselves and others and how they would like others to see them. In the consultation it is reflected in what the patient wants it to be like but is unable to name in the therapeutic agreement, i.e. what they want to happen but can not contract for (see Chapter 25).

A patient's fears and delusions mirror each other and although some patients more easily show one or another, in a well received case aspects of both will be seen. The more fundamental the state that is revealed the more directly these two aspects can be seen as balancing or compensating each other. For example a patient may have a fear of falling (from an elevated position) balanced by a delusion that they are unworthy (need to be kept down), or a fear of animals with a desire to (or delusions they should) let out their animal desires. Allowing these fears and delusions to be seen clearly is vital to working with the deeper aspects of patients. Not expressing them leads the patient to further re-enactment of their deepest pathology; not perceiving them yourself leaves you vulnerable to the patient's projections (see Chapters 23, 25).

Sleep and Dreams

Sleep plays a vital role in the maintenance of a balanced state; the body is able to 'catch up' and repair and the 'batteries are re-charged'. If sleep is disturbed then the pattern of disturbance gives a useful pointer to remedies; sleep position gives helpful totality and constitutional information. Often the general well-being and energy a patient feels is closely connected to sleep quality.

Frequently an improvement of the sleep pattern is an early sign of a significant healing reaction. Sometimes patients experience excessive but pleasant and natural sleepiness in response to a remedy that can be clearly distinguished from an unhealthy sleep.

Many patients may not remember or are initially reluctant to share their dreams. Some suppressive treatments, especially those, like sleeping tablets, that are used to promote sleep, often block dreams. Getting a patient to remember and talk about dreams can take some encouragement and it needs to be made safe for the patient to reveal these 'gems of the case'. After explaining that dreams are important a rich 'dream world' sometimes emerges. Some patients benefit from being asked to note their dreams before coming and it can help to even encourage or invite patients to dream and to record them. For some patients who are alien to the homeopathic process it feels strange to be asked this in a questionnaire or before they meet you and understand the process. A sign of a practised homeopathic patient is often how they volunteer information, including dreams. In these 'expert patients' it is often possible to receive a wealth of information, including dreams, fears, delusions, generals and mentals in addition to the local symptoms. Indeed, careful time management can be required, especially if time is constrained, in order to cover all aspects of the case.

Through dreams the patient may 'discharge' or compensate for unwanted thoughts (excreting unresolved emotions) and explore unfulfilled ones. Dreams may simply reflect transient disturbances of the day's events, or more deep-seated psychological states that are important to the case. They may reflect fears or delusions that the patient has. Dreams are particularly important to the homeopath when experienced the night before the consultation as they may reflect the patient's unconscious desire to reveal information they want to contract to work with but are uncertain about. Dreams after taking a remedy often indicate a shift of symptoms; dreams on an anniversary of an important event are one way of revisiting unresolved issues.

Some dreams are recurrent and more memorable, sometimes revealing not only information that may be repertorised and matched to a remedy but that expresses important and central aspects of the case that, when named, can permit access to the case at a more psychologically perceptive layer, as Sandra's case illustrates.

CASE STUDY 13.1

Sandra, age 33, years presented with asthma. She had recurrent dreams of being pursued. Inviting her to talk about what she thought was pursuing her enabled her to talk about a previous unmentioned abusive relation and was part of the indication for Medorrhinum that helped her allergic symptoms and also made her feel 'better than ever'.

Social History

Occupation, partner, car and home, like all things, are important parts either of totality or constitution.

The social history is often the area where patients will describe their significant relationships to others – including to their parents, partners, children, community and culture – and significant life events such as redundancy, separation and bereavement. These relationships are important in their own right and because they provide a vital awareness of the family, social, community and cultural influences. This in turn describes the context of a patient's life, including what is permissible, normal, encouraged or defended against. This is essential as we seek to understand aspects of the case that are otherwise hidden or masked.

It can be difficult to move directly from features in the social history to the materia medica, although the constitutional picture of many remedies includes how they interact with others and how they behave in social situations. It is often while exploring the social history that a patient begins to grasp the implications of the illness within the wider context of their life, and to

Totality and Constitution

understand the potential for change that being well might bring.

Family History

Often a detailed family history can be prepared by the patient before the consultation; it should include not only parents and grandparents but also any children and grandchildren as susceptibility is indicated by both. Siblings and their children also add information. In addition to knowing the major diseases that run through the family it is helpful to know whom the patient 'takes after' either in appearance or temperament. This is particularly important in children and babies; the younger they are the more important it is likely to be. There is often a stronger maternal influence in very young babies and the paternal influence often increases between ages 4 and 10 years. Asking about the family (or social situation) is often one of the introductions needed for patients to describe their major life events and psychological state. Often susceptibility is shaped by the family history; sometimes this provides much of the information we have to prescribe on, as Frank's case illustrates. While each family member is a separate case there are many occasions when improvement and deterioration of family members seem to follow one another.

CASE STUDY 13.2

Frank, age 38 years, was the oldest of four children. He went to boarding school age 8 and suffered from 'no illnesses whatsoever'. He had two children, one of whom was having treatment for malaise following glandular fever. Frank developed angina at age 36, for which he gave very little symptoms of note. Conventional medication helped at first but he was gradually becoming increasingly lethargic. There was a strong family history of cancer and diabetes. He was prescribed Carcinosin, which helped his lethargy, and at follow-up he gave a much fuller case and was able to talk with feeling about his childhood and relationship with his parents for 'the first time'. As Frank felt better, so his son's health improved!

Moving Deeper Towards Confused and Hidden Cases

The symptom picture may be confused when there is lack of clarity, order or hierarchy of symptoms. Many factors that can cause this, most notably suppression, have already been discussed.

Patients with chronic disease may also be taking conventional drug treatments that alter the way symptoms are expressed. When starting as a homeopath, if it is possible to treat cases that have not had 'much dosing' then these cases are often easier to interpret and prescribe for. As symptoms become less characteristic because of the suppressive effects of conventional treatment so the case is harder to see and therefore to treat. A chronic case with no suppression, e.g. eczema with certain time aggravations and contact aggravations, is much easier to cure than one that has been suppressed and the modalities lost.

Two other major reasons why symptoms may not transparently reflect the totality also need to be considered – hereditary and cultural factors. These and how they bias the clear expression of the case are explored further in Chapter 26 and Section VI.

REFLECTION POINT

- How can you know that what you see is all that can be seen? If the case is not static, and until the patient is cured new information is always surfacing, how often should the case be retaken?

Styles of Consultation

'. . . the heart of all healthcare is a therapeutic meeting between bodies'

Kellas 2006

In most complex cases the complete case requires elements of both taking and receiving the case. While taking the case lends itself to a fairly uniform style of consulting, the style of receiving the case is more likely to reflect the homeopath's individual approach. In addition to developing your own preferred style of consultation, you are likely to want to develop a range of styles to suit different approaches to treatment and different methodologies of prescribing. Your style will change with different patients as the consultations unfold. The style of consultation that will allow a Nux Vomica patient to reveal most will be very different from the style of consultation that will allow a Pulsatilla patient to be similarly revealing. Just as we have certain preferences of learning style, and prefer teachers with a compatible style, so different consulting styles may suit different patients. Both knowing your own 'default' style and being able to adopt other styles when needed will broaden the range of patients with complex cases from whom you can receive a 'three-dimensional' case. There is no one 'right' style; rather, different factors will determine the best approach in each case. If you are fixed to one style then some remedy types will be more difficult to observe.

The most useful ways of developing consultation skills and styles are experience and reflection. One of the best ways of learning is by watching yourself and others in practice; both by sitting in and by watching videos of others and yourself.

Starting

Most individuals make a rapid and often accurate assessment of each other within seconds of meeting.

By the time the patient is sitting opposite you, you may have noted how they booked their appointment, met them in the waiting room, seen a referral letter or received information from a questionnaire. You may already know them or the family; you might recognise their address or know something about where they live, their occupation, age, and gender.

The unspoken agenda of a consultation is often formed very quickly when the homeopath first meets the patient; it is influenced by your body language, your dress, your behaviour and your emotional state. The patient will gauge how seriously you are taking the consultation, whether you are trustworthy, how strongly you have your own agenda to follow and how you are likely to respond to what they want to say.

Through experience and training you should be intimately aware of what pushes your buttons, how you respond at different times of the day, on different days of the week, and to different people, including people of different social, age and ethnic groups.

Time

A totality approach to a complex case is likely to require a great deal of information. Many patients and homeopaths are anxious about having too little or too much time. Once the homeopath has decided on the practicality of appointment times then it is possible to contract clearly around the time available for the consultation. If the patient has particular needs for more time this can be discussed and perhaps accommodated either through a longer appointment or returning sooner.

If patients have particular needs to cover complicated or detailed aspects of the case then asking them to do some 'homework' on it can help. As deeper issues emerge it can be a powerful reflective exercise for patients to write down their feelings and document their experiences. It is also a way to sensitise patients to noticing or remembering information they might not otherwise recall. For example, they may be able to note dietary preferences between visits, or to note dreams first thing in the morning, or to record reactions to treatment when they happen.

Eye Contact

Some patients are self-conscious of eye contact. Some find it easier to express themselves more freely when there is a level of disassociation from the homeopath (like psychotherapy patients talking on the couch with the therapist behind or beside them). If patient or homeopath is uncomfortable with eye contact it may point to a need to clarify the contract, reviewing issues about intent, confidentiality, time, money, etc. It almost certainly reveals some unease that needs to be understood and resolved. Making good eye contact can be difficult while keeping appropriate records or referring to texts or computer. Care must be taken not to allow these activities to detract from the quality of the homeopath's 'presence' and attentiveness to the patient.

Pace

Many patients need to be invited to expand on the history but in a way that does not interrupt them. If you feel a symptom is incomplete then holding in your mind the question you want to ask will sometimes and, at first, rather surprisingly get it answered without you having to verbalise it. Silence is also one of the most powerful tools as it can invite more information, give permission for reflection and deepen a case. Restating what the patient has said, using the patient's own words or in paraphrase, allows information to be checked out and triggers the patient to recall more.

Flow

The consultation can be considered as a flow of energy or information between patient and homeopath. The patient's information or energy blocks will often be apparent in the consultation, and what is not expressed or spoken of is important in understanding complex cases. Often a hint of what is being avoided or not spoken about in the consultation can be picked up in the early stages of the consultation, and will influence how the consultation evolves. Recognising where the energy or flow is blocked is central to understanding the case. A homeopath who wishes to work at a deeper level than the presenting symptom has to be sensitive to where the energy is in a consultation – what they and the patient are drawn to, what they and the patient are avoiding. In the pattern of the case, what is not there that might be expected, or what is there but not expected, become the 'strange, rare and peculiar' symptoms of the confused or masked case.

When the flow of a case becomes 'stuck' often a different style of consulting or noticing something different will allow it to move on. A sign that the case is 'flowing' is often that the patient is able to express and flow though different feelings in the consultation, perhaps shown by a sigh, a tear or laughter.

Paradox

Paradoxes or seeming contradictions often reveal important areas of a case. They may be suggested by being 'over stated' or by the release of emotions when something is discussed. For example, a patient may say, 'I'm really not like...' often when they clearly are. Wherever appropriate, investigating a paradox will reveal a deeper symptom. This is why the noticing of Freudian slips or contradictory information is so important, and why many deep cases only start to be expressed when the patient is confident to reveal themselves even if only unconsciously. Being able as the homeopath to be 'emotionally present' is vital to establishing deep rapport and to modelling the expression of feeling. Sometimes the emotional paradox is important such as the patient talking about a pain or upset in a trivial way or while smiling, as Peter's case illustrates.

CASE STUDY 13.3
Peter, age 48, had attended several times to talk about his chest pain. He would talk about his symptoms in a light-hearted way and when describing his chest pain he smiled. Asked how he felt when he had the pain, he said it felt as if he deserved the pain. Peter gradually got in touch with the feeling and started talking with tears in his eyes about a deep-seated guilt that he had felt since childhood. When asked about his childhood he spoke about 'being sent away to school' and feeling 'inadequate.' This pointed to the remedy Aurum, for which there were several keynotes and to which he responded well.

Often at first sight the paradoxical expression is confusing, but this confusion is because something different and often deeper is touched on. For example, the Ignatia patient will often want to be loved unconditionally. To test out how much they are loved, they will say things that might cause the object of their love to push them away. A typical Natrum muriaticum patient in love wants to love from afar so will sometimes choose a completely unsuitable and unavailable person to worship.

Matching

If everything the patient does reflects part of the remedy state then even background noise or movement the patient makes reflects that remedy state – the more it is repeated the more important it is to the case. The patient might not regard it as a symptom, or even be aware of it. For example a Staphisagria patient may blink or grimace, a Sulphur patient may scratch, a Kali carbonicum patient may clear the throat, a Phosphorus patient may have a background cough and a Lycopodium patient may have a furrowed brow. If you are in doubt what a particular feature, movement or mannerism might mean then try copying or matching it yourself until you are clear of the feeling that you get from doing it. By repeating and matching it you may gain insight into what the feature, movement or mannerism is expressing for the patient. You may not need to actually make the movement and still find it helpful to reflect on why something happens at a certain point in a consultation. It may at first appear a novel suggestion to match a patient's movement, mannerism or choice of words but it often happens unconsciously when developing rapport (see 'Projection', Chapter 23).

Understanding what the patient is expressing through a repeated action, such as using a hand gesture or touching part of the body, can give a key pointer to a case as Jon's case illustrates. While

CASE STUDY 13.4

Jon was big and quite threatening in his manner. He was sitting with arms and legs crossed, with what might be called very closed body language. By 'matching' the same body language I gained some insight into his vulnerability but it seemed to allow him to start talking about his partner, who was threatening to leave him unless he resolved his drink problem.

matching can be thought of as how the homeopath passively receives information, then the same behaviour has an 'active' component that is part of a more dynamic communication. This more 'active' side to matching is distinguished by calling it 'enacting'.

Enacting

A particular behaviour that is frequently repeated can be thought of as representing an aspect of the case that stops something else from being expressed – a sort of 'stuckness'. In consultation this 'stuckness' can seem like an interruption to the sense of 'flow' in the consultation; in this way the exact posture, mannerisms, words and expressions the patient uses can present a block to the natural flow of the case.

Enacting the behaviour, mannerism, sound or movement can help shift these blocks to reveal other aspects of a patient's case. By mirroring or actively matching the patient's movements, mannerisms, words, etc. several things can happen. Not only can the rapport be deepened and the homeopath gain an insight into what it is like to be the patient, but also the patient can, through connecting with why they are behaving in a certain way, reveal deeper aspects of the case – often leading to greater clarity for both patient and homeopath. One of the easiest places to start using this is to enact hand movements or a mannerism the patient makes when describing a symptom, as Sue's case illustrates.

It requires confidence and some practice to integrate these skills into a consultation, most easily gained from supervised experience and trying them out in careful and controlled ways (see Chapters 23, 28). Often the matched and enacted action, experience and feeling happen spontaneously in you and can inform you not only about your situation but also the patient's. I am aware of many cases where noticing a cough, drowsiness, and a movement in my own hands or feet has drawn my attention to something that is happening. When these behaviours remain unconscious and become routine they can account for your fixed response to particular or groups of patients, such as the routine nodding of the head or tapping

CASE STUDY 13.5

Sue had many different symptoms coming on over a decade. She kept swallowing and holding her throat when talking about her dead father. At first she resisted talking about him. By repeating her movement I realised something was not being said. When I invited her to talk some more about her father and said I wondered what was not being said, Sue revealed that she had been unable to come to terms with his death 10 years before and thought of him every day. She still had his clothes. She had other Ignatia features, a remedy that might have helped with her loss. When I pointed out the hand movement she was making when talking about him she repeated it and started to cry. She then described how angry she was with how little care her father had received and how she had never told her mother how angry she was. After Staphisagria she 'found her voice' and her various problems started to improve and her case moved on.

of the feet; saying 'Yes', 'Um' or 'Oh'; or persistent feelings of wanting the patient to hurry up or slow down. These can all be thought of as compensated behaviour and can run not just through an individual but also through a whole section of a professional group (see Chapter 23).

Enacting and matching can reveal important but otherwise unconscious and unexpressed symptoms, especially linked to strong emotions. They can be, and often are, used spontaneously by parents to describe their children's behaviour and expressions, or by owners describing pets.

Disassociation

Inviting patients to imagine, in the safety of the consultation, how they might respond to different situations can reveal aspects otherwise unexpressed, e.g. asking patients to imagine conversations: 'I wonder how you would feel if your partner said this' or 'Is there anything you would like to say to X about this?' One technique frequently used

(although often unconsciously) is the incomplete sentence. For example, 'I suppose often people do this because…' or 'I wonder if…' or 'What would it take to…' or 'I suppose it feels…'. This is often combined with words the patient has previously used. So if a patient has been talking about a hard pain the homeopath might try 'and a hard pain might mean… or feel like…?'

Withdrawing eye contact, when writing notes or looking things up, often gives patients a chance to disassociate and talk more spontaneously. Some apparent 'inattention' within a consultation is not always a bad thing. In many cases when the homeopath looks something up in repertory or materia medica some new information emerges.

Other manifestations of this 'disassociated behaviour' include the patient's doodles and tunes they hum. The different style can be combined so that patients might ask to bring a picture with them or talk about the music or art they like. Using projective techniques may also bring otherwise hidden thoughts forward. For example, using 'ink blots', doodles or practising disassociation in supervision when talking about the case may help you improve your own projective techniques and help you when you want to use them with patients.

Drawings

What children draw often communicates significant information and I find it helpful to both ask children to draw in the consultation (as in John's case) and to invite artists to bring copies of their work with them.

CASE STUDY 13.6

John was 8 years old and described as hyperactive. On taking the case his mother commented that he was often anxious and agitated. He was interested in 'machines' and I asked him to draw one. Figure 13.1 is a copy of what he drew. John said that the plane 'is flying straight at me and firing its guns at me'. This is how he saw it. He responded to Stramonium.

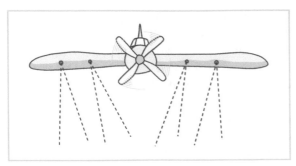

Figure 13.1 John's drawing

Where the Energy Is

If we see symptoms as an expression of a block in the free flow of an individual's vitality, then where this block lies in a case, including any resistance to enquiring about it and the difficulty the patient has to access or recall symptoms, provides information about the block. Talking more abstractly about 'energy and blocks', rather than symptoms, allows some patients to explore sensitive issues that might otherwise be difficult to name. Similarly we may be aware that something has changed as a patient comes into the room, and just observing the change without the need to name or comment on the shift can be an important part of receiving the case.

The Use of Metaphor

Metaphors are often used by patients, e.g. 'I feel all at sea', 'It sticks in my throat', 'I feel I am on a roller coaster', etc. When patients use these phrases it reveals something about the case and projects it on to something else. When strong, unusual or persistent, a metaphor can provide access to information that is otherwise masked. You might 'play dumb' and invite the patient to describe what exactly the metaphor means, e.g. 'What do you by mean "being at sea"?'. The feelings associated with it and what they might feel or imagine feeling in that situation are relevant, e.g. 'How would you feel at sea?'. The metaphor itself may directly or symbolically have something to do with the remedy.

Provocative Approaches

In some cases – often due to lack of an emotional language, low esteem, low emotional competence or failure to assert themselves – a patient finds it difficult to engage emotionally with their problem or to reflect on their feelings. This is often the case where there are especially negative feelings or where someone is emotionally closed or attached to particular mindsets and feelings. By matching the patient's behaviour and words and then taking them further, to over-emphasising them, we can bring about a reaction in the patient that unblocks the emotional or intellectual 'stuckness'. This provocation, of course, needs safeguards but can add significantly to the case picture and enhance the therapeutic consultation (Farrelly & Brandsma 1974).

Finishing

When patients become aware that the consultation is ending, then symptoms they were reluctant (consciously or unconsciously) to include in their agenda might surface – the so-called 'doorknob' symptoms. Being clear at the outset about the length of a consultation is an important part of allowing these to come up. Of course, the whole dynamic of the consultation can be thought of as encouraging these to emerge. They frequently point to the unconscious or non-contracted agenda of the patient and indicate where the consultation might go. Sometimes the moment when they emerge is the critical moment to respond; at other times they need at least to be acknowledged and a deliberate intention to address them at the next appointment expressed.

Endings are an important part of the homeopathic consultation and treatment process. In addition to the end of each consultation a broader end-point of the whole treatment process needs consideration. It may be articulated in the impression and plan in each case, even though this is reviewed and may be modified at each consultation. Like the doorknob syndrome, only after dealing with one problem and coming to the end of a treatment process might another set of symptoms and agenda emerge.

The ending of each course of treatment is important and should allow a review of all the treatment, and review the expectations and outcome of a particular treatment process. It should also permit discussion and decisions about any further treatment, especially how the patient will cope with any residual symptoms and how to maintain the improvement.

In some ways it is helpful to recognise that all our cases, especially our interesting and challenging cases, stay with us as part of our 'knowledge and database' to inform our experience and later work. This is why we need to talk about difficult cases and those we are struggling with, rather than (or at least as well as) the inspiration we take from our successful cases. By sharing difficulties and failures we can support and learn from one another (see Chapter 25).

REFLECTION POINT

- Think of a recent consultation. How have you used some of the techniques detailed here to help you in that consultation? To what extent are you aware of how the patient makes you feel and how they feel during the consultation? Reflect on your consultations and consider what your consultation style is like. How does your consulting room or other contact the patient has with your practice complement this?
- How are matching, enacting and the provocative approaches mentioned following homeopathic principles of like treating like?

Summary

This chapter attempts to blend the science and art of homeopathy into a cohesive approach in the consultation. It explores how the case can cover both those symptoms and causations so important to the first two models of health and how it can be extended to receiving the case through aspects of the totality and constitution.

The ability to form a holistic impression of a case has to precede the ability to manage the case using totality or constitution. The homeopath who extends the case into these areas must remain centred and able to build on all information in the case. This chapter builds on the work done on learning styles (Chapter 12) and extends this to thinking about your own style of consulting. No one style is 'right', but there is often one style which will enable you to see a particular case more clearly. With experience, it is possible to 'pick up' a style of working and mix it with others that fit a particular patient, aspects of their case, model of health or approach to treatment. While it helps for the homeopath to separate out the different skills and approaches that might be used in their consultation, what is vital is experience in using these techniques so they can be blended into a coherent and personally effective way of consulting holistically.

As the case deepens so the importance of rapport and empathy increases – we explore this and working with difficult cases later (see Chapters 23, 25). As we will see in Section V, in more confused and hidden cases, those aspects that are not offered up consciously and spontaneously by the patient become increasingly important. A homeopath who uses some of the techniques mentioned here will realise that it is in the relationship between the homeopath and the patient, including the homeopath's own internal processes, that much valuable information emerges about the confused and hidden case.

References

Farrelly F, Brandsma J 1974 Provocative therapy. Meta Publications, Capitola CA

Kellas A 2006 Working with movement and dance in healthcare. J of Holistic Healthcare 2006 3:24–28

Mercer S, Reilly D, Watt G 2002 The importance of empathy in the enablement of patients attending the Glasgow Homeopathic Hospital. Br J Gen Pract 2002 52:901–905

Bibliography

Kaplan B 2001 The homeopathic conversation, the art of taking the case. Natural Medicine Press, London

Neighbour R 1989 The inner consultation. MTP Press, Lancaster

Totality and Constitution

III

CHAPTER FOURTEEN

Reaching Towards the Totality

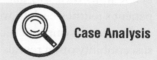 **Case Analysis**

David Owen

Introduction

Chronic illness can benefit from treatment based on causation and presenting symptoms. But generally, as cases become more complex, so causation appears multifactorial and frequently becomes obscured and presenting symptoms reflect only part of the case. In these cases a prescription matched to the patient on their totality or constitution, or a mix of both, will act more deeply and give more reliable results. The repertory is a vital tool for finding which remedies fit which symptoms and constitutional features in complex cases. This chapter explores several different strategies of repertorisation. The confidence in any strategy and the likely response to treatment based upon it is always a consideration for the homeopath. How well indicated is the treatment and how might treatment progress?

Of course, case analysis still takes place within the context of the patient's overall management, involving several important stages of case assessment (see Chapter 4), before matching the case to a remedy picture. Different approaches to case analysis reflect different ways of looking at the hierarchies of information in a case, and in turn provide strategies for exploring more difficult cases. Exploring some of the different strategies at this stage will prepare you for working with the more confused and hidden cases covered in later sections.

Case analysis frequently indicates several possible, similar remedies, and this 'differential diagnosis' needs to be worked through to identify a best-indicated remedy, the simillimum. As case analysis proceeds information may emerge about unfamiliar remedies that may fit the case better than more familiar remedies. In this way the case analysis is a dynamic process interwoven with the study of materia medica and the development of the case.

Case Analysis of Complex Cases Using Totality and Constitution

The job of science is to explain observations by way of the relationship of one thing to another. The role of the artist is to portray observations by way of the observer's relationship to it. As cases become more complex so the homeopath requires both the art and the science of homeopathy to make sense of what is observed, its uniqueness and its complexity.

When you have taken and received a complex case you are likely to know your patient in a way that not many other people do. Often this process sheds new light on the symptoms for the patient, who may know themselves better after the case than before. Once you understand what is wrong with the patient you begin to understand what has led to what is wrong – and this in turn can lead you to understand what needs to happen for the patient to put right what is wrong. Remember that sharing a holistic impression of the case with the patient, including what they are really suffering from, how it evolved, and what can be done about it, is therapeutic in its own way and frequently a start in the patient's journey back to wellness (see Chapter 25).

The total symptom picture and constitutional susceptibility often reveals a structure and order to the case. Matching this picture (with its structure and order) to the remedy picture (with its own story and pattern) is at the heart of case analysis. As we have discussed before, the materia medica is written with much greater emphasis on symptomatology than in terms of the constitution and susceptibility. Some constitutional features are described in the materia medicas and a little are included in repertories. One of the strengths of materia medicas that look at families of remedies is that they often identify themes that run through the susceptibility and constitution rather than just the symptoms when ill. In an attempt for clarity I have separated constitutional and thematic approaches while, in fact they are frequently used together and the materia medica overlaps.

Differential Diagnosis

Although it is helpful to consider prescribing on causation, presenting symptom, constitution and totality separately, in practice several approaches may be used in a case and may point to the same remedy. Deciding which approach to use and when depends on many things. It helps to be able to move between them and draw from each what lends itself best to the particular patient you are treating in that particular situation. The aim is to end up with a list of possible remedies that each fits as much of a case as possible – referred to as the differential diagnosis of similars. There may be strong confirmatory or exclusion indications for a remedy or group of remedies; by considering each remedy in turn the case may reveal new previously unnoticed symptoms. Looking at the remedies in more detail in the materia medicas or provings may provide the fine detail necessary to distinguish between these similar remedies. hopefully leading to the simillimum.

Which Symptoms to Choose?

In the holistic model no one symptom gives the whole picture. Not only is it impractical to seek remedies for every one of the patient's symptoms, but it is also unlikely one remedy will 'cover the whole case'. There are two solutions. First, the symptoms that are strong or characteristic of the patient or the illness are most likely to point to 'characteristic' remedies that cover broader aspects of the case. Second, choosing remedies that cover a balance of symptoms from the local, general and mental aspects of the case points to more 'representative' remedies. A mix of these two methods often provides a shortlist of remedies that include the simillimum. The more deep-seated the illness and the more complex the case, the greater the relative importance of 'characteristic' or 'representative' symptoms to the analysis.

Different homeopaths give primacy to different 'characteristic' and 'representative' symptoms and to some extent the layout of different repertories reflects the priority of the compiler; each has their following. Boenninghausen, for example, gives primacy to the generalised modalities and concomitant symptoms. Kent does rather the opposite and prioritises the psychological symptoms; Box 14.1 shows a common interpretation of his hierarchy from the most important to the least. As you will appreciate from earlier chapters there are several different ways of assessing hierarchies in

---

BOX 14.1
Kent's Hierarchy
1. Emotional and feeling symptoms
2. Disorders of intellect dysfunction such as, delirium, confusion
3. Symptoms of memory disturbance
4. 'Peculiar' symptoms which are not expected as part of the pathology, e.g. 'sensation of something alive in the abdomen,' a keynote of Thuja
5. General symptoms
6. Modalities concerning reaction to bodily environment, e.g. temperature, time, position, motion, etc.
7. Peculiar symptoms
8. Common, particular and pathological symptoms

different patients (see Chapter 6). Part of the art of case analysis is deciding what the appropriate hierarchy is in a particular case.

Cautionary Note on the Primacy of Mental Symptoms

Using Kent's idea of the supremacy of the mental symptoms, even when there are strong and clear physical symptoms, can lead to problems. Although mental symptoms are often more individualising, it can be difficult to be really clear about the symptom from the proving or to be confident all remedies that have that symptom are in the rubric. Many of the provings took place before detailed psychological types and profiles were documented, hence a strong clear modality is worth many half-guessed or poorly matched mental symptoms. Less definite mental symptoms can then be used as concomitants in the case, to distinguish between the similar remedies.

Remember when treating patients with mental illness that the presenting symptoms are equivalent to the local pathological symptoms of the 'mind'. Other symptoms that guide you to the individual susceptibility may be more important.

Using Food Desires, Aversions, Aggravation and Ameliorations

Kent considered food symptoms less useful than other 'generals' and modalities. In his repertory a rather incomplete list of food symptoms appear in the stomach section – perhaps in Kent's time the available choice of food, and therefore the individuality expressed by food symptoms, was much less. In most repertories now they are more complete and included as generals. A good case can also be made to consider them as mentals – often they are expressed clearly and easily even when other mental symptoms are hard to establish and they may tie in with other areas of the case. For example, in Sulphur cases the high body temperature may need a high energy, high fat diet. In Argentum Nitricum the high state of mental arousal will need 'brain food' provided by the sugar that is craved. Weighting any food desires and aversions needs to take account of fashions

and normal exposure and consumption, and to be truly marked they need to be distinctly different from the average population.

In some patients a food may both produce an unwanted symptom and meet in some way a need the patient has. In those patients who continue eating the food, chronic symptoms develop and the 'food sensitivity' becomes masked. Indeed, it is not uncommon for the patient to crave a food that is contributing to their symptoms. In this way foods can be a maintaining cause; only after or during treatment might a patient find it possible to identify and give up a culprit food. In the provings and clinical experience, remedies frequently have both a craving and aversion to the same food. This, and the incompleteness of rubrics based on foods, has led some homeopaths to include all remedies that have an affinity (craving/desire, aversion, aggravation/agg or amelioration/amel) with a particular food.

Which Rubrics to Use

Once the hierarchy of symptoms is clear, choosing which of these to look for as a rubric is next. This will depend on the repertory available, the exact rubrics and how closely they match the symptom. Box 14.2 lists factors (in no particular order) that might be considered when selecting rubrics depending on the hierarchy and approach to treatment being used. Sometimes a compromise is needed between choosing the most significant symptoms and a manageable spread of rubrics. Often the more individualising modalities of a specific symptom will not translate exactly into a rubric and a less specific symptom might need to be used. This is helped by more modern repertories being hierarchically accurate so that each rubric always contains all the remedies in its sub-rubrics. In some cases several rubrics may each describe the symptom – in these cases the rubrics can be combined, requiring attention as to how the remedies in the resultant rubric are weighted. In other cases a particularly individual characteristic or unusual symptom and rubric can be weighted more strongly because of its uniqueness. Knowing conventional diseases can help identify which rubrics are unusual for a particular patient.

BOX 14.2

Considerations in Selecting Rubrics

- Spread the rubrics between mental, generals, physicals
- Choose some rubrics that pertain to the disease, those that are part of the totality and have come on since the patient has been ill – especially those things that have changed most significantly
- Where appropriate include causation factors and strong symptoms or keynotes – both as confirmatory and exclusion rubrics
- Consider less specific rubrics if they contain a more representative collection of remedies; also consider 'permissive' rubrics (see below)
- Consider, depending on how repertorisation is taking place, the size of the rubrics
- Consider rubrics that cover structural signs, functional processes and sensations, as these are another way of getting a balance to the totality; if there is a strong indication in one of these areas, seek confirmation in other areas
- Distinguish between rubrics that pertain to strong features of the individual's constitution, i.e. those that have always been there and others that have come on since the illness and fit the totality

The more similar a match between symptom and rubric, the more likely a successful outcome to treatment will follow. A useful check on the individual value of the rubrics you have selected is to ask, if you used these rubrics alone, how easily you could separate out this patient from a group of patients with a similar illness.

Limitations Inherent in Rubrics

Rubrics vary hugely in size and are never complete as new remedies are being added all the time and no remedy has been proved on every type of susceptible prover. Different repertories will include different numbers of remedies and weight them

differently. A tension exists between how comprehensive a repertory is versus how easy it is to use.

REFLECTION POINT

- What rubrics might you use to describe any aspects of your own condition?
- Look up these rubrics in some of the repertories mentioned in Chapter 9
- What do rubrics that describe a healthy person tell you about them?
- Reflect on the tension between getting enough data for repertorisation to represent the totality and using only the most accurate data?

Permissive Rubrics

Sometimes a local modality that has no rubric or only a small rubric can be looked up as a general modality. For example, the rubric *Throat, pain, warmth amel.* is small but the general modality *Warmth amel.* is much bigger and could be combined with throat pain rubric to give more remedies than in the rubric *Throat, pain, warmth amel.* Kent rather frowns on this, which is why he has been so careful to include all local symptoms with their own modalities, yet admits these are incomplete. Boenninghausen, however, regards any local modality as reflecting the totality. Caution is needed as in some remedies or symptoms the local modalities are out of step with the rest of the case and these might be keynotes due to this peculiarity, e.g. aggravation from warmth of the Arsenicum headache in an otherwise chilly remedy. It is a question of care and judgement in choosing when it is helpful to 'generalise' a local modality – where possible this should be checked against the materia medicas and a prescription influenced by permissive rubrics more carefully confirmed.

Permissive rubrics also include those used but not offered in exactly the same way in the repertories. For example, a patient may dislike slimy food, like snails – it may be permissive to consider other foods that are slimy and rubrics with aversion to those foods, such as oysters.

Large Rubrics

Some very common features of a patient can be represented by large rubrics that might not be particularly individualising but can still point towards some remedies and away from others. Including these in repertory analyses has become easier with computer repertorisation (see Chapter 19).

Repertorisation

In every prescription there are aspects of the remedy that aren't in the case and aspects of the case that aren't in the remedy.

Basic repertorisation has been described in Chapter 9. In this chapter, to reflect the analysis of more complex cases, different strategies for repertorisation are considered. Most of these calculate the relative strength of a remedy indication based on the frequency of its occurrence in the repertory, the weighting of the symptom that the rubric is related to in the case, and the weighting of the remedy in each rubric. The scoring and ways of viewing and comparing different remedy scores is illustrated by the display of a computer repertory analysis in Figure 19.6 (p. 257) and Figure 21.1 (p. 287). This scoring has several limitations which are noted briefly in Box 14.3 and which are important to understand if the homeopath is to make informed decisions based on repertorisation results – bearing in mind, despite sophisticated computer programs, the art that lies behind case analysis.

Analysis Using the 'Three-Legged Stool'

Given the number of different possible symptoms, rubrics and strategies there is much to be said for including the most significant symptoms in the three main areas of the case – the physicals, generals and mentals. Both this and other broad approaches rely on using large but representative symptoms, like casting a net over possible remedies. Their success depends on casting the net widely enough, and checking a wide range of possible remedies in the differential diagnosis of remedies.

Some homeopaths feel many symptoms relating to the totality should be included; others that a few well chosen symptoms better represent the

---

BOX 14.3

Limitations to Strict Numerical Scoring of Rubrics and Remedies

- Symptoms may not always accurately translate into rubrics
- Symptoms may not be accurately weighted, and weighting itself seeks to give a fixed numerical score to something that is descriptive – for example, if a remedy is weighted 3 it does not mean that the symptom is three times as strong, or the remedy three times as likely to have that symptom, as a remedy weighted 1
- Symptoms and therefore rubrics are not all of the same importance; weighting rubrics as 1, 2 or 3 is only a very rough approximation of this
- If a remedy is not in a rubric it is not scored but it may actually be an important eliminatory symptom (perhaps in these cases the remedy should be given a minus score)
- Rubrics are often incomplete, in that they do not have all the remedies present that can cause and therefore cure each symptom
- Some remedies, such as Sulphur, are better proven and therefore have more occurrences in the repertory and are more likely to occur in case analyses of many rubrics – without this being taken into account polychrests like Sulphur are always likely to be favoured

---

'centre' of the individual case. It is not always possible to find strong or reliable symptoms in all three areas, and the choice has to be made whether to take several strong symptoms in the mental sphere, e.g. against less strong symptoms in the generals or locals. Judging this balance is part of the art of the homeopath. The different strategies below are mostly variations on this strategy; the exact strategy chosen may use elements of a number of these depending on the case, the symptoms and rubrics. It is not uncommon to find homeopaths (particularly, but not exclusively, those new to repertorisation in complex cases) using many different symptoms and many different strategies of analyses, giving many indicated remedies.

Where it is difficult to see the well-indicated from the partially-indicated, it is useful to have in mind the use of the minimum number of symptoms with the maximum characteristic and representative value to the case. Choosing the right analysis strategy is similar to finding your optimum style of consulting. Some strategies are better suited to some cases than others but it is equally important to find strategies you are most comfortable with and with which you can most rapidly gain expertise, while remaining open to what other strategies might offer.

Number of Rubrics

If covering breadth of case is important, then for each remedy the total number of rubrics covered by a remedy, rather than its absolute score, is more important. So a remedy in three rubrics as a 1 would be more important than a remedy in one rubric with a score of 3.

Small Remedies

Small remedies may be emphasised either by disregarding the polychrests or by weighting remedies inversely to their frequency of occurrence in the repertory. This will emphasise small remedies that have few symptoms in the repertory. The fewer the total occurrences of a remedy in the repertory, the more it is emphasised.

Small Rubrics

The smaller the number of remedies in a rubric the more peculiar (strange, rare and peculiar symptoms) that symptom might be, and so the more it can be weighted. The smaller the rubric the more the remedies in that rubric are emphasised.

Prominence

This emphasises remedies that are unusually strong in a rubric, e.g. one remedy in bold while the other 20 remedies are in plain type. Such a symptom is likely to be a keynote of that remedy.

Families

It is possible to emphasise family groupings of remedies – so the occurrence of one remedy in a family brings other family members forward in the analysis. For example, five different Carbon-containing remedies may each occur only weakly in the repertorisation. Using this strategy the carbon remedies each emphasise each other and the relative importance of each carbon remedy is enhanced. It might lead to closer examination of each of them or other carbon remedies that are little known.

Themes

Different rubrics that represent a single theme in the case might be combined, e.g. all the rubrics that have a quality of hardness or all those that are linked to over-sensitivity – which might be mirrored in physical, emotional, intellectual or general symptoms. All the rubrics in one theme can be collated together, pointing to remedies that represent that theme. Then several different themes can be compared with each other to see the remedies (or families of remedies) that share these themes.

Some themes are clearly indicated in the repertory, others used by some homeopaths are more permissive. For example, a patient who wanted at any cost to escape their symptoms, even if it means doing something they strongly object to on principle, might be found in the rubric 'desire for escape'. A patient high up in an organisation but frightened of being displaced and 'falling from grace' might fit the rubric 'fear of high places or fear of falling'.

Elimination

A sure, highly graded symptom that may be a local, general or mental symptom, is used to select a rubric (or combined rubric) that is assumed definitely to contain the indicated remedy. If a remedy is not in this rubric it is not considered further. It is helpful when working without a computer repertory (see Chapter 19) when including many large rubrics or when there are many similarly well indicated remedies, to distinguish between them. It is, however, only as accurate as the symptom is important and the rubric is complete!

Other Analysis Strategies

While the importance of repertorisation should not be under-played, there are many other ways to achieve a shortlist of remedies; some of these are explored in later chapters. A case may be divided into different aspects, e.g. different pathology, constitutional features, hereditary influences or themes, and a remedy shortlisted for each. This may be used singularly or combined. In parts of the world where there was for many years an absence of a well-translated repertory, other sophisticated strategies of case analysis not dependent on repertories have been developed.

Limitations of the Repertory, and Compensating for This

In addition to the limitations above there are two other general limits. First, the repertory loses an element of context and detail compared to the materia medica that themselves have already lost some detail from the provings; they are inevitably an 'abbreviation' of the materia medica. For example, several remedies may have anticipatory anxiety but each has slightly different things they are more or less anxious about, and will manifest the anxiety slightly differently. Indeed, the difference between an anxiety, fear and phobia is not just determined by the word the patient or prover uses but has qualities about wide or narrow focus, known or unknown cause, intensity and whether it is always there or only at times in response to a particular situation.

Second, the rubrics are laid out according to a particular structure and hierarchy determined by the author of the repertory. This helps us know where to find the particular piece of information, but also can shape and constrain how we think of a symptom and rubric. It is a testament to the insight of previous generations that we have such valuable and versatile repertory tools. Although becoming familiar with one repertory is enough for most homeopaths at the start of their studies, beginning to look at others that are structured differently both broadens your analysis options and opens you to interpreting what you observe in other ways not constrained by one structure or another.

Rubric Studies

It is helpful and important at this stage to understand why different remedies share the same key rubrics. For example, if the patient is very anxious about their health and their anxiety is out of proportion to their illness, then there is a strong likelihood that the rubric 'anxiety about health' or 'hypochondriacal' is going to be useful. Understanding the reason why each remedy has this symptom and how the quality of the anxiety is expressed differently in each remedy, will help choose between them. When reading the materia medica or studying the repertory it is helpful to reflect on why and precisely how a remedy expresses a particular symptom. You might like to look through the rubric 'anxiety about health' and 'hypochondriacal' and from reading the materia medica consider why each remedy is in the rubric – how uniquely does it get anxious and what particular situation is likely to trigger it?

Materia Medica Searches

Given the limitation of the repertory, searching original materia medica and provings may suggest possible remedies for more unique symptoms. With computers it is possible to search many materia medicas to find all occurrences of a particular word, e.g. to look for the words 'fear' and 'height', when they occur next to each other within a set number of words, sentences or paragraphs (see Chapter 19). This generates a list of remedies, weighted according to frequency of occurrence, which may be exported to a repertory program or cross-referenced to the original materia medicas. It is also possible to add different synonyms, so we could compare fear of heights with anxiety, vertigo or panic in high places. The ability to search large amounts of materia medica and compare different symptoms and rubrics have allowed a clearer perception of the pattern behind symptoms that different remedies have and so has encouraged the thematic understanding of remedies and this in turn has helped the observation of themes running through cases. As the technology has improved, so the ability to work thematically has improved.

Thematic or 'Related' Rubrics

As the disturbance in the patient that relates to a remedy state expresses itself in many aspects of the case, it can be thought of as a quality or combination of qualities that may express themselves through many different symptoms (like an archetype or symbol that is expressed in many aspects of the conscious and unconscious world of the patient). It may be easier to identify this quality in some symptoms than others, e.g. a patient who is fearful of black dogs may be helped by remedies that have dreams of black dogs, anxiety around dogs, or imagines seeing or has fears of dogs of any colour. If this approach is extended, then they may also be helped by remedies that have blackness in other symptoms, or in the source of the remedy, or the mythology associated with the remedy. While these approaches appear quite far removed from traditional repertorisation they are valuable in difficult cases where they may point to a much deeper-acting remedy than would otherwise be found.

Active, Passive and Compensated Symptoms

It is not always possible to identify the most important symptom in a case. This is one of the reasons why cases are confused and hidden and is discussed fully in Section VI. It is helpful to think of these cases as made up of several themes, that each intertwines in several layers and where one symptom is often connected to another. How the symptoms are connected reveals as much and often more than a single symptom, e.g. if all symptoms appear on the left side of the body the sidedness may be most important.

In remedy pictures, several symptoms can appear as if they are on an axis that runs from polar opposite symptoms. Often what apparently seem opposite symptoms in fact have a correspondence. They may be thought of as primary and secondary actions, inner or outer expressions, or as mirror or parallel images. It is these axes that the themes describe and include apparently polar symptoms that can be thought of as active and passive. These run through both cases and the materia medica. A patient with, for example, anticipatory anxiety may have found expression of their symptom by forcing themselves into situations, perhaps sporting or performing, where it is acceptable to be anxious and where their anxiety is expressed. They may 'passively' hold the symptom by being anxious about a sport or situation where they might suffer anticipatory anxiety.

A third way is also possible, that is to 'compensate' for the 'anticipatory anxiety' and to effectively avoid all situations where they might experience it, e.g. keeping to a very safe group of friends and experiences. It is as if they withdraw from expression on that axis and instead express themselves tangentially. In these cases the more peripheral symptoms and expressions of the themes may be all that point towards the underlying state and right remedy (Sankaran 1991).

You will see from this that one reason a case might appear confused is that the symptoms are presented in a way that does not directly reflect the deepest aspects; they may be passive or compensatory symptoms. It may require the removal of several layers to see the active aspects of the case, although if the passive and compensated symptoms are known a remedy may be found that ties in many aspects of an otherwise confused case.

The Four Elements

Different philosophers have attempted to define the fundamental polar states. The idea of man 'crucified' on the two primary axes, vertical and horizontal, spiritual and material, light and dark, is not new. And the idea of the four poles or elements occurs in many teachings including those of Paracelsus, Empedocles (fire, water, air and earth), Hippocrates (melancholic, phlegmatic, choleric and sanguine – gall, bile, phlegm, blood) and Jung (intuition, thinking, sensation, feeling). Each of these poles, and the axes they create, reveals the way symptoms can be seen as an active or passive expression (Nux Vomica, for example, has both an active choleric expression but also a phlegmatic need to relax). Understanding how different poles relate helps clarify and is another way of analysing what would otherwise be a complex and confused mix of symptoms in both cases and remedies (Reves 1993).

Repertorisation in More Difficult Cases

Repertorisation and repertory data are only ever a guide to the possible remedies. They never cover all the totality or all the constitution. Indeed, as the data are predominately derived from proving symptoms they include few constitutional features, and many remedies often share those that are represented. In difficult cases, repertorisation provides 'pointers' in the direction of remedies. Repertorising during the consultation may reveal lines of enquiry to follow in the case, and becomes a part of the case-taking, in helping to clarify and develop symptoms. Sometimes it is this process that starts to reveal the essence, themes and patterns running through a case. Extensions of the normal repertory that describe themes and their relation to different remedy groups are starting to emerge in some books (Sankaran 2002).

Clarifying Rubrics

By looking at rubrics and the remedies in a rubric during case-taking, ideas may emerge that allow you to explore or clarify the symptoms and rubrics that you might use. For example, scanning the rubrics about chest pain may inform you about the variety of modalities that exist and that should be enquired about. Care must be taken that this does not bias the analysis towards preconceived ideas. One way to reduce this possible distortion, particularly useful when first in practice, is to give the patient a list, e.g. the different types of pain, and let them choose the best description. Another is to have a period of time, perhaps without the patient present, to start analysing and repertorising the case, then to ask the patient back in to clarify and explore symptoms – it is at this time that confirmatory and eliminatory factors can be considered.

Different Analysis Strategies

It is useful to have different methodologies for analysing a case as each will explore or 'explain' the case in a different way. When different strategies of combining and weighting rubrics and different methodologies point to, or away from, the same remedy or group of remedies it can clarify a case analysis. In some cases the symptoms that can be repertorised are not always the deepest or strongest symptoms; while a remedy indicated on this basis may act deeply, it is more likely to lead to the emergence of other and hopefully deeper-acting remedies at future consultations (see 'Treating using several sequential remedies', Chapter 15).

When the Totality Is Not Enough

When viewing the case holistically, with the whole case not expressed in the totality, we are already seeing the first signs of a confused and hidden case. As a case becomes more difficult, then it is more likely to comprise several 'layers'. This leads to both confused and hidden cases – confused where different symptoms (some that may be passive or compensatory reactions) appear contradictory and no clear hierarchy is seen, hidden where the deeper aspects are masked either by the overwhelming disease process or because the deeper disturbances are culturally masked (see Chapter 30).

When an aspect of a case is not expressed clearly it instead shows itself in the unconscious of the patient. It is the unconscious and unseen aspects that contain much of the 'potential susceptibility' of the patient and that determine so much of the 'constitution'. Revealing and understanding the unconscious therefore holds the key to exploring these cases, initially by understanding the patient's constitution, then by looking at what the patient projects onto others, and then by exploring what others project onto the patient. The constitution is discussed further below; projection is explored in Section VI.

Plan of Treatment

Illness is what the patient has on the way to see the doctor; disease is what they have on their way home.

A plan of treatment is likely to indicate a preferred homeopathic approach based on the impression of the case. It will also include ideas about the overall management of the patient related to the 12 stages outlined in Chapter 4 (page 40). In some cases it is possible to see a differential diagnosis that is several remedies deep, with one remedy being most clearly indicated, nearer the surface, but some showing a deeper partial picture and others offering just a glimpse of their potential. The deeper possible remedies are worth noting as they may become clear when a new hierarchy emerges and give information about the direction and remedies indicated in subsequent consultations. This is particularly important when we consider that in many complex cases there is likely to be a course of treatment that is going to need several remedies. An awareness of how the remedies are related to each other, and how one remedy might follow another, is vital to managing these more complex cases (see Chapter 15).

The exact plan of treatment may be influenced by quite practical factors such as the complexity of the case, the time available, how acute or chronic the illness is, if the patient will be able to attend for follow-up, if the patient is using homeopathy as a one-off or as a therapy throughout their life. The expectation that one prescription will solve the majority of chronic diseases at a single intervention is unrealistic and a potential cause of dissatisfaction with, and disappointed expectations of, homeopathy. Some patients may present with an acute illness or local symptoms that they require treating. The homeopath may see that the case is deeper, but until the acute problem or local symptoms have responded to treatment the patient may be reluctant to contract to work more deeply. It can sometimes seem that the patient needs first to experience the benefits of homeopathy before undertaking deeper treatment. This education and development of the homeopathic patient and the cultural awareness of what a deep homeopathic prescription entails is an important part of helping patients reach a level of awareness where they can obtain the deeper benefits that homeopathy can offer.

The Totality Vs Constitutional Approach

While the totality and constitution are two sides of the 'holistic approach', and are usually used together in some way, there are times when one approach or the other may be favoured – the totality if just the symptoms since the patient became ill are to be considered; the constitution if considering the state of the patient before any symptoms developed. For example, a patient may want to be treated constitutionally before they enter a situation that might make them ill, or when pregnant to reduce the susceptibility of the child. In practice, as symptoms, even if only acute ones, are always happening, and constitutional features may be due to previous (or inherited) illness, there are always connections and overlaps between the two methods. Understanding the different focuses of the totality and constitutional approaches will allow you to see the relative merits of both. How these are brought together in different situations will shape how you work in the holistic model (see Chapter 11).

Each constitutional type prefers certain environments and is predisposed to certain illnesses. Some homeopaths see treating your constitution as like having your car regularly serviced. It is more likely to keep going in different environments and to have fewer problems. In this way constitutional prescriptions may be a way of maintaining the body in optimum health. However, even a constitution that is completely healthy in one environment may find itself susceptible in another. No one type will be healthy in every situation!

While there may be a typical constitutional picture for a remedy not all patients who need that remedy will fit the typical picture. So constitution can be a good positive indicator but not as useful as an eliminator.

Many patients share common susceptibility, and so share some constitutional features. Not surprisingly these often correlate with frequently indicated remedies (polychrests). As you treat more difficult cases it may be helpful, rather than thinking of there being a single remedy that suits all aspects of an individual at one time, to think of there being several remedies, each of which may cover some aspects of the case. Identifying these respective pictures often helps clarify the case and reveal new symptoms or hierarchy that allows the remedy that covers most or the deepest part of the case to be teased out. When a case falls between two or more remedies that are quite different there is likely to be a third (often smaller) remedy that is indicated. This raises the question of when to use a sequence of remedies or to seek a more specific remedy, often a small remedy that might not have been well proved (see Chapter 15).

What is a Healthy Constitution?

A constitutional type will have characteristics that are habitually present in good health, but also be prone to particular symptoms when ill. For example, while a Sulphur patient may need the fatty foods they crave, over consumption may lead to digestive problems. Those who need sugar might become diabetic or hypoglycaemic. When the constitution of an individual has all the characteristics they need (or the majority of them) to function well in their present environment, then we refer to them as having a healthy or strong constitution. It is likely that if they find themselves in an environment that is only slightly different their vitality will be high and they will be able to generate a response that will enable them to cope with the new situation.

Previously Well Indicated and Effective Remedy

The right constitutional remedy may help a patient in a number of different acute or recurrent illnesses. If a remedy has acted well before it should be considered again.

The Central Disturbance

In some cases and with some remedy pictures there is a clear pattern to the whole picture that stems from a single central issue or disturbance. Prescribing on this is more akin to prescribing on the essence or central theme but when there is a clear link between the central disturbance and the peripheral symptoms the essence and constitution may effectively be seen as one.

Classical Prescribing

Many homeopaths describe a whole person, totality and constitutional approach as 'classical homeopathy', meaning that prescribing is based on strict principles (usually those of Hahnemann but with significant influence from others, most notably Kent), and they use a single medicine in a single prescription. Classical prescribing can be helpful in many complex cases but as cases become

more confused and hidden so those aspects of the totality displayed by the patient point less clearly to the remedy. Hahnemann noted this difficulty in treating much chronic disease and observed several patterns of symptoms related to the suppression of common major illnesses; he called these 'miasms'. Prescribing on these is sometimes referred to as miasmatic prescribing.

Introduction to Miasms

Section III started by looking at symptoms and susceptibility and how they theoretically determine the holistic picture. In practice, in our current culture of self and prescribed medication for every ill, most cases with chronic illness are almost immediately coloured by suppression and palliation. In these cases, the picture changes and the case can only be understood fully by seeing the deeper layers of the case. This has been recognised for as long as homeopaths have treated chronic disease. If the miasmatic aspects (or layer) of a case are not treated then they provide an obstacle to cure. Homeopaths use the concept of miasms as one of the ways to make sense of and manage these deeper, more difficult, cases. (The word miasm comes from the Greek word 'mianein' relating to a stain or taint; this is covered in detail in Chapter 17.) When a disease is incompletely cured it generates a susceptibility that is passed on to others. These traits are inherited, but may also be passed on through the cultures we evolve and inhabit. The three miasms Hahnemann described relate to three fundamental disturbances of degeneration (destructive), over-activity (autoimmune) and disorder/proliferation (tumour).

Miasmic Constellations

Different patients, disease processes and remedies belong to each of these miasms. One model that is helpful when considering miasms is a pattern that connects different remedies and symptoms – rather like a constellation of stars in the night sky that are connected by a pattern. You might struggle to remember every star individually but find it easier to remember the constellations it relates to. In the same way that a constellation of stars has key

Totality and
Constitution

or central stars, so the miasms have key remedies. Several constellations can overlap and one remedy can be part of more than one. As the homeopath becomes more experienced they see more patterns in the remedies and more connections to each other.

Three Main Miasms

In Chapter 17 we look at the overall themes running through the main miasms including examples of mental, general and local features of these different miasms. The miasms tie in with both the constitutions of different patients and to themes that run through certain remedies. They provide a useful pointer to the relevance of important constitutional features in a patient, e.g. patients with a saddle-shaped or turned-up nose (syphilitic), too big a nose (sycosis) or a sharp and straight nose (psoric). It raises the consideration that the constitutional features and susceptibility of one generation are shaped by the illnesses of a previous one. They indicate the important effect that suppression of a disease can have, leading to the development of susceptibility. Ultimately any disease that is not completely cured gives rise to new susceptibility – acquired and hereditary illnesses are in fact closely related and differ only in the time frame or time line over which they manifest. Miasms are also used by some authors to convey something about the general expression of groups of remedies in terms of fundamental types of reaction that are less directly linked to disease process but provide one way of looking at how remedies are related to one another (see Chapter 22).

Summary

Looking in detail at the analysis of complex cases we can recognise the important role of the repertory, for which an accurate and full case with weighted symptoms is central. We are also reminded that analysis cannot be isolated from the study of the case, the patient as a whole and the materia medica.

For the homeopath, finding the way around the repertory and learning how to repertorise is part of the apprenticeship. Understanding and mastering the structure and strategies for using a repertory, whether paper or computer, is like mastering the tools of any trade. Remember, the finest painting is made from perceiving clearly, knowing the fundamental colours, a range of brush strokes and experience.

As cases become more difficult, so a range of analysis strategies using the totality, constitution and reviewing what is unconscious in the case is vital. This is explored further in subsequent chapters. General guidance about the hierarchy of information in a case and the weighting of symptoms has been given, but there is always a tension between the emphasis we give to very characteristic small individualising symptoms and more representative symptoms that are seen to express themselves in many areas of the case. This is reflected in the tension between using predominantly broadly indicated polychrests and the specific and focused small remedy.

Although the ideal situation in every case would be to identify the totality and constitution, the reality is that we can only approximate towards this. In practice this means that patients will often zigzag from one remedy to another as they move towards wellness. How to support patients and maximise the ease of this journey back to well-being requires compassion, insight and perseverance. In the next chapter we will look in more detail at the practical tools of applying and using a constitutional and totality approach.

References

Reves J 1993 24 chapters in homeopathy. Homeopress, Haifa

Sankaran R 1991 The spirit of homeopathy. Homoeopathic Medical Publishers, Bombay

Sankaran R 2002 An insight into plants, 2 vols. Homoeopathic Medical Publishers, Bombay

Bibliography

Norland M 2001 Origins of the Mappa Mundi. Am Homeopath 7:102–105

Saxton J 2006 Miasms as Practical Tools. Beaconsfield, UK.

CHAPTER FIFTEEN

Managing Complex Cases

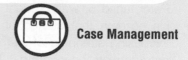 **Case Management**

David Owen

Introduction

This chapter explores first the practical management of complex cases in the context of chronic illness, and second the 'journey' back into health as the treatment proceeds. The more complex the case the longer the journey and the more steps it is likely to entail. The different ways in which a complex case can be analysed may suggest a number of different remedies. Each might only partially fit the case and which, if any, of these are used is determined by the knowledge of the homeopath, the case, what is being treated and the analysis strategies used. These all contribute to the context in which decisions about management are made (see Chapter 5).

Each prescription is a stage in that journey and is informed by the overall impression of the case and the overall plan of treatment being used. As we have seen, the impression is informed by the model of health, the plan is informed by the approach to treatment and the prescription is determined by the methodologies being used. All these factors will influence the remedy selected, guide the optimal potency and frequency of dose to use, and affect the possible and likely reactions to treatment.

The Journey into Illness

There are many different ways of summarising the impression of a complex case. It might include a pathological or structural diagnosis, a description in terms of sensation (I feel, I sense, my senses tell me) plus emotional and intellectual impressions, and a functional diagnosis in terms of physiology (I do this, I'm too hot, I perspire). The impression is expressed as a summary of the narrative and may include an idea of how deep the illness goes, what is happening now and is likely to happen if untreated, and how it has evolved and what has to happen to reverse it. The impression is often closely tied in with the eventual remedy prescribed. This has led to the practice of using the name of the remedy prescribed in the place of the diagnosis, such as diagnosing someone as a 'Phosphorous' patient. This shorthand fails to reflect the full nature of the patient and their management.

The reality is that, with rare exceptions, chronic illness and complex cases are rarely perceived completely accurately at first – when they have had suppressive treatment they often are partially confused or hidden. So it is unlikely that a single remedy will match the totality or constitution and cure completely without the need for further prescriptions.

The case, and therefore the choice of appropriate remedy, may appear to change as the case unfolds over time – both in our understanding of its evolution prior to treatment and in the response to treatment. This may be seen as the patient's 'journey into illness' and, as they start to recover, their 'journey into wellness'. In Chapter 3 we discussed the 'time line' of a patient's illness; it is also possible to think of a 'time frame' for a

Totality and
Constitution

CASE STUDY 15.1

Peter, aged 5, was brought for treatment of his eczema that started at age 9 months. Increasing strengths of steroid creams were not adequately controlling it. He had also had asthma, controlled by inhalers, since he was two and a half. He had unsuccessfully tried a dairy exclusion diet. Treatment based on the presenting eczema symptoms was difficult as there had been suppression and modalities were unclear. There was an apparent absence of general, mental and constitutional features – making a totality prescription difficult. There was, however, a family history of allergic disease and of tuberculosis in the maternal grandmother.

Prescribing the nosode Tuberculinum bovinum led to an initial aggravation (helped at that time by reducing dairy intake), followed by a clear picture of Phosphorous emerging in aspects of the totality. This gave further improvement of the eczema and, in time, a gradual reduction in the need for steroid creams. The parents remained happy to use inhalers for his asthma, which he appeared to grow out of at age 9. He re-presented age 14 with hay fever and a relapse of his asthma; at this time he had a clearer general and mental picture of Phosphorous that helped his hay fever and asthma. After several prescriptions his respiratory function improved and he cautiously reduced his inhalers.

patient's recovery. Peter's case illustrates some of these points.

Frequently one remedy is observed to 'unlock' another. In more difficult cases the treatment may take some time to reveal the deepest aspects of the case. In some confused cases several different remedies might be needed over a period of time and in hidden cases a remedy or several remedies may be needed regularly to 'unmask' the case (see 'plussing' and 'LM potencies', Chapter 20).

Over time much can be achieved by moving things on one step at a time in the journey towards health. Patients may have expectations of dramatic cure from a single prescription, and explaining to them the idea of 'journeying back to health' can help them have a more realistic view of the management of more difficult cases. It also allows the homeopath to point out that the journey is for the patient to make, and to invite the patient to participate consciously in this process and to accept that it may take some time. Of course, if the picture is clear and the remedy is strongly indicated it can happen much more quickly.

It is common for a patient to ask how long it takes to recover from an illness. One way is to consider it as a proportion of the time over which the illness has developed. It may well take one-tenth of the time that the patient has been ill for them to make a full recovery – if there has been significant suppression it may take longer. Part of the planning and the process of follow-up is identifying significant points along the way that indicate the patient is improving.

Does the Constitution Change?

The observation that a patient requires several remedies, including constitutional remedies, raises the question of whether the constitution changes or whether none of the remedies accurately enough match the underlying constitution or susceptibility. While many basically healthy individuals appear to maintain what appears the same constitution for many years of their lives, those who suffer chronic disease and who have deep-seated cases, especially when suppressed, seem to move through different but linked constitutions. Rather than being represented by a single remedy, the constitutional picture is perhaps better thought of as being represented by a group of remedies with overlapping susceptibility. Another way of understanding the constitution is that it reflects the simillimum – how the constitution evolves and changes in response to life experience reflects how the simillimum changes.

In the holographic model we can understand the case as a series of themes that run through different layers – so important to understanding confused cases. As such, different layers or parts of the constitution come into focus at different times in a person's life. Often an apparent change in the constitution corresponds with when the life situation changes most; such as when first going to school, at adolescence, when leaving home, getting a job, getting married, having children, suffering bereavements, redundancy, etc. Perhaps such events and life stages tend to bring forward different susceptibilities within the constitution. For example, pregnancy may make certain remedy pictures more likely. There are different views as to how much different constitutions may partially co-exist or over-lie each other and whether these follow clear patterns. My own observation is that there is frequently an order to this and that this reflects the commonly observed remedy relationships – and also a connection between remedies of different families and kingdoms (see 'Related remedies', Chapter 27).

Constitution and Environment

If the patient's apparent constitution changes when exposed to different situations and environmental factors, then to understand the constitution it is helpful to see the connection between the remedy and the situation in which it is required. This is why certain remedies often suit people in certain professions or jobs, not that this is used as a major indication, but it may be a confirmatory. The homeopath who is aware of the major environmental and situational changes affecting a patient should also be aware of the types of constitutions that may become ill in these environments. This awareness presents homeopaths (and indeed all health care practitioners) a responsibility to inform society of the health consequences of environmental changes.

As patients move between diverse environments due to rapid social change, travel or living longer, so the constitution is increasingly challenged. Some individuals who maintain the same constitution for many years of their lives do so because they are good at maintaining a healthy environment and life style. Likewise a shift in the patient's situation and life style can be a sign that a remedy has acted. Understanding what situations make different constitutional types ill and what symptoms they typically get is an important part of studying the materia medica and is a form of causation and local picture that each remedy has.

What sort of Patients Respond to Totality and Constitutional, Homeopathic Treatment

Patient decisions about what treatment to follow is often based on an incomplete picture of both their condition and what treatment entails. The totality and constitutional approach suits those patients who realise the importance of taking into account all the symptoms and their susceptibility, and who are prepared to spend time revealing the whole case. Patients who choose to see life holistically might do this even though they have quite localised symptoms. In some patients the motivation comes because they have conditions where there is no conventional well-indicated treatment. Other patients may have tried conventional treatment that either has not worked or has caused intolerable adverse effects.

Those patients where there has been (or is) much suppression or many different disease processes often present confused cases and are likely to benefit from the insight that the thematic approach to treatment brings (see Sections V and VI). They include patients with several systems, organs, or tissues affected by deeper functional or structural disturbance. For some patients with co-existing syndromes, realising that a treatment that seeks common ground to all their symptoms makes sense, is the start of a long but worthwhile healing process. In patients with gross structural changes including tumours and disease of more vital (or central) organs, including those who have had much surgery and deep-acting suppressive medication, their cases are more likely to be confused and hidden – often requiring thematic, miasmatic and reflective approaches.

The Plan of the Journey Back to Wellness

Planning a patient's homeopathic treatment is central to both the patient and homeopath having realistic expectations of what can be achieved. It sets objectives of the treatment in terms of medium and long-term goals and allows realistic short-term goals of a particular prescription between each consultation. It allows the role of a single consultation to be understood in the context of the treatment process as a whole. Attempting to manage cases without a plan is like setting off on a journey with no idea of where you want to go, no directions of how you are likely to get there, and no idea of what you are likely to pass on the way.

A common mistake is to think that treatment can be completed in a single consultation. That way lies the mistaken belief that there is 'a magic bullet' for every case; it leads to unrealistic expectations and disappointments for both patient and homeopath.

Treatment and Maintenance

If the homeopath or patient is unrealistic about treatment they may become disillusioned before they have seen the journey through to its conclusion. Newcomers to homeopathy often fail to plan adequate follow-up. The number of appointments that a patient will need will vary greatly depending on many factors; an average for a patient with a complex (but not confused or hidden) case having an illness that has gone on for 4–5 years is between four and six appointments over 6 months. In more deep-seated cases treatment may go on for much longer, with the treatment sometimes going through phases of just maintaining the patient and the improvement they have had so far. It may take some time for a confused or hidden case to unfold and reveal new information. The patient still requires support during this time until a new prescription becomes clear.

The speed at which a case unfolds is influenced by many things and it is not always possible for the patient or homeopath to progress a case as fast as they would like. There can be issues about the type and level of support a patient needs, life style changes that need to be made, the speed at which suppressive medication can be stopped, and the depth, time and cost of treatment with which the patient or homeopath is able or comfortable to work. Unfortunately many patients (and some homeopaths) see a partial improvement as all that is required or desirable. If these patients stop homeopathic treatment part way through they are likely to relapse.

Suppression and Palliation

A homeopath in planning the course of treatment is aware that the patient may need to work through symptoms that have been suppressed and to let symptoms move in the direction of cure. Enabling patients to work through these symptoms is both a function of rapport with the patient and of understanding the palliative and suppressive forces that are at play. Management includes, as appropriate, reducing suppressive medication and making life style changes.

Understanding and managing palliation and suppression is an important aspect of the homeopath's role in more deep-seated cases. For example, a patient brought up in an environment where everyone suppresses grief may need to 'get in touch with' their grief – which is why homeopaths need to be aware of the culture and society that has shaped the patient's life or that they now inhabit (see Chapter 30).

Secondary Gain

That a patient may gain some benefit from particular symptoms or illnesses is well recognised. Understanding how illness interfaces with the patient's needs is an important part of managing the patient, as Jan's case illustrates.

Somatisation/Sensation, Function and Structure

It is well recognised that psychological illness affects the physical body – the holistic model is a means of observing and treating both aspects. In the holistic model all sensations, functions and bodily structures are connected and can be thought of as different but interconnected realms of symptoms.

CASE STUDY 15.2

Jan, age 48, presented in a wheelchair with arthritis – she had found out that her partner had been having an affair shortly before she had 'worsened' and had to start using the wheelchair. While this might be completely coincidental, it was thrown into focus by her refusal to have any artificial drive to her wheelchair or to have anyone but her partner pushing her. When this was explored in the case, her need to always know where he was indicated a theme around control and betrayal.

So a patient who initially suffers from anxiety (sensation) might start to fiddle with their hands and bite their nails (function), and eventually their nails might weaken and split (structure). In some ways the anxiety can be thought of as being held in the functional and structural changes of the fingers and nails. To treat the nails, the anxiety will need to be addressed; if it is not, then it will effectively be transposed onto other symptoms. In this way it can be helpful in some cases to think of symptoms as a form of 'projection' of something that is unable to be held or integrated within the healthy individual (see Chapter 23). Whatever realm the symptom is expressed in, it expresses something of what is being projected.

For some homeopaths the origin of what is being disturbed is outside the patient, ultimately more 'spiritual'; for others it is understood as coming predominately from choices the patient makes about their environment and life style. One way extrapolates health matters into religious belief; the other extrapolates all causes as a consequence of the patient's choice. Both perceptions need to be balanced in understanding and working with the totality.

One Remedy or Several Remedies

Many homeopaths aspire to selecting a single remedy that covers the complete case and will heal the patient from presentation to discharge. In practice this is frequently not possible and there are various

reasons why many prescribers use several remedies at different times (see unicist, inter-current and combined remedies – Chapter 30).

In many simple cases a single approach and methodology may be clearly indicated. There is often comprehensive information available in the materia medicas about causation and local symptoms to choose a remedy from. However, some prescribers will mix several remedies together; sometimes because each covers an aspect of the case, e.g. a mixture of Aconite, Belladonna and Chamomilla (ABC) in a fretful child; at other times to provide a 'spread' of remedies when the modalities are unknown or the prescriber is unsure what to give. These mixtures are usually used in the same potency. In some areas of practice closely related to homeopathy, such as Bach flower remedies and the tissue salts, using some mixtures of remedies is normal practice.

Sometimes different remedies indicated from different approaches and methodologies are mixed together. For example, in France and Germany many clinically indicated prescriptions include a mix of remedies for organ stimulation combined with those for presenting symptoms, usually in different potencies.

As cases get more complex so it is often possible to see several models, approaches and methodologies each pointing to aspects of many remedies. A best-fit prescription in one methodology or approach might not cover all the case. This leads to some prescribers using remedies in close succession or in parallel with each other, often using different potencies depending on the approach being used (see Chapter 20). These preferences are sometimes well established by different homeopathic schools such as that used by the Eizayaga school (Box 15.1).

In the thematic and reflective approaches the materia medica knowledge and how to represent this in repertories is still evolving. This can make confused and hidden cases hard to prescribe for with confidence unless there are good confirmatories. An awareness of how remedies can interact with one another (see Chapter 27) and how poorly indicated remedies, especially high potency ones,

BOX 15.1
Eizayaga's Combined Approach

Developed in Argentina by Dr Eizeyaga, this is offered as a well-tried way of combining different approaches and methodologies into a coherent management strategy. He categorised symptoms into 'lesional', 'fundamental', 'miasmatic' and 'constitutional' and then analysed them separately, seeking a remedy for each. Each is treated in its own right and may require a different remedy. The lesional aspect correlates to the local disease that might be acute, chronic, periodic or permanent, and may be reversible, irreversible, curable or incurable. Prescribing is based on local modalities, concomitants, and including mental and general symptoms that have come on since the onset of the disease.

The fundamental is based on features which have developed during a person's life and which relate to the person rather than the disease process (the totality minus the local). It overlaps with the constitutional picture and includes significant life events. After treatment at the fundamental layer the patient will return to their original constitutional picture.

The constitution is based on healthy characteristics that have mostly been present for a long time and include genetic factors, body hair, body type, hair colour, basic personality etc. Features that are taken here relate to the compensated or socialised or normal behaviour of the patient. Often a few basic polychrests, particularly mineral remedies, are used for this layer and a patient moving towards this layer is perhaps a sign that they are moving away from the confused case to a more straightforward chronic disease.

The miasm as a deep-set theme remains even after the presenting problem is cured; treating this helps to consolidate a cure to prevent a relapse. It relates to the weakest and most susceptible aspects of an individual – and that susceptibility may be active, exposed or dormant.

can further confuse a case is necessary to prescribe sufficiently cautiously (see 'Treatment of confused and hidden cases' – Chapter 29). As a general rule most homeopaths are correctly cautious in prescribing high potencies and reluctant to combine high potency remedies.

When a remedy is well indicated by totality and constitution a homeopath can confidently prescribe a single remedy. As the indications move to either end of the range of models and approaches so confidence often decreases – it is here that mixtures of local remedies and two remedies, one for the person (or 'inside') and one for the illness (or 'outside'), are more often used. As these cases 'clear' so a single remedy covering the totality and constitution at that time often emerges.

In practice seeing an 'inner' and 'outer' remedy is more often the case if you are attempting to work simultaneously across the different models of health with no one clear totality or constitution. It leads frequently to the prescription of a single high potency remedy for the inside nature of the patient using themes or miasms, followed by a low potency remedy for the outer symptoms of the illness on local symptoms or causation.

The Treatment Cycle

Healing is a process that takes time.

The different layers and realms of symptoms create a multidimensional picture of the case that builds and presents sequentially. Working through this is not a linear process but may helpfully be thought of as requiring a number of stages over a cycle of a number of consultations and treatments. Although not every consultation will require a prescription, the stages of the consultation and treatment process and what is learned from them are very important. Patiently allowing the case to unfold over time, and paying close attention as it

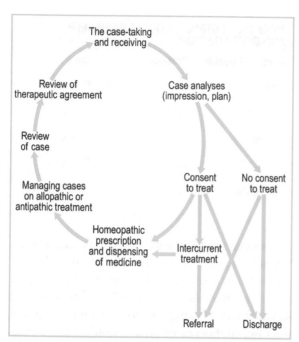

Figure 15.1 The treatment cycle

does so, calls upon a number of different models of health to reflect and interpret what is happening, and employs a number of different approaches to treatment – leading to a number of possible prescriptions based on different methodologies. Figure 15.1 illustrates this as a series of stages or phases.

Sometimes there is a single central disturbance that runs throughout the treatment cycle. At other times there can be many different dimensions to the case that each need to be resolved. Some of the deepest cases will only unfold over years or decades, sometimes there will be phases of active treatment where the case is changing, interspersed with maintenance phases where the case appears static but may well be consolidating improvements already made, before being ready to move on and tackle deeper issues.

Case Analysis

Case analysis involves forming an impression, making a plan and giving a prescription. In complex cases there are several possible ways of analysing a case – matching the depth of the analysis and methodology to the depth of the case is as much homeopathy as matching the remedy within a methodology. When no one impression, plan or

prescription covers all aspects of the case a choice has to be made on what is to be treated first. It is informed by both the patient's and homeopath's preference, and determines the therapeutic agreement (see Chapter 25). Not uncommonly, patients who fail to appreciate the potential depth at which homeopathy can work request relief for their most distressing presenting symptoms. Only when these symptoms have been addressed might they be prepared to work more deeply. In other cases a prescription may focus on just one or two aspects of the case; as these are resolved others emerge or become the priority.

Consent to Treat

Once the plan of treatment is clear, the purpose and probable effect of any prescription becomes clear. With this information the homeopath can meaningfully ask for consent to treat. In order to give informed consent the patient needs an idea of the possible reactions to a management strategy including the remedy. As the holistic treatment will ideally take into account all aspects of the case including the symptoms (totality), the susceptibility (constitution) and suppression that has taken place, these three areas each need to be considered. In practice they are not separate entities but are dynamically connected, so advice will cover not only the indicated prescription but other (suppressive) medication being used and also life style.

Referral and Discharge

Patients also require information about 'other treatment options', so the homeopath requires a familiarity with other health care systems the patient may benefit from. Deciding when to refer a patient is often difficult and, despite realising why it is advisable, the patient may experience feelings of 'rejection' and the homeopath feelings of 'failure'. Developing and feeling part of a team of different practitioners and advisers is often an important part of a homeopath's professional support and in integrating homeopathy in a patient's care.

Discharging a patient includes situations where no clear consent to prescribing exists and no follow-up is required. If the patient is to be followed up by phone 'to see how the treatment goes' this is not a discharge – the homeopath and patient remain 'in relationship'. When discharging a patient it is helpful to clarify who is now clinically responsible for the patient, whether the patient has all the information they need about their treatment, and to invite the patient to give feedback to you.

If a patient relapses sometimes after an initial improvement then it may relate to a deterioration in their condition, a lowering of the vitality (or increase in susceptibility) or a wearing off (or antidoting) of the remedy. In many cases it is because the initial treatment and arrangements for maintenance were inadequate.

Inter-Current Treatment

Although ideally a patient will only need or receive one homeopathic remedy that covers all their symptoms, in practice, especially in more complex cases, patients seek out different inter-current treatment for particular symptoms. This may be provided by other systems of medicine or by prescribing homeopathically using a different approach. This may be because a particular symptom needs controlling or because of an overlying acute picture. What these inter-current treatments should be, when they should be used, and their possible interactions with totality and constitutional treatment, is the subject of much discussion.

Potency and Administration of the Remedy (See Chapter 20)

It can at times appear critical to choose the optimum potency and there are cases where one potency acts while another does not. However, at other times the potency seems very much secondary to choosing the best remedy and 'if the remedy is right, the potency doesn't matter'. Historically, higher potencies were developed to avoid toxic effects with the guideline that the minimum dose was all that was required. To try to reduce the variability and confusion to those new to homeopathy I invite you, when you start in practice, to consider using the potency that matches the model of health you are using.

Table 15.1 POTENCY, MODELS OF HEALTH AND DEPTH OF CASE

Modes of health	Potency	Case
Relational	200c, 1M or 10M	Hidden
Holographic	200c or 1M	Confused
Holistic	200c	Complex
Biological	30c	Simple
Pathogenic	12c/6c	Straightforward

As a general rule the treatment approaches often, but not always, correlate with the depth of the case that is being treated and therefore the most appropriate potency (Table 15.1). When this is not the situation then selecting the potency on the depth of the case, confidence of prescription or, more pragmatically, what is available to you may be indicated.

Other prescribers use other criteria, such as when dealing with an illness that presents purely on a physical level using a 12 potency, for functional disturbance a 30, and a disturbance of sensation a 200 or higher. For example, causation such as an insect bite might be treated with a 12c, while causation or symptoms of shock/fright might be treated with a 30 or 200c.

Some remedies are described as working best in different potencies. This is often due to how the remedy is most commonly used. Lycopodium is sometimes talked about as working best as a 12c, which is true when used in local prescribing – but when indicated by totality or constitutional a 200c is more appropriate. As a general rule deeper treatment for deeper cases indicates higher potencies.

Frequency

How frequently the remedy needs repeating depends on how high the patient's vitality is and how frequently it needs stimulating to respond. Generally, the higher the potency and the clearer the match to the complete case the less often it needs to be given. Frequently, high potencies are given in a split dose, often two or three doses at 12-hour intervals. While in some cases a single

Totality and Constitution

remedy given once may be sufficient, in other cases the same remedy may be needed several times particularly with more entrenched functional or structural disturbance. When to repeat a remedy at follow-up is something that taxes many homeopaths and is covered in more detail in Chapter 16. As a general rule when a maintaining factor is still likely to be present, then a dose may need to be repeated on a more regular basis. Remember if the maintaining factor is a causative factor, as they often are, the patient may need to be encouraged to address this or else a long lasting cure will be elusive. The homeopath does more than just find a remedy and an illness is often part of life's therapy.

When a maintaining factor is likely still to be present, or the illness is particularly structural, then a dose repeated on a more regular basis may well be indicated – 12c potency twice a day is not uncommon. A 30c potency is often only needed as an initial treatment, although repeating it for functional disturbances twice a week will sometimes give more consistent responses. In the realm of sensation a single split dose is usually adequate.

Administration

Remedies can be antidoted by strong smells and tastes, including some foods. The need to avoid these can be explained in terms of the potentised remedy being a subtle energy whose action can be inhibited. It is therefore advisable to take the remedy on a clean mouth, dissolved under the tongue, and to avoid coffee, mint, etc. Remedies often appear more easily antidoted when first taken but once they have acted they are harder to antidote accidentally. I find it particularly important to advise patients to avoid potential antidotes when taking high potency remedies.

Managing Cases on Allopathic or Antipathic Treatment

Homeopaths need not be discouraged from treating patients with a history of allopathic or antipathic treatment, although the treatment cycle needs to take this into account at every stage. The effect on the case and analysis is covered in the detailed

discussions in earlier chapters on suppression. Knowing what symptoms are due to adverse effects of conventional and recreational drugs is important in establishing the hierarchy of a case. Patients who have predominately used homeopathic remedies, especially if over many years, are often more sensitive to conventional drugs, respond to lower doses and are more susceptible to adverse effects.

Some patients use allopathic or antipathic treatment for discrete symptoms while using homeopathy for others. The management implications include understanding the potential interactions of different treatments and the need to communicate with those supervising other treatments. It is likely to alter both how deep and clear the case is and possibly the action and duration of both treatments.

Other patients will try several treatments for the same symptoms. This can make both the case and interpreting any response to treatment difficult – such patients are therefore not for the inexperienced. As homeopaths become more experienced they may feel freer to experiment with different models, approaches and methodologies in these situations and be more able to interpret the responses to the different methodologies.

There are often several prescriptions that will shift the case in some way but knowing how these might relate to the overall plan of treatment, including non-homeopathic interventions, is often the mark of experience.

Reviewing the Case

During treatment, as rapport develops and in response to a remedy, new aspects of the case may become apparent, leading to more of the case being revealed. More complex, multidimensional cases with symptoms on many levels and themes running through different layers gradually become clearer during treatment. This can make it appear at first as if the disease is getting deeper and new remedies are required. It is important to distinguish between seeing more of the case and the actual disease getting worse. Once the 'full' case is appreciated and the correct treatment started, the case will start to 'clear' and move towards a simpler picture. This is indicated by a change of the existing symptoms following the laws of cure. Sometimes one remedy can help the case over many stages of healing. In other cases the focus of the treatment can change significantly, and the impression of the case and plan of treatment will require regular modification.

In cases where a seemingly well indicated remedy fails to act then a number of factors have to be explored. Most often this happens because the remedy is not similar enough to the patient but other reasons include obstacles to cure, antidoting, insufficient vitality and, occasionally, a failure in potentisation or preparation.

Review of Therapeutic Agreement

At the end of each consultation it is worth being specific about what has changed, and what is being treated. For example, if a patient presents with an apparently simple illness which, when the case is retaken, proves to be more deep-seated and complex, the treatment plan needs to reflect this. The patient should be made aware of the implications of this and that it will lead to re-analyses and new consent etc. The agreement is not a static, legal document – it is a dynamic expression of the relationship intentions of the patient and the homeopath and contains the hopes, expectations and possible remedy reactions. Like the treatment cycle itself, it is evolving and changing.

REFLECTION POINT

- Reflect on a complex case you have seen and think about the different components of the treatment cycle. Which stages are easy and which are hard or unclear? How, as a case gets increasingly confused or hidden, might this change?

Remedy Reactions

When a remedy acts, although symptoms may appear to shift subtly there is invariably a deep and significant shift in the patient's vitality – it is clear to those around the patient that something has moved.

There are many different ways in which a patient may react to a treatment, but the key responses are that the patient is getting better, worse, or staying the same. To decide between these it is important to be clear about how closely the case reflects the patient's true state, and to distinguish between the disease and the patient's well-being. We have already seen that some treatment may help reveal a deeper disease that was not seen before – even though it was there.

Aggravations

It is only possible for a remedy in potency to unveil and reveal a state that already existed in some way before the treatment.

Aggravations, or more properly therapeutic aggravations, are not uncommon phenomena in homeopathic prescribing. They indicate that the individual is responding to the medication by generating or increasing the symptoms, which in homeopathy are seen as part of the body's way of coping with an illness. They normally consist of a worsening of existing symptoms.

This understanding within homeopathy that the symptoms are the body's effective response to the illness, rather than a failure of that response, is central to our understanding of illness and healing. The duration of any aggravation depends on the time the symptoms have been present, the degree to which they have previously been suppressed or blocked, and the overall vitality or ability of an individual to heal. In acute conditions these aggravations will usually last for minutes or hours; in chronic conditions for days or weeks or, rarely, even months.

Aggravations must be distinguished from deterioration of the patient's illness according to the natural history of the disease process and a worsening of symptoms due to reduction of other medication. Strictly speaking aggravations are a worsening of symptoms already present and must be distinguished from a return of symptoms from the past, a change from a chronic to an acute picture, and proving symptoms (see Chapter 16). In a true aggravation the patient will often give some indication of being better in themselves, either emotionally, mentally or generally, often with an increase in energy or better sleep. This is why it is so useful to establish and record the basic energy state of the patient at the first consultation.

Suppression and Aggravations

One way of thinking of aggravations is the clearing out of things which are stopping the person from being well, e.g. a patient who had been smoking for many years developed catarrh, going on for several months, after taking a remedy. In patients with much suppression or contributory life style factors there is likely to be prolonged aggravation. In the treatment of drug addiction a period of detoxification can go on for some time, during which the patient may need a great deal of support. Patients with inhalant, contact or food sensitivity will have less aggravation by minimising exposure to the substances to which they are sensitive. After the homeopathic treatment has been completed, they can often tolerate exposure without reaction. It is as if the remedy initially 'unmasks' sensitivity – indeed, this unmasking is similar to the revealing of hidden cases that is discussed in Section VI. In cases with much suppression or that are likely to aggravate, using LM potencies (see Chapter 20) lessens the likelihood of an aggravation.

The key thing to understand homeopathically is that, as a general rule, an aggravation is a sign that a remedy has acted. When a patient comes and says 'Since I took this remedy this, this and this have been worse' the first response of the homeopath is 'Good!'.

Some patients will seek relief for aggravations with modest medicinal and life style palliation. Others may use a great deal of palliation and suppressive medication and in these cases, it may lead to the expected improvement from a homeopathic medication being lost. This is particularly noticeable in higher potency remedies prescribed on subtler indication and may lead to a well indicated remedy being considered to have failed to act. Following an aggravation, new symptoms may emerge, and it may be necessary to retake and re-analyse the case. If patients are not expecting or are unable to tolerate an aggravation they may drop out of treatment – and when they later get an improvement, they fail to attribute this to the remedy.

Managing Aggravations

When patients have a severe aggravation, first seek to understand if the reaction is one that fits with your understanding of the case. If so, support the patient and encourage them to work through it. Second, review the different causative and contributing factors; if advice has not already been given on these then suggest environmental and life style modification, particularly if there are maintaining causative factors. Third, consider local symptomatic (homeopathic) treatment for the aggravation, e.g. Calendula tincture in an eczema flare-up or Valerian tincture for an anxiety state.

It is in such cases that good rapport and contracting enable the patient to come back to the homeopath, rather than give up on a treatment they feel made their symptoms worse. It is not uncommon for a patient who has had an aggravation to 'give up' on a homeopath, only to then try another therapy or homeopath. And when the aggravation settles and they get better they often fail to attribute it to the first homeopath!

If the aggravation symptoms do not settle then it may represent a remedy that has acted only partially or not deeply enough. In this case repeating the remedy at a much higher potency may complete the action of the remedy.

In a small minority of patients where aggravations cause significant and or prolonged distress with no sign of abatement then the aggravation may be antidoted. This may be achieved either with a specific homeopathic antidote, different for each homeopathic medicine, or by using a general antidote – either material or homeopathic doses of strong aromatic substance like Eucalyptus, Camphor, Mint or strong coffee. Different practitioners seem to favour different ways of antidoting and I suggest initially it is helpful to get advice in management of cases that have a prolonged aggravation.

My personal experience is that about 10% of cases get an aggravation that causes them concern and may need some short-term support. Of these, about 10% require treatment, mostly either simple life style modification or local treatment. A small number may require the use of the same remedy in higher potency, which completes the action of the remedy (see Chapter 16). In those where it does not, then using strong aromatic substances can 'switch off' the aggravation. While diminishing the activity of the remedy and reducing the aggravation, they do allow some subsequent improvement.

For the newcomer to homeopathic prescribing in chronic diseases one of the most frequent causes of spoiling a case, when all the hard work has been done, is to move from a correct remedy because of an aggravation or healing crises.

Follow-up

Remedies provide the information needed by the individual to heal. After a first prescription has acted then the case will have changed. If the remedy provides all the information then a complete recovery is possible, although the journey back to health may go through several stages. If the first remedy does not provide any information that resonates with the case then nothing happens – and the case needs re-taking and re-analysis to find a first prescription that will act. If it provides some of the information needed there is a partial recovery and a picture of the new state can be seen. Sometimes symptoms become clearer and others are brought to the surface, in which case further time may continue to improve things. If and when this process fails to progress in a healing direction a second prescription is needed (see Chapter 16).

If the new state that is revealed is deeper after the first prescription then the case is still being clarified and in some ways the first prescription can be understood as part of revealing the full case before the case is clear. This often has to happen in confused and hidden cases. The aim of the homeopathic treatment process is the gradual reduction of symptoms and return to health. This involves a clarification of the case, a surfacing of old, often suppressed, symptoms, and gradual recovery. It is important to remember to take account not only

of the response of the presenting symptoms but the overall well-being of the individual.

Remember that when a patient feels better at the deepest level do not change the treatment until it has fully acted. That is, do not give a second remedy unless a symptom picture is clear – this usually requires the previous remedy to have completed its action. It may take as long to reverse the case as it has taken to build up.

Obstacles to Cure

'Man's freedom to enjoy consciousness is affected by disease. Life's aim is to get rid of self made obstacles to health.'

James Tyler Kent

When a well-indicated remedy fails to act, something effectively blocks the remedy from acting – this is referred to as an 'obstacle to cure'. A common obstacle is a maintaining cause, but a number of other factors commonly influence a remedy's action. While in different patients and for different remedies these can be diverse and idiosyncratic, there are some general or common obstacles (Box 15.2). One practical way of categorising them is as physical, emotional or psychological. Obstacles to cure can also cause a well-indicated remedy to act slowly or incompletely. When a remedy acts partially, it may help its full action to be seen if the relevant obstacles can be reduced or removed. This is another reason why the homeopath is advised to have a broad understanding of those factors that influence a patient's health.

At times illness may remove the patient from the obstacle; it is only when they start getting better that they come into contact with it again. The illness may be the patient's way of making the changes necessary to avoid a cause or an obstacle to cure. This can lead to a relapsing pattern of illness, e.g. a patient who is stressed at work may relapse whenever they are well enough to return to work. In this way illness is one way that we monitor our lives and seek out a balanced state with our life situation. At other times it is when we get ill that we are brought into contact with obstacles to cure, so a patient who is taking

BOX 15.2
Common Obstacles to Cure

Physical Obstacles
- Mechanical – such as trauma or poor posture
- Antipathic or allopathic drugs
- Exposure to harmful or antidoting chemicals
- Caffeine
- Poor diet or nutritional deficiency,* over-eating
- Inadequate or excessive exercise
- Sexual restraint or excess
- Use of recreational drugs
- Lack of fresh air
- Extremes of temperatures, weather, draughts etc.

Psychological Obstacles
- Sabotaging any treatment (patient does not want to be well)
- Secondary gains
- Fixed ideas
- Patients unwilling to admit they have been helped
- Psychotherapeutic work running counter to laws of cure
- Intolerance of any remedy reaction
- Pride and arrogance often masking the true depth of the case
- Fear of the unknown leading to reluctance to explore the case

Emotional Obstacles
- Dependency
- Deep insecurity
- Deep emotional traumas
- Bullying behaviour (victim or persecutor)
- Over sensitive people who suffer constant calamity
- Ostracised by society
- Emotional exhaustion or 'burnout'

*Using the analogy of a building, for healing to take place it requires both the information of what goes where (the architect's plan), provided by the remedies, and the actual building materials, that might include such things as adequate nutrition, etc.

antipathic drugs will not fully respond to the correct homeopathic remedy. Hence the need for the homeopath to have an overview of all treatments a patient is likely to be taking.

If a maintaining cause or obstacle continues over much time it can traumatise the body or mind to the extent that it takes a significant time to heal, even after the cause or obstacle is removed. During this time a cure will not be possible and the vital force can become depleted. For example, post-traumatic stress can cause problems for some time after the stress and it may require this aetiology to be specifically treated before other remedies can act. Even after they have been corrected some causes, such as nutritional deficiencies may continue to influence the body for years. Animal studies show that the effects can carry on for generations after the deficiency is corrected. This gives a hint to the long-term treatment necessary for hereditary illness and the benefit for future generations of treating illness fully in this generation!

In many cases it can be difficult to distinguish between factors that prevent the case from being seen or factors that in some way block the remedy from acting. In practice these can be considered as much the same. For example, a patient taking corticosteroids for asthma may lose many of the modalities that would help indicate a remedy. It is this, more than the absolute obstacle or antidoting factor, which makes prescribing the simillimum difficult.

Managing Patients With Obstacles to Cure
While identifying and reducing possible obstacles to cure is an important part of managing patients, it must be remembered that it frequently takes time for a remedy to act fully. In many cases it is important for the patient to be supported in their symptoms while a deep-acting remedy acts. Such support needs to be offered in a way that minimises the potential obstacles to cure. This may involve treatment using more than one model of health at the same time. If the models of health are clearly distinguished and appropriate potencies of remedies used, my experience is that patients may

Totality and Constitution

III

receive symptom relief with homeopathic remedies while undergoing concurrent deeper treatment. If local homeopathic treatments are likely to block deeper-acting remedies or make interpreting the response to treatment unclear, it is preferable to use herbal or naturopathic remedies – or even conventional treatments. How patients are managed using inter-current treatments is one of the most controversial areas of practice.

Sometimes aggravations and healing reactions can be sufficiently strong to necessitate support for the patient in their own right. So a patient with eczema may get an increase in discharge or a flare up of symptoms when a deeper allergic sensitivity is being dealt with. Patients will often need supporting through such temporary deteriorations of symptoms and there are several ways of doing this – including the use of local treatments for support of eczema such as Calendula or Graphites cream and reduction of causative factors.

New Symptoms

There are a number of reasons why patients might experience new or modified symptoms in response to taking a course of homeopathic treatment; these are described below. After prescribing a remedy it is important to note any new symptoms.

Perception of the Case Deepening

Initially new symptoms might become visible because the case is being seen more deeply; these are not new symptoms or constitutional features to the patient but become newly recognised. At times the degree of suppression is such that too much of the case is masked to see it clearly – so the suppression and state it sets up needs to be treated first. It can involve organ support for organs required to clear the suppression or repair of organs detrimentally affected by the suppression (often the same organs) using organ remedies. Or it may mean specifically working to reverse the suppressed state by reducing or stopping the suppressive medication (with appropriate care) and prescribing on the suppressed state, e.g. using isopathic treatment (see Chapter 5).

Coincidental Symptom Changes

New symptoms may arise during the course of any treatment, coincidental to any medication being taken – these occur for a variety of causes unrelated to taking the medication. An indication of whether symptoms might be unrelated to any medication taken will be obtained from any chronological link between new symptoms and whether events taking place at the same time could possibly cause those symptoms. Understanding the natural history and epidemiology of disease, and knowledge of pharmacology, are important aids to interpreting the possible causes of change unrelated to the homeopathic intervention – or indeed the failure to respond to it.

Curative Changes

There may be a change of existing symptoms following the laws of cure, including the return of previous symptoms. As the case becomes simpler and clearer it can give a more acute presentation, particularly if those acute symptoms have been a precursor of the case. Chronic illness healing after, or being displaced by, an acute illness is well documented. This phenomenon is sometimes known as 'syndrome shift'.

Proving Symptoms

At times new symptoms emerge that were not seen in the case before or are a more superficial manifestation of a previous deeper symptom. If these symptoms are in the materia medica of the remedy given, then they may be similar to 'proving symptoms' – and indicate a close affinity between case and remedy. More patients show proving symptoms the more a remedy is repeated, but if used judiciously then the stronger or more peculiar the reaction, the stronger the indication in favour of that remedy. Proving symptoms can also develop when a remedy is a close match to a case but not close enough to bring about a therapeutic reaction. The longer the remedy is repeated the more likely this is to happen. They may indicate that the prescription was close and that a related remedy may be a more accurate prescription.

Totality and Constitution

If new symptoms are not a return of old symptoms or proving symptoms then they are revealing a shift in the case that needs re-taking and re-analysing to include the new symptoms.

Return of Old Symptoms

When old symptoms return it is invariably a good sign and the patient can be reassured. If the hierarchy of the case is understood it will be clear why old symptoms have returned. While the picture is still emerging it is prudent to wait, as sometimes the symptoms will clear of their own accord, leaving the patient substantially improved. If the symptoms become fixed, then this will indicate a new remedy that may be related to the previous one.

Summary

In this chapter we have explored homeopathic treatment as a process and journey back into wellness. We are starting to move from homeopathy in relation to tasks and towards seeing it as a process. As we move on to explore strategies to help with difficult cases, we extend this further. The vital role that suppression plays in the manifestation of the totality in establishing the constitution has been further explored in this chapter.

The chapter went on to look at the 'treatment cycle' and to identify those stages or phases of treatment that are repeated often cyclically (or perhaps spirally) over the course of time. Some patients may only attend for a single consultation and not even receive a prescription; others will go through the cycle several or many times, using one or many different prescriptions and using various models of health and approaches to treatment. Although the separating out into stages creates an artificial perception of the treatment cycle, it is a valuable way of examining the component parts, so that you can explore and develop each in turn.

This naturally leads us to consider the remedy reactions that a patient may manifest and whilst some of these were included in this chapter, they are discussed in more detail in the context of the second prescription in Chapter 16.

Bibliography

Chappell P 2005 The second simillimum: a disease-specific complement to individual treatment. Homeolinks, Haren, The Netherlands

Eizayaga F X 1992 Treatise on homoeopathic medicine. Ediciones Marecel, Buenos Aires

Hahnemann S trans Dudgeon R E 1852 The lesser writings of Samuel Hahnemann. W Headland, London. Indian edition 1995. B Jain Publishers, New Delhi

Henriques N 1998 Crossroads to cure, the homeopath's guide to second prescription. Totality Press, St Helena

Norland M, Robinson C 2003 Signatures, miasms aids: spiritual aspects of homeopathy. Yondercott Press, Cullompton, Devon

Speight P 1961 A comparison of the chronic miasms. Health Science Press, Rustington

Totality and Constitution

III

Section IV

Broadening our Understanding

CHAPTER SIXTEEN

The Second Prescription

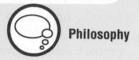 **Philosophy**

David Curtin

Introduction by David Owen

Chapter 15 considered the remedy reaction within the context of managing the complex case, although the principles to following up a case are the same for all cases. In this chapter I have invited David Curtin to look in more detail at the second prescription – and by implication the, third and fourth prescription, etc. We move beyond the realm of one prescription fitting each case from start to finish. As you tackle increasingly complex, confused and hidden cases you will face the challenge of moving from finding a single intervention to understanding and guiding a treatment process. Grasping the principles of the second prescription is about understanding what happens to a patient and their vitality when they receive a remedy that acts. Like the thread through a necklace made up of a series of precious stones, the process holds the remedies together as a whole. Conceptualising and navigating through a plan of treatment opens up the management of cases that would otherwise be incurable.

The First Follow-Up

At the first follow-up consultation the prescriber has the opportunity to assess the progress the patient has made and whether or not the remedy given has acted. The timing of this consultation must be carefully chosen. Sufficient time must be allowed for the remedy to produce some changes and allow the case to shift if it is going to. Waiting too long allows the patient to forget any early changes or, if the illness is not improving, to become impatient. If an explanation of the interval between consultations is not given, the patient may lose confidence in the homeopath. A period of 3–4 weeks will be about right for most complex cases and chronic illness, but acute illness may respond quickly and simple cases may only require a much shorter time scale in order for the picture to change.

Follow-Up of the Complex Case or Chronic Illness

Many cases are spoiled or confused by inappropriate prescriptions at the first follow-up, usually due either to a lack of understanding or not taking proper care. There are a number of questions which one needs to ask oneself:

1. What has the effect of the first prescription really been?
2. Has the remedy acted, and if so has it acted curatively?
3. Was it the simillimum or a partial similar?
4. Which symptoms have improved? Are any symptoms worse? Are there any new symptoms?
5. Does the patient feel better? Has the patient's energy improved?
6. Has the remedy completed its action? If not, no remedy may be needed at this point.
7. Was the action good enough to warrant a repetition of the remedy? Should the remedy be changed? Or is no remedy needed?
8. Does the potency need to be changed?

Taking the Case at the First Follow-Up

As at the first consultation, the patient must be given the opportunity to speak freely – questions asked should initially be open questions. If this approach does not give you all the information you require you may need to ask increasingly specific questions. You need to know whether there have been changes to the case at any level including feelings, behaviour, thoughts, energy, sleep, desires and aversions, as well as specific symptoms.

It is then helpful to ask for a day by day, or week by week account of the changes of symptoms in order to establish a clear time line – it is especially important for the first few days after the remedy was given. Explaining this and asking patients to note these early changes at their initial consultation can help. It is useful to give this in writing as verbal instructions are frequently forgotten in the intensity of the first visit. It can also help if the patient writes a daily record, like a diary, of the response. Without this, patients will often jump about in time when recounting their symptoms, making it difficult to get a clear view of what has actually happened. Asking for a score out of 10 for each symptom (for example, when zero would be no problem and 10 would be the worst imaginable) at each consultation, enables a comparison with previous consultations. It can help to actually record changes 'over' or 'alongside' the original case record, possibly in a different coloured pen, building a sort of three-dimensional record.

Analysing the Information

Knowing whether the remedy has truly acted curatively requires careful assessment of all the information the patient gives you. You cannot simply take what the patient tells you at face value.

Change or No Change?

It is surprising, when getting better, how a patient can forget they ever had a symptom, so distressing when they first presented.

Some patients will report that the remedy has definitely worked and that they feel a lot better when, after detailed questioning, you discover that nothing much has changed. This can be because

the patient has great faith in homeopathy or in the prescriber, and is convinced that the treatment is working. Others may report that nothing has happened, that everything is the same, when in fact there have been major shifts. Perhaps even the presenting symptoms are no longer present. This can be because the patient is sceptical and reluctant to admit that the treatment has had any effect. More commonly it is simply that the symptoms with which they presented have gone and they have forgotten about them often because other aspects of the case have been revealed. This may seem strange, but the curative process can be so subtle that sometimes the patient is unaware that the remedy is acting or the picture 'evolving'. Vithoulkas' (1978) description of this process, 'The follow-up interview', is excellent and is essential reading.

Inter-Current Events

Other factors which must be taken into consideration when assessing changes include any substantial deviation from the patient's usual routine. Going on holiday after taking the remedy, or a crisis in the family such as a death, or any other major change planned before the patient took the remedy, or an external event beyond the patient's control all make assessing the effects of the remedy difficult. Any major change initiated after the patient has taken the remedy must, of course, be considered a possible reaction to the remedy, such as the patient suddenly deciding to take a holiday, or buying something they have always wanted, or ending a relationship, or perhaps starting a new relationship. Careful consideration of every event is important as even something seemingly beyond the patient's influence – such as getting the sack at work, or getting a new job, or meeting a new partner – may be the result of the action of the remedy and indeed may be central to the curative process. Changes in prescribed or over-the-counter (OTC) conventional medication and changes due to the natural history of the disease process must also be considered.

Thus in order to make a valid assessment of the effect of a remedy it is necessary to have a clear understanding of what constitutes cure in general, and also in this patient in particular. This means you will need to understand what needs to be cured in the patient, and also how cure may proceed under the influence of a homeopathic medicine. It includes an understanding of the hierarchy of symptoms, and the nature of an organism's reaction to homeopathic medicines – of which aggravation, amelioration, and direction of cure are all a part. These issues have been covered in preceding chapters.

Re-Taking the Case

If it becomes clear that you do not have the information you need to find a good remedy for the patient you will need to re-take the case. What this will involve will vary hugely from case to case and the model of health you are using. It depends what is missing – it could be a simple modality or it could be something profound. If you think that the patient may have withheld some important information you will need to elicit this somehow. The patient may not know what it is that you need to know, so it is not necessarily just a question of asking them what they have left out. Sometimes, however, this may be what you need to do. It is not surprising that a patient may have not told you some deeply personal fact about themselves at the first consultation. It may take time for them to trust you enough for this to happen. All your case-taking skills will be needed for this.

Follow-Up of Simple Case

The principles are exactly the same here as for complex cases. The only difference is the time scale. Hours become the equivalent of weeks, so whereas you may have the first follow-up in a chronic illness after 4 weeks, in an acute illness you may have the first follow-up after 4 hours. The exact timing will depend on the case and may be shorter or longer than this. Certainly you can expect to see changes within minutes or even seconds in some cases such as a child with a high fever due to otitis media or tonsillitis, or a teething child that is screaming. In the case of a cough that has been going on for a few days you may follow-up after a day or two.

Remedy Reactions

Having taken the case and analysed the information, the prescriber must come to a conclusion regarding what the effect of the remedy has been (see Chapter 15) and make a decision about what the second prescription (if any) should be, taking into account the plan of treatment they had in mind. There are many possible scenarios, and it is impossible to describe each and every situation. A clear understanding of the homeopathic process is essential for the prescriber to make an informed decision at this point. It is possible to give some general guidelines – I will do so under some broad headings.

No Reaction

If there has been no change at all the homeopath must consider the following possible reasons for this.

Dud Remedy

The remedy has not been medicated for some reason (pharmacy error). Or the remedy may have been exposed to strong sunlight over time and been inactivated

The Patient Did not Take the Remedy

This could be for a number of different reasons. They may have forgotten to take it, it may not have arrived in the post, they may have lost it, or they may have been suspicious of the remedy and not wanted to take it. There are many other possible reasons and it is always worth checking the patient's compliance.

Slow-Acting Remedy

Some remedies are known to be slow to act, and may be especially likely to be slow in certain cases. Kent describes a case where Silica produced one of the best homeopathic reactions he had seen, but it took 6 months before there was any effect. In modern life it is unlikely that either the homeopath or the patient will wait this long, but fortunately such a long wait is rarely needed although some remedies, e.g. Silica, do often take longer to act than others.

Wrong Remedy

If you suspect this is the reason the next step is to go back to the case and study it again. It may be that you already have a shortlist of close remedies and it is then simply a matter of choosing the best remedy on the list. Otherwise you may need to re-analyse the case. You may decide that the case you have is inadequate and you may then have to re-take the case (see below).

Wrong Potency

Most patients will respond to some degree to any potency if the remedy is correct or at least a close similar, even though the ideal potency will work best. Occasionally a patient may be sensitive only to a narrow potency range but this is fairly unusual.

Remedy Antidoted

The remedy may be antidoted either by accident or on purpose. Antidoting factors may include a visit to the dentist, strong coffee, other medicines, a big shock or accident. None of these will always antidote, and even if they do the effect of the remedy may pick up after a day or two.

Types of Curative Reaction

Prescribing the most closely matched remedy (or simillimum) is ideally what the homeopath aims for in every case, although finding this can be difficult for a number of reasons. The case may not be clear, or may not be properly understood by the prescriber. There may be no remedy in the homeopathic materia medica that closely matches the case as it may have been inadequately proved or not be properly represented in the repertory. Different methodologies may point to different remedies, several of which might be close, but only one is the simillimum. When the simillimum is prescribed it will, if it is not blocked, produce a reaction. The patient may just get better or may experience a homeopathic aggravation usually followed by amelioration.

The nature, intensity and duration of an aggravation will vary from case to case. It will be influenced by the potency of the remedy given, the sensitivity of the patient, and also on the nature and duration of the pathology. Where there are structural changes in important organs, there is a greater possibility of serious or prolonged aggravation – in these cases I usually prescribe a lower potency in order to minimise the aggravation. In some cases it may take longer for the aggravation to begin after the remedy has been given, in others if the aggravation is only slight it instead goes on for longer. Some of the possible different reactions are summarised in Figure 16.1.

Aggravation

The true simillimum could be said to be exactly the right remedy in exactly the right potency. In such a case the aggravation (see Chapter 15) may be so subtle as to be hardly noticeable. A higher potency may produce quite a strong aggravation of symptoms, but even so the patient may not mind as they will say that they feel better despite the aggravation and the aggravation is over more quickly.

A potency that is low may also produce an aggravation. This may occasionally be prolonged or happen each time the low potency is repeated and a higher potency may be needed to complete the cure. This may seem paradoxical. One way of looking at it is to think of the remedy as stimulating the patient sufficiently to react but not strongly enough that this reaction is followed by amelioration. John's case illustrates this.

CASE STUDY 16.1

John, age 9, was brought to see me with behaviour problems. He also had warts. His health had otherwise been good for the previous two years. Mother and father were separated. He was a very intense boy. According to his mother, he would go totally berserk if he was angry. He was very jealous, particularly if his mother had a friend round. He was also jealous of his younger brother whom he bullied and would thump very hard. At school he was bullied. At home he was the bully. He was cautious, and fearful, especially of being alone. He was given Nux Vomica 200, single dose.

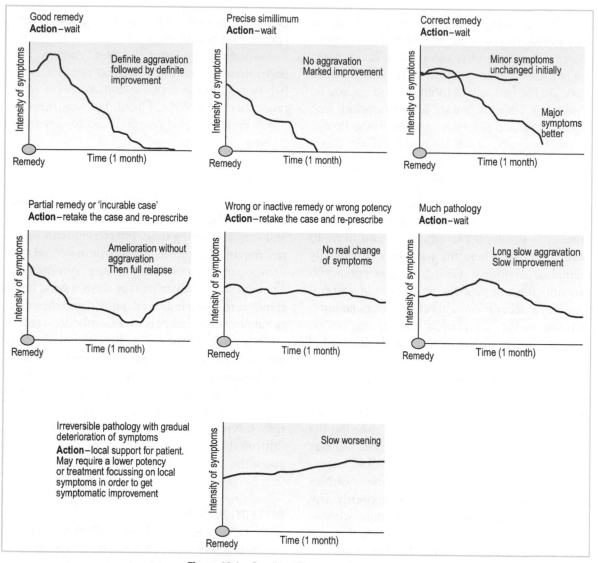

Figure 16.1 Possible different curative reactions

First follow-up was two months later. He was much better emotionally, was full of energy. He was 'glowing', as his mother put it. His warts had gone. One got much bigger and then fell off, the others disappeared.

Nine months later in mid-September his mother brought him back to see me as he had been getting angry a lot – screaming furies. He was wetting the bed, which made him cross. He had been fine until he started school. He described his new teacher as being a pain. He was given Nux Vomica 200 single dose. Two weeks later his mother phoned and said that he had been worse after the remedy with no sign of improvement. I suggested that she give him four doses of Nux Vomica 6. She phoned again 10 days later to say that he had been temporarily better after the Nux Vomica 6, but worse again since. I prescribed Nux Vomica 1M. He was even angrier for 2 days after and then became very much better.

The following October, one year later, he began wetting the bed every night. He was really angry about it and would not talk about it. He used obscene language as if he was trying to shock. He had lots of tantrums and socially he was shy. He was grubby and dishevelled, also lazy, but could not bear disorder in the house. Everything was unfair. He had been very much better for a long time after Nux Vomica 1M. I prescribed Nux Vomica 1M.

He was worse after the Nux Vomica 1M and remained so, but I had no contact with him or his mother until 1 month later. He was prescribed Nux Vomica 10M. He was quickly much improved and remained so for another 2 years.

The main learning points from John's case are that you can get a prolonged aggravation if the potency is not high enough. It is more likely to occur in a case where the pathology is primarily mental or emotional. Giving a higher potency in this situation will push the patient out of aggravation into amelioration. This at first seems counter-intuitive to the observation that an aggravation is more severe if the potency is higher rather than low.

If you do get a prolonged aggravation in a case, you may rightly be concerned that giving a higher potency may make the situation worse. If there are maintaining causes or the remedy is close but not close enough then this may be the case. You may have noticed that before giving a higher potency of Nux Vomica, I first gave a few doses of Nux Vomica 6 which relieved – albeit temporarily. This is a useful strategy to help you determine whether more of the remedy is needed, or whether you have already given too much. If a few doses of 6 or 30 potency aggravate further then you should give no more of that remedy. If you get amelioration, even if it does not last, you then know that more of the remedy is needed. I use the words 'more' and 'less' here simply to indicate that further doses are required, and you can be confident that higher potency will work better.

The patient's vitality is another factor that will influence the nature of the aggravation. A patient with a strong vitality may have a strong aggravation, which comes on quickly (hours to a few days), lasts a relatively short period of time (again hours to a few days) and without long-lasting ill effects. A patient with a weak vitality may have a difficult aggravation that they do not tolerate well. It may come quickly, or it may take some time to appear and may last a long time. Interfering with such a reaction by making other prescriptions could spoil such a patient's possibility of cure. Alternatively, a patient with low vitality may show a good initial response to a well indicated remedy, and then deteriorate because vitality is so seriously depleted.

In severely ill patients, where the aim of care may be 'terminal care', a patient can get a dramatic improvement in symptoms (mentals, generals and locals) and find a more contented state. This improved state may be at the expense of long-term survival with worse symptoms. Weighing this difficult balance raises important ethical issues about the intention of treatment.

REFLECTION POINT

- How will you respond to the ethical dilemmas such as how fully will you warn patients about an aggravation and will you always tell the patient what you are prescribing? How do you feel about treating patients for terminal care? These and other questions will benefit from being fully discussed with colleagues and teachers.

It is important to understand that cure is a process and may take some time and several successive prescriptions to complete – if indeed complete cure is possible. In difficult cases the remedy can act to clarify and reveal a case, showing a new picture and the need for different simillimum. There is much discussion about whether this means a first remedy is just a similar, not the simillimum, and if, in a confused and hidden case, it is possible to find at the first visit a simillimum that covers all aspects of the case – even those disguised or hidden in the case. Perhaps it is more useful to think of the simillimum as a dynamic state that can evolve in the individual as a confused or hidden case becomes clear.

Aggravations need to be distinguished from healing reactions that might include the case being expressed through more superficial symptoms or from previous unresolved symptoms. Skin eruptions in particular may return or occur as healing progresses at a deeper level. Mental and emotional symptoms frequently improve alongside or before physical symptoms. Symptoms disappearing in the reverse order to which they appeared sometimes bring a transient return of old symptoms.

Remember the importance of differentiating between return of old symptoms and the appearance of new symptoms (see Chapter 15). The patient may not always clearly remember old symptoms – it is helpful to ask the patient specifically when a symptom appears to try and remember if they have had it before. Often the return of old symptoms is fleeting and may even appear in a dream. This kind of recall can include emotional symptoms and the patient may dream of the original cause of an emotional upset or fear, after which the problem may be resolved. Old symptoms which reappear may be the revealing of a deeper layer or other level that will not go so quickly if it is not also covered by the remedy.

Partial Relapse

When some time has passed after a successful first prescription and the patient gets a slight return of one or more symptoms – but overall remains well with the main symptom remaining better – you may wonder whether to repeat the remedy. In such cases, rather than waiting for a full relapse a few doses of the same remedy in a lower potency may be all that is needed to restore the patient to health.

A Changing Picture

If repetition of the original remedy no longer has an effect, despite having tried different potencies

or if a new remedy picture has emerged then it is the time to change the remedy. But be cautious unless or until a different remedy picture has become clear. The symptoms of the first remedy will mostly have gone, so long as that remedy was the simillimum at that time. You may have had glimpses of this remedy earlier, but it is better to wait for this picture to become clear in order to avoid choosing the wrong remedy, and also to get the maximum benefit from the previous remedy. This will make your work simpler in the long run. Changing the remedy is discussed in more detail later (see Chapter 27).

Partially Curative – Partial Similar

In much homeopathic practice it is probable that the majority of prescriptions are partial similars, also known as just 'similars'. Frequently this is all that is possible when time is limited or in a confused or hidden case as not all the symptoms are apparent. Similars can assist the healing process just as the simillimum can; however, it may take several such remedies to complete the process. Homeopathy would probably die as a profession if this were not the case. The following are characteristic of the effect of a similar remedy:

1. Cures some symptoms and not others.
2. Action weakens when the remedy is repeated
3. Symptom picture may be different when the effect of the remedy wears off.
4. Partial proving – new symptoms appear that are in the materia medica of the remedy given (as opposed to old symptoms returning).

How well the remedy will act will depend on how closely similar the remedy is to the case. A remedy that is a very close similar may act almost as well as the simillimum. A remedy that has only a slight similarity to the case may have little or no action. Working with similars is slower, more complex, and involves several changes of remedy but it may be all that is possible with some patients, and with the repertoire of remedies available to or known by the homeopath. It requires close observation of the patient and careful thinking over a period of time in order to make good progress.

Broadening our Understanding

IV

It is helpful to think of the match of remedies as a spectrum between no match and complete match. If the remedy is closely similar the overall effect should be beneficial and there may be the classic homeopathic aggravation followed by amelioration of symptoms. There may be one or two new symptoms appearing, but they should not be troublesome and will soon pass off. The patient will usually be pleased with the result.

If the remedy has only a slight similarity to the case there may still be improvement in some symptoms. There is less likely to be an improvement in overall well-being of the patient except possibly for a day or two. This can be confusing for the inexperienced prescriber as the patient may report that they felt a lot better for the first couple of days and then relapsed to the previous state. The patient's view may then be that the remedy was good but it didn't last. The patient may ask for a stronger or more frequent dose. In such a case repetition is unlikely to be of much benefit. On the contrary, new symptoms may appear after such a partial similar, not necessarily after the first dose but if the remedy is repeated new (proving) symptoms, typical of the remedy but not of the patient, may appear. In some cases these proving symptoms may be burdensome and persistent, requiring an antidote. Patients who are sensitive and react easily to stimuli are more likely to develop proving symptoms.

One way of looking at similars is to think of an archery target, the bull's eye being the goal, which is equivalent to the simillimum. Close similars are in the ring surrounding the bull's eye, partial similars in the outer ring. Remedies that have no effect whatsoever have missed the target completely. While the bull's eye or simillimum is the goal it cannot be achieved in every case. Hitting somewhere within the target range much of the time is a reasonable expectation. Remember also that the remedy is only part of the homeopathic process. Every aspect of the patient's encounter with the homeopath can be therapeutic, including taking the case, and discussing life style options and other management strategies (of which homeopathic intervention is only one part) with the patient (see

Chapter 25). However, the goal of the simillimum can keep the homeopath focused at all times on the best match of remedy to patient.

Deterioration – Negative Change

The most common reason for a patient deteriorating is the natural progression of the disease, but it is important to be aware that a homeopathic medicine can occasionally be responsible for the worsening of a patient's condition. This may take the form of a prolonged aggravation of specific symptoms or a decline in the patient's energy and well-being if vitality is already compromised. In these cases a choice has to be made whether to wait to see if a new picture emerges or if the remedy should be antidoted (see 'Antidoting' in Chapter 15). A general decline can also be brought about by prescribing too high a potency in a patient with a very weak vitality – usually associated with prolonged, severe and suppressed chronic disease. Care is always needed in prescribing for such cases. While homeopathy is a subtle form of treatment its effects are very real and it is not helpful to patients or the student homeopath to think that indiscriminate prescribing can do no harm.

Prescribing the Next Dose

If the first remedy was the simillimum then when the patient relapses the remedy may be repeated either in the same or a different potency. In my experience the same potency will usually act well for two or three repetitions (more in long-standing cases if the remedy suits the case deeply) after which the potency may need to be changed. One indication when to change is how long each repetition of the same potency acts. If it lasts longer than the previous one, the remedy is still accurate and acting deeper. If shorter, another remedy state may be emerging. Common practice is for the potency to be increased, usually by one step, e.g. from 200 to 1M, or from 1M to 10M. Usually this will work well. Occasionally I have found that increasing the potency has not worked, as Jean's case illustrates, but I think this is the exception rather than the rule.

CASE STUDY 16.2

Jean, age 49, had presented with rheumatoid arthritis and had responded well to Sulphur 1M, single dose. She felt better in herself quite quickly, and there was a gradual improvement in her joint symptoms until they were about 60% better. The improvement lasted nearly five months, after which she relapsed. She felt flat and the joint pains were getting worse.

I repeated Sulphur 1M and saw her 1 month later when she reported, 'Everything has gone wrong'. She had a headache like she had never had before, and then 3 hours after the remedy she vomited, which made the headache worse. She was then fantastic for a week, joint pains were very much better, but it was downhill from there on. This scenario suggests, of course, that the remedy was a similar and not the simillimum so I studied the case again to see if another remedy might be more appropriate. Sulphur still seemed to be the best choice so I decided to increase the potency to 10M.

One month after Sulphur 10M Jean reported that she had a slight improvement in the first week, and then she felt worse again. She also said that she felt on the verge of a cold all the time, always tired. At this point the case for changing the remedy is growing stronger. However, in view of the excellent response of the first dose of Sulphur 1M, and the lack of an obvious new remedy to give her, I decided to persist with Sulphur and gave her a 200 potency.

After the 200 potency Jean had a remarkable improvement. She felt much better within 2–3 days and her joint symptoms were 90% better for the first 2 weeks. She remained a lot better for 8 months, although not as good as 90%. After 8 months she was relapsing again. Sulphur 200 was repeated, with no effect after 6 weeks. I then gave her Sulphur 1M which worked very well, all symptoms much better within 2 days. 'You have hit the nail on the head' she said. The improvement lasted 7 months, albeit with a few ups and downs along the way. Sulphur 1M repeated – no effect. Sulphur 10M given – no effect. Sulphur 200 given – better for 1 month. Sulphur 1m given again, no effect. Sulphur 200 given again – slight improvement for the first 10 days, then a lot better: 'I've improved nicely – lovely' she said. This improvement lasted for several months.

The pattern of prescribing in Jean's case continued for a further 2 years, after which I lost touch with the patient. The main learning points from this case are:

1. Increasing the potency is not your only option and is not always the right thing to do. A lower potency may be needed and may act better. Ideally the potency of the remedy should be matched to the patient's need – this need can move in either direction.

2. Do not be in too much of a hurry to change the remedy. The overall outcome of this case was good although not perfect. At no time after the first dose of Sulphur 1M did the patient's symptoms relapse by more than 50%. Her relapses were relative and she never went back to her original state.

If Sulphur had ultimately failed then re-taking the case would have been the next option (see above). Another action I might have taken would have been to prescribe a nosode as an inter-current remedy.

When to Repeat

The patient will often not be permanently cured by the first dose of the simillimum. If this is the case, then when the reaction to the remedy finally wears off some or all of the symptoms will gradually relapse – when they do they will be the same symptoms as before. However, they will usually be less severe than before. J T Kent describes this very clearly in his *Lesser Writings*:

'After the curative impulse has entirely subsided, the symptoms will appear one by one, falling into place to arrange the image of the disease before the intelligent physician for the purpose of cure. If the first prescription was

the simillimum, the symptoms will return, and when they return, asking for the same remedy.'

When the effect of the remedy has clearly worn off it is then time to give another dose of the same remedy (see 'Getting the timing right' below). There is some difference of opinion as to whether the potency should be the same as the first prescription or whether it should be slightly different. Certainly in *The Organon* Hahnemann says that potency should be slightly different – this, however, refers particularly to the LM method of prescribing. Kent is clear that the same potency can be repeated, so long as it continues to act. Certainly in my experience a repetition of the same potency will act well in most such cases, usually for at least two or three repetitions. Any aggravation following the first prescription is likely to be less on repetition, if the simillimum was prescribed.

Change of Potency

After a few repetitions (as and when indicated by the symptoms of the case) the remedy may not act so well, or the duration of action may be shorter. This is the time to consider changing the potency. If the relapsing symptoms remain the same then only the potency, and not the remedy, should be changed. It may be that some new symptoms will appear – these can be the first indication of a new remedy picture emerging. However, the remedy should not be changed at this point; the original remedy should be given in a different potency, usually higher, and will usually work well.

'When the picture comes back unaltered, except by the absence of some one or more symptoms, the remedy should never be changed until a still higher potency has been fully tested, as no harm can come to the case from giving a single dose of a medicine that has exhausted its curative powers. It is even negligence not to do such a thing.'

J T Kent, *Lesser Writings*

Getting the Timing Right

The general rule is that you repeat the remedy when the previous dose has completed its action, that is, when the symptoms recur. But how precise do you have to be with getting the timing right? What happens if you repeat the dose too soon? If you repeat too soon you may cause a proving. This can be a problem because the proving symptoms may make you think the patient needs more of the remedy if you don't understand what is happening. If you wait too long you simply delay the cure – better than prescribing too soon. But you don't have to wait until all the symptoms have returned.

In my experience you can repeat the remedy when the symptoms are beginning to return without causing any harm to the patient. But you need to wait long enough to be sure that the patient is not just having a bad few days or that a different picture is emerging. Most people's symptoms wax and wane a bit and there is no harm in waiting a few days to be sure. The time scale will give you another clue. If it is 3 months since the first prescription and the symptoms are returning then it is highly likely that a repeat is needed. If it is only 2 or 3 weeks and the patient has had a bad week then it may be only a temporary relapse of symptoms and it is better to wait.

Some patients will plateau. That is to say their symptoms have improved, and they feel better, but they have reached a point where they are not making any further progress. After some time has passed the case needs re-taking to ensure there are no blocks to cure and new symptoms have not emerged. If not, then it is reasonable to repeat the remedy. The exact timing of this will vary from case to case.

Changing the Remedy

There are some cases in which one remedy is sufficient, and repetition of the same remedy, perhaps in different potencies, as and when called for by the symptoms, is all that is ever needed. However, many cases will need a change of remedy at some stage. The less the similarity of the first remedy to the case the sooner this will be. I have always strongly expressed the view that if you have given a remedy that is working well, do not be in a hurry to change it (even if it is not the simillimum) as a new remedy picture can take some time to be seen clearly. Often the first remedy will be 'good enough' and over time a cure can be established. I have seen so many cases, some my own, where the remedy has been changed and the second remedy given was not as good as the first. Often the first remedy has not been given enough time to complete its beneficial action. It is easy then to lose sight of the first remedy and keep on changing to yet another remedy – the case then becomes confused. It is not necessarily the patient's symptoms that become confused, but rather the prescriber becomes confused and may end up giving so many different remedies that he cannot see the wood for the trees.

Suppose that you want to drive from London to Leeds and you choose to take the A1. This is not a bad choice, but after 10 miles and several roundabouts you may get impatient with the A1 and think that the M1 would have been better. You may then take the next exit heading towards the M1. This is all well and good and you may reach the M1, which will take you directly to Leeds. However, you may find that the road you have taken passes directly over the M1 and you end up meandering down side roads for ages. You may end up completely lost. At least if you had stayed with the A1 you would have been making good progress towards Leeds. Eventually, of course, the A1 bypasses Leeds, but it will have brought you quite close and at the right moment will give you clear signposts to direct you the rest of the way. This is the equivalent of the perfect time to change the remedy. The A1 will take you no closer. The symptoms of the patient will at this time clearly call for a different remedy.

The next remedy will often be related to the first remedy in some way. It may be a complementary remedy, or one that is known to follow well. Studying the related remedies will usually make it easier for you to find the next remedy when it is called for by the symptoms.

Summary

My intention in this chapter has been to give you clear guidelines that you can work with and which I hope will make your work as a homeopath easier. They are guidelines – not hard and fast rules. Some cases will be simple and require few prescriptions. Others will be more complex and require many prescriptions over time. Every case is unique, and although many will follow the patterns that I have described, there will always be some cases that will be different in one way or another. If you take a logical approach to your work, finding what these differences are and responding appropriately will enable you to find your way through.

Bibliography

Hahnemann S 1842 Organon of the medical art, 6th edn. Based on a translation by Steven Decker, edited and annotated by Wendy Brewster O'Reilly. 1995 Birdcage Books, Washington.

Kent J T 1926 New remedies, clinical cases, lesser writings, aphorisms, and precepts. Ehrart & Karl, Chicago

Vithoulkas G 1978 The science of homeopathy. ASOHM, Athens

Broadening our Understanding

IV

CHAPTER SEVENTEEN

The Chronic Miasms

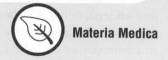 **Materia Medica**

David Lilley

Introduction by David Owen

Recognising that there are traits and patterns that run through patients and that link together remedies was, and still is, a turning point for homeopaths. For the homeopathic profession it enabled an approach to cases that would not respond to prescriptions based solely on presenting (disease) symptoms. For individual homeopaths it provides the tools to move from seeing cases from 'the outside', focusing on the disease state, to grasping the meaning of more complex and otherwise confused cases 'from the inside'. For many, the outer manifestations of disease including the cause, presenting symptom, even the totality, is more familiar than the inner world of the patient's suffering. This inner world touches the patient's constitutional susceptibility, patterns of susceptibility shared by many, and even our own inner state. To help navigate this transition, I am delighted that David Lilley has agreed to share his insight into the miasms – the most historic and useful of the patterns that homeopaths can tap into.

Previous chapters have already introduced the idea of themes within a case and remedy, reflecting and linking together aspects that might otherwise not be seen as clearly. We revisit other thematic ways of looking at cases and remedies in later chapters, but first, it is part of a homeopath's common understanding to see the major miasmatic themes that influence our patients and ourselves. Understanding how unique remedies relate to each other is the next stage in developing a dynamic understanding of the materia medica. These are fundamental to understanding susceptibility, and it is no coincidence that they are linked to the suppression of deeply ingrained, disease states. David sets the groundwork for further study of the miasms (see Chapter 22) and provides a model for seeing miasms as a fundamental and evolving tool for the homeopath ready to take treatment to the inside.

Miasmatic Theory

The highest calling of the homeopathic physician is the facilitation of the individuation process of the patient by harmonising homeopathic therapy with the spiritually healing power of illness.

Possibly the most precious jewel in the homeopathic philosophical crown is the theory of the chronic miasms. It provides us with a profound understanding of the evolution of chronic disease within the animal kingdom, and proves of inestimable value in the clinical assessment of the patient, in planning a strategy of therapy, and in the evaluation of therapeutic response. It also gives clarity, meaning, and relationship to all the many and varied manifestations of disease and their erstwhile arbitrary and disconnected, generic classifications. It invites you to see the essentially beneficent and creative role of disease in the destiny of humanity and its catalytic affect in the unfolding of the spiritual qualities of the individual.

I shall commence by introducing you to the theory of miasms, building on the brief introduction given in Chapter 14. Historically, the concept of the miasms was the chief element in determining and understanding the homeopathic management of chronic disease. Despite modern developments in homeopathic knowledge and diverse methodologies, miasmatic theory remains a major factor in case analysis and a major methodology for prescribing. In elucidating the miasms, I shall take you through the evolution and the cardinal characteristics of the five miasms that play a critical role in how chronic illness manifests. Although only a few remedies can be mentioned here, these do reveal how the materia medica can be understood in the light of the miasms, and illustrate a way of discerning how themes and patterns run through a case. Finally, I wish to show how the miasms relate to each other dynamically, and how perceiving miasmatic evolution as a spiral permits us to anticipate and recognise therapeutic strategies likely to be central in the treatment of new and evolving diseases, such as Aids.

Hahnemann's Miasmatic Theory

Hahnemann observed that despite removing all hindrances to cure, and successfully treating acute conditions, such cases showed a repeated tendency to relapse – presenting either a recurrence of similar or more severe symptoms or, in many instances, the emergence of a changed or different clinical picture. It was as if some underlying condition, which had remained unaddressed by even the most carefully selected and successful remedy, continued on its inexorable course. His experience with cases of chronic disease proved similar – initial improvement would be followed by relapse and previously successful remedies inexplicably lost their efficacy.

Intrigued by these experiences, and still convinced of the validity of the homeopathic principle of cure, with his characteristic thoroughness he set about searching for patterns of disease in patients and in their family histories to explain and solve the problem of this phenomenon. After a period of intensive investigation, his conclusion was that, like waves on a vast ocean, both the manifestations of acute illness and the symptoms and signs of chronic disease were superficial expressions of

a deeper, hidden, destructive force – and that only treatment which addressed this underlying condition would prove permanently curative.

Hahnemann called this a 'miasm', describing the concept of an undermining, pervasive process of contamination or pollution of the system, a blight or stigma, acquired or inherited, which renders the individual susceptible to certain patterns of illness. He identified the presence of three major miasms: the *psoric* miasm, presenting externally by way of an itch or eruption, such as scabies, and the *sycotic* and *syphilitic* miasms, related to the sexually transmitted diseases gonorrhoea and syphilis. After Hahnemann, other researchers identified the *tubercular* miasm, perceived as a combination of psora and syphilis, and *carcinosis*, the cancer miasm – a mixture of the other four miasmatic traits, with one or other miasm dominant.

The Disease Continuum

These fundamental miasmatic patterns are present within all of us in varying degree, influencing our feelings, thoughts, inclinations and behaviour. The miasmatic influence may be subtle or starkly apparent. Other factors that contribute to the unique make-up of the individual, and which are intermeshed with the miasmatic attributes, are endowed and inherited qualities and the effects of situational imprinting and conditioning. These all combine to form filters through which the individual perceives a distorted image of reality. Conclusions, prejudices and responses based on distorted perception or delusion account for much of humanity's strife and misery.

Homeopathic philosophy regards disease as a continuum, or miasmatic sequence, which began in our distant, ancestral past, extending down to us through countless generations. 'The sins of the forefathers visited upon the children' – each generation adding its contribution to the disease legacy. Palliative and suppressive methods of therapy can only add to the continuum and its complexity. Our constitutions may be considered as vessels of water removed from the ever-flowing river of life. Water drawn from the river has been polluted upstream by the fears, grief, angers, jealousies,

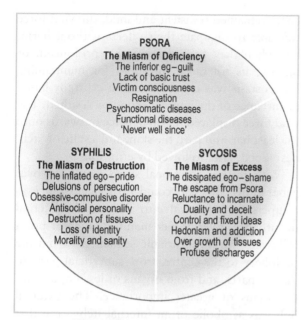

Figure 17.1 The three main miasms

resentments, and hatreds of our forebears, including those of our parents. Our miasmatic state is the product of this pollution, and of our own dysfunctional acting and thinking.

By the same analogy, if the individual is the vessel, the family is the stream, the community is the river and humanity is the ocean. Pollution of the vessel will inevitably pollute the stream, the river, and ultimately the ocean. Conversely, by addressing the causes of pollution in the individual, we are able to modify the distorting, miasmatic filters and positively influence the health, not only of the patient, but also of the family, the community and ultimately of humanity – bestowing a legacy of improved health upon those who come after us. Figure 17.1 gives a diagrammatic representation of the three main miasms.

The Psoric Miasm – The Miasm of Deficiency, Deprivation, and Despair

The name 'psora' derives from the Hebrew word *'tsorat'* meaning a groove or a fault; a pollution or a stigma. These words accurately describe the nature of the psoric miasm. Box 17.1 names a few of the main features of the psora.

The Origin of Psora

'The oldest history of the oldest nation does not reach its origin. Unless it is thoroughly cured, it persists in the organism until the last breath of the longest life. Not even the most robust constitution, by its own unaided efforts, is able to annihilate or extinguish Psora.'

S Hahnemann

BOX 17.1

Major Characteristics of Psora

- Psychosomatic disease; emotions cause functional disease
- Disturbed homeostasis
- Functional disturbances without structural change
- Psora and deficiency are synonymous:
  - food intolerances
  - inability to thrive
  - hunger and food cravings
- Weakness of the vital force – debility, enervation, and lack of stamina
- Lack of vital heat
- Lack of vital reaction:
  - impaired immunity and impaired powers of repair and recuperation
  - well-selected remedies fail to relieve or permanently improve
- Alternating states
- 'Never well since': conditions dating from some previous, sometimes remote, mental, emotional, infective or physically traumatic event
- Conditions following suppression of eruptions or discharges, or suppressed function
- Hypersensitivity of the immune system: the atopic state
- Hypersensitivity of the faculties
- Psoric cases are relieved by skin eruptions and by natural eliminative processes

*'The greatest force to arouse the evils of the psoric dys-
crasia is grief and sorrow.'*

H A Roberts

Psora represents the origin and foundation of disease in the human species, and is reflected in the
animal world, especially in those species which
have been closely associated with humankind. The
miasm is of ancient origin. It is the most fundamental taint and hence has been described as 'the
mother of all disease'. It is the presence of psora
that makes all other diseases or miasms possible. It
is the beginning of the disease continuum.

When archaic man first evolved from his homi-
nid predecessors, he was still an innocent child of
nature, living in harmony with nature's processes
and protected by the instinctive, animal will. There
was no *dis-ease* of miasmatic form. Some 100 000
years ago a vital transition point in human intellectual and emotional evolution was reached –
evidenced by a vastly more sophisticated tool
technology and anatomical changes required for
complex speech. It was this expansion of emotional capacity and cognitive ability that provided
the soil for *dis-ease* and subsequently for psora.

While all animals experience what we understand as basic emotions, it is the ability to feel
and suffer these emotions subjectively, vicariously,
empathetically, and sometimes for an extended
time, which distinguishes the emotional life of
Homo sapiens. Interwoven with these profound
changes came that most wonderful human attribute: the *capacity to love* in that singular and
special way that only humans can. Such a love
intensifies fear of loss, and the grief and bereavement that follow loss. Psora is the inevitable price
of innocence without enlightenment.

Psora and the Vital Force

The cause of psora, and therefore of all endog-
enous, miasmatic disease, originated in the mind
of man with thoughts and emotions, which were
out of step and in conflict with nature's harmony
and balance. These incrementally impinged on
the ordered frequency of the homeostatic vital
force of the body. While these negative influences remained transient and mild, the vital force
was able to dissipate their effects without harm,
but when they proved recurrent, prolonged, or
intense, its tolerance threshold for maintaining
homeostasis was exceeded, and a centrally based
disturbance of the internal economy resulted. The
vital force displaced this imbalance outwards onto
the least harmful part, the skin, and a state of 'itch'
developed, later followed by eruptions.

With further emotional stress, extended over
generations, the skin could no longer suffice as
a superficial safety valve to alleviate the internal
disturbance. Ever-deeper manifestations of psora
followed – in an invariable sequence – from the
periphery to the centre, from superficial parts to
deeper parts, and from organs of less importance
to organs of greater importance. The external
itch was symbolic of an internal itch – the first
susceptibility or vulnerability to disease. All subsequent disease builds on this susceptibility, which
remains as part of the human condition, is inherited, and displays itself in all the many and varied
forms of functional and psychosomatic disorders
characteristic of psora. Only later, with the suppression of these disorders and the admixture of
other miasmatic influences, would disease become
structural.

Because the vital force always seeks to exter-
nalise any dysfunction, diverting it away from
critical organs and systems, the manifestations
of psora are highly vulnerable to suppression.
If suppression should take place, the implosion
of morbid energy will prove detrimental to the
future health of the patient. This is very much the
present situation of humanity – and the consequences are alarming. Modern medicine, heedless
of nature's healing methods, and yielding to expe-
diency, is continually designing ever more sophisticated means of suppressing the manifestations of
disease. The disease continuum is constantly being
intensified.

The Advent of the Sulphur and Psorinum Archetypes

The evolutionary unfolding of the human mind
created circumstances fraught with the potential

for psychosomatic disease. Archaic *Homo sapiens*, like other primates, was at one with his environment and compatible with his peers. Dominance was strictly hierarchical; aggression and submission were ritualistic and essential for the propagation of the strongest genes and for preserving the integrity and the security of the troop. On to this idyllic stage stepped the first psoric archetype Sulphur: alpha man – aggressive, assertive, domineering, competitive, territorial, selfish and egotistical. His advent commenced the subtle and insidious process of empowerment of some at the expense of others. Released from instinctive control, the egocentric nature of Sulphur asserted itself and behaviour contrary to the welfare of the tribe, and eventually the species, was gradually initiated.

Knowing the workings of the Sulphur mind and with the annals of human history before us, we can anticipate that domination became oppression and eventually persecution; that aggression became violence and eventually murder; that submission became deprivation and eventually slavery. With the emergence of the entitled alpha-type and the disentitled beta-type, as revealed in the ancient texts, mankind arrived at the Cain and Abel stage of emotional evolution. Cain and Abel – alpha and beta man – Sulphur and Psorinum – perpetrator and victim. A study of the materia medica of these two remedies will provide further insight into this critical relationship. The major psoric remedies are given in Box 17.2.

The Psoric View of Life

For the psoric being, birth onto the earth plane may be likened to expulsion from paradise and descent into chaos. Common feelings, often unconscious, are of being alone, abandoned, forsaken, isolated, inferior, insignificant, puny and vulnerable. They are at the mercy of an unfeeling, unthinking, remorseless, clockwork universe. Life is not benign, nor does it have positive intent. Tormented by legions of fears, frequently about security and survival, they are pessimistic and filled with foreboding, always borrowing trouble and anticipating failure and misfortune. Troubled by a heavy sense of responsibility and duty, they are easily moved to feel guilty, unworthy, and even beyond redemption. Resignation is more common than acceptance, and a sense of martyrdom may offer them consolation. Some features of a psoric view of life are given in Box 17.3.

The causes of psora remain with us to this day and are ever multiplying. Most important is the lack of a loving, holding environment in early childhood, and hence the failure to develop basic trust. Other causes are: intense, prolonged or suppressed emotions; the stresses of modern life; conditions that threaten the security and stability of life; conditions that break the spirit; poverty, squalor, overcrowding, malnutrition, and lack of education; loss of freedom; discrimination and victimisation. On the physical plane the deprivation of psora is manifested in a state of malfunc-

BOX 17.2

Major Psoric Remedies

Many remedies, but especially all the *carbons* and *carbonates*; the psoric triad – *Sulphur, Calcarea carbonica, Lycopodium* – all remedies derived from elements and molecules vital for normal physiology.

The nosodes: *psorinum*; the bowel nosodes: *dysentery co*; *Gaertner*; the *Morgan* group; *mutabile*.

BOX 17.3

The Psoric View of Life
- Lack of basic trust
- Lonely, isolated, disconnected
- Vulnerable, defenceless
- Inferior, unworthy
- Abandoned, rejected
- Pessimistic
- Depressed, despondent, despairing, suicidal ideation
- Apathetic, purposeless
- Self-pitying

tion – usually, but not always, an under-reaction, resulting in deficiency, malnutrition and susceptibility to infection and infestation. Psychosomatic disease and disturbed homeostasis are the basis of psora. Despite all its negativity, psora is the beginning of the individuation process of the evolving human psyche. The individual is a spiritual being on a mystic quest, in search of his, or her, divinity; their disease is a mystic experience with mystic significance, it charts their course, their ascent to perfection. Working with disease and not against it, *deep homeopathy* facilitates the process of self-realisation. This objective is the highest calling of the homeopath.

The Sycotic Miasm – The Miasm of Excess, Escape, and Decadence

'Sycosis' was the name Hahnemann gave to the chronic miasm that is linked to gonorrhoea. It is derived from the Greek '*sykon*', meaning fig. Sycosis therefore means fig-wart disease, which describes the frequent external manifestation of the otherwise concealed miasm.

Sycosis: the Escape from Psora

The oyster, the source of the remedy Calcarea carbonica, metaphorically portrays the psoric response to a life experienced as inherently threatening and hostile. It produces a shell or shield to protect itself and anchors itself firmly to its rock. However, the evolutionary thrust in molluscs is towards emancipation and reaches its greatest freedom of expression in the cephalopods: the cuttlefish, squid and octopus. Likewise in the individuation of the human psyche there is an inevitable and unconscious urge to escape from the negativity of psora. Psora is human life under duress, existing in a delusion of separation, vulnerability, and mortality. It is intolerable. *The desire to escape the psoric delusion lies at the heart of the sycotic miasm.*

We now live in a sycotic age, dominated by escapism: an escape into distraction, denial, disso-

ciation, entertainment, indulgence, sensual gratification, excitement, excess, ecstasy, and lust. By saturating the senses we attempt to ease or numb the pains of our reality and proverbially lose ourselves in 'wine, women, and song'. To aid us in this quest, we have food, tea, coffee and tobacco, and more ominously, alcohol, cannabis, and other mind-altering substances. In our flight from psora we invoke Dionysos (Roman: *Bacchus*) the god of wine, feasting, revelry, sexual rapture, ecstasy, debauchery, and psychotropic drugs. Though we may temporarily escape the doom and gloom of psora, instead of liberation, we induce dependency, addiction and destruction. In sycosis the tendency for progressive emotional deterioration through habituation to vice is highly characteristic. Although the concept of original sin is a typical example of psoric thinking, sin began with sycosis not psora.

Sycosis and Gonorrhoea

Another layer of susceptibility is added to that of psora and the predator – waiting opportunistically in the wings is the *Neisseria gonorrhoea*, the pathogenic organism responsible for the sexually-transmitted disease gonorrhoea. However, just as scabies is not the cause of psora, but a consequence of the psoric state of mind, so gonorrhoea, though intimately related to the sycotic miasm, is not the cause of sycosis, but a consequence of a promiscuous, delinquent, and reprobate mind. Reflect on the sycotic view of life in Box 17.4.

Gonorrhoea has a history going back into the shadows of antiquity. Transmission occurs almost exclusively by direct sexual contact. Remarkably, the gonococcus is only pathogenic to humans. Our inner nature provides the susceptibility; hence, immunity to re-infection is negligible. Psora must be present in the constitution before gonorrhoea can be contracted. This susceptibility is not only linked to psora, but also to the degree of sycosis already present in the constitution and an absence of virtue or morality. Its contagious power is at its highest in promiscuous, illicit, and clandestine sex; in sexual congress without a relationship,

BOX 17.4

Major Characteristics of Sycosis

- Escapism
- Autism: refusal to incarnate fully
- Duality: false front, closed, private, secretive
- Control: perfectionism, fastidiousness, obsessive-compulsive disorder
- Fixed ideas
- Hedonism: high sexual energy, sexual perversions, creatures of the night, 'wine, women and song', self-abuse: alcohol, recreational drugs, excess, extremism, fanaticism
- Passionate, intense
- Addiction and habituation
- Jealous, possessive, suspicious
- Vindictive hate
- Deceitful; manipulative; exploitative
- Overgrowth of tissue, infiltration, thickening, adhesions, tumours
- The mental state is relieved by the appearance of warts, growths, or abnormal discharges and aggravated by their suppression
- Sycotic discharges are green to greenish-yellow; fish-brine odour
- Herpetiform eruptions
- Streptococcal infections and their complications
- Sycosis attacks tissues of mesodermal origin: reticulo-endothelium, connective tissue

companionship, bonding, mutual respect, or love; and where alcohol and cannabis are involved.

The toxicity of the gonococcus appears to be entirely due to an endotoxin. Therefore, even successful antibiotic therapy results in the release of endotoxin into the system and causes a thorough gonorrhoeal intoxication. When a cure is affected by appropriate homeopathic stimulation of the body's defence systems, this complication is prevented. Acute infections that remain untreated, or are chemically suppressed, add further sycotic contamination to the existing miasmatic load. Sycosis

permeates the entire constitution and becomes a progressive, pathological influence throughout life, and is capable of transmission to sexual partners and offspring.

Sycosis may be defined as a constitutional, miasmatic state that is either inherited or transmitted sexually and which is exacerbated by a neglected or suppressed gonorrhoeal infection.

The Duality of Sycosis

Nature is the grand creator of symbols, through which she transmits her silent knowledge. The gonorrhoeal organism is a diplococcus, symbolising in its twinning the duality and duplicity of the sycotic mental state. The symbol is of two kidneys, which points not only to these organs, but also to the entire genitourinary tract, the pelvic organs, and the water metabolism. These are the particular targets of sycotic disease. The sycotic may be the victim of sexual abuse. An unconscious survival strategy of victims is splitting, disassociating, or disconnecting from the body with a sensation of being split in two, of being double, or floating. These are symptoms to be found in major anti-sycotic remedies.

Another example of sycotic duality is the opening up of psychic awareness to other dimensions. The hedonism intrinsic to the escapism of sycosis magnifies the inherent duality of the human psyche: the saint and the sinner, the wholesome and the perverse, the ego and its shadow. Conflict between the moral and the corrupt ensue. The sycotic personality is ever in contention with itself. In the Anacardium archetype this sense of duality and conflict is experienced as a devil on one shoulder and an angel on the other. They are often creatures of the night, drawn to the bright lights, throbbing music, sleaze, sensuality, and places of ill repute where they can indulge their hedonistic preferences. As dusk approaches their complaints recede and they come alive, their minds energised, brimming over with creative thoughts. This state continues into the early hours of the morning. They are passionate, intense, and extreme, always seeking new sensual thrills, often the forbidden and the taboo, to stimulate their jaded appetites.

The Shame of Sycosis

Whereas the psoric sense of responsibility and duty encourages guilt, the devious, clandestine life of the sycotic fosters shame. The sycotic feels soiled, blemished, and unclean, and may experience self-loathing. This is a rejection of self and is pathologically reflected in autoimmune disease, which is essentially sycotic. They are closed, private, and secretive. Whereas the fear of psora requires a shield, the shame of sycosis demands a mask. The mask we wear to conceal our rejected shadow-self is the persona. Under the influence of sycosis we see the structures of the psyche becoming more clearly delineated. Despite appearances, the individuation process gains momentum.

Sycotic Emotions

The psoric being views the world as chaotic and out of control, the sycotic compensates for this by the rigid control of perfectionism, often in every aspect of their lives, and these qualities become an important part of their mask. Taken to the extreme, they may develop obsessive, compulsive tendencies. The sycotic is egotistical, selfish, and insecure, and is inclined to feel jealousy, envy, suspicion, resentment, and vindictive hatred. In relationships they can be terribly heartless and cruel. By nature manipulative, seductive, and deceitful, they comfortably move into politics and crime.

Sycotic Manifestations

The excesses of the sycotic mind and emotions are reflected in the excesses of the miasm's physical manifestations. There is overgrowth, thickening, and induration of tissues (warts, cysts, growths, adhesions, keloids) and profuse yellow-green discharges, all of which relieve the inner miasmatic state and must not be suppressed. The nosode prepared from a gonorrhoeal, urethral discharge is Medorrhinum (mother of all discharges) and two major sycotic remedies are Thuja and Nat-sulph (Natrum sulphuricum). Other major sycotic remedies are in Box 17.5.

> **BOX 17.5**
> **Major Sycotic Remedies**
> *Alumina*; *Anacardium*; *Antimonium crudum*; *Argentum nitricum*; *Cannabis indicus*; *Cannabis sativa*; *Cimicifuga*; *Lachesis*; *Lilium tigrinum*; *Lycopodium*; *Natrum muriaticum*; *Natrum sulphuricum*; *Nitric acid*; *Platinum*; *Pulsatilla*; *Sanicula*; *Sepia*; *Silicea*; *Staphysagria*; *Sulphur*; *Thuja*; all the *Muriatics* (chlorides).
>
> The nosodes: *Medorrhinum*; the bowel nosodes: *Morgan-Pure*; *Sycotic co*; *Proteus*.

Syphilis – The Miasm of Destruction, Degeneracy, and Barbarism

Venereal syphilis probably arose many thousands of years ago in the Middle East or North Africa from a continuum of non-venereal spirochaetal infections. It is regarded as a disease of advanced urbanisation and it is possible that sexual transmission of the spirochete only occurs when a critical mass of the adult population are involved in multiple-partner sex. Such a proposition emphasises the association between non-bonding, non-loving, casual, and illicit sex and the destructive energy of the syphilitic spirochaete. The breadth and destruction that exist in this miasm are represented by some of the characteristics observed in patients expressing this miasm (Box 17.6).

The Cradle of Syphilis

The history of Europe re-enacts for us the evolution of miasmatic disease. After the fall of the Western Roman Empire, Europe descended into the psoric desert of the Dark Ages, a culturally and intellectually barren period, which persisted for hundreds of years, characterised by severe winters, poverty, famine and misery. Towns were overcrowded and filthy. In the 14th century the continent was continuously ravaged by war; life was difficult and precarious. In 1348, out of the East, the Black Plague, spread by black rats and their fleas, descended upon Europe, destroying

BOX 17.6

Major Characteristics of Syphilis
- Systems:
  - the skin and mucous membranes
  - lymphadenopathy
  - cardiovascular – endarteritis, arterio-sclerosis, aneurysms
  - central nervous system – conditions affecting the parenchyma of brain and spinal cord
  - the eyes and optic nerves
  - the bones
  - congenital abnormalities
- Destructive lesions – ulceration, necrosis, gangrene
- Staphylococcal infections; recurrent boils and abscesses
- Inflated ego – delusions of grandeur; ego-tism; megalomania; narcissism; love of money and power; ambition; avarice
- Paranoia – delusions of persecution
- Fixed ideas
- Monomania
- Obsessive-compulsive disorder; ritualism; constantly washing hands, compulsive checking
- Lack of identity
- Perfectionism, fastidiousness
- Need to control, dominate, dictate
- Intolerant of contradiction, reproach, reprimand; easily take offence
- Quarrelsome; insolent; defiant; rebellious
- Fear: *the night*; sleep, insanity, disease, death, evil, of perpetrating violence, loss of control, falling

millions, and leaving havoc, political disarray, and anarchy in its wake. Law and order were overthrown, religious faith was shaken, and sycotic corruption and sensuality prevailed. The stage was set for the emergence of the Great Pox: syphilis.

In 1495, the siege of Naples by Charles VII of France provided the match that fired a pandemic of horrific proportions. The tragedy was peopled by armies, soldiers, prostitutes, abused and starving populaces, and enacted against a backdrop of violence, burning, pillage, rape, debauchery, death, and destruction. Such is the cradle of syphilis. The syphilis of those early years was much more virulent and florid in its manifestations than the disease we know today. It could rapidly prove fatal and the pustular skin lesions were far more gross and repellent. With all its repulsive hideousness, syphilis soon supplanted leprosy as the brand of pollution and sinfulness. From Italy, like wildfire, it spread worldwide, killing and maiming hundreds of thousands and leaving a permanent miasmatic legacy in its wake.

The word 'syphilis' derives from a popular, epic poem written by the Veronese physician, Girolama Fracastora, or Fracastorius. The pastoral tells the unfortunate story of a shepherd, named Syphilis, who having blasphemed against Apollo was cursed with a loathsome disease.

The Pale Thread

The organism, which found the suffering, excesses and depravity of humanity ideal for its spread and survival, was the inconspicuous, feeble *Treponema pallidum*: the 'pale thread'. An almost transparent bacterium with a body twisted into a spiral – the symbol of the serpent. It is as fragile as it looks, totally dependent on its exclusive, intimate relationship with man. Despite its fragility it is one of the most virulent organisms known. It possesses remarkably few genes, and hence contains so few proteins in its cell membrane that it remains undetected by its host's immune system. This tenuous membrane is also able to bind proteins derived from the host's blood. The resulting camouflage permits the organism to remain invisible, free from attack, and able to survive in its victim's body for years.

The psoric needs a shield, the sycotic wears a mask, and the syphilitic, like the 'pale thread', often remains hidden, the little grey person who blends with the environment. The syphilitic pervert often successfully remains undetected and invisible in society. They are able to adopt the outer semblance and conservative customs of the society they move in, ensuring their anonymity.

Broadening our Understanding

IV

Syphilitic Manifestations

The primary lesion of syphilis is the chancre. Its appearance occurs after the disease has become systemic and is a demonstration of the externalising power of the vital force. Unless natural healing is brought about, as with sycosis, the further development or chemical suppression of syphilis result in a miasmatic condition in the patient, which will be transmitted dynamically by inheritance and sexual contact, even in the absence of the infecting organism.

The clinical pictures of primary, secondary, and tertiary syphilis give to us a clear indication of the organ affinities of the syphilitic miasm, which often provides a clue in selecting appropriate anti-syphilitic remedies or Syphilinum, the nosode. Most important are mucosal ulceration (e.g. Mercurius), lymphadenopathy (Phytolacca), cardiovascular disease (Aurum), neuropathies (Causticum), skeletal disease (Mezereum), ophthalmic diseases (Kali-iod), congenital abnormalities and the deterioration of the emotional, moral and intellectual life. Other remedies of the syphilitic miasm are given in Box 17.7.

The classic picture of general paralysis of the insane (GPI), a severe form of neurosyphilis, which often exaggerates previous personality traits to even grotesque proportions, provides a template for recognising the presence of a dominant syphilitic, miasmatic influence in patients. These characteristics may be expansive – even grandiose, depressed, paranoid, schizophrenic, or dementing.

As previously noted, psora must be present in the constitution before the venereal diseases gonorrhoea and syphilis can be contracted. It is significant that these organisms are only pathogenic to humans. Whereas sycosis is a marriage of psora and constitutional gonorrhoea, the syphilitic miasm is primarily (sycosis is invariably present) a combination of psora and constitutional syphilis, in which the syphilitic influence predominates. When psora is predominant in this combination the tubercular miasm manifests.

Syphilis, Fire and Hepar Sulphuris Calcareum

Syphilis spreads like wildfire. Like fire, the disease consumes, dissolves and destroys the tissues, the morality, the identity, the intellect, and the sanity. Fire is a symbol of syphilis. In a unique experiment, which produced a unique anti-syphilitic remedy, Hahnemann took flowers of Sulphur (fire/syphilis) and the middle layer of the oyster shell, Calc-carb (psora), and burnt them in a crucible. The resultant liver-coloured compound he called Hepar sulphuris calcareum.

Syphilis and the Sociopath

The profile of the syphilitic mind is a disturbing one. We see an awful potential for antisocial behaviour, criminal activity, extreme violence, cruelty, brutality, murder, sexual perversion, and moral degeneracy, often aggravated by substance abuse, and presided over by a chilling lack of conscience or remorse, paranoia, and megalomania.

When society descends into war, and anarchy and lawlessness prevail, out of the woodwork of the community emerge the previously pale, hidden, silent syphilitics, able at last to consort with their evil brethren, and to indulge and gratify their dark, dread fantasies and impulses in the light of day. In sycosis, the ego and shadow are in contention; in syphilis, the ego and shadow are one, and the night is their nemesis.

Tuberculosis – The Miasm of Resurrection, Revolution, and Genius

By the middle of the 16th century the original florid severity of the syphilitic pandemic had begun to subside with milder skin lesions, less

BOX 17.7

Major Syphilitic Remedies

Arsenicum album; *Arsenicum iodatum*; *Asafoetida*; *Aurum metallicum* and its salts; *Causticum*; *Fluoric acid*; *Kalium-iodatum*; *Lachesis*; *Mercurius*; *Mezereum*; *Nitric acid*; *Phytolacca*; *Silicea*; *Stillingia*, and all the *Halogen* salts.

The nosode: *Syphilinum*; the bowel nosodes: *Bacillus no. 7*; *Gaertner*.

IV

Broadening our Understanding

pain, less bone destruction, and fewer deaths. It was as if a truce had been established as spirochete and host became more tolerant of one another. Nature, however, had achieved her objective. Humanity had been thoroughly impregnated with the syphilitic poison. The remission in severity signalled the beginning of a miasmatic change, which would lead to the next wave of communicable disease – tuberculosis.

When we contemplate the deficient nature of psora, it is clear that to achieve expansion and drive without the decadence of sycosis or the degeneracy of syphilis, a critical stimulus and change was needed to urge the individuation process of humanity forward. The change involved a receding of syphilitic dominance and the re-emergence of psora, now vitalised by the admixture of syphilitic energy. The stimulus was the modified fire provided by the embers of the syphilitic pandemic.

Tuberculosis – the Offspring of Psora and Syphilis

The organism that profited from the conflagration of syphilis was the *Mycobacterium tuberculosis*. We know that the evolutionary, miasmatic cycle we have traced so far has been enacted before in civilisations of the past. Tuberculosis (TB) is a disease of ancient origin. From rural areas TB spread to the densely populated cities and found its ideal circumstances among the crowded poor, preying especially upon the young, the malnourished and the overworked, who often existed without sunlight and fresh air. Later it affected all levels of society. The incidence became extremely high, resulting in a thorough permeation of European genetic stock with this chronic miasm. Anti-tubercular therapy may kill the bacillus and seemingly cure the patient, but the miasmatic contamination persists and may be handed on by inheritance, but, unlike sycosis and syphilis, not by sexual contact.

TB targets certain organs. *M. tuberculosis*, being primarily inhaled, especially involves the respiratory tract, while *M. bovis*, being ingested, especially involves extra-pulmonary organs and tissues:

lymph glands, bones, joints, serous membranes, central nervous system, intestines, genital organs, kidneys, adrenal glands, eyes, and the skin.

The Tubercular Constitution

The miasm frequently creates a person who is inclined to elegance, refinement, and aesthetic sensitivity. In keeping with this the features are often aristocratic, finely drawn, and beautiful. Their eyes are magnificent, expressive, and framed by long, silky eyelashes. In health, they are well proportioned and athletic – fine-boned, lean-muscled, tall, long-limbed, and graceful. They can be fair or dark, blonde, brunette or redhead. When the constitution is weak, they are often too thin, narrow-chested, with bad posture, round shoulders, a sway back, and lax muscles. Their energy and stamina are poor. The least exertion leaves them exhausted. Though they are chilly and seek the sun, they long for cool, fresh air. They may suffer from night-sweats. Anaemia is common. There is a lack of resistance to infection and they are slow to convalesce. Reflect on Box 17.8 to help you appreciate the positive as well as negative qualities of the TB miasm.

The Tubercular Mind

The tubercular mind is right cerebrally dominant: romantic, idealistic, imaginative, artistic, and creative. Tuberculosis was known as the pining or wasting disease. The tubercular individual often longs and pines for an ideal love and suffers terribly from unrequited and disappointed love. Yet they are also fickle, soon become bored with a relationship, and need to move on to new pastures. The intellectual development and creative ability are often precocious and prodigious, but with a tendency to burn out prematurely. The mind tends to be stronger than the body. The tubercular nature is rebellious and defiant and will fight for justice, freedom, and reform. They have an intense love for animals, which they will defend and protect. Likewise, they are deeply concerned for the welfare of the planet. Often, like the sycotic, they have psychic awareness, are highly intuitive, and pick up on others' thoughts and feelings. Their lack of

BOX 17.8
Major Characteristics of Tubercular Miasm

- Ailments from: unrequited, disappointed love; betrayal, infidelity; jealousy; bereavement, grief, sorrow; loneliness; homesickness; boredom
- Right cerebral dominance: artistic, creative, imaginative, intuitive, romantic, idealistic
- Precocious, prodigious, gifted intellect, which may burn out prematurely
- Refined, sophisticated, cultured
- Altruistic: active concern for human, animal and planetary welfare
- Intolerant of injustice, will fight for social reform
- Challenge tradition, convention, authority; rebellious, defiant
- Psychic awareness
- Hypersensitivity: to ambience, surroundings, people, climate

- Bipolarity: alternating, changing moods; cyclothymia; manic-depressive
- Fickle; short-lived enthusiasms; unreliable; unpredictable
- Need for change; restless, unsettled, discontented; need to travel and see the world
- Recurrent, relapsing states; at every return of complaints they have altered, calling for a new remedy
- Changing symptoms and states
- Ailments jump from one area, organ or system to another; pains shift and wander
- Periodicity and intermittency
- Insidious, indolent conditions
- Hedonism; hyper-sexuality
- Fears: dogs, dark, solitude, thunderstorms, disease, suffering, the future
- Indifference; withdrawn, reclusive

boundaries may prove stressful and exhausting. Sensitivity is present on all levels of experience and to all sensory impressions.

There is restlessness, a need to escape boredom, and a constant desire for change and for travel, to go somewhere new, and to do something different. They are curious and enthusiastic. Life seems to hold so much promise and there seems so little time to enjoy all that is on offer. They wish to drink every cup of experience to the very dregs. They are adventurous, experimental, and innovative. They will try anything at least once, but are not as inclined to become snared by addiction as is the sycotic. Dangerous activities, which stimulate the flow of adrenaline, are irresistible to them. Recklessness is a danger. The limelight attracts them like a moth to a flame.

Naturally dramatic and expressive, they love centre stage and the applause of an audience. They are not handicapped by modesty or inhibition. Indeed, they often possess a surfeit of

self-esteem and vanity, and have a flamboyance, which they and others find captivating. They are often at the cutting edge of fashion, opinions, and trends. Their minds overflow with an abundance of ideas, expressed through irrepressible verbosity and unbounded creativity. They sparkle and shine with energy, exuberance, vivacity, and even ecstasy – but always with the danger of fizzling out and plunging into melancholy and despair. Typical tubercular remedies are Phosphorous and Calc-phos; others are given in Box 17.9.

Tuberculosis and the Romantic Age

Fire, like speech, has always been a catalyst for man's evolution and creativity. It is a powerful, multi-facetted symbol: divine energy, purification, revelation, transformation, resurrection, transcendence; patriotic, sexual and religious ardour; inspiration and creative power; passion and love! As syphilis, it illuminated the human psyche. Out of the long psoric night of the Dark Ages and the

BOX 17.9

Major Tubercular Remedies

Arsenicum album; *Arsenicum iodatum*; *Bromium*; *Calcarea carbonica*; *Calcium phosphoricum*; *Causticum*; *China officinalis*; *Coffea crudum*; *Drosera*; *Ferrum metallicum*; *Ignatia*; *Iodum*; *Kalium carbonicum*; *Lachesis*; *Lycopodium*; *Manganum*; *Phosphoric acid*; *Phosphorus*; *Sepia*; *Silicea*; *Spongia*; *Stannum*; *Sulphur*; and all the *Phosphates*.

The nosodes: the *Tuberculinums*; *Bacillinum*; *Psorinum*; the bowel nosodes: *Bacillus no. 7*; *Gaertner*; *Morgan-Pure*; *Mutabile*; *Sycotic co.*

medieval period dawned the Renaissance, followed by the Age of Enlightenment, which blossomed into the prodigious creativity of the high romantic period. Now, there was fire in the mind. This was the world of Chopin and Keats, the world of tuberculosis, and the tubercular miasm.

The period of high romanticism in the arts coincided with the rapid and devastating spread of TB in Europe. Throughout history artists, poets, writers, and musicians have shown romantic tendencies, but the Romantic Movement usually refers to the period from the late 1700s to the mid 1800s (almost the entire lifetime of Hahnemann). Romanticism in the fine arts and literature is a style, which emphasises emotion and passion rather than reason, and imagination and inspiration rather than logic and intellect. It is usually a revolt against the rigorous restraints and formalism of classicism. It was also a revolt against a society which had become abhorrent to the artistic mind; a society that seemed to be governed by science, commerce, industry, power, and wealth. Artists escaped into exotic worlds of fantasy and imagination, the medieval and the ancient past, and the realms of myth and legend. Politically, romanticism opposed tyranny and fought for freedom and equality through revolution, liberalism, and social reform.

Genius flourished in the romantic period. Manic-depressives were numerous amongst the most gifted and creative of the romantics. Many of the symptoms of mania and depression became accepted personality traits of the romantic genius. Whereas the sycotic mind is characterised by duality, the tubercular mind is characterised by the ebb and flow of bipolarity: cyclothymia – hypomania and depression.

The Tubercular Quest

The fire of syphilis has refined and inspired the tubercular individual, filling an unsettled, dissatisfied spirit with interminable restlessness, a sense of unfulfilment, and an insistent need for change. The constant searching and longing, often without a specific goal or objective, but sensed as an impelling need, brings a quickening to the individuation process of the individual. The final sublimation will bring the realisation that what they have sought for all their lives actually lies not in any outer world, or other dimension, but within themselves. All they have suffered and enjoyed, all the longings and strivings, and all the successes and failures were designed to bring them self-knowledge, in which the limitations of ego-personality are transcended, and oneness with all is experienced.

Carcinosis – The Miasm of Transcendence, Sublimation, and Individuation

Disease is an expression of creation's perfection; it has meaning, deep significance, and is essentially beneficent. The vital force is always working at its optimal best. Even malignant disease is a manifestation of the vital force's efforts to bring about the least harmful result in a profoundly disturbed constitution. It would rather produce a cancer than permit a process that impacts upon the emotional and intellectual spheres and impedes spiritual unfoldment. This is not always possible. However, when successful, the inherited legacy of disease is concentrated and encapsulated in a malignant lesion or process. Constitutionally a cleansing of the miasmatic state is achieved, which is manifested particularly in the emotional life. Individuation is accelerated. When the cancer miasm is dominant it often brings with it a state of increasing spiritual awareness, empathy, and a greater capacity for unconditional love.

Pointers to the Presence of the Cancer Miasm

The characteristics of the cancer miasm, carcinosis, are to be found in the remedy picture of the nosode, Carcinosin – a remedy prepared from breast cancer. The remedy was defined and developed by Dr Donald Foubister. Carcinosis is a multifaceted miasm, which derives from a combination of the four other chronic miasms, often exacerbated and compounded by suppression. Foubister recognised that certain physical characteristics pointed to the presence of the miasm, particularly multiple moles, café-au-lait complexion, and blue sclerotics. In such cases there was often a higher incidence of cancer, TB, and diabetes in the family histories. Other features, which later became apparent, were a history of many acute infections in childhood, especially pneumonia or whooping cough, or the complete absence of the usual children's diseases, or the suffering of these only after puberty.

The belief that psychological and emotional states such as grief, depression and stress can foster the development of cancer has been with us since classical times. It has been observed that a remarkably high proportion of cancer patients have lived difficult lives, had much misfortune, or have experienced a particularly traumatic event shortly before cancer was diagnosed. The loss of a loved one, the termination of a close relationship, and depression have often been linked to cancer. Homeopathic clinical experience with Carcinosin has given weight to these conclusions. The nosode is of particular use in the treatment of those who have a history of dysfunctional parenting; an unhappy, often over-responsible childhood; emotional trauma and abuse, whether emotional, physical or sexual; and long continued domination by others. Suppressed emotions are particularly destructive, especially grief, anger and resentment.

Carcinosin has a wide spectrum of indications and it is one of the most frequently indicated nosodes in homeopathic practice. Given the exploding incidence of malignancy in most societies, this is not surprising. Box 17.10 lists some of the pointers to this miasm.

Carcinosis and the C-type personality

By far the most common and defining face this complex miasm presents is the psoric component. When dominant, it produces the well-recognised C-type personality profile and the characteristics of the so-called 'disease to please'. This type suppresses strong emotions, is diffident and self-effacing, ever yielding sacrificially to the wishes of others, avoiding conflict and confrontation, and behaviour that might impose on others or offend them. Outwardly they appear controlled, unemotional and stoical, within they are a seething mass of anxieties and emotions, which they repress. They are nice people and their niceness borders on the pathological. Taking a strange satisfaction in denying their own needs, they equate selflessness with love and caring. Proper and conservative, always conforming to established norms, they never complain, lack assertiveness, and maintain a docile passivity. They are conscientious, fastidious, meticulous perfectionists, and workaholics, who have a heavy sense of duty and responsibility, are self-critical, and easily take on blame and guilt. Remedies linked to this miasm are Natrum muriaticum and Lac caninum; others are noted in Box 17.11.

The Syco-Tubercular Cancer Type

However, this compliant, meek, subservient type is not the only face of the cancer miasm. The admixture of sycosis and tuberculosis often gives it a far more powerful and passionate expression. The syco-tubercular types are high-energy people: active, intense, emotional, excitable, and passionate, very expressive, open, and communicative. If the sycotic energy is dominant, they may show a tendency to extremism, high sexuality, and a love of 'wine, women and song'. If the tubercular energy is dominant, they may show a restless

BOX 17.10
Major Characteristics of Carcinoma Miasm

- History of cancer in the patient
- Family history of cancer, diabetes or TB
- The presence of blue sclerotics, café-au-lait complexion, birth marks, dark or excessive moles
- History of dysfunctional parenting, emotional trauma, abuse
- Long history of domination by others
- Prolonged anger, resentment, grief, fear
- Suppressed emotions, esp. grief, anger, resentment
- When a number of polychrests seem equally well indicated
- Lack of response to well chosen remedies, or when response is short lived
- Constantly changing symptomatic picture
- Paradoxical and alternating states
- Symptoms and signs alternate from one side of the body to the other
- Chronic insomnia; insomnia from birth; insomnia since broken sleep, night-watching
- Compromised immune system:
  - Suggestive evidence:
    - no history of children's illnesses
    - children's illnesses experienced after puberty
    - never well since viral infection (chronic viral fatigue syndrome):
      - glandular fever
      - hepatitis
- Overtaxed immune system:
  - recurrent severe infections in childhood
  - severe whooping cough or pneumonia
- Iatrogenic breakdown in resistance:
  - recurrent or prolonged antibiotic therapy
  - corticosteroids
  - excessive immunisation
- Strong emotions are suppressed – anger, fear, grief
- A veneer of calm, unemotional composure
- An inward seething of anxiety and emotions
- Compliance with the wishes of others; passive subservience
- Sympathetic, compassionate
- Tales of suffering affect profoundly
- Weeps from sympathy with others; yet averse to sympathy
- Anxiety for others

BOX 17.11
The Carcinosin Remedies

Arsenicum album; *Arsenicum iodatum*; *Asterias rubens*; *Bellis perennis*; *Cadmium metallicum*; *Cadmium sulphuricum*; *Carbo animalis*; *Conium*; *Cundurango*; *Graphites*; *Hydrastis*; *Kalium iodatum*; *Kreosotum*; *Lac caninum*; *Lachesis*; *Lycopodium*; *Mercurius*; *Nitric acid*; *Phosphorus*; *Phytolacca*; *Silicea*; *Sepia*; *Thuja*.

The nosodes: the *Carcinosins*; *Psorinum*; *Scirrhinum*; the bowel nosodes: *Dysentery co*; *Mutabile*.

discontentedness, romantic longings, a desire to travel, and a need for adventure, thrills, and new experiences. The cancer miasm has elements of both, but in its highest form it reveals a beauty of spirit that is unique.

An Elevated Being

The Carcinosin subject has an abiding love of nature, of animals, and of humanity, which moves them to altruism of the purest form. Their minds and senses are aesthetically attuned to all that is elevated, noble, and splendid in literature, music, and dance. Their love and compassion are intense,

Broadening our Understanding

IV

selfless, universal, and unconditional. The miasm of cancer facilitates the ascent of the human soul towards its divinity.

The Miasmatic Spiral

Our study of the miasms commenced with psora, followed by sycosis, syphilis, and tuberculosis, giving us the first loop of a spiral. With the consideration of the cancer miasm, the disease continuum comes full circle (Fig 17.2). The carbons, which typify the psoric miasm, are carcinogenic and we can easily recognise the similarity between the emotionally deficient state of psora and the weakness of the C-type personality. After cancer, in the next sweep of the spiral, we should expect another wave of sycotic energy in the genesis of disease, once again linked to escapism, sensuality and profligacy. This has proved true in the widespread Aids epidemic. Following this we should

anticipate new evidence of a destructive, syphilitic-type energy appearing. This is evidenced in the serpent-shaped, haemorrhagic filoviruses. Finally, in the wake of Aids, we are witnessing, especially in Africa, an alarming resurgence of tuberculosis, and everywhere in the world cancer is on the increase. Disease ever recapitulates.

Summary

Knowledge of miasmatic theory is a powerful tool. It gives the physician better understanding of the patient's disease process, provides guidance in remedy and nosode selection, and helps in the interpretation of remedy response. It can even give insight into the emotional patterns and potentials of the patient. A miasmatic diagnosis is often vital to therapeutic success. Despite good case-taking and thorough case analysis, it is common experience during the course of constitutional treatment for the physician to stand on pause and in doubt as to which remedy to prescribe, how to deal with lack of response or the failure of a previously successful remedy, and how to remove unseen obstacles to cure. When in such doubt, it often pays to prescribe miasmatically by choosing an appropriate miasmatic remedy or nosode. Such a choice may sometimes provide the simillimum, but more frequently a reaction will be elicited, which opens the case up. New emotional or physical symptoms emerge, significant dreams may be experienced, and the patient's constitution becomes responsive. Even in more straightforward cases, the occasional dose of the indicated miasmatic or bowel nosode may facilitate the healing process.

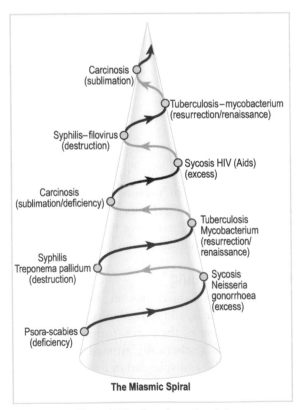

Figure 17.2   The miasmatic spiral

Bibliography

Allen J H 1908 Chronic miasms: psora, pseudopsora and sycosis, 2 vols. Privately published, Chicago. Reprinted 1950 as 1 vol, M V Kulkarni, Bombay

Banerjee P N trans Banerjee P N 1931 Chronic disease: its cause and cure. P C Chakravarty Homoeopathy, Prachar Kavjalaya, Calcutta

Foubister D 1991 Tutorials on homeopathy. Beaconsfield Publishers, Beaconsfield

De Schepper L 2001 Hahnemann revisited. Full of Life Publishing, Santa Fe

Jamison K R 1994 Touched with fire: manic-depressive illness and the artistic temperament. Free Press, New York

Leakey R 1992 Origins reconsidered. Little Brown, London

Roberts H A 1942 The principles and art of cure by homoeopathy, a modern textbook, 2nd edn. Homoeopathic Publishing Company, London

Van der Zee H 2000 Miasms in labour. Stichting Alonissos, Utrecht

Wills C 1996 Plagues: their origin, history and future. Harper Collins, London

Ziegler P 1998 The black death, 2nd edn. Penguin Books, London

Broadening our
Understanding

IV

CHAPTER EIGHTEEN

Veterinary Prescribing

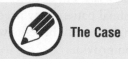 **The Case**

Peter Gregory

Introduction by David Owen

Many students of homeopathy might wonder how a chapter on veterinary prescribing is going to influence their training – in several ways, I hope. First, there is a need for non-human animals to receive non-suppressive treatment. Man is not alone in either his environment or illnesses. Many illnesses that affect mankind are also an expression of diseases that run through all animals (reflected also in the diseases of plants and imbalances in the environment). If homeopaths recognise and rise to these broader challenges, not only may they see illness in a new light, by being aware of influences on patients, but also they may contribute to reducing the reservoir of illness that exists outside mankind. Reflect on whether, given animal husbandry practices, it is surprising to be facing illnesses that animal groups hold or mediate – such as 'bird flu' or prion infections.

Second, I have for 10 years been teaching with and to veterinary homeopaths. Their approach to the case and treatment has taught me a great deal and I believe Peter Gregory reflects some of this in his chapter. Often what human homeopaths might call 'the inside' of the case in terms of mental, emotional and relational symptoms might appear absent but to the attuned homeopath the inside and outside reflect one another. Seeing the deeper aspects of the case revealed through what is carefully observed of a patient's behaviour and relationship to others is a key homeopathic skill that veterinary homeopaths such as Peter are champions of.

Third, homeopathy for pets covers many of the essential features of homeopathic treatment of babies and children, including non-verbal communication, the socialisation they go through (including the not uncommon abuse) and the relationship with third parties – in pets, owners and, for children, parents.

Fourth, and finally, veterinary homeopathy has developed a range of prescribing strategies that can both challenge and inform human homeopaths.

Veterinary Prescribing

Homeopathy represents enormous opportunities for improving the health of animals. Many conditions for which there is no conventional treatment available can improve with homeopathy, and since the latter half of the last century demand from the public has burgeoned. Not only does homeopathy add an extremely useful modality to the skills of a trained veterinary surgeon, it is also enormously empowering to the informed animal owner, who is able to effectively treat simple ailments. Many veterinarians attempt to integrate homeopathy into their general practice, using it as the sole form of treatment or in conjunction with conventional medicine; however there are others, like myself, who concentrate on second opinion or referral work.

Veterinary homeopathy is practised in a broadly similar way to that in humans, but individual species variations may require that a specific approach to homeopathic prescribing be made for an individual animal. This may simply be a matter of a different emphasis, but at times an approach unique to the animal patient may need to be employed if it is to enjoy the full benefits which this form of therapy can provide.

For instance, as a consequence of the non-verbal nature of the patient, the homeopathic history is wholly dependent on the observational powers of the owner. Furthermore, some animals, such as free-ranging sheep, have minimal contact with their keepers.

Many of the more subtle symptoms, so useful in the field of medical homeopathy, are of necessity absent from a veterinary history. For instance, the quality of sensations, in particular of pain, is unavailable to the veterinary homeopath; indeed the very presence of pain can often only be inferred rather than directly described. Consequently, most animals are presented for ailments which have progressed beyond the stage of changes in sensation. Modalities, too, may be dependent on subjective interpretation of observations, e.g. the symptom described by the rubric Generals Heat – 'lack of vital heat' – may be exhibited in a dog by its propensity to lie by the fire, but this behaviour might equally be taken to mean that the animal's symptoms are ameliorated by heat, thus 'Generals – heat ameliorates'. Careful history-taking and observation coupled with experience in the normal behaviour of the species and individual may be needed to make the appropriate distinction. While a veterinary repertory will undoubtedly offer some assistance in selecting rubrics for animals, it is unlikely to overcome this problem completely.

When it comes to the mental and emotional symptoms, the subjective nature of the symptoms is exacerbated. In essence the animal patient is incapable of providing a single direct mental symptom; the best that the veterinarian can do is to try and interpret its behaviour in terms of human emotions. Close observation can certainly yield much which can be useful to the veterinary homeopath, but in the final analysis, the prescriber simply does not know what emotions the animal is experiencing. When one considers the emphasis that most homeopaths place on the mental and emotional symptoms in case analysis, it might appear that veterinary homeopaths are at a disadvantage compared to their medical colleagues. But as will become clear later in this chapter, most veterinary homeopaths simply take such issues into account when deciding on which approach to use in any particular case.

In relation to the issue of obstacles to cure, the veterinary homeopath has to face problems unique to this field of expertise. The feeding and management regimes which are imposed upon domestic animals frequently create a situation where homeopathic medicines struggle to act with any consistency; this is discussed in more detail later in the chapter.

In spite of the foregoing issues, homeopathy brings enormous benefits to animals wherever it is practised. This is due in no small part to the ingenuity of its practitioners in overcoming the challenges described above, and much of this chapter is devoted to describing the approaches which veterinary homeopaths embrace in order to achieve success with their patients.

Categories of Veterinary Patients

It is common practice to divide veterinary patients into four basic categories, each of which reflects the differing situation of the animals within it. There are inevitably areas of overlap, but as the needs of each category vary so significantly it is helpful in a discussion such as this to use the following categorisation:

- There are companion animals ('pets') that range from the ubiquitous dogs and cats to small furry creatures such as hamsters, and exotic species such as spiders and reptiles ('small animals'). However, this category also includes 'large animals' such as horses, when they are kept primarily as pets, or for leisure.
- Second are performance animals, including race horses, racing greyhounds and working sheepdogs.

- Third, there are food-producing animals. In the UK this category is confined to the cloven-footed animals and poultry but in other countries, particularly in the European Union, horses are included.
- Finally, there are wild animals that include exotic wild animals, e.g. captive in zoos, or native animals, either rescued or free.

Companion Animals

As veterinary medicine, certainly in the affluent West, has increasingly devoted its energies to the treatment of companion animals, it is in this sphere that homeopathy is perhaps most commonly practiced. Here the human–animal bond is at its strongest and hence the influence of the owner is at its greatest. It is also important for the human homoeopath to recognise the role of a pet in a family, and hence the intensity of the emotions which surround its welfare. The diseases of dogs and cats in particular are in many ways similar to those experienced by humans and it is not surprising that the homeopathic treatment of their ailments mirrors the medical model most closely.

Referral practices dealing with small animals are presented with a preponderance of animals suffering from the chronic conditions which afflict aged dogs and cats, such as osteoarthritis, urinary incontinence and posterior paralysis. However, chronic skin disease is another common reason for seeking homeopathy – many such patients arrive as 'desperation cases', frequently after prolonged courses of corticosteroids, and very often dependent on them when presented. The symptomatology may be confused and vague, and consequently these complicated cases are not easy to treat; indeed, a proportion of them prove to be incurable. For a few the best that can be done is to effect a reduction in the dose of corticosteroids (though this in itself can be life-saving) but in the majority the symptoms can be relieved – and many cases of chronic skin disease can be cured completely. Other conditions for which homeopathy is commonly sought include colitis and associated bowel disorders, chronic respiratory disease and so-called 'behavioural disorders'. In these cases success rates are considerably higher.

Performance Animals

This category represents such animals as race horses, racing greyhounds and working sheepdogs. If they are to perform to their full potential they must be in peak fitness, and homeopathy can play an important role in maintaining this state. In addition, the prompt homeopathic treatment of injuries can promote rapid resolution of the condition and consequent early return to work. Many performance animals in work are functioning at the limits of their capacity and when these limits are exceeded damage to the physical body ensues. Homeopathy can help speedy resolution and return to the racetrack. Compare this to the situation of the human athlete or bodybuilder who is working for fitness rather than health. In some cases preventative action may be taken; e.g. some thoroughbred racehorses suffer from epistaxis when over-exerted. The condition is viewed seriously by the Jockey Club and repeat episodes will lead to disqualification of the horse from the racetrack. One of the homeopathic snake remedies, usually Vipera, will not only treat the condition but also reduce the propensity for it. Similarly, many racehorses suffer from a chronic fatigue syndrome, possibly as a result of adrenal exhaustion from the stress of racing. Homeopathy can be highly effective in treating this condition.

The stabling or kenneling of large numbers of performance animals in a restricted area renders these populations particularly vulnerable to epizootic diseases – an outbreak of kennel cough, for instance, can cause the complete closure of a dog track. Homeopathy can not only aid in the rapid recovery of the affected animals but can also bring the outbreak rapidly under control – either by the use of homeopathy alone or by the use of isopathy in the form of nosodes. Further discussion of this issue will be found in the following section on food-producing animals.

The horse as a species seems to be extremely sensitive to homeopathy, no matter under what circumstances the treatment is given. This may be due to an innate sensitivity to homeopathy, but horses do often present with a very clear remedy picture that reflects the deepest state of the organism. As such, while they will often respond extremely well to medium potencies such as 30c, the symptomatology can be so clear if there is no suppression as to allow single dose prescriptions of M potencies with relative confidence.

The strict training and feeding regimes inevitably followed in racing establishments may limit the management changes which may be made in aid of the animal's recovery, but an injured animal has to be rested, and an animal with digestive problems has to be fed appropriately if homeopathy is to be fully effective. Similarly, due to the rules which govern racing, no flexibility in vaccination regimes is allowed. The homeopathic veterinarian thus simply has to operate within these limitations, taking them into account in making the prescription.

Food-Producing Animals

In recent years the burgeoning number of farms using organic management regimes has resulted in an increasing utilisation of homeopathy on farms throughout the world, nowhere greater than in the UK. Here the ruling body for organic farming is the Soil Association and their regulations oblige the use of homeopathic or herbal preparations wherever possible. In order to meet the demands of their clients an increasing number of veterinarians are, therefore, finding the need to obtain training in homeopathy. Many farmers are themselves attending courses designed to help them understand homeopathy and use it effectively as an integral part of their management systems. Advantages of homeopathy in livestock rearing systems include the low cost of the medicines and the fact that there are no residues.

The food-producing animal, however, perhaps presents the most challenges for the veterinary homeopath, for it is here that the concept of individualisation is least relevant. In most modern systems of management animals are identified by numbers rather than name, and an individual is seen more as an economic unit rather than as a sentient being. This impersonalisation is imposed to a degree which varies from farm to farm but the notion holds true to some degree for the vast majority of food-producing animals. In addition a herd or a flock may number in the hundreds, so the veterinarian simply does not have sufficient time to individualise every animal for treatment, even if the necessary information were to be available in the first place. Most of the following strategies for prescribing for groups of animals were developed in food-producing animals.

Wild Animals

Homeopathy represents an ideal form of medicine for wild animals whether rescued after injury, or subjected to capture and transport for welfare reasons such as drought or flood. Not only are the medicines cheap, but their availability is not restricted in the way that most orthodox drugs are. This makes them ideal for welfare organisations, most of which operate on limited budgets. In addition, many of the problems such as shock and bruising which manifest in rescued wild animals can be readily treated with homeopathy. Problems with administration are overcome by dropping liquid remedies onto the nose of a rescued animal, or by the use of aqueous sprays – though with a dangerous animal administration by the water supply can also be used. It is my opinion that all such organisations should at least have Aconitum and Arnica readily available for use in their patients.

The Practice of Veterinary Homeopathy

The Importance of Causation

Many veterinarians embark on their homeopathic journey with the first aid remedies, based on causation. The treatment of the ubiquitous skin lacerations and road traffic injuries with remedies such as Arnica and Hypericum is often their first experience of homeopathy.

In comparison with their medical colleagues, veterinary homeopaths perhaps tend to view cases in the pathogenic model, as homeopathic histories in animals often present with quite clear aetiologies. In my experience the most commonly identified mental causality in animals is grief. Companion animals often create extremely close relationships with their family members, be they human or animal, and this leaves them particularly vulnerable to the effects of grief. The relationships may also cross other species barriers; friendships are commonly reported between dogs and cats, dogs and horses, rabbits and guinea pigs, and even dogs and sheep.

The loss of one of these companions can be devastating to an animal and after such an experience many such patients will go into a grief state corresponding to the remedy pictures of Ignatia or Natrum muriaticum, among others. A history of having been re-homed, be it privately or through a rescue kennel, should alert the practitioner to the possibility of a long-standing grief state in the patient, and raise the possibility of prescribing one of the remedies with a reputation in this area. Such a state is also commonly found in leisure horses; it can be heart-rending to hear, in the process of taking a homeopathic history, how many changes of owner a horse may have experienced.

Where the animal itself does not appear to have suffered a loss, sensitive questioning of the owner may elucidate that it is the grief state of the owner which is being played out in the patient. For instance, a cat belonging to someone who has just suffered a bereavement may pick up on the owner's emotions and develop symptoms corresponding to the Natrum muriaticum state.

The specific reaction to grief is also important in the analysis of the case. A normally placid family pet will sometimes apparently become aggressive after the loss of the head of the family, be it from bereavement or divorce; when the dog is presented for arthritis and weakness of the hind legs, the Causticum state, with its emphasis on protection of the family unit, is easily identified from the aetiology alone.

A clear aetiology may also be recognised as being an assault on the physical plane – in this context a common aetiology in veterinary histories is that of vaccination. It was James Compton Burnett who, in 1884, alerted the medical world to the ill-effects of smallpox vaccination in his book 'Vaccinosis'. The title consists of the term he coined to describe the clinical syndrome induced by vaccination, and the substance of the book details how the majority of these cases would respond to homeopathic Thuja occidentalis. Ever since this time, homeopaths have been cognisant of the importance of vaccination as an aetiological factor in chronic disease.

In veterinary homeopathy the issue takes on added importance. Domestic animals, in particular dogs and horses, are routinely vaccinated against a number of infectious diseases, using multiple vaccines administered from an early age. It has long been standard practice to repeat the injections annually, although recently there is a move to increase the interval in some cases to three years. While there is little doubt that the control of such serious diseases such as canine distemper and feline panleucopaenia has owed much to vaccination, veterinary homeopaths consider that there has been a cost to the general health of the animal population as a whole. Such conditions as atopic dermatitis, colitis and epilepsy seem at the very least to be exacerbated by vaccination. Veterinary homeopaths will invariably scrutinise the histories of their patients for any such correspondences which would imply a causative role. As a rule of thumb, any condition appearing within three months of a vaccination is considered to be suspicious; within one month, even more so. As a consequence of this, veterinary homeopaths tend be very careful in the way vaccines are administered, and frequently employ techniques to minimise their use. Such procedures include the measuring of antibody titres to assess protection levels, and the use of nosode regimes for protection (Saxton & Gregory 2005).

REFLECTION POINT
- The reader is invited to consider the implications to the immune system of frequent and intensive stimulation (or assaults) on the immune system represented by repeat vaccination.

Local Prescribing

One way of overcoming the difficulty in collecting a complete history from the patient is to rely on prescriptions based solely on the directly observable physical signs of disease. In a profession where 'they can't talk can they?' veterinarians are well versed in the diagnostic arts; certainly the powers of observation of the veterinarian are finely honed. It is but a short step to the extension of these skills to encompass the fine detail necessary for a homeopathic prescription – though now a 'full examination' must, for instance, include the perineum and the footpads (or hooves), despite the fact that the patient has been presented with influenza.

In many aged patients there is much pathology and it is at this level that the disease process is exhibited. In such cases mental symptoms may be even more obscure and it is here that local prescribing can be particularly appropriate. If a local symptom is 'strange, rare and peculiar', then the prescription is made with an even greater degree of confidence.

Concomitant symptoms may also be vital in the case analysis and the owners of pets are frequently very good at describing these; similarly with time modalities and the characteristics of symptoms. Homeopathy thus brings the owner wholly within the process of making a diagnosis and prescribing the medicine. As a result, the owner's feelings and observations are often validated, for it is the very minutiae which are considered to be irrelevant in conventional medicine which are of such value to the veterinary homeopath. When a dog has diarrhoea vital pieces of information may include the colour and consistency of the stool, the precise time of waking the owner in night, and the reaction of the dog to being scolded – the proffering of this information to an orthodox veterinarian would be seen largely as a waste of valuable time, but the homeopath seeks this information and is grateful for it.

REFLECTION POINT
- Reflect on the challenge of treating a patient who cannot speak.

Working Holistically ('Getting at the Mentals')

As previously discussed, the interpretation of behaviour in terms of mental and emotional states is problematic for the veterinary homeopath. This can be exacerbated when the patient is a small furry animal such as a mouse, or a reptile such as a tortoise. In practice, careful observation of the patient's behaviour and listening sympathetically to a sensitive owner can provide an assessment of the patient's character and emotional state which is certainly adequate for an effective homeopathic prescription to be made. However, it is important to make use of every opportunity to assess the animal's behaviour – to this end it is useful to start by observing the patient as it is taken from the owner's car, and as it enters the waiting and consulting rooms. In the case of a cow, watch it as it comes into the collecting pen and how it interacts with other members of the herd.

The history-taking must explore interactions with other animals and people in detail, along with any obvious fears such as thunder or other loud noises. Nevertheless it should always be borne in mind that the interpretation of this behaviour is subjective, and to some extent dependant on the emotional state of the owner – and indeed that of the veterinarian. One observer may attribute a particular pattern of behaviour to a completely different mental state from that attributed by another – a dog's apparent fear reaction to thunder may be due to a general sensitivity to noise or a reaction to the atmospheric changes involved; alternatively, it may simply be reflecting the fear of a companion. An accurate interpretation may also depend on a knowledge of the behaviour patterns which normally occur in a particular species in a particular situation. It is normal for a small prey species such as a rabbit to fear any object flying overhead as it will be interpreted as a predatory bird, but this is not so normal in a cat – such behaviour in the latter would be accorded greater significance in the case analysis.

There is much debate among zoologists as to what emotions animals are capable of feeling, but suffice it to say that for the effective use of

Broadening our Understanding

IV

homeopathy in animals, it is necessary to accept that they experience the same range of emotions as do humans. The section on 'Mentals' in the repertory may at first glance seem of little relevance to the veterinary homeopath, but it is the imaginative use of this section which often holds the key to a successful prescription in an animal.

Constitution and Breed

In more complex cases of chronic disease, especially where the symptoms are clear, a prescription on constitutional lines is often sought. Putting this concept to use can be another way of circumventing the difficulties inherent in veterinary homeopathy. Even if no other information is available, an assessment of the general physical attributes of the patient can lead to an accurate constitutional prescription. For instance, a Labrador Retriever who is fat, chilly, reluctant to exercise and suffering from swollen joints will probably respond to Calcarea carbonica – the susceptibility of the patient being to exhibit that remedy state. Further questioning of the owner should produce confirmatory information – good appetite, aggravation by cold and damp weather etc. – but even without this a reasonably accurate prescription could be made. The more chronic the disease the more a constitutional approach is likely to be successful compared to local prescribing.

All domestic animals are the product of selective breeding. In the companion animals, sadly, the fashion for showing has resulted in the selection of animals with attributes which, while cosmetically desirable, limit the functionality of the animal as a whole. Examples include the exaggerated skin folds of the Shar-pei dog, which compromise the integrity of the cornea, and the flat face of the Persian cat, which limits its ability to breathe. These physical attributes may represent serious obstacles to cure; it is, for instance, often impossible to completely resolve the hind-leg lameness in a German Shepherd with hereditary hip dysplasia, and symptom reduction may be the best that can be achieved. However, on the positive side, the development of distinct breeds of companion animal has resulted in the selection of individuals with mental and physical attributes which are relatively consistent through generations.

In homeopathic terms this has resulted in a specific breed tending to exhibit features of a specific constitution. Thus the majority of Golden Labradors exhibit features of the Calcarea carbonicum constitution described above, the majority of Irish Setters the exuberant nature of Phosphorus. Relying on these breed–constitution correlations alone is, of course, decidedly unsafe; while many German Shepherds do respond to Lycopodium there are many who do not – so this approach should be viewed critically and used with careful confirmatory and exclusion information.

This raises the issue of how important one should consider the characteristics of the patient which are considered normal for the breed. For instance, if most Cavalier King Charles Spaniels are timid and affectionate, how should these traits be weighted in the case analysis of a specific patient of that breed? It is clear to veterinary homeopaths working on this level that as breed tendencies represent an essential aspect of the patient they must be of significance to susceptibility (constitution) – but also of great importance are those characteristics which run contrary to the breed norm (totality). These latter should be afforded greater significance, and weighted more heavily in the repertorisation of a case to find the totality.

Where animals have been selected for food-production the concept can also be useful, e.g. in dairy cows who can be observed as they wait in collecting yards before and after milking. Sometimes a whole herd will exhibit the same constitution, and in this case a constitutional remedy may be chosen which will beneficially affect every individual in the group. This technique has merit when dealing with any type of herd, and I have even used it successfully in a pack of sled dogs.

REFLECTION POINT
- Reflect on the influence of family, race and gender on the symptom picture presented by any individual patient. Is this different for different species?

Broadening our Understanding

IV

Multiple Prescribing

In view of its deeper effect, most trained veterinary homeopaths would consider prescribing on the totality, and constitution, to be the 'gold standard'. The goal of most practitioners will be to administer such a medicine in a single dose of a high potency preparation. This will be followed by a fairly lengthy period of observation before repeating the dose. However, this is often not possible, and it is therefore quite common for more than one remedy to be given at the same time. This may be to cover aspects of the totality or for different local symptoms. Or it may be different remedies are indicated by different approaches and methodologies (see Chapter 30).

In my experience these situations most often occur in aged animals – it is as if the vital energy is too low to exhibit a coherent picture of a single remedy and instead only makes obvious the local signs of the disease, each one relating to a different remedy. In other cases treatment may start on a single remedy, but new symptoms appear which necessitate a different one. In this way many aged patients seem to 'collect' remedies and may finish their days on a cocktail of homeopathic medicines, each covering a different aspect of the case.

In this context there are many commercial mixtures of homeopathic remedies, designed for use in specific diseases. These sometimes are effective but they focus on treating the local symptoms, not dealing with underlying susceptibility.

Removing Obstacles to Cure

Many animals are presented for homeopathy either following or in the midst of conventional medication. Their symptomatology may be highly suppressed and it may be necessary to employ such techniques as isopathic/tautological use of potentised drugs, or 'clearing remedies' such as Sulphur or Nux Vomica before the picture is clear enough to prescribe on more classical lines. This is particularly true of companion animals. Bowel nosodes are also useful in this context. These are potentised remedies prepared from organisms cultured from normal human bowel contents. They

are particularly useful when a case covers more than one remedy or if well selected remedies are not having the desired effect. Reference to the literature (e.g. Saxton & Gregory 2005) will guide the prescriber to the correct bowel nosode, based on keynotes, or the remedies which appear to be indicated, or on the provings of the bowel nosodes themselves. Administration of the appropriate bowel nosode will usually create a clearer picture of the case and allow a more accurate homeopathic prescription to be made.

Then there is the issue of commercial diets – the widespread promotion of processed (usually dried and pelleted) pet foods has resulted in several generations of dogs and cats who have been reared exclusively on such foods. While it is beyond the scope of this chapter to examine all the possible consequences of this, it seems obvious to many veterinary homeopaths that such foods cannot possibly support optimal health. As such, the continued feeding of processed foods represents a most important obstacle to the patient's recovery – wherever possible the veterinary homeopath will seek to change the animal's diet onto a more 'natural' plane. Having said this, it is not always easy to persuade the owner of the patient to change the feeding habits. Often a compromise has to be sought, either by accepting a partial change in feeding regime or by the use of supplements to fill some of the nutrient gaps left by processing. The more recent introduction of commercial foods for horses raises the same issue in this species.

In performance animals the stresses associated with the high performance expected can certainly affect the response to homeopathy. However, this is counterbalanced by the general health and fitness of the patients, so in practice racing animals respond very well to this form of medicine.

Prescribing for Groups of Animals

Animals are frequently kept in groups – in the case of dog boarding kennels they may number in the tens, a dairy herd may consist of 200 or 300 cows, whereas a flock of poultry may number in the thousands. Prescribing for such groups presents certain challenges, not least of which is the difficulty in individualisation. The following strategies have been designed to overcome these.

Simillimum for the Group
Epizootic/Enzootic Disease
Many of the problems affecting groups of animals are viral diseases, such as infectious bovine rhinotracheitis (IBR) in cattle, orfe in lambs, or kennel cough in dogs. The effects of these on the vital force are frequently so strong as to produce a uniform response from a group of animals. In these cases a single simillimum may be selected to be administered to all the animals in the group. In the case of orfe this would probably be Thuja, as the symptomatology of this remedy corresponds to the majority of cases of orfe. Following this, any individuals who do not respond may be given more specific medicines.

Non-Infectious Disease
Some functional conditions may appear as herd problems, affecting each individual in an identical way. In such instances, once again a single remedy may be selected for the group. Examples of this approach can be found in a trial on the prevention of stillbirths in sows given Caulophyllum (Day 1984) and in others using Sepia to improve the calving-to-service interval in a herd of dairy cows (Williamson et al 1995).

Several metabolic disorders of cattle also lend themselves to this approach. Examples include copper deficiency, hypomagnesaemia and milk fever. Administration of the appropriate mineral in homeopathic potency can have a positive effect on the incidence of the problem in the herd.

Combination Remedy for the Group
Most commonly, an outbreak of disease will affect individuals in a group in different ways, depending on the individual's response to the pathogens. This individuality is further exacerbated by the fact that many infections are multifactorial, with a combination of viral and bacterial pathogens implicated. In an outbreak of pneumonia in calves, for instance, the symptomatology can vary markedly, depending on the individual response of the animal to challenge, and perhaps on the mix of pathogens involved. In any group of animals there may well be three or four distinct symptom pictures apparent, each one indicating a different remedy. In this case, after making the homeopathic diagnosis for each type of individual, the selected remedies may be mixed together and the resulting complex administered to the whole group. Often this is done on the basis of the local symptoms exhibited by the patient; however, an experienced practitioner can make the prescriptions on an approach nearing the totality of symptoms, using general and mental symptoms as well as locals.

This method of treatment should be distinguished from the use of 'off-the-shelf' complexes, many of which may contain tens of remedies in various potencies. These preparations can certainly be effective, but the more specific the selection of remedies to the symptoms actually exhibited by the animals under treatment, the more effective homeopathic medicine is likely to be. A mixture of Kali bichromicum, Bryonia and Phosphorous, prescribed on the basis of observed symptoms, can be expected to be more reliable than a commercial mixture which may or may not include these specific remedies, along with another 10 or so remedies not indicated in this particular group of animals.

Single Remedy Based on Group Totality
With this approach all the symptoms exhibited by individual members of the group are collected, and analysis is performed, if necessary with the help of a repertory, as if the group were a single organism. On the basis of this analysis a single remedy is selected and administered to all members of the group.

REFLECTION POINT
- The reader is invited to reflect on the dynamics which exist in a group to explain the effectiveness of this approach.

Broadening our
Understanding

IV

Nosodes

The use of isopathy does not necessitate the gathering of any information on the patient's symptoms; all that is required is knowledge of the causal agent. Where a specific pathogen is involved, this form of therapy is therefore ideal for the treatment of a herd of animals. While strictly speaking isopathy is a form of therapy distinct from homeopathy, nevertheless it is generally included in the armoury of the homeopath and hence covered here. Several trials have been performed which demonstrate the efficacy of nosodes in the control of mastitis in dairy cattle (Day 1986) and the routine administration of such products is becoming widespread in the UK. However there is a great deal of variation in the type of product and in the response when they are used. By and large it seems that the most effective nosodes are those which have been manufactured using material specific to the farm in question ('isonosodes'). There is also a body of opinion which holds that, in the case of mastitis, using whole milk as opposed to bacterial cultures as the source of the remedy is more effective. Having said this, where pure cultures of specific, properly identified pathogens are used, these 'off-the-shelf' nosodes do seem to be highly effective.

It is, however, important to be aware of the aggravations which can appear after a nosode is administered to a herd of animals suffering from a chronic, subclinical disease. This is of particular significance in the case of mastitis in dairy cows, where stimulation of the defence mechanisms of the udder can result in a flare-up of clinical cases of mastitis and an increase in somatic cell count (a parameter used by commercial dairies to determine the suitability of milk for human consumption). These effects are usually transient but on occasion they can be so great as to necessitate the treatment to be abandoned until the general udder health of the herd has been improved by other means.

Administration of Homeopathic Medicines to Animals

In companion animals, homeopathic medicines may be administered by all the same routes as those used for human patients. However, tablets and pillules have to be swallowed by the patient, rather than sucked – and in any case oral administration is not always possible, especially in cats. For this reason, liquids and powders (or crushed tablets) are popular in veterinary homeopathy, and the use of liquid remedies, as drops or sprays to be applied directly to the oral or nasal mucous membranes, is widespread.

Occasionally mixing in food is the only practicable method of dosing, and as long as bland food is used as a vehicle (e.g. bread for dogs and apples for horses) the effect appears to be adequate.

However, more problematic is the administration of homeopathic medicines to large numbers of animals. Not only is the oral administration of solid medicines to cattle and sheep for the most part impracticable anyway, the considerations of time and stress on the animals of herding large numbers through the necessary handling facilities make individual dosing an impossibility. One exception to this is the dairy cow. At milking time, animals become accessible for individual treatment and spraying a liquid medicine into the vulva is a feasible method of administration. Occasionally an injectable form of the remedy may be used, but the extra equipment required, coupled with the fact that there seems to be no advantage in this approach over other methods of administration, means that it is only rarely used. A liquid potency may be sprayed onto the muzzle of sheep and goats. However, by far the most common method of overcoming the problem of administration in farm animals is to mix the (liquid) remedy in the water supply. This may be accomplished either by dosing individual troughs or by adding the remedy to a header tank.

Repetition of Remedies

It is the experience of many veterinary homeopaths that animals generally seem to need more frequent, and sometimes more prolonged, repetition of remedies than do humans. Opinions on the cause of this vary – some veterinary homeopaths see it as a consequence of the routine neutering of cats and dogs, which somehow renders the patient more refractory to homeopathy; others consider it to be an innate characteristic of the animal metabolism per se, perhaps due to their higher metabolic rates which 'consume' the energy of the remedy more quickly. Whatever the reason, an initial course of homeopathy in an animal can often consist of a 30c potency given daily for a week. This will be repeated when necessary, but may well require repetition a month later. Where there is a risk of interference with the action by concurrent orthodox medicine the homeopathy may be given continuously for some weeks, while gradually weaning the patient off the orthodox medicine.

It should be mentioned, however, that there are veterinary homeopaths who find the sort of dosage regimes prevalent in medical homeopathy to be perfectly adequate in animals – a single dose of a 30c potency or a single divided dose. As so often with homeopathy, there is the opportunity to find a regime which suits the individual practitioner. It is increasingly popular to prescribe the LM potencies in animals; in particular, the continuous dosage régimes of a liquid remedy are found to be well complied with by owners.

REFLECTION POINT
- Why do you think animals might need more prolonged courses of homeopathic treatment than humans?

Miasms in Animals

There is much debate over the validity of the concept of miasms in animals. An understanding of Hahnemann's miasmatic theory leads one to realise that the named diseases which he chose to represent the three major miasms do not directly equate with the miasms themselves. Thus the absence of these specific diseases in animals in no way negates the value of the concept of miasms in veterinary homeopathy. Certainly patterns of chronic disease can be identified in animals which correspond closely to psora, sycosis and syphilis.

In addition, the newer miasms of tuberculosis and cancer are also well represented, mirroring their prevalence in the human population. Given the energetic relationship between animals and man described previously, it would be surprising if this were not so. It is also interesting to note the prevalence of the tubercular miasm in dairy cattle. The disease itself is still not completely eradicated from some parts of the UK, and the inheritance of this miasm leaves its mark in the ringworm, mastitis, pneumonia and chronic scours which so often afflict animals in the dairy industry

The diagnosis of miasms in animals presents no more difficulty than that in humans, and similarly can be an essential step in case analysis. Furthermore, an observant veterinary homeopath can generally identify the mental and emotional basis of the various miasmatic patterns in animal patients, as well as the physical symptoms. Thus the delinquency of tuberculosis and the suppressed emotions of cancer are represented perfectly well in the animal kingdom, along with the chronic respiratory disease or post-viral syndrome with which these miasms are often respectively associated. As an example, cancer miasm is often evident in dogs that have been highly trained for a specific purpose – its preponderance in Border Collie dogs that have been 'trained to perfection' in agility or even sheep herding is a reflection of this.

The Veterinary Relationship

From a psychodynamic point of view the veterinary consultation represents a complex triad, illustrated in Figure 18.1. It behoves the veterinary homeopath to be aware of the opportunity for projection (see Chapter 23) between owner and patient – understanding this dynamic can be vital in assessing the case, as can the dynamic between owner, patient and veterinarian. Not only must the veterinary homeopath be aware of personal feelings – such feelings must also be interpreted in terms of the owner and of the patient. It is not always easy to disentangle the one from the other, but attempting the process can be invaluable for

Broadening our
Understanding

IV

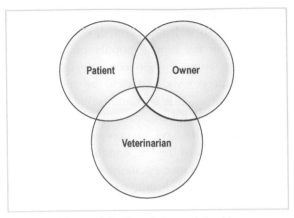

Figure 18.1 The veterinary relationship

all parties concerned. Often the remedy state of the patient is reflected in that of the owner. Indeed, where there is obviously a close emotional relationship between the two, a degree of correspondence may be considered as necessary before a prescription on a fundamental level can be made with any confidence. Whether the animal is reflecting something about the remedy state of the owner or whether the owner is simply projecting it onto the companion is a matter of debate – but either way the relationship does often exist, and understanding this can yield useful and reliable information to the homeopathic case.

Notwithstanding this, such interactions must still be viewed critically. It is, for instance, necessary to establish whether the relationship is as close as it appears – the dog may have been brought in by the neighbour, or it may be presented by the parent of the adolescent with whom it has the closest relationship. However, in the veterinary situation, where direct mental symptoms are lacking, understanding these issues can be of immense help.

Following on from this, it is worth reflecting on what response the patient is likely to show if the owner does not receive corresponding homeopathic treatment or otherwise deal with their problems – be they emotional or physical. For this reason some veterinary homeopaths have been stimulated to gain experience in human homeopathy, or seek the co-operation of a medical homeopath in order to deal with that side of the dynamic.

The psychodynamics of the homeopathic consultation are dealt with in detail elsewhere in this book. The concepts are equally valid when dealing with animals but it must always be remembered that here the homeopath is dealing with an energetic triad – hence the interpretation is that much more complex. While it is in dogs and cats that this dynamic is most obviously relevant, the concept is just as true in the case of so-called 'leisure' horses, or indeed any species of animal where the opportunity exists for the formation of such a close relationship as that described above.

In relation to the above, many veterinary homeopaths are uncomfortable with the concept of ownership of companion animals, and prefer to use such expressions as 'steward' or 'companion' to denote the person responsible for the animal's welfare. For reasons of simplicity, I have chosen to remain with the conventional expression of 'owner', but experience in this field has certainly challenged my preconceptions of the role of animals in a human's life. Treating animals with homeopathy provides a learning opportunity of immense value for the practitioner and one which can indeed change one's world view markedly.

Summary

The use of homeopathy in animals presents certain challenges which, if not irrelevant in human homeopathy, at least have a different emphasis. Overcoming these challenges is not always easy but veterinarians worldwide have engaged with this form of therapy with passion and vigour, with the result that modern veterinary homeopaths enjoy remarkably high success rates in their patients.

There is still much opposition to homeopathy within the veterinary profession. However, as homeopathy is placed on a more scientific basis, more studies attest to its efficacy, and demand from the general public grows further, there is no doubt that in the future this invaluable form of medicine will be truly integrated into general practice, so that the patients of veterinary surgeons worldwide will benefit fully from this remarkable therapy.

References

Day C 1984 Control of stillbirths using homoeopathy. Vet Rec 114:216

Day C 1986 Clinical trials in bovine mastitis using nosodes for prevention. Int J Vet Hom 1:15

Day C 1995 The homoeopathic treatment of beef and dairy cattle. Beaconsfield Publishers, Beaconsfield, UK

Saxton J, Gregory P 2005 Textbook of veterinary homeopathy. Beaconsfield Publishers, Beaconsfield, UK

Williamson A V, Mackie W L, Crawford W J, Rennie B 1995 A trial of Sepia 200: prevention of anoestrus problems in dairy cows. Br Homoeopathic J 84(1):14–20

Bibliography

Hamilton D 1999 Homeopathic care for cats and dogs. North Atlantic Books, Berkeley

Hunter F 2005 Everyday homeopathy for animals. Beaconsfield Publishers, Beaconsfield, UK

Day C 1998 The homeopathic treatment of small animals, 3rd edn. C W Daniel, Saffron Walden

Information Sources and Training

British Association of Homeopathic Veterinary Surgeons *www.bahvs.com*

International Association for Veterinary Homeopathy *www.iavh.*

Academy of Veterinary Homeopathy (USA) *www.avh.org*

Recognised courses of training in veterinary homeopathy are found all over the world. The Homeopathic Professionals Teaching Group (www.HPTG.org) based in Oxford, UK, currently provides UK Faculty-accredited tuition for veterinarians in the UK, Australia, Ireland and South Africa. Elsewhere in the UK the Bristol and Glasgow Homeopathic Hospitals provide accredited courses *www.hptg.org*

In the USA the Academy of Veterinary Homeopathy (AVH) runs courses and provides certification. Several other countries have their own frameworks for accrediting veterinary homeopaths

A list of IAVH accredited courses is available on their website *www.iavh.org*

Broadening our
Understanding

IV

249

CHAPTER NINETEEN

Homeopathic Computer Programs

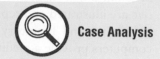

Case Analysis

Phil Edmonds

Introduction by David Owen

Homeopaths have always made use of innovative ways of presenting and searching detailed and extensive information – whether from the detailed and structured materia medicas or the paper and card repertories. At the same time a person's ability to conceptualise something is always connected to how others in that culture think and how those thoughts are expressed. It therefore should be no surprise to realise that computerisation has shifted fundamentally how we think about and the tools available to practice homeopathy. The ability to recognise themes and patterns in different remedies and correlate them to botanical families or the ability to search large libraries of materia medicas are just two such examples. Phil Edmonds has used computers in his practice as well as training others to use them; he brings a practical and clear method to where and how computers can be used. I particularly invite you to reflect on how computers can serve you in the analysis of your cases. In each model of health and approach to treatment they bring important resources that allow the homeopath to focus on what only they can do while broadening, speeding up and making more accurate the process of case analyses. Some student homeopaths and colleges feel that studying paper repertories and doing longhand repertorisation establishes the principles and orientation for repertorisation that can then be applied to computer repertories. Others feel that computerised repertories can be used from early on in the training to gain familiarity. Hopefully after reading this chapter you will be in a better position to weigh up the pros and cons of computerised repertories and materia medicas.

In causative approaches the breadth of data showing association between symptoms and causative or contributing factors allows new ideas and patterns of causation to be considered. For example, searching for all aggravations from milk, cheese and dairy throws up remedies that are susceptible to dairy allergy/sensitivity. Under local symptoms the ability to identify small rubrics that equate to possible 'strange, rare and peculiar' symptoms can increase the confidence in which local prescribing is made; it is also easy to add confirmatory and eliminatory symptoms.

In totality prescribing, the ability to include large rubrics and search for particular symptoms that may require combined rubrics allows the net to be cast wide for possible remedies. The use of small remedy filters to emphasise small remedies or remove polychrests from the analyses can then ensure small but indicated remedies are not discarded without consideration. The rapid cross reference to materia medica eases the important comparison of the remedies in the differential diagnosis. For constitutional factors, features recorded in cases and that run through remedies can be teased out and searched for more quickly than in paper texts.

Thematic approaches have perhaps been most greatly helped by computerisation. The development of thematic patterns in patients and themes in the remedy pictures track each other in a way that is perhaps more than coincidence. The patterns of families that make the use of themes so effective are illustrated and represented through materia medica and repertory searches. In addition, computers provide a medium for rapid growth of information in a way that builds on existing information. Relational prescribing is partly informed by the possibilities of a more dynamic and interactive way of studying remedies and by the recording and searching of key emotional and sensation words that might otherwise be lost in the minutiae of the printed texts.

I encourage you to read this chapter, if at all possible, in conjunction with looking at and trying one of the homeopathic computer programs, of which there are several. Most offer student demonstration programs and as long as you are realistic about how you use the programs then you will find they can aid your homeopathic studying.

What Can a Computer Do for The Homeopath?

This chapter explores what a homeopathic computer program can do and Box 19.1 lists the main features that are covered in this chapter – the most important being how it helps in analysing a case. I look at three main programs and illustrate using screen shots of each. This is not meant to be a detailed comparison of these or a 'training' session. Rather it is a familiarisation of what is available and should stimulate thinking about how computers might help in each of the five different approaches to treatment that run through this book and in each of the different methodologies to prescribing (see Chapter 5).

Storing Rubrics in the Computer Memory for Analysis (Fig 19.1)

All the programs use the drag and drop feature to move data from a search screen to a clipboard for storage and analysis. There is effectively no limit to the size of rubrics or number of rubrics that can be used – but more rubrics does not always more accurately reflect the case.

BOX 19.1
What can a Computer do for the Homeopath?
- Store rubrics in the computer memory for analysis
- Search the repertory for a known symptom (you know where it is in the repertory, e.g. 'mind fear dark')
- Search for keywords in the repertory (you don't know where the rubric is for the symptom you are trying to repertorise)
- Look at cross references (find a more appropriate rubric for a symptom)
- Combine rubrics
- Analyse a list of rubrics
- Extract symptoms of a remedy from the repertory
- Search for themes/concepts, e.g. animals, accidents, otitis media
- Check repertory sources
- Edit your analysis (change or delete rubrics)
- Weight symptoms (underlining/selecting intensity)
- Analyse with expert systems
- Analyse and search families
- Search the materia medica from the repertory
- Search and analyse materia medica
- Patient database
- Multimedia (sound clips and photos)
- Help

Search the Repertory for a Known Symptom

MacRepertory and Radar use a pictogram (Fig 19.2) to find the chapter you wish to select your rubric from. Say, for example, you want to search for 'fear of the dark'. Use the mouse to point to the relevant chapter. Clicking on this brings up a box in which all or part of a search word is typed, e.g. fe for 'fear'. This generates a list of sub-rubrics for fear. Scrolling down the list to 'dark' allows the rubric 'fear of the dark' to be displayed, showing all the remedies contained within it.

With any of the programs it is very easy to drag and drop symptoms onto a symptom clipboard and save it in the memory, and/or print out the analysis. Indeed one of the disciplines you need to learn with a computer is not to put in too many rubrics, as it is now so easy to do. Helping with this is the facility of having multiple clipboards – you can copy all your rubrics onto one clipboard, then select essential symptoms one at a time onto another clipboard, and see how the case builds up.

This is especially useful in cases where you take too many rubrics initially. Figure 19.3 shows the Isis Explorer tree used to guide you to the rubric you want, by book, chapter, and rubric.

The different ways of entering the data, i.e. keyboard or mouse, suit different people so it is advisable to try different programs to see what suits your style best.

Figure 19.1 Drop and drag rubrics

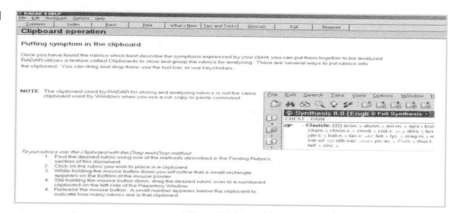

Figure 19.2 MacRepertory pictogram

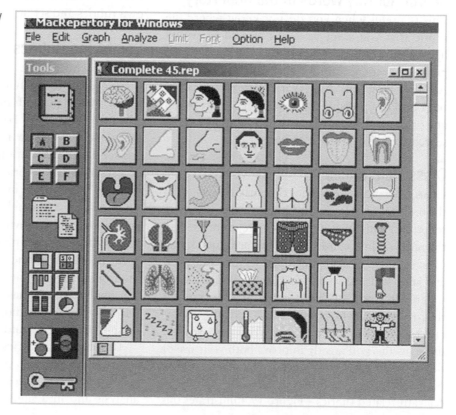

Figure 19.3   Isis explorer tree

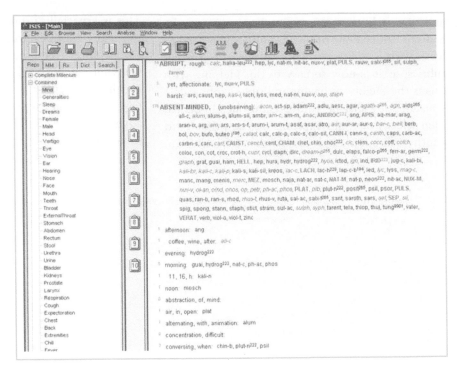

Search for Key Words in the Repertory

This is useful when you do not know where the rubric that you want to use is located or would like to find a list of potential rubrics. In each program you can rapidly search for 'key words'. All the programs have various repertories on offer and it is possible to use several repertories in any one case. It is particularly helpful to be able to search for rubrics and key words.

Cross References

Cross references are rubrics that may be related to the one you are searching. They can help guide you to other, sometimes more accurate, rubrics than the one you first considered. They are a quick way of navigating around the repertory but can skew any analysis if many rubrics representing the same or similar aspect of the case are used. To prevent this, rubrics can be combined. It remains important to know the structure of the repertory you are using, as this will greatly improve both your use of the computer and your choice of rubrics. All the programs greatly improve the ease of identifying relevant related rubrics – Figure 19.4 illustrates this

cross referencing. Additionally, you can add your own rubrics and set up your own cross references.

Combining Rubrics

A very useful feature of the computer repertory is the facility to easily combine symptoms – you lessen the chance of missing the right remedy when you combine. For example, a keynote of the remedy Alumina is to take a long time to answer a question. In one repertory it might not be present in the rubric 'mind answering reflecting long' but will be in 'mind answering slowly'. The advantage of combining rubrics, rather than just adding them individually, is that it widens the net, without overemphasising the remedies that occur in several rubrics. For example, if you take the rubrics 'dreams murder' and 'dreams killing' you might overemphasise Aurum sulph, which is the only remedy common to both. If you combined these rubrics this would not be the case.

Different repertories have different strengths and weaknesses. It is possible to combine different rubrics from different repertories both in an analysis and in a single rubric – if you use these

Figure 19.4 Radar cross references are hypertext (13 shown)

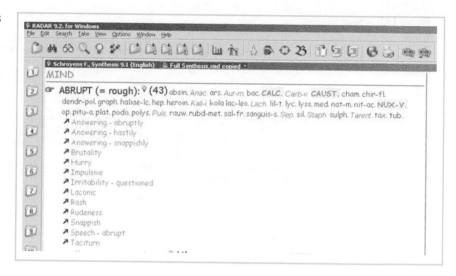

regularly they can help to modify your personalised version of a repertory.

Analyse a List of Rubrics

This technique makes handling large amounts of data much easier, e.g. when using the largest rubrics. With a computer, rubrics, irrespective of size, can be used, weighted, modified and combined at the click of a mouse. The rubrics are entered into a selection of clipboards that can, separately or in combination, be analysed and reviewed. If you want to work thematically you might, for example, put all the rubrics that link to a particular theme in one clipboard. It is easy to weight the rubrics according to their emphasis in the case and look at how a change in emphasis changes the score and relative position for each remedy in your analysis.

This makes repertorising the case as part of the consultation, or immediately after, much easier – providing a shortlist of likely remedies and the opportunity to explore these with the patient at the time, thus confirming the prescription. Rather than hold several possible remedies and rubrics in your head they are recalled accurately from a saved analysis and can be studied at your leisure or built up successively over several visits.

All the programs use a standard 'rubric score' to calculate the most well represented remedy, sometimes referred to as the 'sum of symptoms', adding together the total occurrence of remedies – scoring 3 for a bold type entry, 2 for italics and 1 for normal type.

This can be easily personalised to reflect a variety of analysis strategies including the use of weighting of rubrics, prominence (e.g. taking into account where a remedy is the only bold type remedy in a rubric) and eliminatory rubrics. The information is displayed on a range of graphs (some that look similar to Fig. 19.5) but various graph styles can represent the results of the analysis very differently which suits those who like visually displayed information – helping to identify remedies that might otherwise not be picked out. Having entered the rubrics you want to use in a case, you can easily change from one analysis strategy to another and look at the case from different perspectives, e.g. small remedies, exclude polychrests, small rubrics etc. (see Chapters 9, 14). Figure 19.4 shows the Radar analysis screen, with three symptom clipboards open in the left foreground and the remedies from left to right – showing which remedies occur in which rubrics.

It is possible to speedily move from your analyses to the materia medica you want to use or if you want to set up your personal keynotes (adding things from lectures) – it is up to you. You may alternatively like to see what rubrics a particular remedy features in and how strongly and/or uniquely it features (see below).

Broadening our Understanding

IV

Figure 19.5   Radar analysis screen

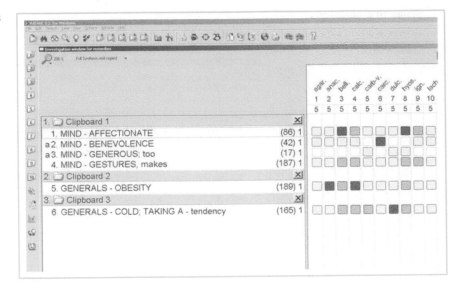

Extracted Symptoms of a Remedy from the Repertory

Sometimes you may want to look at all the rubrics that contain a particular remedy. This can be useful in a number of different situations:

- To differentiate between remedies, e.g. look at all the food desires and aversions of Phosphorous compared with Natrum muriaticum.
- You are considering a small remedy and cannot find any materia medica information.
- You want to study a remedy and want to look at, for example, all the bold type mentals, all the unique rubrics, all the rubrics where the remedy is the only one in bold type.
- You want to check the rubrics of a particular remedy such as Bothrops lanceolatus. It is not in the rubric 'weakness of memory for words', but is bold type in 'forgetful for words while speaking'.

Searching your materia medica and repertory is an excellent example of how you can rapidly store data from a variety of sources in one place and display it in a way that is relevant for you.

Search for Themes/Concepts

Computers now offer another new possibility – searching for themes, rather than just rubrics. This opens up a whole new world of possibilities for searching, e.g. you can search for

- animals, rather than dogs, cats, wolves, etc.
- all the rubrics containing any reference to time, rather than morning, etc.

There is also the possibility of making your own new rubrics to represent themes, e.g. all remedies that have issues with money, rather than just taking fear of poverty, or avarice. Plus you can create rubrics for the main organ remedies and limit your analysis to filter out remedies that do not, for example, have a strong liver affinity. Examples of rubrics you might create to act as filters include 'money', 'liver' or 'obsessive'.

Each of the programs is keen to encourage reflection about cases thematically and each does so in a slightly different way – perhaps reflecting the absence of one clear mechanism or tool for this approach that, while it uses the information in the repertory and materia medica, also looks for dynamic, living relationships and patterns. In Radar you can search for all the rubrics that contain information related to an idea, e.g. lack of self-confidence. In Isis there is a list of predefined themes, and in MacRep themes and concepts can be displayed graphically.

Check Repertory Sources

All the programs allow you to find out where an addition to the repertory comes from. You might trust one source more than another or you might also want to verify a particular addition, or check the context in the materia medica.

Edit Your Analysis

Once you have chosen your rubrics and placed them on a symptom/rubric clipboard you can then modify the selection in a number of ways (Box 19.2).

Underlining or weighting a symptom will change the way a computer deals with the rubric in the analysis. For instance, if you underline a rubric twice the program will treat the rubric, for analyses and scoring, as if you had entered it twice. Underlining helps to give 'light and shade' to a case and is therefore an important tool, as it helps you express your patient's symptoms and the emphasis of the case more accurately. If you find you have taken too many rubrics, then by copying all the rubrics to a spare clipboard you can rebuild the case from scratch with the most essential features – noticing how the analysis changes as you add more rubrics.

There are a variety of ways you might allocate rubrics to different clipboards to reflect how you are approaching the case. If you want to use the 'three-legged stool' methodology you might put mentals in one, generals in one, and physicals in another. If you want a local treatment for a particular problem you might put all the relevant symptoms in a specific clipboard. Using the clipboards is one of the easiest ways of using themes and may enable the analyses of different levels of symptoms or layers of themes.

BOX 19.2

Modifying Rubrics Selected
- Change underlining (intensity or weighting)
- Move/copy rubrics to a different clipboard
- Delete a rubric
- Combine rubrics into a group or a single rubric
- Eliminate remedies that do not occur in that rubric from the analysis
- Mark the rubric as a causation
- View one or more clipboards at a time
- Save or delete the clipboard

Expert and Personalised Systems

All the programs have the option for advanced users of defining their own way of working or using expert analysis strategies based on the methodologies of experienced prescribers. This, and ways of emphasising little known or used remedies, can prompt consideration of smaller remedies that might otherwise not be considered.

Analysis Strategies Using Families

There are various 'filters' you can apply around the general idea of remedy families (see Chapter 22). For example, the computer can show you:
- only psoric (or sycotic, etc.) remedies
- only plant remedies (or mineral or animal)
- only solanacea remedies (or any plant family)
- only salts
- only remedies from a particular part of the periodic table.

This is certainly made easier using computers in homeopathy – you can look at all the plant/animal/mineral remedies with just a click of the mouse. For instance, in Figure 19.6 the graph particularly highlights the usefulness of a limitation to mineral remedies, in a case of frightful dreams of choking, that did well on Calcium carbonate and then went to Calcium silicata – a limitation to just salts makes Calcium silicata a stronger contender still.

Search the Materia Medica from the Repertory

In many ways the traditional role of the repertory is being challenged by the ability to search large libraries of cases and materia medica. There are some clear advantages to being able to do this:
- The repertory always lags behind provings, as symptoms need to be organised, and put into the repertory structure – they can be made available to homoeopaths much more quickly in materia medica format.
- Because the materia medica is less structured you can search for the exact language of the patient.
- The repertory was originally intended to be a dictionary of materia medica, now we can access the material directly.

Figure 19.6 MacRepertory analysis limited to minerals

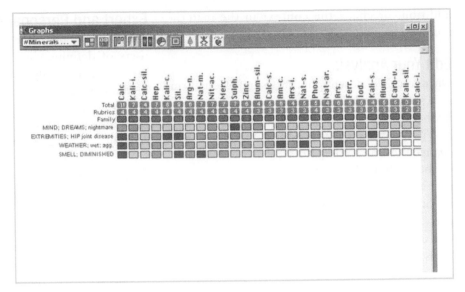

- The libraries of materia medica and cases vary slightly from program to program but each offers what would otherwise be shelves full of materia medicas and journals.
- You can search a whole library for a word or group of words in a few seconds, and view the results.

Limit Your Search in Variety of Ways

It is possible to search for words that are definitely linked, e.g. next to each other; separated by a specified number of words; in the same sentence, paragraph or section. Equally you can search for words that are not linked, e.g. desire for fat but not meat.

Patient Database

In the programs you can view a summary of all the consultations, make brief notes, and look back over a summary of past repertorisation. Computers ease the possibility of searching for certain cases you have seen, e.g. asthma cases, and looking at cases where you have prescribed a particular remedy or cases with a particular outcome. There are many practice management programs available if you wish to extend the use of computers in your practice.

Multimedia

All the programs have sophisticated displays of illustrative materia medica, help screens and other information that often reflects recent developments in homeopathy – where innovation is often easier and quicker to present in a computer program than to publish in writing. Figure 19.7 illustrates such a screen.

Help

Help comes from both printed manuals and online help screens with audiovisual programs.

Summary

Computer programs are able to repertorise big or multiple rubrics much quicker than is possible with a book. They provide you with the resources to analyse your cases in a variety of ways, using a variety of methods and strategies. Each program is well supported and training and familiarisation are recommended before using any of them in practice.

Figure 19.7 Isis multimedia screen

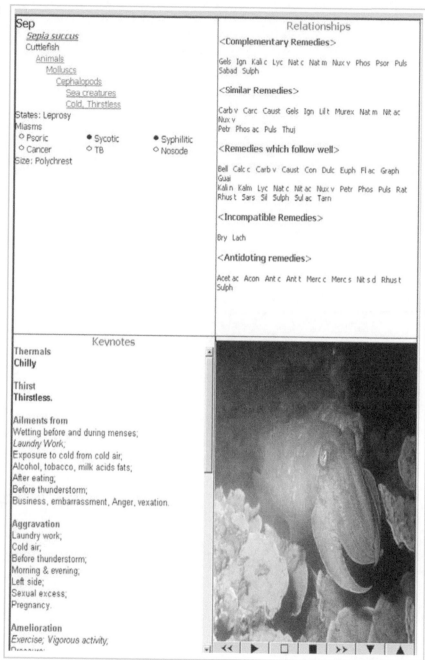

CHAPTER TWENTY

Homeopathic Pharmacy

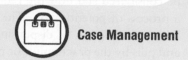

Case Management

Tony Pinkus

Introduction by David Owen

It may seem strange to wait until this far into the book before tackling the question of homeopathic pharmacy – particularly potency and administration. However, I have found too many homeopaths distracted, confounded and constrained in their study of homeopathy by different nuances in the use of different potencies. I have in previous chapters made some very general and rather sweeping statements about the use of potency such as recommending the novice homeopath confine themselves to low potencies of 12 or 30 in straightforward or simple cases. In practice, different homeopaths develop different ways of using potency depending on the case, methodology and their own experience. To enable you to better develop your own view on potency, we spend some time going through the basic principles of homeopathic pharmacy and the preparation of remedies so that you can make informed choices about potency.

I hope by this stage in the book you can understand my concern for patients being given frequent high potencies and that managing patients is made harder by the inaccurate administration of remedies. By now I hope you are able to both appreciate enough of the different models of health and have an insight into your own competencies to match cases accurately to remedies through respective methodologies – to both handle and prescribe the higher potencies with the care they warrant.

As you will appreciate, the choice of potency is influenced by the clarity of the case, the model of

health, the approach to treatment, the methodology used and the remedy. Additionally, the risk of aggravation, the certainty of the prescription, the aim of the treatment, the likelihood of any antidoting factors and the ability to follow the case up will all shape the decision regarding potency.

I am grateful to Tony Pinkus for providing the background to how remedies are prepared and dispensed – so that you might conceptualise how a patient can hopefully be matched not only to their simillimum but also to their optimum potency. Tony is equally at home talking about the material sources of our remedies as when reflecting on their subtle energetic qualities – homeopathic principles hold true in whatever model they are used. I have found a helpful analogy in matching potency to an individual is to think of the remedies as 'falling' through the patient's subtle body. Different potencies resonate at different depths, hence the recommendation that (generally) the deeper the case and model of heath used to understand it the higher the potency.

Homeopathic Pharmacy

The object of this chapter is to introduce all aspects of homeopathic pharmacy, from the preparation of remedies from raw materials, to the description and administration of dosage forms and over-the-counter (OTC) prescribing. Homeopathy employs ultra-high dilutions, rendering its mechanism of action difficult to describe in the normal medical models of biochemistry and physiology. Instead the concept of the remedy as an 'energy' or 'vibration' will be considered and how the remedy is prepared by a process of potentisation. The chapter concludes with a description of dispensing of drops, tablets and pills by the practitioner or pharmacy.

Originally homeopathic remedies were prepared by the early practitioners themselves. Hahnemann's *Organon* is divided into three major areas: 'principles', 'practice', and 'remedy preparation' – thus giving equal prominence to homeopathic pharmacy. Knowledge of how remedies are prepared and used is crucial to the practice of homeopathy.

Pharmacopoeia – How Remedies are Made

In order to make a homeopathic remedy we require knowledge of the properties and origin of the source material together with a method of preparation. Materia medica, mentioned in other chapters, are clinical texts and contain detailed descriptions of usage but no methods of production, standardisation or testing of the raw material and finished product. This information is encompassed within a homeopathic pharmacopoeia. Standardisation is critical for manufacture – it tries to ensure the remedy will be identical irrespective of whoever makes it, providing they use the same starting material and follow the same method. It is crucial that a remedy matches its monograph in the materia medica, otherwise the clinical response will be at variance with that expected by the homeopath. The homeopath therefore relies on the integrity of the homeopathic pharmacy to provide remedies which are not only standardised but also conform to the original 'proven' substance.

Conventional methods of standardisation are limited to measurable physicochemical properties, and while these are important there are other equally relevant considerations for the preparation of homeopathic remedies. It is possible that how the person making the remedy feels and behaves has an effect on the remedy being prepared. The intention and feeling may mirror the sensitivity of practitioners and influence not only the choosing of a remedy but also the choice of homeopathic pharmacy to dispense that remedy. This 'having the right feeling'

is an ineffable factor accepted without question and underplayed within our culture, but clearly important when considered from both a pharmacy and practitioner's viewpoint. It is the attention to detail beyond the measurable that requires such integrity by the homeopathic pharmacist.

Conventional pharmacy use pharmacopoeias to manufacture and standardise medicines. A small number of homeopathic pharmacopoeias exist, although they are limited in the number of remedies listed. In Europe there are German, French and British homeopathic pharmacopoeia and outside Europe others such as the United States, Mexico and India. Currently the European Pharmacopoeia is incorporating homeopathic monographs harmonised from the pharmacopoeia of its member states. Pharmacopoeias are used extensively in the manufacture of remedies, although there is still a large gap between the number of pharmacopoeial monographs and the number of remedies in use – the main reasons being the proliferation of new remedies and the extensive range of small, rarely used ones.

Standardisation of remedy preparation is practical in most cases but almost impossible in others. Where a monograph describes a plant, the parts used and when to harvest them, it is relatively easy for everyone to make an equivalent remedy that matches the expectation of the practitioner. However, there are wonderful anomalies in the materia medica that delight and surprise us. For example, the original proving of Tarentula hispanica was conducted with a remedy made, unintentionally, from a decomposed spider. The single spider, sent across the Atlantic by ship, arrived dead and mouldy. The remedy is invaluable but to replicate the original material and thereby standardise production is impossible. Similarly, Causticum is made from burnt lime – a potash preparation whose exact composition is unknown.

The challenge for homeopathic pharmacy is to make remedies that faithfully match their corresponding picture in the provings. Calcarea carbonica could be made very easily from a plentiful commercial source of anhydrous calcium carbonate. However, the proving was conducted with a

Broadening our understanding

IV

remedy prepared by painstakingly scraping out the calcified inner layer of an oyster shell. One is a mineral, even if it was originally derived from ancient bones, whereas the other is clearly an animal from a specific source – do these feel the same to you? Changing the source of starting material is clearly unwise.

Colour is a form of vibration and we all have different responses to different colours – an example encompassing both points is Cantharis made from Spanish Fly. The proving was conducted with *Cantharis vesicatoria*, a beautiful green iridescent flying beetle, native to Spain and northern Africa. The beetles nest in trees overnight and are caught by shaking the trees early in the morning, before the sun's heat has inflated their wings. A selective predator, they survive solely on a rare burrowing bee, which, in becoming extinct, has threatened the beetle's existence, making the remedy difficult to produce. Many types of the drab brown and black striped Mylabaris beetle, being also Cantharis species, are plentiful in Asia. We could save a great deal of effort by accepting the Mylabaris as an alternative source material, but the remedy would clearly be at variance with that used in the proving. The remedy may have similar chemical content but its complete picture be different in important ways.

Range and Source of Remedies

Remedies are prepared from all three kingdoms of Nature, plants accounting for about 65%, minerals 30% and animals 5%. In addition, there are a host of new and miscellaneous sources including allopathic drugs, allergens, chemicals, and foods. In my own company, we have made over 3500 remedies over the last 25 years – each in three potency scales, with numerous potencies within each scale. Whereas we are all familiar with plants, animals and minerals, there are some unusual remedy categories employed by homeopaths.

Nosodes

Nosodes are prepared from diseased biological material. A nosode is a remedy made from raw material of diseased origin containing a mixture of foreign and host matter. With the advent of bovine spongiform encephalitis, autoimmune disease and hepatitis this is a now a controversial area. A French manufacturer has established with the Pasteur Institute that 8x or 4c (1 part in 100,000,000) is the lowest non-pathogenic potency that could be guaranteed to be non-infective. The method currently used is to prepare nosodes from purified and inactivated cultures of the pathogenic organism. This satisfies many safety issues and ensures we and our clients know exactly what the remedy is prepared from. The plethora of commercial vaccines can also be prepared as nosodes, popular for antidoting vaccine reactions, being purified samples containing the killed or live organism with a mixture of preservatives and antibiotics. Not all nosodes are made from infected tissue. Some are made from diseased tissue, e.g. Carcinosin and the large number of cancer nosodes are derived from tumours such as breast, testicle, lung and bowel.

Bowel nosodes isolated from stool cultures in the 1950s by the Pattersons – emulating the work of Edward Bach – are a discrete group that cannot be replicated today. The over-use of antibiotics and the changing classification of types of bacteria mean we cannot identify with any certainty from which organisms each was isolated. Although most nosodes are obtained from animal tissue some are derived from plants, with examples such as Secale (ergot) and Ustilago (corn smut).

Sarcodes

Sarcodes are obtained from healthy tissue such as thyroidinum (sheep's thyroid), folliculinum (rat ovaries) and secretin (a gut hormone). Remedies have been made from healthy tissues such as ligament, cartilage, bone, artery and hormones – some have been proved, many are used speculatively in an attempt to restore normal structure and function. You might like to reflect on the use of oestrogen in potency in the menopause or using potencies of TSH, thyroidinum or tetraiodothyrinine in thyroid dysfunction.

Broadening our understanding

IV

New Remedies

The side effects of allopathic and antipathic drugs are sometimes used to give an indication of their action in homeopathic form. However, this will be considerably less informative than a proving (see Chapter 2). Often new remedies follow a typical fad curve, practitioners being naturally inclined to explore the latest discovery yet consistently returning to tried and tested polychrests. In recent years a tranche of new remedies have appeared, accompanied by new provings, with well-reasoned extrapolations from known materia medica or clinical observations. Some have enjoyed wide success, such as Jan Scholten's 'Elements of the periodic table' and Peter Tumminello's 'Twelve jewels', whilst countless others remain obscure. A new classification of Imponderabilia is the term employed to describe the oddities that do not fit elsewhere, e.g. Tlacote water, obtained from a well in a small Mexican village and reputed to be a panacea, or vibrational remedies from the Nile temples, pyramids and ancient sites, electricity, moonlight and colours all fall into this category.

Veterinary Remedies

Many enquiries received by homeopathic pharmacies are requests for remedies for cats, dogs, rabbits and horses (see Chapter 18). Large numbers of cats and dogs receive homeopathic remedies instead of conventional vaccinations and treatments. The demand to treat livestock is also considerable – many UK farms use homeopathy routinely to treat and prevent disease in cattle, sheep, pigs and chickens. The advantage of a residue-free treatment makes homeopathy an economical imperative for farmers. Remedies are administered to a cow by spraying her vulva during milking or added to the water troughs to prevent common herd problems.

Constitutional treatment of cattle is similar to that in humans and equally successful. A herdsman who knows his cows can learn the major constitutional remedies surprisingly quickly. Sheep are sprayed on the nose as they run by a race or the remedy is sprayed on grass being grazed. Pigs are

treated in water troughs or aerosoled in their pens. Chickens are treated via drinkers fed from overhead medicated water tanks – chickens treated for stress-related conditions like feather pecking produce browner eggs with thicker shells as the stress reduces. Many new nosodes have been prepared by making remedies from animal diseases; this avenue is becoming increasingly popular as an easy introduction to prevention and treatment for the novice prescribing on causation.

Over-the-Counter Prescribing

Whereas a handful of dedicated homeopathic pharmacies supply a vast range of remedies in a wide spectrum of potencies, most retail pharmacies and health shops offer over-the-counter (OTC) ranges in a 6c or 30c potency The manufacture and marketing of OTC remedies within the European Community requires licensing in accordance with the Homeopathic Directive (see p. 272), although unmarketed remedies are excluded from licensing. Many countries outside Europe have adopted some form of licensing based on the European model. Where access to a homeopath is restricted, rare or too expensive, the availability of OTC remedies is an important option for the public. Many countries benefit from thriving homeopathic OTC markets and the remedies form an integral part of their cheap and available self-medication products.

OTC prescribing is necessarily restricted to minor self-limiting conditions and limited to the ability of the shop staff's knowledge and experience of homeopathy (Box 20.1). The usual scenario is truly one of self-help with the aid of a flyer or booklet – teaching yourself homeopathy and self-prescribing in a busy shop is not easy for anything but the most straightforward or simple case. Unfortunately many people try to self-treat inappropriately and when it does not work think homeopathy has let them down or failed!

The success of homeopathy on the high street is variable, there being numerous competing products and services in a conventional pharmacy. However, the greatest barriers to the spread of homeopathy

Broadening our understanding

IV

- Approach a homeopathic pharmacy/manufacturer who can supply both remedies and advice. The latter should be able to offer both OTC products and an extensive range of remedies in a wide potency spectrum required for individual prescriptions. Many homeopathic prescriptions will need to be individually prepared for you.
- Stock a limited range of remedies for common OTC complaints, ensuring this is provided with adequate sales support. Consider this range carefully, taking advice from practitioners and suppliers.
- Consider studying an appropriate introductory or foundation course.
- Train your staff to provide homeopathic advice on minor self-limiting conditions, without going beyond their level of competence. Make use of self-help sheets and provide registers of qualified practitioners.
- Acquaint yourself with local homeopaths for referral and your own support. Be aware that many local groups arrange meetings for discussion and continued professional development.
- Knowledge comes with experience and your progress will increase markedly with customer feedback. Great satisfaction will be gained in broadening your awareness of the remedies by simple prescribing.

are the lack of knowledge from the shop staff and poor education of the public. Frequently, the driving force is an enthusiastic assistant whose interest, borne of personal experience, has inspired an entire community.

OTC Versus Practitioner Prescribing

There is a world of difference between acute OTC prescribing and a consultation with a homeopath with access to a homeopathic pharmacy. Many homeopaths disparage the commercialisation of homeopathy because of the wish to prescribe for everyone holistically. In practice many patients can be helped by prescribing on the cause (such as Arnica for injury, Aconite for acute infection or panic attack) or on the presenting symptom (such as Drosera for whooping-type coughs, Cuprum for night cramps, Hepar sulph for very tender boils).

From a manufacturer's point of view, mass-produced remedies have to be actively marketed. If you have invested in a manufacturing site, employees, licenses, etc. you clearly have to sell products in order to survive, as opposed to waiting for patients to arrive with individual prescriptions. In this respect manufacturing and marketing a particular product can grow the general awareness of homeopathy but is limited (like all OTC prescribing) to certain, often self-limited conditions. Inappropriate OTC or self-treatment can delay and sometimes complicate treatment.

Manufacture

Method of Trituration

Remedies made from minerals are often insoluble and the initial phase of grinding the source material with lactose using a pestle and mortar, called trituration. Although considered to be an inert medium, like water, lactose is perhaps less inert in our age of milk allergies. Hahnemann, who was devoted to consistency and accuracy, dictates a method of triturating to 3c that embraces dilution and succussion called C3 trituration used for all source material to manufacture the starting potency for LM potencies. He cunningly includes rest periods to allow recuperation between stages, so ensuring the same energy is employed from start to finish. Aphorism 270 states:

'Divide 99 parts lactose into three aliquots. Add one third to mortar, add one part substance to be prepared. Mix for a moment then triturate strongly for 6–7 minutes. Scrape mass in mortar for 3–4 minutes to make homogenous. Repeat trituration for 6–7 minutes with the same

force, followed by scraping for 3–4 minutes. Then add second aliquot of lactose mix for a moment and repeat the stage above exactly. Then add the third aliquot and repeat again. Finally decant the triturate into a bottle and tightly seal and protect from light. Label with the name of the remedy and the attenuation 1c.'

Mother Tinctures

The starting point for any remedy of vegetable origin is the preparation of its mother tincture (MT), similar to any herbal tincture prepared by herbalists. The quaint expression 'mother' reminds us this tincture will soon give birth to a family of potencies. Calendula and Hypericum are used topically in the form of tinctures and creams for healing wounds, Thuja mother tincture is applied to warts and veruccas, Euphrasia tincture is diluted in freshly boiled and cooled water before bathing sore eyes, and Crataegus mother tincture is used in some cardiac conditions.

A pharmacopoeial monograph provides the method for mother tincture preparation. In the absence of a monograph, an in-house method is created from knowledge of the material's physicochemical properties. The first consideration is solubility of the raw material in water and alcohol. If insoluble it is prepared by trituration.

In plants, fresh material is used whenever possible as they seem to produce superior remedies to dried ones. Plant material is not completely soluble and requires mincing and soaking in alcohol (a process known as maceration) for the active elements to be released into solution. The active soluble parts of the plant are separated from inert cellulose structures, which are filtered off. Many substances are soluble in either water or alcohol, the primary solvents used in homeopathy, providing a simple method of mother tincture production. A notable exception is Carbo vegetabilis (vegetable charcoal), a common remedy originating from a plant but prepared like a mineral. Carbo vegetabilis is made from beech wood chips, which Hahnemann decided to carbonise to an insoluble charcoal, which has then to undergo trituration.

The Role of Water

The preparation of a mother tincture involves transferring the information or qualities of a plant into solution. Water and alcohol have fascinating roles in this process. Water, a simple liquid, is highly organised and much has been written about its complexity and its importance as a liquid, but, in my mind, none demonstrate how it absorbs vibration more clearly than Masaru Emoto (1999). This Japanese scientist became fascinated by the individuality of snow flakes, and decided to photograph ice crystals of water from a variety of sources and exposed to various messages. He observed that vibration uniquely shapes frozen crystals of water. In two beautiful volumes he features stunning photographs demonstrating how gentle, loving vibrations create harmony and beautifully complex crystals, whereas destructive vibrations, pollution and obscenities produce disorganisation, simple and chaotic structures. He concludes 'the messages from water are telling us to look inside ourselves'. The message is palpable and crucial from a homeopathic perspective.

Alcohol

Alcohol preserves the information or vibration of a remedy in a solution and has an important role from preparation of the mother tincture to medicating tablets. It is both a preservative of the raw material and of the information and vibrational properties of the remedy. In dispensing, alcohol transfers the remedy, coating tablets, pills or granules, in addition to acting as a drying agent of the coated medication. The alcohol used in the preparation of remedies is 95% ethanol, from a vegetable rather than mineral origin. Plant material varies greatly – some plants are more succulent than others, or contain oily or less soluble constituents. Hence the pharmacopoeial methods and individual monographs vary in the percentage of remedies, for example, ethanol and water to be used in the preparation of maceration of Calendula needs 33% and Crataegus 87% alcohol to obtain a standardised mother tincture.

Preparation of Mother Tinctures from Plants

Composition

Fresh plant material decomposes quickly and must be prepared immediately upon receipt. Raw material, grown organically without chemicals, may be in the form of leaves, flowers, roots, rhizomes, bark, fruit, seeds or whole plant.

Concentration

The German pharmacopoeia specifies an alcohol: plant ratio of 3:1 whereas the French traditionally use 10:1 and their more dilute mother tinctures are D1 or 1x by comparison.

Washing

The first step is to ensure that plant material is free from dirt and insects and to clean it with the minimum amount of water so as not to artificially increase its weight or water content.

Dry Weight Calculation

Mother tinctures are prepared with a specific ratio of alcohol to plant, calculated for consistency as dry weight of plant material. Hence the second step requires a calculation of the dry weight of the plant material to establish precisely how much water is lost and how much alcohol to add. A small sample of plant is retained to calculate the loss on drying. The retained sample is weighed, oven dried and re-weighed to establish water loss and therefore the correct volume of alcohol to be added to make a 3:1 dilution.

Preparation

Plant material is weighed, minced and placed in glass preparation jars to which a small volume of alcohol is added to preserve the material whilst awaiting the result of the calculation above. The addition of ethanol and water is made according to the pharmacopoeial monograph being adjusted for each sample – the percentage of alcohol varying between remedies from 30% to 90% ethanol.

Maceration

After adding alcohol the jar is stored in the dark for a period of one month, during which it is regularly agitated to ensure efficient maceration, before filtration and pressing to remove insoluble components.

Labelling and Storage

The mother tincture is labelled and given an expiry date in accordance with its monograph, generally 5 years. In nomenclature a mother tincture is designated by the suffix MT or by the Greek letter theta (θ). After labelling the container is stored in a cool, dark place to avoid sunlight accelerating decomposition.

Testing

The mother tincture is tested in accordance with its pharmacopoeial monograph to ensure that it complies with the specification. The range of tests for physicochemical properties includes appearance, odour, density, and thin layer chromatography. Ironically no tests are available to assess the crucial, if ineffable, vibration or information quality we associate with a remedy except proving and using it.

Mother Tinctures from Non-plant Sources

Other non-plant source materials vary in their solubility in water and alcohol. Most chemicals have a known degree of solubility listed in reference texts such as the Merc Index. Where the substance is soluble a saturated solution can be prepared as the mother tincture. Soluble biological materials, such as snake, spider and bee venoms, are made in this manner. However, Sepia (dried cuttlefish ink) and most minerals are insoluble and must be prepared by the traditional method of trituration described below. The recent method of Immersion has been introduced to capture the vibration of an insoluble material in water. An example is Diamond (by Peter Tumminello), which can neither be dissolved nor triturated.

Potencies

Potentisation by *attenuation* (dilution) and *dynamisation* (succussion) are descriptions used by Hahnemann to describe the two-phase process employed in making a homeopathic remedy from its mother tincture. They describe the paradoxical enhancement of efficacy as source matter disappears exponentially from the solution. Why a remedy becomes more potent with sequential dilution and succussion is indeed a paradox. To further complicate matters we discover how in some cases relatively inert substances take on new properties as a consequence of potentisation (Aphorism 269). Both dilution and succussion are required to achieve the effect, although historically homeopaths have argued as to which has the more important role.

After his life-changing experience with Cinchona, Hahnemann strove to remove the side effects of his remedies by diluting them. Although this worked, it did so at the expense of efficacy and Hahnemann expended great effort in the pursuit of this goal. His somewhat apocryphal discovery of succussion was said to have occurred when the liquid remedies in his medicine case spilled out and bounced around his carriage as it trundled down a cobbled street. Discovering these agitated dilutions to be more efficacious than his regular remedies was inspirational to Hahnemann, who then had the means to revolutionise medicine with safe and efficacious remedies.

Potency Scales

The original scale of dilution was centesimal (1:100), in which one part of mother tincture is diluted in 99 parts of pure water and alcohol. The corked glass vial in which the remedy is prepared is only filled two-thirds, allowing turbulent flow from the action of succussion to energise the liquid. Immediately after dilution, the remedy vial is vigorously shaken in a particular manner described as succussion or dynamisation. Held tightly, the vial is bounced, through a 90 degree arc, onto a leather bound book or similar rebounding surface. The force employed is that achieved by bending the arm up to shoulder height and striking downward as hard as possible.

Throughout his career Hahnemann experimented with different numbers of succussions used between dilutions, varying from 2, 8, 10, 12, to 100 strikes. Today we use 15 succussions at each stage of centesimal dilution and 100 succussions with LMs (see below). An interesting feature of the centesimal scale is the choice of exponential rather than linear potency sequence, with a range of 3, 6, 9, 12, 30, 200, 1000, 10,000, 50,000 and 100,000 dilutions of 1:100. The initial part of this sequence was developed by Hahnemann, the higher potencies by his successors.

A decimal dilution scale was introduced by Constantine Herring in which successive potencies are diluted one part in ten at each successive stage. A comparison of centesimal and decimal scales is shown in Table 20.1.

There are 6×10^{23} molecules in a mole of solution (Avogadro's constant). By diluting the mother tincture beyond 12c we exceed this number and know there is unlikely to be a single molecule of source material in potencies of 12c and above.

Table 20.1 COMPARISON OF POTENCY SCALES

Degree of Dilution	Centesimal Potency	Decimal Potency
1:100	1c	2× or D2
1:10,000	2c	3× or D3
1:1,000,000	3c	6× or D6
$1:10^{12}$	6c	12× or D12
$1:10^{24}$	12c	
$1:10^{30}$	15c	30× or D30
$1:10^{60}$	30c	
$1:10^{200}$		200× or D200
$1:10^{400}$	200c	
$1:10^{2000}$	1M	
$1:10^{20,000}$	10M	
$1:10^{100,000}$	50M	
$1:10^{200,000}$	CM	

Broadening our Understanding

IV

Paradoxically these 'higher' potencies are considered more deep-acting than those below, demonstrating that remedy action has little to do with material content. Since the same therapeutic effect is achieved above and below 12c we can conclude that the action is not due to material content.

The decimal scale is more commonly used in Germany and USA with only lower decimal potencies being popular in the UK. An example describing the different effect of potencies is with the treatment of a boil with Hepar sulph. In low decimal potencies it will promote suppuration from a headless boil, having a simultaneously mild anti-inflammatory action. As the potency is increased to 30c the remedy rapidly reduces inflammation at the expense of the slower physiological effect of expelling pus. This is important to remember if we are not to accidentally suppress a discharge. Energetically this makes perfect sense and can be employed to great effect in infections.

Biochemic tissue salts are a popular series of mineral salt remedies prepared by trituration to a 6× potency. Although prepared homeopathically they are prescribed according to a perceived bodily deficiency in one or more of the mineral salts – which they may help the absorption or utilisation of, rather than acting according to the Similia principle, although some have also been proved and so might have 'joint' indications.

The Preparation of High Potencies

The higher the potency, the more it has been diluted and succussed. The centesimal scale of potencies is by far the most popular with homeopaths. Hahnemann made some 200 remedies, all by hand up to the 200th centesimal dilution. Homeopathic nomenclature designates these with a suffix 'c' or 'cH' (centesimal Hahnemannian), indicating that each was prepared in an individual vial in the method described above. This time-consuming process requires many vials and corks and a huge effort to maintain consistency of succussion.

As homeopaths have worked with more difficult cases and subtler models of health so they have wanted not only more and more remedies, but also higher and higher potencies to impact more efficiently at the subtle levels.

The influence of Kent considerably changed the limits of potentisation. Whereas Hahnemann stopped at 200c, Kent encouraged the use of much higher potencies, challenging the pharmacies to become more inventive in their means of producing remedies. Consequently, a variety of potentisation machines appeared in the late 19th century to accommodate requests for potencies of 1M, 10M, 50M, and CM, and higher – all impractical to produce by hand. These machines (Barker 1992), produced between 1850 and 1920 and coinciding with the Industrial Revolution, used various inventive methods for combining dilution and succussion.

Earlier, in 1829, the Russian Von Korsakoff had entered into a dialogue with Hahnemann about a method of producing high potencies with a single vial machine. The vial was filled, mechanically succussed and emptied, leaving the residue of one drop to act as the starting point for the next dilution. This method of 'dry grafting' was approved by Hahnemann, although he was concerned about the consistency of preparation and suggested limiting it to producing no higher than a 30c.

This advice was flaunted by the Kentians who, without access or knowledge of Hahnemann's later work on LM potencies (see below), were exploring the higher end of the centesimal scale. In 1869 Bernhardt Fincke patented his method of continuous fluxion, in which the pressure of water dropping into a one-dram vial performed the dual actions of succussion and dilution simultaneously. In 1878 Thomas Skinner refined continuous fluxion, insisting that attenuation (dilution) and not dynamisation (succussion) was solely responsible for the activity of the resultant potency. This was countered by Julius Caspar Jenichen, whose hand-made potencies were considerably valued. It was Jenichen who believed succussion gave a remedy its strength and introduced the idea of potency as opposed to simply dilution.

High potencies from machines were described by a personal nomenclature, e.g. 10MK (Korsakovian) or 10MS (Skinner) – other machines by Boericke, Swan, Tyrell and even Kent being similarly identified. After Kent's death in 1916 the use of high potencies declined, low potencies and triturated tablets becoming the norm. US homeopathy fell into decline at this point. The machines also fell by the wayside, with only isolated companies supplying the industry – Boericke & Tafel being the notable US supplier of Skinnerian remedies until their demise in the late 1980s.

More recently several machines have attempted to faithfully replicate human hand succussion and embrace both Korsakovian and Fluxion methods to enable realistic production of ultra-high potencies. Korsakovian machines embrace a slow emptying procedure which, when multiplied by the number of cycles, makes the preparation of CMs impractical. The Fluxion process, which makes the process less time-consuming, is used by pumping ultra-pure water into the vial at high pressure and forcing it out after each succussion session.

LM Potencies

The fiftymillesimal scale is described in Aphorism 270 of the sixth edition of the Organon, prepared for publication in 1842 (a year before Hahnemann's death). The introduction of the LM method was so radical that his widow, Melanie, felt unable to compromise his life's work and blocked its publication. This edition remained hidden until its discovery by Richard Hael who published it in 1921 – by which time the Kentian influence had encouraged the alternative path of high potency prescribing.

The LM scale was, in some homeopaths' eyes, the pinnacle of Hahnemann's career, combining the maximum benefit to patients with the greatest uniformity of remedy preparation. Rather than being prepared from mother tincture all remedies are triturated to 3c (1ppm), a point at which all materials are considered soluble. Thereafter the dilution scale of 1:50,000 is followed in a two-step process. One grain of the 3c triturated powder is diluted to 500 drops of alcohol to make

the LM tincture; then one drop of the tincture is added to 99 drops of alcohol and succussed 100 times. This 1:50,000 dilution of the 3c is potency LM01 tincture. Five hundred granules (the smallest granules, of maximum surface area to volume) are moistened with the LM01 tincture and dried on filter paper; this is the LM01 potency. One granule is dissolved in a drop of pure water and added to 100 drops of alcohol and succussed 100 times to produce LM02.

Successive potencies are prepared by repeating the stages above. LM potencies are prescribed in a linear scale starting with LM01, the 0 denoting the single granule dose dissolved in water and succussed by the patient before each dose. Patients are given a 100 ml bottle of the remedy and instructed to take one spoonful daily and shake the bottle vigorously between doses. Different homeopaths often adapt this precise methodology to suit their practice. LMs are often promoted as less likely to cause aggravations. The LM01 bottle taken by the spoonful stirred in water lasts for 20 doses, after which the LM02 is started if required. There is a big qualitative jump from the last highly succussed dose of LM01 to the little succussed LM02; patients sometimes notice the different effect.

Plussing

Before the advent of LM potencies Hahnemann evolved a system of incrementally changing the potency between doses by one degree at a time to avoid repeating the same strength, e.g. 200 to 201, or 1M to 1M+1. The use of ascending potencies in a powder sequence is relatively similar, although the differences in potencies are greater, i.e. 30, 200, 1M. This is used by some homeopaths when treating very stuck cases or those, like cancer, with much structural damage. The remedy may be prepared in drop form and succussed and diluted slightly after each dose.

Practitioner Dispensing, Building a Dispensary

The methods described above yield medicating potencies in 95% alcohol that can be supplied directly to practitioners or used to prepare prescriptions on their behalf. Potencies are run in either ultra-pure water or alcohol, with all but the final potencies and their immediate predecessors being discarded. Potencies are made in 95% alcohol and stored in corked neutral glass vials protected from light. Neutral rather than soda glass is chosen to prevent residues leaching into the remedy; unbleached corks are used for the same reason. Light and strong odours such as camphor, menthol and eucalyptus are considered to antidote remedies, so are avoided.

A homeopath can easily equip themselves with a kit of remedies to dispense to patients. The convenience of being able to dispense in acute situations cannot be underestimated and portable kits of polychrest remedies are invaluable. A range of essential remedies and potencies are instantly available for emergencies, enabling prescriptions to be dispensed quickly.

Dispensing Remedies

Dispensing is extremely simple and involves medicating a blank vehicle (pill, tablet, granule, powder or liquid) with the desired potency in 95% alcohol. The shelf life of medicating potencies is infinite but the product prepared in tablet or pill form is given a 5-year shelf life. This is more arbitrary than accurate, no measure of potency being available. The remedy is dispensed by adding several drops of medicating potency into a pre-filled vial of tablets, pills or granules, or onto individual powders. The alcohol carries the potency and dries the remedy on the surface of the tablets or pills. Hence it is imperative not to handle the tablets or otherwise disrupt the film on their surface. By medicating in the final container there is no contamination from extraneous sources; no additional heat drying is required since the alcohol evaporates to dryness, coating each tablet in turn.

The 'vehicle' used to carry the remedy is composed of an inert medium such as lactose or sucrose. Various pharmaceutical forms of the vehicle are available; powders are pure lactose, tablets are a lactose/sucrose mixture, and pills and granules of various sizes are pure sucrose. The choice of pharmaceutical form is largely subjective with some preferring tablets to pills or vice versa. Certain situations demand a particular form, e.g. an ascending series of potencies is ideally delivered with a numbered powder sequence. In the example below the first four doses are medicated as indicated and the remaining powders are unmedicated (sl standing for sac lac or sugar of milk):

Rx Aurum 30, 200, 1M, 10M in 1–4, sl to 30

Important information can be gleaned from patients with such a prescription of numbered powders, e.g. exactly when and for how long the remedy worked. Placebo doses can be helpful in some cases in improving compliance, reassuring the patient and clarifying at what stage in a treatment programme the case starts to react. Some homeopaths will use a placebo 'lead in' to separate reactions due to the consultation and reactions due to the active treatment. Prescribing pattern change and historically placebo was used more commonly and many patients were not told the name of the remedy they were taking. Patients are now much keener to know what they are taking and why, they may well look it up in the materia medica.

Routes of Administration

Oral dosage forms are the most usual presentations, although other routes are employed. Topical preparations such as creams and ointments containing 5% mother tincture are useful for external use in a variety of symptoms such as bruises, haemorrhoids, eczema, sprains and warts. Eye drops, nasal sprays, suppositories, pessaries and injections are also available. Injections are very common in Germany, where marketing directly to doctors ensures a steady demand. In addition, the remedy can be delivered by inhalation of alcoholic tinctures or applied to acupuncture points on the skin. Remedies for babies can be given in freshly boiled and cooled potable water. Eye washes made up in freshly boiled and cooled potable water can also be used to dilute Euphrasia or Cineraria mother tinctures.

Patient Instructions

Advice to not handle the remedy, but tip tablets or pills into the cap and then onto a clean, dry tongue, is important. These, and other instructions, can be given to all patients on a simple instruction sheet, perhaps combined with practice information such as how to find out what to do if there is an aggravation, etc.

Remedies should be stored in a cool, dry place away from strong odours, mentholated sprays, and perfumes. Certain substances antidote remedies although some patients, despite ignoring advice about correct administration and antidoting, still get good reactions to remedies! Many homeopaths advise that peppermint and toothpastes containing mint should be avoided when taking remedies. Coffee is considered to deplete the action of many remedies and should be avoided during treatment and for some time after higher potencies.

The Homeopathic Directive

After the thalidomide crisis, the 1968 and 1971 Medicines Acts introduced three classifications – POM (prescription only), P (pharmacy only) and GSL (general sales list) – to control the marketing of medicines. Medicines that did not fit into these three categories were assigned a temporary status, called PLR (product license of right), in which they could continue to be marketed until new legislation found them an appropriate home. This was fine for companies that had PLRs but has made it difficult for new companies to develop new medicines within the Medicines Act. Different countries have different challenges with their own particular legislation.

European homeopathic manufacturers deplored the absence of licensing for homeopathic medicines across Europe, resulting in an inability to market unlicensed products in other member states. The only way this could be achieved was to establish separate manufacturing bases in each country. The activity of supplying an individual remedy to a practitioner is exempt from the Directive; this protects the supply of many thousands of remedies that have little market demand.

Bach Flower Remedies

Bach flower remedies are flower essences prepared according to a different method to homeopathic remedies. Dr Edward Bach discovered a means by which everyone can treat themselves according to how they are feeling. His 38 flower essences from indigenous trees, shrubs and flower species, encompass the spectrum of human emotions familiar to each of us. By honestly identifying and accepting how one is feeling, a number of Bach flower remedies corresponding to the feeling can be selected and mixed together. The resultant mixture is taken orally by adding drops to water.

Bach discovered each flower's natural gift by feeling the vibration of the plant on field trips. He observed dew drops and felt how they captured and irradiated the essence of the plant. Originally he collected them early each morning but soon evolved two more practical methods – solarisation and boiling.

The sun method achieves what sunlight does with dewdrops. The essence of the plant is captured in water by floating flowers of the remedy on a glass bowl of spring water for several hours in bright sun. The remedy is made in situ so that water accepts the vibration from both flowers and the growing plant. After the flowers have wilted the essence is strained and diluted with equal parts of brandy.

The boiling method is employed when the flowering period is less sunny, as with trees. The flowers are collected, brought to the boil and simmered for 30 minutes, then strained and preserved with equal parts in brandy. Bach flower remedies are then prepared by diluting the preserved essence above 1:240 in brandy. Several drops are taken in water and sipped as required. Water is required to release the vibration and allow it to be accepted into our body, the alcohol holds the vibration in solution ready for release.

Material Dose

Ironically, homeopathy has become over-associated with the use of highly diluted medicines. A remedy acts because it is homeopathic to the case, not because it is highly diluted. A remedy works in material dose, as Hahnemann's initial proving with China officinalis demonstrated. The potentised form of the remedy was introduced as a significant and necessary refinement to overcome side effects and toxicity. Paradoxically, the remedy is known to be considerably more efficacious and safer through potentisation (dilution and succussion).

Summary

I hope you have gained an awareness of the scope of the homeopathic pharmacy and pharmacopoeia, and the importance of integrity in preparing remedies that correspond to their monographs in the materia medica. An understanding of the process of preparation, from raw material to mother tincture and potentised remedy, should provide you with a clear idea of how the final remedy is prepared and aid you in selecting the optimum potency or making informed choices when potency needs changing.

References

Emoto M 1999 Messages from water, vols 1 and 2. Hado Kyoikusha Co, Tokyo

Barker R 1992 LM potencies, 2nd (revised) edn. The Homeopathic Supply Company, Holt, Norfolk

Bibliography

Argumentation for Amendments of Council Directive 92/73/EEC, Nehoma, December 12, 1994

Castro M 1995 The complete homeopathy handbook: a guide to everyday health care. Macmillan, Basingstoke

Hahnemann S trans Künzli J, Naudé A, Pendleton P 1983 Organon of medicine, 6th edn. Victor Gollancz, London

Julian O A trans Mukerjee R K 1992 Treatise on dynamized microimmunotherapy. B Jain, New Delhi

Lockie A 1989 The family guide to homeopathy. Elm Tree Books, London

Medicine and Healthcare products Regulatory Agency 2005 MHRA Consultation letter MLX312 20 June 2005

Broadening our understanding

IV

Section V

Deepening our Approach

CHAPTER TWENTY ONE

Signatures

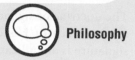 **Philosophy**

Misha Norland

Introduction by David Owen

'As above, so below'

In Sections V and VI we move further to the 'inside' of the case, the remedies, the approaches and methods used homeopathically. As you look into the centre of the case and the fundamental nature of the remedies, and reflect on how to make use of your own inner process in treating patients, it is appropriate to revisit how the inner and outer nature of man reflect each other. This reflection of one thing onto and into another is at the heart of the philosophical understanding of 'like mirroring like', where one part of the body reflects other parts – as used by auricular acupuncturists and in reflexology. I am very grateful that Misha Norland has provided this opportunity to reflect on how all things carry a sign or 'sign-ature'. For those who choose to perceive it, this signature not only communicates one thing's connection to all things, but it is a dynamic part of that connection; it represents its 'sign-ificance'. It is perhaps easiest to appreciate this with the homeopathic remedies where the signature of the source material communicates something of the remedy's potential. For all homeopaths it may aid in remembering a remedy picture. For some, the quality or theme 'sign-aled' in a remedy and its presence in a patient represent a deep connection between the patient and their environment, between the microcosm and macrocosm.

In another way the signs that the remedies give a homeopath provide the very language, ideas and symbols to allow us to perceive and interpret a case. Perhaps they provide a way of encapsulating that understanding then giving it back to the patient in a remedy through the information it holds. There are concepts in this chapter that 'set the scene' for this section and, although challenging, are illustrated in the homeopathic tradition through the case example. Grasping the ideas helps us perceive the case; preserving the case helps us grasp the ideas. Understanding what signs connect different remedies, whether atomic weight or botanical family, lays the foundation for understanding how different remedies may be related to each other and by which pattern and theme.

Finally, signatures offer an insight into how the world of the patient and the world of the homeopath are connected. By recognising, naming and agreeing on what is perceived by you and your patient, connections and bonds are made between you both that reflect the healing process – some might say determine it! The inner process that you experience will, to the extent that you experience the patient, parallel the process taking place in the patient. As all relationships, including therapeutic ones, are subject to this process homeopaths seeking a deep insight into patients are well advised to establish a clear insight of themselves. As homeopaths we share a clear language through the homeopathic remedies, although there are many ways of deepening and clarifying our understanding of them. I wish you well on finding a way that works for you and am grateful to Misha for sharing a method that has informed him.

What is a 'Signature'?

The doctrine of signatures holds that the Creator marked each of His creations with a sign. This signature is an indication of the healing property of the organism. Every ancient culture contains its own version of this doctrine, which was originally not just a medical principle but a way of seeing the world. According to this world view, at the level of the dynamic life force or essence all things are interconnected. This is because the same laws of nature that give form to plants, animals and minerals and their medicinal properties also give form to our bodies and the illnesses that take root in them. By careful observation of the form, behaviour and habitat of a substance, we can learn how it interacts with our own bodies and minds.

Though there are allusions to the doctrine of signatures in the writings of the Greek physician Galen (AD 129–c. 210), it was first applied systematically to Western medicine by the great Swiss physician Paracelsus (1493–1541). Paracelsus was often referred to as the last alchemist and he was undoubtedly a forerunner of homeopathy, though it fell to Samuel Hahnemann to codify and name it as such. Paracelsus said that our soul:

'… intuitively perceives the powers and virtues [of herbs], and recognises at once their signature. This signature is a certain organic or vital activity, giving to each natural object … a certain similarity with a certain condition produced by disease, and through which health may be restored in specific diseases of the diseased part.

'This signature is often expressed even in the exterior form of things, and by observing that form we may learn something in regard to their interior qualities even without using our interior sight. We see that the internal character of a man is often expressed, even in the manner of his walking and the sound of his voice. Likewise the hidden character of things is to a certain extent expressed in their outward forms.

'As long as man remained in a natural state he recognised the signatures of things and knew their true character; but the more he became captivated by illusive external appearances, the more this power became lost.'

Paracelsus, 'The Aurora
of the Philosophers' (Waite 2002)

For those who knew this language of signatures in the natural world, not only was the inward power of a thing similar to its outward form, but also its name reflected its physical form. This was true, so it has been written, because the entire created universe was continuously unfolding out of the infinite source in terms of speech or sound. The Saint James's Bible translation of Genesis, 'In principio erat verbum…' states, 'In the beginning was the word…'. The source of creation was silent but contained the entirety of all the diverse sounds and forms of creation in seed state. From this the name of each object or creature was brought into being. The name was understood as a network of subtle impulses or tendencies in which the entire structure of the physical form is contained in seed form, much as a great oak tree is contained in a tiny acorn.

Signature and Symptoms

Knowledge of a remedy's signature is not merely a theoretical exercise that enables us to speculate about its homeopathic uses. The signature can bring together all the symptoms of a proving into a cohesive remedy picture. For example, why should a person needing Calcarea carbonica have fears about murder, fire and rats, and be worse from exertion? Looking at the remedy substance, Calcarea carbonica is made from the middle layers of the shell of an oyster. After passing through an immature mobile phase of existence, the oyster quickly transforms into a creature that sticks itself to a rock for the rest of its life. It is a filter feeder, taking in passing food particles, and relying upon its thickening shell for protection against crashing waves and predators. Small wonder then, that the remedy made from this creature, weighed down by its ever enlarging and heavy house, is useful for those who are worse for exertion.

Calcarea carbonica types in health feel as safe as houses, while in sickness they feel as vulnerable as an oyster without its shell. Children in particular are wary of leaving the protective shell (their home). They may fear murder, because it endangers their own person; fire, because it endangers their house; and rats and vermin, because they invade their house and eat their food. In this way, the signature pulls together a remedy's many seemingly disconnected physical and mental symptoms to reveal the main themes and essence.

The signature is expressed by the substance's experience of being what it is. This includes the substance's habits, form, and interactions with humans. These elements are revealed by the provers, and are lived out by the patient as a characteristic complex of sensations and functions. Strange, rare and peculiar symptoms can frequently be particularly useful expressions of the signature. For example, Ferrum metallicum's characteristic of 'shall not bend' expresses the strength of iron. Depletion of iron leads to the well-known anaemic symptomatology of lack of strength – bending or 'iron gone soft'.

To put signatures into a useful and practical context, I would like to take you on a journey exploring an ancient map which states that the manner of materialisation of objects from their source into form, from spirit into matter, may be expressed by elemental stages. It shows how objects and their qualities become visible and intelligible. It describes a way in which we experience the world around us.

Quantum physicists have stated that what appear to be particles (matter) are rather manifestations of electromagnetic waves – vibrating fields of energy. Einstein has stated, 'We may therefore regard matter as being constituted by the regions of space in which the field is extremely intense.'

The model of spirit manifesting as ether, or fields of energy, playing out into the world of matter in terms of elemental fire, air, water and earth has been described in the dialogue of Arjuna and Lord Krishna in the Bhaghavad Gita. This informed the ancient Egyptians, while the map was further developed during the classical Greek period – when the four elements were associated with the four temperaments. This map of elements is of the essence in astrology as well as oriental and mediaeval Western medicine.

There are Five Elemental Levels Through Which We Experience the World

The ancient Greek philosopher Heraclitus, referring to the four elements other than ether, wrote:
'each of the elements lives by the death of the others: earth lives by the death of water; water lives by the death of air; air lives by the death of fire.'

In other words, the essence of the superior elemental force must die – that is play out, into the matrix of its inferior elemental force in order to imbue it with vitality and existence. The five elements can be thought of as gradually moving from spirit into matter and are:

1. Etheric energy – which is immaterial, reveals itself as primal non-verbal experience and as intuition.
2. Elemental fire – almost immaterial, the energy of combustion, heat and light, reveals itself as images.
3. Elemental air – dense enough to fly in, reveals itself as thoughts. These are products of the intellect, representing our discriminative awareness 'playing' over experiences and memory.
4. Elemental water – yet denser, to swim in, reveals itself as feelings. These inform us of our likes and dislikes.
5. Elemental earth – solid, to build with, reveals itself as sensations. These are experienced in the body directly by the five senses. Physical pathology is the final outcome of derangement of the above elemental levels.

First Level – Elemental Ether

Elemental ether is apprehended as direct, non-verbal experience. Like a telepathic resonance, ether is more related to the 'vibrating fields of energy' referred to by quantum physicists, than to the lower levels of manifestation. At the etheric level we experience directly what is there. In the therapeutic setting, it is understood to arise out of the 'seed-state' of the disease and communicates its primal being, its disease signature. This is analogous to a remedy's signature, which is expressed by the substance's experience of being what it is. This is, of course, the 'like cures like' principle in action; more than that, it is why homeopathy works – because the signatures of the substance and the disease match up in their original 'seed state' as 'vibrating fields of energy'. In health, elemental ether manifests as intuitions and clairvoyance and gives us insights into interior 'seed states'. In diseases these are the characteristic distortions which we are in search of. Gestures often arise at this level (that is from etheric energy manifesting in lower levels), as do images (that is from etheric energy manifesting in the second level).

Second Level – Elemental Fire

Elemental fire links to images. It is primarily through intuition and clairvoyance (literally, 'clear vision') that the etheric level unhesitatingly expresses itself in elemental fire as image and the spirit world manifest to us. This can be seen because fire illuminates, as well as heats. The heating aspect is related to passion and desire, such as are enacted in religious rituals, where the holy image is revealed upon the altar. There is an equally compelling sexual aspect, where the imagery is erotic. It is also in the form of images – many experiences and their associated sensations and feelings are stored as pictorial memories.

References to images are mostly found in the homeopathic repertory in dreams, fears, delusions and delirium, where the boundaries of consciousness and sub-consciousness are blurred. Our dreams 'talk to us' in pictures, while we literally talk in images whenever we use a simile or a poetic analogy. In drawings, especially children's fantasy sketches, images abound. They are also expressed in adults' doodles when exacting attention upon an object's form is quiescent. As with dreams, their significance can be revealed using association and imaginative amplification. Intuition and

clairvoyance are differentiated by reason. This leads to the next level.

Third Level – Elemental Air

Elemental air links to *thoughts*. These are products of the intellect, that discriminative faculty which decides that something is this and not that. Examples of malfunction include confusion, being lost in thought, and deviations of memory. Delusions and delirium states give rise to distorted thoughts and confused awareness, while clear thinking helps us stay in touch with, and navigate according to, the higher purposes of our existence (see paragraph 9 in Hahnemann's Organon).

Once we have established the truth of our intuition, we can respond appropriately – that is, in the way of *Homo sapiens* (thinking humans) – and then cross the threshold (with human confidence) into the more primitive, survival-oriented, world of feelings. Feelings ascertain whether a thing suits us or not, whether we wish to accept it or not. This function has been developed and championed by animals.

Fourth Level – Elemental Water

Elemental water links to *feelings* that arise in response to energy, sensations, thoughts and their associated images and memories. Our empathetic resonance with each other and with animals is a feeling response brought to us by elemental ether. Feelings include love, joy, rage, grief, jealousy, isolation – they manifest as emotion giving rise to actions (primary emotion). When suppressed, emotions turn inwards upon themselves (secondary or compensated state). Secondary feelings and emotions are complex derivations of the primary, uncompensated source – this can make them difficult to navigate and of lesser value to the prescriber.

Just as intuition mediated by thinking and feeling takes care of the soul, so instincts take care of the body. Instincts are experienced as sensations, which in turn drive actions and gestures. The organs of locomotion and, in humans, the hands, are directly expressive of instinctive will and of feelings as 'e-motions'. For this reason, gestures and body language are worthy of the case receiver's closest attention.

Fifth level – Elemental Earth

Elemental earth is experienced in the body physically as *sensations*, directly by the senses or indirectly through body memories. Sensations include descriptions of pain, such as clawing, shattered, as well as experiences of the other organs of sense, such as red, shrill or putrid. The material level or corporeal earth is where the five different elements all meet and manifest. As they play out into the body, if each is not balanced, physical pathology is the result – its exact expression depending upon the imbalance of the different elements.

The Four Kingdoms and the Five Elemental Levels

The kingdoms considered here are animal, plant, bacterial and mineral.

Etheric energy (level 1) is common to all things in nature and represents their lowest universal, shared spiritual connection, which at the highest and undifferentiated octave of being is pure spirit. Another common denominator of all four kingdoms is the level of sensation, obviously, because they and we are formed of matter in the material world. So, top (level 1) and bottom (level 5) are in common for all the kingdoms in nature.

To examine this further, we understand that a mineral or bacterium or plant does not generate feelings or thoughts as an animal or human would. However, they do 'share' primal sensations with us because we all have bodies and physical structures as well as an etheric field through which common experiences are mediated. These experiences, supplemented by imagery, arise in the beginning. Images, before they are grounded in the physical realm, are energetic representatives of forms and structures – they are precursors of physical forms in much the same way as an architect's plan is the precursor of the building. Because these are the common denominators, they are worthy of our particular attention. To put it another way, when

we boil the fat off the bones of a case, what is most striking is the energetic, etheric experience in the body, because this is how the disease expresses itself at its bed-rock, bodily interaction with the organism's spiritual vital force. This energetic experience, or 'vital sensation', as Rajan Sankaran calls it (see Chapter 22), is the uncompensated expression of the disease's 'seed' state and is its characteristic form signature.

After this initial distortion of the etheric energy by the disease (primary action), the vital force fights back in an effort to restore homeostasis (secondary action). The complex of secondary actions is what we call compensation. It is the coping mechanism adopted by the organism in order to survive, while labouring under the unvanquished influence of the disease. Only when the simillimum is administered will total cure occur, referred to as 'permanent eradication of the disease,' in paragraph 2 of Hahnemann's Organon.

So this is the rub – how do we accurately match the remedy to the patient? I would argue that the signature most closely expresses the uncompensated state. As we have noted, etheric energy and sensation, along with associated imagery (often articulated through gestures and drawings), most closely expresses the uncompensated disease 'seed' state. Thus the simillimum is found when the remedy's signature equals the signature of the patient's diseased state – the seed matching the seed. As an example of signature, consider the remedy Falco peregrinus (from a captive, stud peregrine falcon), which has the characteristic sensation of feeling trapped, hooded, required to do things against its will and numb, versus the mobilisation of vital aggressive energy to be the free spirit, which at their essence, they are – an energy and sensation that may be encircled by flying imagery.

Animal Signatures

Patients experiencing the world in animal remedy states experience competition for resources and the need to establish their own territory. Key expressions include: to stay alert; sexual display; to be attractive; to make a performance and to be seen as the best; avoiding humiliation and shame. Relationships are typically experienced as challenging, vying for dominance and position (predatory), or feeling subjugated and submissive (prey) – feeling ugly, unattractive, used, abused and worthless.

Plant (Including Fungal) Signatures

Patients experiencing the world in plant remedy states exhibit enhanced sensitivity to their surroundings, they relate how they are affected by their environment, by others; they often express how they are hurt, injured, easily influenced; they may like to actively explore their feelings and inner realities; relationships may be struck to protect against a perceived violation of inner vulnerability. In short, plants are at the base of all food chains, they are eaten, they are passively responsive and sensitive. Often they protect themselves, becoming actively responsive, e.g. by developing thorns and poisons, while flowers are attractive to pollinating insects, developing colour, scent and nectar. Here their outward expression may mimic that of an animal remedy and express as active and aggressive. To tell them apart, we must look to the inner state: the animal experiences the world as a place to go-get in, the plant as a place to adapt to, the mineral as a place to find a bed rock of certainty.

Viral and Bacterial Signatures

Patients experiencing the world in viral and bacterial remedy states, on the one hand exhibit features of invading and destroying (living off plants, animals and humans) and, on the other hand, co-operating and developing interactive communities. In this respect there are similarities with plant issues – finding a safe place within which to adapt.

Bacterial evolution represents the first 400 million years of life. These organisms were responsible, amongst other feats, for developing mitosis and radically changing the entire chemical composition of the atmosphere. Co-operation is the key to survival and symbiotic relationships the key to evolution. While this may seem contrary to Darwin's theory, it is of course its necessary corollary. Once co-operation evolves into symbiosis, one species, or in the case of the cell, one organelle, cannot survive without the other. They are locked together. Patients who need remedies from this vast and little explored kingdom have features of co-operation/maintenance/growth versus destruction/contamination at the heart of their case.

Mineral Signatures

Patients experiencing the world in mineral remedy state have issues with material structure and maintenance of order. These patients tend to be systematic; questions arise such as: how can I organise and secure my goal?; what is my place and role in the family? Relationships are forged to fulfill a yearning for completion. This is analogous to compounds, in which elements bond together. Elements and compounds, being the building-blocks of matter, form the structural components of all living systems. Laws have been devised which allow us to predict chemical reactions with accuracy. It is this capacity for ordering and structuring which is the signature for these patients. The fears are of breakdown and weakness; lack of stamina; lack of the support of others; lack of stability and security.

Which Signature

Establishing into which kingdom signature a patient falls, narrows down remedy choices and helps establish what the issues for a patient are. For example, we may note, 'This patient is acting like a plant remedy because they are so passively sensitive to their surroundings, so easily influenced and hurt.' Therefore, we would look at plant remedies before considering remedies originating from other kingdoms, this is discussed further in Chapter 22.

Establishing an individual's characteristic expressions (function or output) is useful in differential remedy analysis, however their characteristic key signature (sensation or input) gives us primary data for remedy selection. This is where the levels come in, because the schema indicates what is most useful in a comprehensible hierarchy.

To recap: in the beginning, as the disease entered the patient and made a take-over bid for control of the vital force – attempting, as it were, to impress the host organism with its will – the host submitted more or less passively to the disease. This is represented by the primary, acute response, which, should the disease be congenital, is experienced by the mother and may result in miscarriage or distorted functional changes such as unusual cravings or aversions. If the patient survives, then secondary action, unaided by remedies, should vanquish the disease. However, because of innate susceptibility, due to miasmatic and congenital factors, this exteriorisation does not occur often enough (indeed it is usually suppressed by drugs and inoculations) and so the slate is not cleared. Then the disease remains within. Now both it and the patient struggle to be in control.

The disease state may be viewed, quite literally, as a spirit possession. The dialogue between the two entities express as symptoms. Of these symptoms the most idiosyncratic (strange, rare and peculiar – SRP) are our surest guide to a curative remedy. Idiosyncratic expressions are those which originate from the unconscious, automatic responses of mind and body at levels 1 (etheric energy), 1 + 2 (image), 1 + 4 + 5 (unconscious gesture) and 1 + 5 (sensation in the body). When at least two of these levels match up and are expressive of the same state, then we may be pretty sure that we are witnessing the disease entity. This entity is best known by its signature because this is what it is before the complexities of secondary functioning and compensation set in.

In order to see how knowledge of the signature can enable us to find the simillimum, we can now consider the case of Sera.

CASE STUDY 21.1

Sera, age 7, had brown hair, tied back in a long ponytail, spot on nose, blotchy face, missing all top front teeth. Pink and white zipped top. Sits still, one hand in her lap. Turns head away when embarrassed. Finds it hard to talk, looks towards mum most of the time. When mum answers Sera appears uninterested. She does not engage with her. Sera speaks easily and well, once mother is out of the room. Keeps mouth slightly open after talking. Seems bunged up. The corners of her mouth are wet. Sad eyes, cute face. Looks neglected – a bit of an Oliver Twist. She becomes quite fidgety towards the latter end of the case-taking.

Presenting complaints: bedwetting, eczema in folds of elbow joints, head lice and threadworms.

Mum is of thin build; has long black hair. Sera hides behind mum to begin with. Rash in fold of elbow joint. (Mother pulls up Sera's sleeve.)

Mother: 'It itches and she scratches.'

Misha (thinking she will comment on her rash) to Sera: *'How do you feel?'*

Sera: 'I sometimes feel that my house is not my house.' (She sucks her thumb.)

Mother: 'We smudged the house (burnt sage) but it didn't help. She feels uncomfortable in the house. She dreams about a little girl calling to her.'

Sera: 'Sometimes I hear my name, "Sera, Sera" and other kinds of names. I say, "Who said that?" but no one answers, or they say, "No one says it".'

Mother: 'Doesn't like to go to school much, but does well there. Made one good friend, but then she left – that upset her. Her older brother is aggressive and jealous of her. He jumps out on her and freaks her out. He does it on purpose.'

Misha: *'How do you feel?'*

Sera: 'I feel scared. I want to get on with him but he won't let me.'

Mother (butting in): 'She was born five weeks premature into a very tense family atmosphere. A lot of rejection and confusion. Husband had a nervous breakdown – wouldn't go out, afraid someone was waiting and would kill him. Won't communicate with the family, only talks about what others are doing in their lives. Is someone else doing the "right thing"? His father is an alcoholic. He was bullied at school. Sera has been bedwetting quite regularly, started up again after I had my third child. Sera is the best behaved. She gets anxious when we all fall out. We have a lot of arguments in our house. I have a bad temper. When my husband had mental health issues, I took it all personally. I felt horrendous, mad, insane, suicidal. I had feelings of such terror. My husband would be quiet, almost catatonic. I took the withdrawal as rejection.'

Sera dances around the room, like a penguin. Mum says nothing. Then mum comments that Sera has to put up with a lot because she is the middle child. Older one gets attention because he's naughty, got very jealous of her when Sera was little. The younger one gets the most attention because she's the baby. Then mother volunteers that Sera is very concerned about her appearance. Looks in the mirror at lot. She likes drawing animals, and has a dog. Misha takes mum into the next-door room and carries on with Sera alone so that Sera's account is unhindered by her mother's interjections.

Sera: 'I like soft fur. I like puppies – I like holding them. I feel sad because Ruby (the pet dog) can't have puppies.'

'Tell me about being sad?'

'Cry when I get sad, mum says, "That won't work." Cry … When I am upset.'

'Tell me?'

'When my brother took the Halloween hat off me and wouldn't give it back. I felt sad. It made me feel unhappy.'

'What else makes you feel unhappy?'

'When I want something but can't have it. It is really annoying. Then I have a tantrum.'

'How?'

'You're noisy when you have a tantrum. I feel guilty when I have a tantrum – I feel I've done something wrong.'

'You've done something wrong?'

'Yes, because everyone sees me, everyone laughs. I feel they put me down. I feel hurt. I feel like running away. When I'm upset it brings me around to having another tantrum.'

'What do you want to do?'

'I feel like throwing stuff at my door. I feel like hitting and stamping. I feel like making a lot of noise.'

'What else makes you feel upset?'

'When my brother keeps on lying to me and not giving me what I want. I feel like hurting him back, but normally just go and tell mum. Brother is stronger than me.'

'Scared of brother?'

'Especially when he jumps out. Normally call for help. First get angry. Feel like hurting someone. Might try and push him off me.' (She wraps a thread from her sleeve around her fingers – goes into a dazed state.)

Sera has brought along a picture, depicting a blue monster with five ferocious heads with prominent red mouths and teeth. I ask her to show it to me.

'What does it do?'

'It eats everybody and captures a princess. I got the story from a fairy tale. Princess story – it has a happy ending. The monster protects the princess from people getting her, but the princess doesn't want that, she wants to get free.'

'How does the princess feel?'

'She feels sad. She feels lonely – she's been forgotten. There is no one to care for her.'

'Tell me your favourite stories?'

'I like ones about lonely dogs, but then they get a family and it has a happy ending.'

'How does it go?'

'The dog gets to run off and then some other family gets to look after it.'

'Tell me more about this?'

'The people and the dog were always arguing and they were looking after the babies and not the dog, then someone left the door open and the dog went to another family. The people didn't have enough money to sell it. The new people didn't mind that it was an annoying dog. The happy ending is that the dog got a happy home and was well looked after.'

'Any dreams?'

'They are about the sea, about crabs and dolphins. The crabs are trying to pinch me, the dolphins are trying to come back to see if they can stop the crabs from pinching me.'

'I had a scary one, has a bit of Harry Potter in it. I go to the toilet and there is a troll, and he chases the girls and he got me. I went into my mum's bed. The troll looks big and blue, strong, massive feet, he can crush people, and he can squeeze you really hard. He has no hair.'

'Anything else that scares you?'

'Dark in the room. Thought something might jump out and get me, a monster or something.'

'What is it like?'

'It is like a normal person and has really sharp teeth.'

'How do you feel if you are alone?'

'Feels scary. If someone pops out to get you, there is no one to save you. If you're alone and you're walking down to school by yourself, you don't know if anything will get you. I'm afraid of the finger eater. You should never shake hands with a troll. It has razor sharp teeth.'

'Favourite things?'

'I like the way penguins waddle about. I like crystals, especially rubies – shiny and red. I like fairytale books. Exciting stories. I like the princess and the pea.'

'Tell me about your favourite one?'

'All these princesses, Queen says, they are not real. Then a person comes and they think she is a pretend princess, so they put a pea under 20 mattresses. She is sensitive enough to feel it, she is a real princess – the prince marries her.

'Polly and the stupid wolf. Polly is clever, the wolf is stupid. Wolf thinks he can get her but he can't.'

'Any other problems?'

'Waking up is a problem. Don't want to wake up and go to school. Had lie-in today because I'm not going to school. Saturday and Sunday are our sweetie days. If I'm bad only get one chocolate, if really bad get nothing.'

'What food do you love?'

'Chicken and I love the chicken bones. I like chicken noodles. I use chopsticks. Nanny taught me how to use them. Two in one hand. I don't like Brussels sprouts.

'Get travel sick in the car when stress is going on.'

'Stress?'

'If we are having an argument or my sister is being manic.'

Case Discussion

Sera's case shows an essential feature of the plant kingdom: sensitivity (to hostile surroundings). In Rajan Sankaran's miasmatic schema discussed in the next chapter, the case falls into the typhoid miasm, characterised by an intense short-term effort to survive in a 'do-or-die' situation. After such an effort, it is usual to rest, after which a full return to optimism and health is the expected outcome. The dog story is by far the most important of all the stories because it is Sera's invention. If we swap the word 'Sera' for 'dog', we get a vivid impression of her situation. Let's try it:

The family and Sera were always arguing and they were looking after the babies and not Sera, then someone left the door open and Sera went to another family. Sera's family didn't have enough money to sell her. The new people didn't mind that she was an annoying girl. The happy ending is that Sera got a happy home and was well looked after.

The dog/Sera is not being looked after; indeed, the family wishes to sell it/her, but not for a profit – they have to pay to get rid of it/her! The dog/Sera is worth less than rubbish, or perhaps it is a situation similar to that of a traditional oriental daughter, sold off with a dowry. Later, Sera volunteers that her favourite food is chicken bones. Usually mums throw these into the garbage, while a dog, given half a chance, would heave them out and eat them! In contrast to the story of the dog, Sera tells a princess story, but it too is sad.

Misha: 'How does the princess feel?'

Sera: 'She feels lonely – she's been forgotten. There is no one to care for her.'

Sera is neglected and lonely in her home. She looks forlorn, like a lost puppy.

Sera: 'I sometimes feel it is not my house.' (She sucks her thumb.)

Mother: 'We smudged the house (burnt sage) but it didn't help. She feels uncomfortable in the house. Dreams about a little girl calling to her.'

Sera: 'Sometimes I hear my name – "Sera, Sera" – and other kinds of names. I say, "Who said that?" but no one answers, or they say, "No one says it".'

Here a similar element enters in. Sera dreams and hallucinates voices calling her name, yet when she responds, no one answers or she is told, 'No one says it'. And there is also the reverse aspect to this: the voice calling out to her in her dream is giving her attention, perhaps assuaging her feelings of rejection. I use the word 'rejection' because it is how Sera's mum described her feelings during her husband's psychosis. When Sera's mum described her husband's nervous breakdown, she said:

'… he wouldn't go out, afraid someone was waiting and would kill him. Won't communicate with the family, only talks about what others are doing in their lives. Is someone else doing the "right thing"? … I took it all personally … My husband would be quiet, almost catatonic. I took the withdrawal as rejection.'

Sera's father felt paranoid about being murdered and was almost catatonic.

In cases where information from the primary carer is available, and certainly in cases of children, I take the parental situation as paramount. It is the crucible within which the children are fused. Sera's situation at home has led to her feeling neglected and threatened by omnipresent danger of a sudden, unexpected, menacing type. This is an intense type of danger, requiring outside help to ensure survival.

'If someone pops out to get you, there is no one to save you. If you're alone and you're walking down to school by yourself, you don't know if anything will get you or not.'

And a little later:

'I'm afraid of the finger eater. You should never shake hands with a troll. It has razor sharp teeth.'

Sera dreams of crabs trying to pinch her, and of being crushed by trolls. Another real danger comes from her brother:

'Scared of brother?'

'Especially when he jumps out. Normally call for help. First get angry. Feel like hurting someone. Might try and push him off me.' (She wraps a thread from her sleeve around her fingers – goes into a dazed state).

Sera's response to her brother, and also her tantrums, fall within the typhoid miasm: an intense short-term effort to survive in a 'do-or-die' situation. After the effort, it is natural to rest, however, going into a dazed state (as Sera does after telling her story) is indicative of trauma. Is the finger winding, dazed state like her father's catatonic state? Speaking about tantrums, Sera says:

'I feel guilty when I have a tantrum – I feel I've done something wrong.'

'You've done something wrong?'

'Yes, because everyone sees me, everyone laughs. I feel they put me down. I feel hurt. I feel like running away. When I'm upset it brings me around to having another tantrum.'

'What do you want to do?'

'I feel like throwing stuff at my door. I feel like hitting and stamping. I feel like making a lot of noise.'

We are reminded of the story of the annoying dog who makes trouble. Worse, we are told that she feels put down and hurt because she has done something wrong. (It is interesting that Sera's mum reports that her husband asked, 'Is someone else doing the "right thing"?' because 'right thing' and 'wrong thing', being exact opposites, express the same concern.) There's no running away for Sera – small wonder she feels that her home is not her home. It is a hostile home, which contains a psychotic father, a dangerous brother and a mother who tells her that crying 'won't work'.

Deepening our Approach

V

Receiving the Signature

When receiving and probing a child's case it is often difficult to penetrate into the vital sensation (where etheric forces act out in the material body) along a verbal track of association, but it is easy to do so with drawings. In children's art, where imagination is not constrained by habits of recording, it is often easy to read the subconscious subscript. Sera obliges us by bringing along a drawing (requested by me), depicting a blue monster with five ferocious heads, prominent red mouths and teeth. The feeling which emerges is consistent with her stories of danger and imminent attack. When we rake though the case, looking for key impressions, we get: attack, pinching crabs, razor sharp teeth, crushed by trolls, scared, I have done something wrong. In response to these 'inner' impressions (sensations), her active expressions (functions) are to run away or to have a tantrum. She feels like throwing stuff at her door, hitting and stamping, making a lot of noise.

There are also passive expressions in the form of dreams and hallucinations of voices calling her name and she wraps a thread from her sleeve around her fingers while going into a dazed state. These sensations and passive and active expressions fall into the picture presented by the family Solanaceae, although a case can be made for other families also. However, when we examine Sera's drawing with its five biting heads, then the choice is narrowed down to the Solanaceae. The trio of Belladonna, Stramonium and Hyoscyamus are all disposed to bite and strike when in delirium. They act out in this way because their inner impressions are of being attacked and bitten (e.g. 'I'm afraid of the finger eater. You should never shake hands with a troll. It has razor sharp teeth.').

This case might have been solved using several different methodologies; however, signatures offer an insight into the inner nature of Sera and a remedy that matches this is likely to act deeply. A repertorisation of rubrics derived from Sera's statements leads to the need for differential analysis between contesting remedies, shown in Figure 21.1. Here, knowledge of the signature comes to our aid because our repertorisation throws up three members of the Solanaceae family alongside other remedies. We need to plumb the depths of remedies to find the true fit:

MIND; DELUSIONS, sold; being (1): hyos.

The chosen remedy was Hyoscyamus (henbane) in 1M potency.

The Signature of the Remedy – Hyoscyamus

This plant's favorite habitats are middens, waste ground, and old dumps. Here too it is that Hecate (queen of the Underworld and protector of witches) lurks and the dogs and strays of the

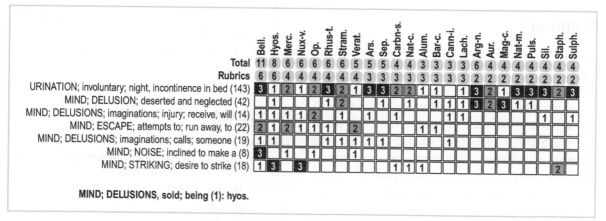

	Bell.	Hyos.	Merc.	Nux-v.	Op.	Rhus-t.	Stram.	Verat.	Ars.	Sep.	Carbon-s.	Nat-c.	Alum.	Bar-c.	Cann-i.	Lach.	Arg-n.	Aur.	Mag-c.	Nat-m.	Puls.	Sil.	Staph.	Sulph.
Total	11	8	6	6	6	6	6	5	5	5	4	4	3	3	3	6	4	4	4	4	4	4	4	4
Rubrics	6	6	4	4	4	4	4	3	3	3	3	3	3	3	3	2	2	2	2	2	2	2	2	2
URINATION; involuntary; night, incontinence in bed (143)	3	1	2	1	2	3	2	1	3	3	2	2	1	1	1		1	3	2	1	3	3	2	3
MIND; DELUSION; deserted and neglected (42)		1			1	2			1			1		1	1	1	1	3	2	3	1	1		
MIND; DELUSIONS; imaginations; injury; receive, will (14)	1	1	1	1	2		1		1		1					1	1					1		1
MIND; ESCAPE; attempts to; run away, to (22)	2	1	2	1	1	1		2							1	1							1	
MIND; DELUSIONS; imaginations; calls; someone (19)	1	1				1	1	1	1							1							1	
MIND; NOISE; inclined to make a (8)	3		1		1		1																	
MIND; STRIKING; desire to strike (18)	1	3		3							1	1	1										2	

MIND; DELUSIONS, sold; being (1): hyos.

Figure 21.1 Repertorisation of Sera's case

community seek scraps of food or plunder what others have rejected. (We are reminded of the dog in Sera's story.) In European witchcraft lore, the juice of henbane mixed with lard was rubbed into the armpit and groin to produce the infamous flight of the witch. Waste ground and witches tell us a story of exclusion from society – those who are thrown out, reviled, destroyed, or simply rubbished (the opposite of the princess in Sera's fairytale). In Shakespeare's *Hamlet*, the old king was betrayed and killed by henbane juice being poured into his ear while he slept.

The patient for whom Hyoscyamus is the remedy feels deeply endangered; they may have been betrayed or otherwise devastatingly injured. The feeling most often is of having been neglected, rejected and rubbished by loved ones. Thus this remedy is famous for the treatment of jealousy (when one feels dumped) and for old people who have been dumped in a home. One often hears stories of double incontinence or sexual exposure which single out such individuals as problematic – a particularly negative form of attention-seeking!

In Sera's case these trends are as yet lightweight; yet one can see that, untreated, the roots of the henbane pathology would surely strike deeply into a fertile soil of threat and neglect. Sera's mother reported that one week after the remedy the bed wetting had ceased. One month after the remedy, the nits had gone and the skin eruptions had healed. Sera felt much calmer and happier about going to school.

Summary

As we saw in the case of Sera, knowledge of the signature helps us cut through the stereotypical portrait of Hyoscyamus (the jealous nymphomaniac). As another example, knowledge of the signature of Platina can help us cut through the stereotypical portrait of that remedy (the haughty nymphomaniac). Platinum is the most-used catalyst, a property that implies the most intimate involvement with reactive substances but also the capacity to return as if unchanged to its former state after the reaction is over. Platina

demonstrates the mineral kingdom theme of yearning for a partner to complete itself, but this yearning is enhanced by its catalytic quality of remaining alone and unchanged. Hence such rubrics as:

- MIND; DELUSIONS; alone, she is alone in the world
- MIND; DELUSIONS; great person, is a (above others and therefore alone).

On the physical level, the sensation is hyperaesthesia and its opposite is numbness, especially of sexual organs and lips – the most intimate (catalytic) of organs. Hence the primary polarity is between isolation and intimacy. Therefore, this has to be the marked feature in a case for Platina to be the simillimum. This polarity is consistent with the rubrics:

- MIND; KILL, desire to; sudden impulse to; husband, her beloved (leaving her alone)
- MIND; KILL, desire to; child, her own (the ultimate estrangement).

Imagery consistent with the Platina picture is bright and unreactive on the surface, a polished front, while inwardly the imagery is dirty or corroded. The story could be one of sexual abuse.

We all need a good working knowledge of materia medica, complete with proving symptoms. But as these examples show, knowledge of the signature gives us the clearest view of the interior, the uncompensated state of a remedy. Looking for the prevalent sensation and imagery in a case gives us an insight into the uncompensated (primary) disease state of the patient, which is matched by the remedy, which is in turn best known through its signature.

References

Hahnemann S 1842 Organon of the medical art, 6th edn. Based on a translation by Steven Decker, edited and annotated by Wendy Brewster O'Reilly. 1995 Birdcage Books, Washington

Waite A E 2002 Hermetic and alchemical writings of Paracelsus, vol. II. Bertrams, London

Deepening our Approach

V

CHAPTER TWENTY TWO

A Journey of Discovery into Kingdoms, Families and Miasms

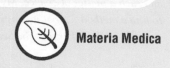
Materia Medica

Helen Beaumont and Maggie Curley

Introduction by David Owen

For many students of homeopathy the move from the useful but outer and disease-orientated approaches of treatment towards the inner person-centred approaches is a challenging one. In the materia medica it can at first appear that whole new areas of information about the remedies need to be learnt thematically, while in fact what you learn about the inner qualities of the remedies connect and complement the outer detail. While learning the remedies often presents a challenge to the memory, you will find it much easier if you can see the plan or pattern that underlies each remedy. Studying these, like all materia medica studies, does far more than just provide the tools of the homeopathic trade; they allow us to see and recognise our patients, they inform the concepts through which we analyse our cases and reveal how different remedies relate to each other in differential diagnosis, and guide in the navigation of cases that might require management over a number of years and remedies.

I am grateful to Helen Beaumont and Maggie Curley for undertaking the important task of clearly and succinctly drawing together some of the different ways the themes and patterns that run through the materia medica can be understood. These represent some of the most recent developments in homeopathy and will build on the idea of remedies having a key signature that is reflected in the material from which the remedy is made (see Chapter 21). The remedies and patients can be understood from the perspective of their key themes. Two of the axes

that represent these themes are the vital sensation and the quality that is expressed by the miasmatic state (see Chapter 28 page 386).

One plan, or map, does not suit every remedy. It should come as no surprise to you at this stage in your studies to find the plan that is most structured and based on the atomic make up of the source material fits the mineral remedies that have themes so connected to order and 'structural relationships'. Plant and animal remedies equally have plans that reflect their respective 'sensitivity' and 'relationships'. Some homeopaths will find some models, like some remedies, easier to study, learn and recognise; the challenge and opportunity for you in this chapter may be to reflect further on your materia medica strengths and weaknesses. Helen and Maggie do a superb job of reflecting something of the rebirth that has happened in homeopathy over the last 20 years – and which the homeopathic profession has been moving slowly towards over the last 200 years.

Kingdoms, Families and Miasms

Rajan Sankaran describes the state of homeopathy 20 years ago as:

"… likened to a man with an air gun, standing in a field and shooting up in the air randomly. Once in a while a bird flew in the path of his aim and was shot. The homeopath would say 'What a great shot that was!' Patients had to struggle to get in the line of fire! There was lack of consistency … one case would be a success and the

next five were failures ... prescribing cannot be so arbitrary and such a matter of chance. My effort all along has been to find a method ... that is consistent and reproducible",

R Sankaran, 'The Sensation in Homeopathy'

The recent developments in classical homeopathy would appear to provide a three-dimensional map to get to the centre of the case, the simillimum, by using the concepts of kingdoms – animal, plant, and mineral – families and miasms. Over the last two decades, original thinkers such as Massimo Mangialavori, Jan Scholten and Rajan Sankaran have realised that remedies fall naturally into groups based on criteria of their natural kingdom, botanical family and symptom themes. This chapter explores the work of these contemporary homeopaths who have made such huge advances in the development of these concepts. It will look at the three kingdoms, how the theory of miasms has been extended, case-taking, and the source of the remedy. This chapter will illustrate how it is possible to move from a position of 'shooting randomly' to one of a more precise aim that more consistently leads to an accurate prescription.

Miasms

In the search for maps in homeopathy Sankaran studied Hahnemann's theory of miasms and concluded that each miasm represented one way of experiencing a situation. In 'The Sensation in Homeopathy' he describes the miasm as a *'measure of how much or how intensely or how acutely or chronically or how deeply or desperately the situation is perceived'*. The miasm is identified by how a person copes with situations, their perception of the problem, their reaction, the level of hope and despair, and the pace and pattern of their pathology.

Taking the five previously described miasms of psora, sycosis, syphilis, tuberculosis and cancer (see Chapter 17), Sankaran has expanded the miasmatic spectrum by adding acute, typhoid, malaria, ringworm and leprosy. He identified which remedies belonged to which miasm by studying the rubrics of a well known remedy from that miasm. If the syphilitic miasm is looked at, the key words include

destruction, despair and suicide. Alumina is a syphilitic mineral remedy from the third row of the periodic table, with main issues around identity. Some of the well known symptoms include suicidal thoughts of killing self with a knife, despair of recovery and delusions of personal identity.

After receiving a case, having explored what the patient means by their expressions and descriptions, it is useful to underline words that belong to the miasm and kingdom. When looking at the acute miasm it will be possible to identify times of extreme panic – where the patient will describe how 'all of a sudden' terrifying events happen where they feared for their life and they have had to get help or escape. When this episode passes, their life then returns totally to normal with no sequelae, until the next time. An example of this would be the Stramonium child who wakes all of a sudden, screaming, terrified, inconsolable and clinging to their parent – and who has no recollection of the event in the morning. To start identifying the miasms it is helpful to review a successful case where the remedy is known and pick out expressions and words associated with that miasm. It is possible to very quickly see the pace of the case from the words the patient uses and how they react to their situation.

An abbreviated explanation of the 10 miasmatic states is given in Table 22.1 but further reading of Sankaran's work is recommended.

The Kingdoms

Our remedies are derived from the natural world of plants, minerals and animals. The whole aim of the practitioner is to understand and find the source of that remedy as expressed by the patient. The art of arriving at the correct prescription has relied heavily on knowledge of materia medica and mechanical repertorisation. Both of these tools are essential but are greatly helped using recognition of the themes or patterns running through a case and a remedy.

This 'pattern recognition' in turn benefits not just from themes and essences but from a system or map of these patterns. With the new work on kingdom classification, such maps have been

Table 22.1 AN ABBREVIATED EXPLANATION OF SANKARAN'S TEN MIASMS

Miasm	Sensation	Reaction	Key Words	Remedy Examples
Acute	Sudden life-threatening dangerous situation	Instinctive flight or fight response. Child-like clinging, helplessness	Acute Sudden Panic Violent Terror Fright	Aconite Belladonna Arnica Stramonium
Typhoid	There is a feeling of a critical situation which if properly handled will end in total recovery but there is a threat of death or collapse	An intense struggle needing concentrated effort for a short duration	Crisis Emergency Sub-acute Sinking Recover	Bryonia Rhus Tox Nux Vom Baptisia
Malaria	There are episodes of acute intermittent attack with an underlying fixed feeling of being deficient	This sensation is experienced at a depth of being fixed and permanent like sycosis	Intermittent attack Stuck Unfortunate Harassed Hindered Persecuted	Colocynth Capsicum Cina
Psora	A difficult situation but there is hope and the problem is solvable. Failure would not be the end of the world	A struggle to succeed but make the effort	Struggle Confidence Difficult Hope Anxiety	Sulphur Psorinum Calcarea carbonica
Ringworm	Lies between psora and sycosis, sharing characteristics; a difficult situation beyond easy reach	Alternating between struggle and resignation, constantly trying, then sits inactive before trying again	Trying Struggle Irritation Discomfort	Calcarea Sulph Teucrium Dulcamara Sarsaparilla
Sycosis	There is a fixed weak spot within me which I must hide or cover up	Keep weak spot hidden from others. Fixed ideas or ritualistic behaviour	Fixed Avoid Accept Hide Secretive	Thuja Medorrhinum Natrum Sulph Pulsatilla
Cancer	Chaos which is going out of control and heading to destruction. Task is beyond the individual's limit	Total control of self and environment. Everything is going out of control and it is impossible to do anything about it	Control Perfectionist Fastidious Order Chaos	Carcinosin Arsenicum Album Staphysagria Nitricum Acidum
Tubercular	Feeling of intense oppression and desire for change. Suffocating and time is short	Hectic activity. Put all efforts into getting out leading to burn out and destruction	Hectic Trapped Closing in Desire for change	Tuberculinum Drosera Phosphorus Many insects and spiders
Leprosy	Hunted down and isolated, feels dirty, disgusting and as is shunned or cursed	Avoids the sight of people. Despair	Disgust Contempt Isolation Repulsion	Hura Aloes Iodum Curare
Syphilis	There is no hope. Have committed an unpardonable crime	Complete despair. Suicidal or homicidal	Destruction Despair Murder	Mercury Aurum Platinum

Deepening our Approach

V

developed which we believe more reliably lead the practitioner in the direction of the simillimum. Much as a strong Parisian accent is an indication of French nationality, so each kingdom has its own language, its own themes and its own sensitivities to situations. To understand these concepts more clearly, each kingdom will be described.

The Mineral Kingdom

The mineral patient feels something is lacking, that their structure is incomplete and something is missing within them. This can be clearly seen in the Kali salts with their backache – their structure will not support them. Patients requiring mineral remedies will often quantify, categorise and analyse situations in a very organised and systematic way. General themes and language of the mineral kingdom are as follows:

- *Structure* Key words: Backbone, foundation, cement, crumbling
- *Complete–incomplete* Key words: Fragile, rock solid, permanent, circle, square
- *Dependent–independent* Key words: Family, partner, husband, nice home, relatives, standing on your own two feet
- *Lack–need* Key words: my weakness, so disorganised, loss, failure of exams, financial
- *Stable–unstable* Key words: solidity, stand firm, collapsing, brittle.

The map or a tool that helps define the remedies from the mineral kingdom is the periodic table of the elements. In the 19th century Dmitri Mendeleev put the 65 known elements of his time into a table based on their atomic weight and left unoccupied the places where he was confident other elements as yet to be discovered would ultimately fit. Time proved him right!

Jeremy Sherr has explored the periodic table as a source of homeopathic remedies and this has resulted in some excellent provings, e.g. Iridium, Germanium and Plutonium to name just a few. However, the idea of predicting the qualities of a homeopathic remedy from its position in the periodic table has more recently been defined by the work of Jan Scholten and Rajan Sankaran.

The periodic table is comprised of six horizontal rows, or *series*, and 18 vertical columns or *stages*, each with its own themes. These series have been named by Scholten after their most characteristic element and are outlined in Table 22.2.

He explains the columns as 18 different stages in a continuous process of development. Each element in the row represents a stage in the development of its theme, going from growth on the left, to success in the middle, to decline and decay on the right. These different stages are given in Box 22.1.

Table 22.2 THEMES OF THE ROWS OR SERIES

Series	Theme
Hydrogen series	Conception and existence – do I exist?
Carbon series	Separation – I exist but am I one with the mother or am I separate?
Silica series	Identity, individuality – I am separate but what is my identity as a separate person?
Ferrum series	Security, protection and task – I have an identity, but what is my task in life? Am I secure?
Silver series	Creativity and performance – I am secure, but am I creative?
Gold series	Standing on your own feet, responsibility – I am creative but am I a leader, am I responsible?
Lanthanide series	Disintegration and death

BOX 22.1
Themes of the Stages or Columns

1	Beginning	10	Lord and master
2	Finding a space	11	Preserving
3	Comparing	12	Division
4	Establishing	13	Withdrawal
5	Preparing	14	Pretending
6	Proving	15	Loss
7	Practicing	16	Remembering
8	Persevering	17	Letting go
9	Success in sight	18	Rest

Hence in the Gold series there is the dependence and inability to take responsibility of Barium and the Baryta salts, moving to the obvious leadership of Platina and Aurum, to the downfall and collapse as there is progression across the periodic table, seen in Plumbum and Bismuth. These two axes of series and stages allow each element to be placed in relation to these and each other. In addition, different mineral remedies can be divided into various groups each with different qualities (Box 22.2).

REFLECTION POINT

- Using the above tables and boxes reflect on a mineral remedy you know to see how its materia medica reveals its themes.

The case of a 35-year-old business man who presented with symptoms that had been present for some time illustrates how this approach to treatment and prescribing methodology can be used.

BOX 22.2
Different Groups of Mineral Remedies

Metals
- Concerned with performance and defence
- 4th row more concerned with defence – battle of Ferrum and Cuprum
- 5th row with performance – Palladium and silver-tongued Argentum
- 6th row have very strong issues surrounding both performance and defence – they are not just protecting their family but take on responsibility for the whole world – Aurum the King

Cations
- Elements which give away electrons to become positively charged
- Occupy the left-hand side of the periodic table; the most reactive being the Alkali metals like Sodium, Lithium and Potassium
- Need to bond with negatively charged anions to become complete
- This is reflected in the homeopathic picture of the need for relationships and bonding

Anions
- Elements which accept electrons to become negatively charged
- Occupy the right-hand side of the periodic table, like chlorine (muriaticum)

- Need to bond with a positively charged cation to become complete
- The energy is focused on maintaining relationships, a desire for company (Arsenicum)
- At stage 17, the Halogens have a feeling of being totally let down or betrayed

Salts
- This is the union of cation and anion
- The two bring their own individual characteristics to the relationship and they express qualities of both – although they may also have qualities of their own
- The cation and anion may be from the same row, as in Nat mur (row 3), or from completely different rows, as in Arg Nit (Silver from row 5 and Nitrogen and Oxygen from row 2)

Acids
- The acids show a struggle followed by collapse
- The type of struggle will depend on which element is involved
- In Phosphoric acid the struggle is to constantly care for others in order to be loved and accepted
- In Muriatic acid it is the struggle to avoid disappointment which drives them to be more nurturing

In this case the issues of responsibility and performance are brought out at every level. He talks of being indestructible, challenged, of his business and his achievements. This places him in Row 6 of the periodic table, the metals of the Gold series. However, he is not at the pinnacle – he is not yet supersonic! The element in column 9, just before the top, is Iridium. He was given a single dose of 1M and now feels able to take his business further with less sense of burden of responsibility

CASE STUDY 22.1

(P – Patient; D – Doctor)

P: 'I was as fit as a fiddle. I was indestructible but now I feel sick and there is numbness and a feeling across my upper body. All the tests are normal so I cut out wheat and things improved but I'm not 100%. I run my own business and there have been difficult challenging times. I am responsible for 40 people. I've not got one mortgage I have 40. It is a shock to find I am not indestructible.'

From the outset, the language is in terms of percentages, responsibility, not being indestructible.

D: 'Tell me a little bit more?'

P: 'There is an unpleasant numbness and my body tingles, I have to sit up straight and take a deep breath. [Throughout the interview the patient took deep sighs.] I get a tingling feeling and I just want to get rid of it, I have work to do, a life to lead. I am irritable with inner frustration. I thought I was indestructible, this is not me. Walking is a challenge, I feel I will fall over or collapse.'

Again the theme of indestructible and collapse – mineral themes.

D: 'Any fears?'

P: 'Of being trapped. It would be a nightmare to be buried alive, you could not move in the coffin.'

D: 'Tell me more about being trapped.'

P: 'Business-wise, I feel frustrated; I set things up as a one man band but it has not grown as I hoped, I have not turned it into something supersonic. There is an element of restriction as I can't do what I like. How people think of me is important. I want everyone to love and like me and I have 40 mortgages to think of.'

Trapped for him is not that of being a caged animal or having a plant sensation such as tight and stiff, it is about business, about not being supersonic. He describes 'an element of restriction'.

[Deep sigh again and he shudders as sensation returns.]

D: 'And the opposite of this?'

P: 'To be free, sitting in a café, with people I want to be with, chatting, putting worlds to rights, no one judging me, no guilt, not having to achieve anything.'

D: 'Tell me more about being judged?'

P: 'It's to do with self-esteem. I need other people to say I am good. I use a business excellence model and I am very good at it. I am asked to do talks. It gives me a personal high; these are really big companies, 500 people at the conference. Blimey what a challenge – let's see how good you really are. I rehearsed the first seven words and knew if I could get them out I would be OK. I pictured everyone cheering and in the end I got top marks as a presenter. Bring it on – it was amazing. Next two years I got full marks but then had a group of 50 people, and felt more challenged, I only got average score. Bugger! I wasn't the best; I wasn't the top. I was not good enough because I know I am better than average. Business has not flourished as it should, if people judge the business they judge me. I have more to do, more to achieve. In 20 years time I want to have sold the business for millions, and be widely successful doing talks and helping other businesses grow.'

Deepening our Approach

for his 40 employees. Interestingly, many of the words he used, and the continuous deep sighing, correlated well with the proving of Iridium done by Jeremy Sherr.

The Animal Kingdom

All animals depend on plants or other animals for their existence. Unlike the plants, they cannot make their own food, and in order to survive they have to compete. For the species to be maintained, they have to compete in terms of territory, sexuality, food source and habitat. Some are predators, some are prey, but the issue is always one of 'I versus you'. The issue of the victim or the aggressor, the weaker and the stronger, will be voiced clearly by a person needing an animal remedy, whose 'non-human song' is from this kingdom.

Mention must be made here of the work of Nancy Herrick (1998), Jonathan Shore (Shore et al 2004) and Jeremy Sherr (1997, 2002) and whose animal provings have contributed enormously to the materia medica. Some of the general themes of animal remedies include:

- survival – the threat comes from outside
- competition
- victim/aggressor
- inferior/superior
- sexuality
- jealousy
- dreams of animals, strong like or dislike of animals
- 'something is being done to me'
- 'it is killing me'
- 'he affects me'.

The specific characteristics of each sub-group depend on their mode of existence in nature and it is these characteristics which will be exactly reflected in the patient. The keynotes in Box 22.3 give the main themes which emerge.

The case of a delightful, highly intelligent 6-year-old boy (see Case Study 22.2) who was brought for treatment of eczema illustrates how themes of the animal kingdom can be used in prescribing. Itchy, sore eczema of both elbows had started four months previously, when he been under a lot of pressure to be well behaved at school. It soon emerged that the eczema itself was less of an issue than his behaviour problems.

CASE STUDY 22.2

(D – doctor; C – child; F – father)

 D: 'Tell me about his behaviour?'

 F: 'He was suspended from school five times for lashing out at the teacher, striking and being aggressive. He couldn't behave the way the school wanted him to.'

 C: 'I want to be grown up and independent.'

Already there are some peculiar characteristics – he wants to be grown up and independent at the age of six and is also aggressive and 'lashes out'.

 D: 'Tell me more about being grown up?'

 C: 'I like adventures and grown-up things.'

 F: 'He ran away from home when he was 3 – curiosity led him out, he's a great explorer.'

 C: 'I am the only one in my family who wasn't born in England, so I am the odd one out and I don't like that. Maybe that's how I got my love for animals, it's huge.'

This is extraordinary from a 6-year-old child and needs to be understood more fully.

 C: 'I've always loved animals, cats particularly; I admire them for their stealth. They creep up and pounce with their skill. They hunt and feed and defend their territory. Wild cats kill and hunt. Tigers and leopards are my favourite because they are pretty. Cats like me and they don't like change of routine. I don't like changes either. Cats like being up at night, they are semi-nocturnal. I like being up at night.'

D: 'Tell me more about being grown up?'

C: 'I like making food for myself, like being able to tell people what to do. I don't often get the chance to do what grown-ups do like going out at night. We went bat watching once and I could stay up and have fun in the dark.'

D: 'What would you like to do when you grow up?'

C: 'Something to do with animals. I'm not really like most people, I'm different. I want to put understanding into people about animals.'

F: 'He is very scientific about animals. He was terrified of her grandfather's Alsatian.'

C: 'I got up and looked angry at him.'

F: 'He is very protective of young children but by the time they are 2 or 3 they aren't so attractive.'

C: 'If there is a baby in the house I protect it.'

The strong animal themes are coming through, both in his interests and his behaviour. Nocturnal, independent, aggressive, nurturing young to a certain age, great love of animals, especially cats. Further questioning is needed to lead to the source.

D: 'Tell me more about being at school?'

F: 'It was torture for him, he wants to have his own way and finds it difficult to do things he doesn't want to do. He will scream and lash out and run away. He tried to climb over the wall to escape. He loves climbing trees and is quite fearless, will go up until he gets stuck. He's not by nature aggressive, just lashes out with frustration. He went through a phase of biting when he was three.'

D: 'What things do you like doing for fun?'

C: 'I love pyjama parties; you can do good things in the dark. I want to be nocturnal. I want to be a wild animal. I think my Mum or Dad is a cat, a big cat. I'd love to be a leopard...'

And with patience and a trust in the method, he names the animal – the source!

BOX 22.3
Remedies from Different Animal Sub-Groups

Mammals
- Dependence
- Independence
- Dependence on group or master
- Nurturing young
- Feels he has suffered wrong
- Submissive
- Aggressive
- Usually sycotic miasm

Snakes
- Malicious
- Deceitful
- Scheming, manipulative
- Jealous
- Camouflage
- Attention seeking through music, dance, sex
- Loquacious
- Increased mental activity
- Feel dirty and guilty
- Clairvoyant
- Strong leprosy and syphilitic miasms

Birds
- Desire for freedom
- Opposite sensation of restriction, suffocation, trapped
- Desire to travel

- Dreams of flying
- Responsible, dutiful
- Spiritual
- Caring for young
- Cancer and tubercular miasms (raptors syphilitic)

Spiders
- Predator
- Revengeful
- Impulsive (snakes are sly but not impulsive)
- Hectic, restless
- High sexuality
- Tubercular miasm

Insects
- Fruitless activity
- Rush of flow of thoughts and speech

- Vindictive
- Jealous
- Fear of being crushed
- Feel looked down upon
- Feel small
- Mostly tubercular miasm

Sea creatures
- Suffocation
- Belonging to a group
- Protection (shellfish)
- Water
- 'Clamming up'
- Strong sycotic miasm

He was given Panthera pardus (leopard) 200c three doses. Within a week of taking the remedy, the eczema cleared but, more importantly, his sleeping and his mood were much better and he was able to start at a new school. He said: 'I only wanted to get out of school once. Sometimes I want to live alone, to be completely free. I'd live on the fields behind our house and go from place to place. Indoors seems like a stuffy little shed. Night is when I most like to be out. I'd like to be awake and doing something at night.'

This was an extraordinary case, not only because of the child himself but how it demonstrated the deeper understanding of the homeopathic process; of being able to take the patient right to the energy of the source. He gave the whole description of the leopard – independent, wild, nocturnal, climbing trees – and then for good measure he named the animal!

The Plant Kingdom

Unlike the animal kingdom, where the behaviour of the source material is easily observable, the plant kingdom presents more of a mystery to the homeopath. From the very beginning, when Hahnemann did his first proving on Cinchona

bark, plants have been widely represented in the materia medica. They have been studied from their known effects, from their toxicology and from provings, but never very systematically. There were no maps.

That is until in the early 1990s, when several homeopaths, aided by the computer repertories and materia medica programs available, started to explore plants according to their botanical family, their similar properties and themes and therefore similar clinical effects. Plants are able to make their own food, chlorophyll, by reacting to sunlight and drawing water and minerals from the ground. As this finely-tuned process depends on great sensitivity to the environment, Sankaran hypothesised that each plant family had its own unique expression of that sensitivity. He studied the individual families, and came to the conclusion that it was possible to classify them according to their sensations and reactions.

Refining the map lead to the question of why different remedies from the same family have such differing symptomatology. It seemed that the sensation was common to the whole family but that it was expressed in differing degrees of pace, depth or desperation. In other words, different plants

Table 22.3 SENSATIONS, REACTIONS AND COMPENSATIONS OF TWO WELL KNOWN PLANT FAMILIES

Family	Sensation	Passive Reaction	Active Reaction	Compensation

Compositae	Injured
	Hurt or insulted
	Shocked, burnt or scalded
	Fear to be touched, hurt
	    or approached
		Numb
		Anaesthetic
		Stupor
		Catalepsy
			Insulting
			Hurting others
			Cruel
			Violent
			Strikes
				Tough guy, can take all the
				    beatings
				Protective of others

Liliacaea	Forced out, squeezed Oppressed Constricted Excluded, left out, neglected	Must hold on tight	Must move	Attractive behaviour Belonging, being included, being part of

of the same family belonged to different miasms. It was this breakthrough which initiated the development of a chart of the botanical families and the remedies related to the miasms.

This is a 'work in progress'and therefore necessarily incomplete. A more detailed look at the plant kingdom using two well known families and a clinical case will help to explain the concepts behind the method. General themes and language of the plant kingdom are:

• sensitivity
• reactivity
• impression of the environment
• sensation and action are equal and opposite and experienced at every level
• no importance of predator/prey as in the animals or of the structure/order of the minerals
• I am affected by… 'Things affect me'
• 'I am sensitive to…'
• 'I feel … heavy, compressed, brittle, contracted…'

For every sensation there is an equal and opposite reaction, both in physical and emotional expressions. The reaction can be either active or passive, or in some cases can be seen as compensation. The common sensation of the Anacardacia family for example, is 'caught', 'stuck', 'can't move'. The opposite or active reaction is to want to move, to be restless, while the passive reaction is that of being immobile or unable to move. The compensation is to be constantly on the move. Tables 22.3 and 22.4 are extracts from Sankaran's book 'An insight into plants'. The first illustrates two families and the

second suggests how plants from these two families can be perceived according to their miasm.

You might like to reflect on how the remedies you already know something of can help inform you about the other remedies in these families. The case of a 50-year-old woman with chronic abdominal pain illustrates how this method can be used (Case Study 22.3). She was given Aloe 200c, three doses. On follow up, her exclamation as she walked through the door was: 'It's a miracle! Everything came out of my bowel and I haven't had any pain since. I've lost weight, bought some

Table 22.4 PLANT REMEDIES FROM EACH OF THE FAMILIES ACCORDING TO THEIR MIASM

	Compositae	Liliacaea
Acute	Arnica, calendula	Veratrum
Typhoid	Chamomilla	Paris
Malaria	Cina, Eup. perf	Colchicum
Ringworm	Taraxacum	Sarsp.
Sycosis	Senecio	Crocus, lil. tig, sabadilla, helonias
Tubercular	Abrotanum	Agraphis
Cancer	Bellis	Ornith
Leprosy	Lactuca, inula, lappa	Aloe
Syphilitic	Echi	

Deepening our Approach

CASE STUDY 22.3

(P – patient; D – doctor)

P: 'I've had a desperate weekend. Problem is my stomach ever since hysterectomy 21 years ago. The man who did the operation couldn't give a damn and my stomach was in a terrible state. I've had terrible trouble with my bowel, sometimes diarrhoea, sometimes constipation. Sex was painful. I didn't like myself because of my looks. My breasts are big and heavy. I'm now a size 18 and my stomach is so sore. I just don't like me. I hate dressing myself, I'm huge. I see no end to it. If I could stay in the house I would because I'm so uncomfortable.'

D: 'Tell me about your stomach?'

P: 'It feels so full I have to undo everything; I press my knuckles in to my stomach. [Clenches fist] If I go to the toilet properly I feel clean from the inside and it feels great.'

D: 'Opposite feeling?'

P: 'Dirty, disgusting, horrible.'

These are words of the leprosy *miasm; she perceives everything as dirty and disgusting and hates herself. There is a degree of desperation here which she voices as she comes through the door.*

P: 'I think a lot of my problem is my bowel, I feel if I pushed it down it would be better [clenched fist]. It's a wonderful feeling when I release the bowel movement, I feel clean. I'd love the inside of my stomach to be cleaned out then everything would be pushed out [fist]. When I have a good bowel movement I feel there is a down pressure and I have to sit on something to stop the pushing out. I get the same feeling sometimes after sex, like something is going to fall, it's dragging. When it all goes back to place the feeling is wonderful. I hate the embarrassment of going to the toilet; it's horrible, disgusting, stinks. I have every cleaning product known

in our toilet. At times I get diarrhoea and it pours out of me, it happened in the bed once, I was mortified, it was just horrible.'

The sensation she is describing is of pushing down, dragging, something going to fall out, a pressure – the sensation of the Liliacaea *family. We need to confirm this in other areas of her story.*

D: 'Have you had the same pain in other situations?'

P: 'My periods were agony, unbearable pain, screaming. The pain in the vagina was like a knife being pulled out slowly, I would have to press hard in to it to push it up or it felt it would come away.'

Her active reaction is that she must hold on tight.

P: 'One time I asked Mum to sit on my stomach to push the blood out. As soon as the blood came out it was nice.'

D: 'Dreams?'

P: 'Yes, the most horrendous ones. Snakes, I hate them, they are ugly – my sister put one in the bath once and I stood on it, my whole body felt frozen and I suddenly had a period, everything came out of me. My faith is important to me, I fear God, I have to answer to Him, and I don't want to do bad things. I enjoyed sex a lot but not so much now even when we watch porn. When my husband had an affair and I thought about them having sex it was horrible, disgusting.'

D: 'How did you feel?'

P: 'I felt pushed out.'

Here the miasm and the sensation come together – she feels disgusted, pushed out of her marriage and her physical symptoms also have the sensation of pushed out. The remedy which comes in the leprosy miasm of the Liliacaea *family is Aloe.*

new clothes and I even like looking in the mirror now'. This case demonstrates that using the map of kingdoms and miasms can take us to a known remedy which may well also be indicated by repertorisation of the presenting symptoms.

Case-Taking

The approach to case-taking illustrated in the above cases reveals the deeper patterns that can make sense of otherwise confused cases. When the cause, symptoms of the presenting complaint, and mental and general symptoms (especially the emotional) are described in the same terms, this points to a pattern which links both mind and body, to what Sankaran terms the 'vital sensation'.

Any aspect of the case can reveal this pattern and different homeopaths find different aspects of the patient's case most clearly or easily reflect this theme. On a more cautionary note, this approach to case-taking can often point to a pattern that does not match any known remedy. In these cases either the closest remedy must do or another model may decide which remedy is indicated.

'The chief complaint is the microcosm of the … vital sensation and energy … and having touched this most central point right at the outset, one can see the rest of the case branching from this core.'

R Sankaran, The Sensation in Homeopathy

Reaching the Source

By now, the reader will have gained some insight into the process of 'map reading'– a process which involves both leading and being led by the patient. It is too easy to stop the journey of understanding the patient at a level we are comfortable with. Using our repertorisation to home in on the big rubrics like 'ailments from grief', it is easy not to progress beyond the superficial layers – but it is central to treating confused cases that we do; that we go towards the centre of the case and core of the remedy. We must be open to the patient telling us 'how the grief feels now' or 'my personal experience of it is…'. If it is the most central thing it will relate to every other aspect of their life.

It is much like setting out to find the source of a river, not making do with reaching the widest part rather, patiently taking the windy route to the little village on the hill, carefully looking for the second field on the right next to the church, going through the gate and looking for a small puddle of water – the spring itself.

It is as the patient brings you closer to this source, where the story can appear to be making no sense to you, that each patient will reveal their uniqueness, the world of the source.

Animal cases often provide clear source words. A patient who did well on Lac caninum used the words 'snap,' snappy' and 'bitch' on several occasions throughout the consultation. During the proving of Dama Dama (the fallow deer, J Sherr unpublished), a number of provers came up with words and images such as 'rutting' and 'fallow'. A case of Iridium said 'I always thought of myself as hard and indestructible'– Iridium is the hardest metal known. This expression of the source in the patient is what Sankaran refers to as the 'non-human song', which is out of place and therefore a cause of turmoil.

Summary

Having studied in some depth the developments of the last decade, what conclusions can be drawn as to the value in practice of this three-dimensional map? Once the method is understood, the case received clearly and the remedies known, this is a system which, with experience, is both reproducible and consistent.

It must be emphasised that everything hinges on the case-taking process. When witnessing an experienced prescriber in action taking a live case it can appear effortless. To be confronted with your own patient and have the courage, belief and patience to let the centre of the case unfold is another story. Although some of the concepts are new, this is not a method which dispenses with solid homeopathic teaching. In fact, the foundation stones of materia medica, repertory and philosophy remain at the heart of the practice.

Using this method, the materia medica is expanding as never before – we are able to use remedies we would never have dreamed of using a decade ago. It makes so much sense that when remedies are studied they are done so in the framework of kingdoms and families. To teach Belladonna in isolation, without discussion of the whole of the Solanaceae family, or Calcarea carbonica without mention of the position of its elements in the periodic table, is limiting the range of approaches you have available to treat patients.

Bibliography

Herrick N 1998 Animal mind, human voices: provings of eight new animal remedies. Hahnemann Clinic Publishing, Nevada City

Sankaran R 2002 An Insight Into plants Vol 1 and 2. Homeopathic Medical Publishers, Mumbai

Sankaran R 2004 The Sensation in Homeopathy, Homeopathic Medical Publishers, Mumbai

Sankaran R 1994 The Substance of Homeopathy. Homeopathic Medical Publishers, Mumbai

Sankaran R 1991 The Spirit of Homeopathy. Santacruz (West), Mumbai

Scholten J 1993 Homeopathy and Minerals. Stichting, Utrecht

Scholten J 1996 Homeopathy and the Elements. Stichting, Utrecht

Shore J, Schriebman J, Hogeland A 2004 Birds, homeopathic remedies from the avian realm. Homeopathy West, Berkeley CA

Sherr J 1997 Dynamic provings, vol 1. Dynamis Books, Malvern

Sherr J 2002 Dynamic provings, vol 2. Dynamis Books, Malvern

Deepening our Approach

V

CHAPTER TWENTY THREE

The Homeopathic Relationship

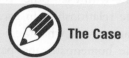

The Case

David Owen

'To heal requires the patient to act with trust and the doctor with integrity'

Dr Lee Holland

'The physicist does not discover, he creates his universe'

Henry Margenea

Introduction

The homeopathic relationship is at the heart of any homeopathic process that sees health and illness as more than external causes and local effects. The therapeutic interaction cannot be separated from the therapeutic relationship. This chapter invites you to see illness and treatment as more than the label of a disease and a medicine. It explores diseases and remedies as aspects of perception and advocacy in homeopathic relationships. It examines the idea of perception and objectivity in the homeopathic relationship before trying to understand the relationship from the points of view of both the patient and the homeopath. I hope that this exploration into the homeopathic relationship will allow you to take a fresh look at the homeopathic process.

Understanding the homeopathic relationship increases the ability of the homeopath to make sense of confused cases and to reveal hidden cases. By 'reframing' these difficult cases in terms of our relationship with the patient, rather than as a prescriber of remedies, we glimpse the case in new ways – making it possible to see themes that run

through a case and how the patient is affected by and effects their environment (including us, their homeopath). Exploring working this way is a natural extension and deepening of seeing patients from a holistic perspective.

A theme we return to throughout this chapter is that there is 'no external reality separate from the observer of that reality'. Any change in the observer, the observed, or the medium through which perception takes place alters what is perceived. This raises fundamental questions about how we understand and explore our reality. For instance, if there is a different reality for each observer, then how legitimate are measurements and experimentations of one observer's reality in interpreting the reality of another? As no two observed events are truly independent of the observer it throws into contention the idea that any event is disconnected from or randomly associated with any other perceived by the same observer.

Relationship

Every patient and every illness has a story. Listening to that story you only truly hear it if, to some extent, you enter into it.

If patients are happy to work with their feeling there are many styles of consulting that can help the patient to be 'physically, mentally and emotionally present'. Many depend on a good relationship between patient and homeopath and its importance increases as cases get more confused and hidden (see 'Style of consulting' in Chapter 13). How patient and homeopath perceive and communicate with each other is an important dynamic of the relationship. In every case there is what the patient says, what the homeopath hears, and what the homeopath and patient think was said and heard. What the patient and homeopath anticipate will be said and heard will determine what they are able to say and hear. It will colour their objectivity.

What is Objectivity?

'A change in the spin of one particle in a two particle system would effect its twin simultaneously, even if the two had been widely separated in the meantime'

A Einstein, B Podolsky, N Rosen 1935

The relationship and interaction between the observer and the observed are always to some extent determined by the attributes, attitudes and experiences that each brings to the encounter – the 'filter' through which you perceive a patient. This is acknowledged in both modern physics and psychotherapeutic practice. Like coloured glass or a lens, the filter through which perception takes place will colour, distort or focus what is perceived. While the ideal may be to see through 'clear glass', in reality the medium is created and tinted by both the observer and the observed. While the homeopath may hope to consult with absolute objectivity, in practice there is always an element of subjectivity. The observer can never be unbiased while there is any anticipation of events or attachment to outcome. The more the observer can be conscious of their subjectivity, the more they can allow for and reduce their bias – the more unconscious the bias, the more difficult it is to account for. By understanding the relationship between the patient and ourselves we begin to make conscious, and allow for, this lack of objectivity.

The Medium of Perception / The Remedy and Disease

'If the statistical predictions of quantum theory are true, an objective universe is incompatible with the law of local causes'

Summary of Bell's Theorem

'It shows that our ordinary ideas about the world are somehow profoundly deficient even on the macroscopic level'

H P Stapp (1971)

Homeopaths perceive patients and patients perceive homeopaths as if through a lens. The lens (as illustrated in Fig. 23.1) allows the patient to focus needs onto the homeopath and for the homeopath to focus healing onto the patient. The 'lens' allows the patient to expresses their suffering and the doctor to relate to the patient's suffering through the symptoms. The patient arrives with an illness and goes away with a disease. The patient brings their case and receives a remedy. The two sides mirror each other, and as we gain deeper insights into one, so we gain deeper insights into the other. The 'lens' also ultimately protects both the patient and homeopath, permitting an openness between each other but also constraining and limiting the influence of one on the other.

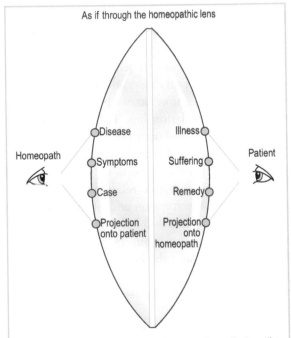

The 'lens' allows the homeopath to see the patient as the homeopathic case and to focus those aspects of the relationship that might not be brought to awareness in another relationship. It also allows the patient to focus their expectations and projections through the homeopathic lens onto the homeopath. It is the lens that allows the perception of both the carer and the patient as respectively the homeopath and the homeopathic patient

Figure 23.1   The medium of perception

The closer the two sides accurately reflect or match each other, the clearer the case is. The more detail that is expressed (in the patient's account of the illness), the more complete a picture it is possible to describe (the more accurate the diagnosis). Using only the conventional (pathological) diagnostic labels of disease often inadequately expresses the patient's illness. By attempting to summarise an overall impression of the patient's case, the homeopath is attempting to express their overall perception – which may include reference to disease, symptoms, remedy and the relationship.

The medium through which the range and breadth of a patient's suffering is communicated is informed by the concepts and remedies the homeopath has to hand. If they know 10 different remedies for claustrophobia they know 10 different ways it can be experienced – and perceive it more accurately than someone who thinks all claustrophobia is the same. In this way understanding the materia medica is fundamental to the homeopathic process. The homeopath aims to see disease in its broadest and most descriptive sense and to develop competencies to receive a wide range of what the patient offers. Reflecting this to the patient gives them permission to share and invites them to reveal more of themselves in the consultation. The effect of any remedies prescribed (specific effects) and the effect of the therapeutic relationship (nonspecific effects) are related – and cannot, in practice, be meaningfully separated (see Chapter 24).

Communication

The more you wish to perceive, the more present you need to be.

Communication is the interplay of the different factors allowing expression and perception, frequently leaning heavily on language and verbal communication. One part of cases being difficult (confused or hidden) is that what is being communicated is not explicitly said or declared, another is that what is being expressed is not perceived clearly.

When talking about allopathic approaches to health care doctors talk about 'fighting illness' and 'the battle to be well', where the illness needs to be 'beaten', the medicines will 'kill' off the disease etc.

The homeopath follows the patient and the symptoms they 'play out' in the case and 'moves' things on. I invite you to think of the homeopathic relationship as like a dance – finding the 'rhythm' and 'steps' to the case and looking for the remedy that 'strikes the right chord' or 'hits the right note'. To extend this metaphor, 'the music' is created by the patient and the homeopath 'tunes in to' the patient. The homeopath can observe the patient's dancing in a detached way – and in many simple cases this may be sufficient. In more confused and hidden cases you may find it helpful to enter into a metaphorical dance with the patient to understand the dance and what the patient is communicating. By mirroring the patient's movements you can glimpse the world from the patient's view and hear the tune the patient is dancing to.

The Homeopath's Ability to be Present

The art of the homeopath is to be able to observe what is happening around them while being fully present in it, to pay attention. You are required to hold the intention of something happening with the possibility that anything could. Attention actually creates possibilities, e.g. noticing that a particular patient uses the words 'right and wrong' in the consultation leads to exploring what these mean to the patient, who may then, for example, start talking about their sensitivity to criticism.

The aim is to become skilled at linking what is happening in 'the here and now' with what has come into the consultation from outside, 'the there and then'. There are techniques for doing this such as working with a tentative statement – 'I notice that…' or 'I wonder if…'. Or by describing what is happening to you as part of the consultation – e.g. 'I notice that when you say this I feel…'. Often by being able to articulate these feelings the homeopath's ability to be present in the consultation is greatly increased. This in turn models the ability for the patient also to become fully present. Inviting the patient to imagine how they might act in other circumstances, or to remember how they have acted or felt in the past, can also reveal things about them that they might otherwise choose not to present to you. For example, 'I wonder how you might feel if…' or 'I wonder how you reacted when…' or 'I wonder if you ever feel this…'.

While the homeopath at one level simply hears the patient's story, engaging and relating to the story often increases the detail and quality of the story being told. However, there are risks in this process if the homeopath is insistent on getting their own story told or if they are unaware of what their own story brings and how it colours what they see (see Chapter 25).

Using the techniques of 'enacting' and 'matching' (see Chapter 13) to mimic the patient's body language or some of their phraseology enables you to meaningfully engage with your feelings. These feelings will, surprisingly often, mirror or highlight the patient's feelings and frequently enable the patient to engage and express them, often allowing deeper symptoms to surface.

The Patient's World and Their Ability to be Present

Observing patients – how they sit, how they move, how they are dressed – gives indications of how open they are to relating to you. Many patients are unfamiliar with the invitation to engage in a 'relationship of this sort' with a practitioner. They need to develop trust in you before they can do this; if you can model this open and trusting relationship to them, it greatly helps and demonstrates some of the values you choose to work with (see Chapter 25).

Inviting the patient to be present and make their feelings conscious requires a rapport and trust that has to be consciously created. If patients are unwilling or unable to share emotions in the consultation it makes observing deeper aspects of the case difficult. If a patient is avoiding emotions it is worth reflecting on why they are doing this. Is this their way of keeping control, do they not trust their own feelings or you? Sometimes the feelings expressed by a third party, like a pet owner or parent, can 'surrogately' point to important aspects of the case. The closer and more exclusive the relationship, the more likely there will be synchronicity or overlap of the remedy states.

Why Cases are Confused and Hidden

There is a close relationship between patients' fear and delusions: their fears concern what will hap-

pen outside, their delusions are how they construct their world from inside to try to prevent their fears.

As illness moves deeper, symptoms often become more structural, unconscious or suppressed. As they do so they express fewer individual nuances of the patient. In deep-seated chronic illness the whole state of the patient reflects how they have adapted to the situation they are in now. Symptoms that were present previously or might have been present in a different situation are hidden or masked. In the consultation it is possible to explore these past symptoms and to see how the patient imagines things might be in different situations. The situations the patient desires to create and avoid are expressed through what we refer to respectively as the patient's 'delusions' and 'fears'. As the case gets more confused and hidden so these become increasingly important; they are a way of seeing what is otherwise masked. In the consultation the skilled homeopath can not only invite the patient to consider what their symptoms would be like in different situations, but also take the patient through their imagination, hopes, dreams, ambitions, fears and anxieties into such situations so they can experience what it feels like. Frequently this reveals new and previously hidden features of the case.

Projection of the Unconscious

Difficulties arise when there are unmet expectations or hopes in either the patient or the homeopath.

It is normal for us all to have aspects of our personality that are unconscious. Some of these are more hidden or 'in shadow' than others but all of them can influence our everyday relationships and everyday lives. This influence can be understood as the unconscious seeking to be recognised or manifest in the conscious, or as the conscious attempting to keep some things 'out of sight' in the unconscious. We can all be considered to be acting out aspects of our unconscious and suppressing aspects of our conscious – with the potential for particular aspects of our unconscious to be brought to the surface (our buttons pushed) by certain people or situations.

If what are acted out or suppressed coalesce around social norms they are considered normal and may not stand out. Others that do not coalesce around social norms might be considered unhealthy, odd – or even mad. While this is more easily observed and described in the psychological realm, the same happens with physical characteristics – some are expressed as symptoms, some are hidden and only manifest in certain situations. In hidden cases often the homeopath and patient share the same cultural and population norms, so making it harder to recognise a patient's symptoms. In these cases the patient's illness reflects the health of the culture and population as much as the patient (see 'Public health homeopathy', Chapter 30).

Projection (Transference and Counter Transference)

Those aspects of the patient that are not expressed explicitly are always reflected in some way in the patient's situation or the people around them. They are important to perceive and can be thought of as the unconscious projected on to others around them (transference). In response to this transference there will be a reaction in those that experience it. The homeopath who realises this attempts to consciously notice this projection and channel it through the treatment process. What is not consciously noticed will be passed on in some way into your situation or the people around you – and is liable to be projected in some way onto the patient (counter transference).

It is normal to experience projections in a consultation. If it is conscious it is less likely to bias the case – and can give important pointers. If projection appears absent it may be that the case is progressing straightforwardly. In a difficult case it is more likely that the homeopath is unaware of it and may be an indication that the patient and homeopath are unconsciously colluding with each other, acting out their unconscious agendas. A case may be difficult due to projection either by the patient or the homeopath (often both!) – perhaps reflecting a cultural predisposition (or miasm) that both the patient and homeopath share.

Staying Centred
'Physician heal thyself'

When working with projection it is important to be aware of where your feelings originate. Part of the personal development of any homeopath is realising the cultural and social factors they are influenced by.

It is important to realise if feelings arise from your own state, and not in response to the patient, they can confuse and confound the case. It is therefore important for you to be centred and in a balanced state. This requires professional support and supervision (see Chapter 25).

Projection by the Patient

Transference is caused by seeing the present situation through an emotional lens shaped by past situations. It relates particularly to aspects of a relationship from the past being projected onto relationships of the present. It is often our significant past relationships, such as with parents and siblings, which affect our present ones and become central to our character. The case of Mary illustrates this and you might like to consider Box 23.1 before you read her case. It lists some of the techniques that can help identify projection, including transference and non-verbal expression of suppressed or unacknowledged feelings.

Transference is strongest while it remains unconscious. The more strongly it is hidden the stronger the emotion (both positive and negative) it can generate, and the more significant to the case. As a general rule a good indication to significant transference taking place is if you register strong feelings in the consultation. Acknowledging these is both therapeutic and provides an essential guide to prescribing – especially in confused cases.

In confused and hidden cases the patient's symptoms do not express all aspects of the disease state. The less the symptoms are expressed, the greater the transference. For the homeopath it is important to understand projection as being generated not

BOX 23.1
Techniques That Can Help Identify Projection by the Patient (Transference)

- Ask patients specifically how they are feeling in the consultation and when discussing aspects of the case – especially if you notice feelings in yourself.
- Look for any signs of feelings surfacing (eyes watering, laughing, avoiding eye contact, touching a part of the body)
- Invite patients to imagine they are talking to the people that they feel generated these feelings in the past. For example, you can invite the patient to talk to you as if you are a parent or a sibling. You might encourage them (give the courage) to think about what they would like to say to them now, how they feel saying that, and what they might need to hear when they say that.
- Consider the feelings behind the patient's language, for example 'heartache' 'under the skin' 'weak at the knees' etc. Feelings have correlations to parts of the body. At times these appear obvious but warrant being stated consciously, such as when a patient with angina describes feeling broken hearted about a relationship, a patient with indigestion feels gutted after a disappointment, a patient with backache talks about a disagreement like being 'stabbed in the back', a patient with a rash saying a person who irritates them gets 'under my skin' or with hay fever describing someone as 'getting up my nose'.

just by unexpressed feeling but also by suppressed symptomatology and from any unexpressed feature of a patient. The sum total of what is unexpressed or unresolved from the past (the there and then) contributes to who we are and how we project ourselves in the present (the here and now).

Some cases are difficult because they initially appear to lack symptoms or modalities. When the case is sensitively received it may reveal additional symptoms (see Chapter 13). In truly confused and

CASE STUDY 23.1

Mary, aged 45, consulted for help with catarrh and postnasal drip. Her husband was a patient and had been disabled from an accident in his teens. She had a history of depression from her 20s and recounted, without obvious feeling, when as a child (she couldn't recall the exact age) her parents separated. While talking about her parent's separation she stroked her throat and kept swallowing. At this moment the homeopath became aware of an increased intensity in the consultation. Mary became angry at the homeopath and asked why she was being asked 'all this'.

The homeopath asked her how she felt and mirrored the same hand movement to the neck back to her. She said she felt she was suffocating when talking about her father. She went on to say she felt very angry and resentful that he didn't leave the family home at an earlier age. She remembered that he had left after she and her sister had 'left home' and gone to university. Some of this anger was transferred onto the homeopath; the homeopath offered to 'role-play' Mary's father and she was able to 'get in touch' with her anger. Encouraging her to talk about and express her feelings of anger provided information to distinguish between those remedies with suppressed anger and this in turn helped the homeopath and Mary see that she had a deep insecurity around men. She responded well to Sepia.

hidden cases, including cases where the vitality is low and where the totality and constitution are not expressed, then the case is revealed through the unconscious behaviour of the patient. The deeper the disturbance, the more forcefully it has to express itself in some way – if not through conscious symptoms then through projection.

Working with projection frequently requires clear emotional communication. The homeopath may find ideas developed in work on emotional intelligence (Goleman 1995) and through non-violent communication (Rosenberg 2003) helpful as

Deepening our Approach

they explore how, when something is observed, it gives rise to feelings that if not expressed generate needs and lead to actions. Likewise the unmet needs a patient has will determine the feelings they are most likely to experience. Patients will recreate situations and relationships that generate the unexpressed feelings and reinforce their unmet needs when that is what they are familiar with. If the consultation and treatment allows insight into those unmet needs, and expression of those feelings, longstanding patterns of behaviour can shift.

REFLECTION POINT

- Consider what different experiences of transference you have experienced in different consultations. How has this affected your relationship with patients?

Projection by the Homeopath

Feelings generated in the homeopath during a consultation fall into three main groups. First are those feelings generated on a coincidental basis in the homeopath at the time. These are likely to vary from consultation to consultation and day to day, e.g. if the homeopath had recently experienced an upset in their personal life.

The second group will be those that reflect the steady state of the homeopath and which may persist over some period of time. For example, someone who is in a deep state of grief will find those feelings emerge easily in consultations. If the homeopath regularly experiences the same feelings it may have more to do with their own state than that of the patient's – and may require some resolution for the homeopath's own benefit.

The third group of feelings is those that emerge in response to the patient's projection (transference) and if they remain unconscious, may lead to a reciprocal projection (counter transference). In confused and hidden cases the patient's projections are frequently strong – as are potentially the feelings generated in the homeopath and the reciprocal projections.

A homeopath who is open to, and indeed invites, patient's projections will find that these affect their perception of the case. The more the homeopath is attempting to identify the themes that run through a confused case, the more useful these projections are. When the case is effectively masked or hidden then even the projections of the patient can be difficult for the homeopath to consciously recognise. In these cases the homeopath's reciprocal projections (including counter transference) back to the patient (or to others) provide vital clues to understanding the case.

Counter-transference, in its psychological definition, relates to what the therapist transfers to the patient in response to the transference the patient is projecting on to the therapist. A much broader interpretation can enable the homeopath to use all that they notice about how a patient influences their own posture, behaviour, choice of words. It also influences their behaviour to others and, if 'unresolved', will unconsciously be acted out on friends, colleagues or family – or helpfully be engaged with in supervision (see Chapter 25).

The case of Sarah illustrates how projection and reciprocal projection shed light on a confused case. You might like to read through the points in Box 23.2 to help identify when projection is happening in the homeopath.

We can see how Sarah's tendency was to project her remedy state onto the homeopath. For some patients and homeopaths this can become a comfortable state of 'collusion', in which both patient and homeopath can become 'stuck'. As homeopaths see these confused cases differently it is often helpful to have a colleague who can help by seeing and advising on difficult cases. Some pointers to help identify when reciprocal projection is taking place include the homeopath fantasising or having strong feelings about the patient, breaking boundaries, behaving differently, making Freudian slips or forgetting things. It can include physical or behavioural changes before, during and after a consultation.

It is also important to realise that by making the reciprocal projection conscious there is a chance to deepen the consultation, e.g. 'when you talk like…, I feel…'. This is one of the best ways of getting patients to address their own projections

BOX 23.2
Techniques That Can Help Identify Projection by the Homeopath (Counter Transference)

- Reflect on who the patient reminds you of. In what way are they similar to this person?'
- Is your relationship with them different from other patients? Are you over-familiar or over-distanced?
- Would you feel comfortable if someone was watching you in the consultation? If not, there is likely to be projection.
- How would you feel if you were watching someone else who was behaving like you?
- What is going on between you and the patient? The stronger the feelings, the more likely the projection is to be unconscious and is going to colour how you see the case.
- How easy do you feel it would be to share your projection, if not with the patient then in supervision? The more difficult it is, then the stronger the projection is likely to be.
- Do you commonly experience a particular feeling? The more common, the more likely it is that this is part of your own state. The more uncommon a feeling is for you, then the more likely it is to be a specific response to the patient.

and to examine where it is coming from. It requires skill and courage for a homeopath to address issues related to projection, although it can be rehearsed in supervision. The less the case-taking and treatment process in confused and hidden cases encompasses the perception and reaction of the homeopath, the greater the homeopath's unconscious projection and the more difficult or even incurable a case will seem. When able to recognise and work with these feelings the homeopath gains insight into the otherwise confused and hidden aspects of a case. If they are not able to work with these feelings then they will often find these patients hard

CASE STUDY 23.2

Sarah, aged 43, presented for treatment of her depression. She had had many courses of antidepressants and the case was confused. Exploring her life history it transpired her father, who treated her very specially, doted on her. When she married, her husband also treated her as very special until her first child was born when she was 27 – after which she felt he was neglecting her. She became depressed and presented with postnatal depression that was severe and persistent. Sarah 'looked down' on her friends and spoke about her 'murderous feelings' towards a previous boyfriend who had rejected her.

She consulted a male homeopath and enjoyed being the centre of attention in the case-taking. She started to flirt with the homeopath. The homeopath noted these 'projections' and prescribed Lachesis that failed to act. Sarah continued on her antidepressants and wanted to consult frequently. The homeopath noticed he would note the days she was due to attend and at times consultations with her would run over. The case became increasingly hidden. When the homeopath presented this case in supervision he realised that Sarah made him feel special.

At the next consultation he observed Sarah's need for special treatment, while noting his own need to give it. It lead to Sarah talking about feeling special and expecting others to see that she was special. The homeopath noted for the first time her haughtiness and that he had had jealous feelings about her husband, perhaps unconsciously leading to the prescription of Lachesis. She responded well to Platina and at a subsequent consultation was able to explore her wish to find a father replacement figure and a need to have someone around who made her feel special.

Deepening our Approach

to work with and may, like many health care practitioners, dismiss them with labels such as heart sink, hypochondriacs, incurable, etc.

REFLECTION POINT

- Reflect on a recent consultation when strong feelings have arisen. What are these and what is being projected? Who did the patient remind you of and how might another homeopath have responded differently?
- Do you draw a particular sort of patient to you? What might this say about you? Do you believe that if you deny aspects of yourself you are likely to find yourself being confronted by patients who have similar issues?
- Think about different remedy types – what projections are they likely to generate and what counter-projections would they generate in you?
- You might have positive or negative feelings in the consultation. Which is likely to be harder to recognise and name? Is one more useful or relevant than the other?

Projective Identification

Patients in a particular remedy state will see the world through that remedy state's eyes. They project aspects of the remedy state onto their environment and select an environment where they feel most comfortable and that matches their remedy state. The projector has the unconscious fantasy of depositing unwanted aspects of themselves in another in the hope that the other person will be able to process what the projector could not (Ogden 1979, 1986). For example, a Nux Vomica patient will seek to create a Nux Vomica world. Patients consciously and unconsciously induce feelings in others that are part of their remedy picture. How you feel with a particular patient will be influenced by your susceptibility to those projections, and you are likely to draw to you patients that create or reinforce familiar feelings. It is therefore quite consistent for patients to be attracted to a homeopath who both suits their particular view of the world and whom they believe they might control and manipulate. The homeopath who unconsciously identifies with what is being projected will

feel a sense of 'possession' by the patient – as if the patient's remedy is proving itself on them.

At its most basic, projective identification is one way of sharing how you feel. But it can also be a way of attempting to deny negative feelings by putting them onto someone else – which can, for a short time, make the person who is projecting feel better. Projection may be a mutual condition that leads eventually to co-dependence and mutual lack of objectivity. While it may distort our perception in a therapeutic situation, it is nevertheless common socially, and contributes to feelings of belonging and security. When dependence is eventually broken there can be strong negative reactions, and care is needed to manage it as a conscious stage in a maturing therapeutic relationship. It is one of the reasons why you should be cautious when treating family or friends becoming increasingly cautious as the case becomes more complex, confused or hidden.

If you spend enough time in the company of someone in a particular state you start to experience that state. When, during a consultation, you experience a particularly strong feeling, e.g. hopelessness, anxiety or uncertainty, it is important to consider the possibility that these feelings exist within the patient. When carefully monitored and observed it allows you to experience the patient's remedy state as if you are proving it – and contributes to the 'feeling and living materia medica' picture it is possible to build with experience. When poorly monitored or handled it leads to being pulled into unhealthy or unprofessional relationships and obscures the patient's case. The more susceptible you are to a particular feeling in many settings, the more likely it is to be part of your make-up and to reflect the remedies you might be most sensitive to.

It is worth considering that in every consultation the patient's remedy state in a way proves itself on us. It is the degree and individuality of that 'proving' and its recognition that indicate the remedy. It is possible to see that in the case of Sarah above. A susceptible homeopath might have moved further into a remedy state (proved it) in response to her projection. Homeopaths needing

Deepening our Approach

V

a particular remedy will find similar patients can move them further into that state.

Understanding Ourselves

'Writing a prescription is easy, but coming to an understanding with a patient is hard.'

Kafka (1949)

The homeopathic relationship is unfamiliar to many patients who are not used to being invited to tell their story in such detail or to being heard with such intensity. Some come with expectations that a pill will allow them 'magically' to return to a previous state, to 'turn the clock back'. If this expectation of magician is projected, the homeopath is unwise to except it. Much is possible but it is for the patient to undertake their healing journey – not for the homeopath to take it from them.

The Homeopath's Perception

'The first duty of the physician is to perceive what is to be cured in the case of disease.'

S Hahnemann, Organon, Para 3

Whatever we perceive is influenced by our own state of mind, emotions, culture, race and family. When we observe a patient it is in the context of the homeopathic relationship, including our part in it. The more confused and hidden the case the more of it is in the unconscious – and the more important the homeopathic relationship is in revealing this.

To be emotionally present brings certain challenges, including developing insight and recognising emotions in you. Identifying and learning to manage issues of projection is a key skill in working with confused and hidden cases. Learning from successful cases is often easy but learning from those cases that have not gone well is often harder – but provides much greater opportunity for growth (see Chapter 25). The case of Simon illustrates how identifying transference and counter-transference can help. If this case had been supervised it may have been recognised earlier.

The homeopath occupies a unique position, being able to incorporate medical models of health

CASE STUDY 23.3

Simon presented because he was fed up with his migraines, and came on the recommendation of his wife – who had been 'nagging him' to see a homeopath. At first he seemed brittle, sharp and irritable and I felt threatened and insecure. Exploring his irritability it became clear that he was frightened of expecting too much and finding it didn't work. This connected with his fear of rejection. The irritability and brittleness was an effective way of keeping people at a distance. This theme of wanting to be alone because of a fear of being let down (or letting others down) is a consistent part of the picture of the remedy Bryonia, a remedy I missed for sometime because my response to the patient's irritability was to withdraw and not probe deeper – concentrating instead purely on the local symptoms. I now know that patients in the Bryonia state of chronic disease often make me feel this way and this can alert me to the possibilities of them being a Bryonia case – something we will return to when we talk about emotional materia medica.

(based on cause and effect) and psychotherapeutic ones. Homeopaths work both with 'process and task' and with 'content and outcome'. It is interesting how development in homeopathy over the last 200 years has run in parallel with the psychodynamic developments so important to an individual understanding of patients.

Monitoring the Projection

'Your psychological and physical reactions to patients provide useful and as you get to know yourself reliable information about the patient's condition and remedy'.

A homeopath may simply experience the projection as a 'tingling in the neck' or a feeling that something is important. At this level these things can guide the homeopath in receiving the case; the more these feelings remain unconscious in the homeopath the more likely they are to lead to 'reciprocal projections' or counter-transference. For many homeopaths and other health professionals, there are certain, sometimes common, situations in which counter-transference occurs. Sometimes these are feelings that the practitioner becomes quite attached to such as feeling special, but they can also produce feelings of being in a rut, going through the same thing again and again or feeling worthless or put upon.

For many health care practitioners, including homeopaths, how projection is handled (or more importantly not handled) is a major factor influencing personal, practice and professional morale and behaviour (see Chapters 25 and 30). Knowing yourself is the key to detecting projection, to prevent it remaining unconscious and you buying into it and making it your reality. Projection and reciprocal projection lies behind much abuse of power and both patients and homeopaths being taken advantage of.

Implication for Studying Materia Medica

'When the patient is ready the homeopath will appear. When the homeopath is ready the patient will appear.'

David Lilley

When studying the materia medica, just as when studying the patient, what you see will depends on the perspective you see it from. Your ability to perceive remedies will be influenced by your own ability to recognise that remedy in yourself. So, for example, from the outside an Arsenicum Album proving may look like fastidiousness and controlling, but from inside the patient it may feel like a need to cope with the insecurity and be clear who is in control. A patient may present with irritability but underlying this state may be an anxiety. Part of understanding the materia medica and the remedy pictures is being clear from where you are seeing the remedy.

If the homeopath is in a particular remedy state at a particular time this will colour how they are able to prescribe for their patients. At times you may think you are attracting patients who need a particular remedy, at other times it is all you can see in patients. If you continue to recognise a single predominant remedy in cases it is quite likely you need this remedy yourself. When you are taught

or studying a remedy, you energetically and subtly prove it. The more depth it is taught in, and the more the remedy is 'brought alive', the more something of the remedy state is projected on to you. The effect of this is to generate reciprocal projections in you to the remedy. It can stay active for some time after your teaching and is why you see that remedy more after you have been taught it.

Once the projection has been processed, and you can distinguish the remedy state arising in yourself, you will have gained a deeper understanding of both the remedy and yourself. Some teachers advise students not to prescribe a particular remedy for at least a few weeks after studying it because you are probably not seeing the patient clearly. Other teachers feel you are more likely to recognise the remedy and patients who need it – and they are more likely then to seek you out!

REFLECTION POINT

- Think of a difficult case you have seen. How does this patient make you feel and what are they communicating but not saying? What types of cases might make you feel 'dumped on' and what can you do to prevent this?
- Reflect on the unique position homeopaths have (with skills in a number of models of health) in understanding the psychological and somatic interface of illness. To what extent does the mind and body each reflect the other and how does disease limit the free expression of mental and physical creativity? How does the artificial separation of them restrict what we can know of others and ourselves?
- How might your consulting room and practice organisation reflect what you are unconsciously projecting, what might this tell you about the patients you will attract and those you won't?

Summary

We are only homeopaths because there are homeopathic patients.

This chapter develops the central role of the homeopathic relationship when working in greater depth with patients. It has looked at how both the

Deepening our Approach

V

perceiver and what is perceived mutually define each other; that each observer has their own unique prejudices and that by understanding and knowing these, you are better able to work with them.

In the same way that we talk about homeopathy as an individualised system of health care where five patients with the same condition might each require a different remedy, so we have to be open to the fact that a patient may present a difficult case to five different homeopaths who each may see and bring to light aspects of several different remedy pictures. These different remedy pictures will often be related, but the way they emerge will be dependent on the dynamic inter-relationship between the patient and the homeopath. The homeopathic relationship in this way is not separable from the description of the remedy, the effect of the remedy and the effect of the consultation.

This chapter has explored how projection from the patient to the homeopath and from the homeopath to the patient provides vital information to the understanding of difficult cases. We go on in Section VI to explore in more detail how to work with confused and hidden cases. Working with projection requires intellectual and emotional competence and links to seeing the remedies as emotional, situational and living materia medica (see Chapter 27). The feelings that patients experience in particular remedy states are an important and significant part of that remedy's materia medica. Equally, patients in different remedy states can generate (or draw out) particular feelings in the homeopath. Depending on the state of the homeopath, these feelings may be different. So, for example, a Nux Vomica homeopath will experience a Pulsatilla patient differently from a Pulsatilla homeopath. However, if the homeopath is aware of their own state and develops an experience of working with different cases, the feelings that they experience in particular consultations can give a reliable indication to the remedy state of the patient. This is explored further when discussing the reflective approach to treatment.

For both the patient and homeopath it invites a shift in how they relate to each other and illness. A patient with a chronic illness can understand that illness is telling them something about themselves and their situation, so they can make the changes that mean they no longer need the illness. In the same way, the homeopath can welcome the difficult case as an opportunity to explore their way of working and of knowing themselves more deeply.

References

Einstein A, Podolsky B, Rosen N 1935 Can quantum-mechanical description of physical reality be considered complete? Phys Rev 41:777

Goleman D 1995 Emotional intelligence. Bantam Books, New York

Hahnemann S 1842 Organon of the medical art, 6th edn. Based on a translation by Steven Decker, edited and annotated by Wendy Brewster O'Reilly. 1995 Birdcage Books, Washington

Kafka F 1949 A country doctor. In the penal settlement. Secker and Warburg, London

Ogden T H 1979 On projective identification. Int J Psycho-Anal 60:357–373

Ogden T H 1986 The matrix of the mind. Object relations theory and the psychoanalytic dialogue. Jason Aronson, Northwale, NJ

Rosenberg M 2003 Nonviolent communication – a language of life. PuddleDancer Press, Chicago

Stapp H P 1971 S-matrix interpretation of quantum theory. Physical Review D3:1303

Bibliography

Kleinman A 1988 The illness narratives. Basic Books, New York

Hawkins P Shohet R 2000 Supervision in the helping professions, 2nd edn. Open University Press, Buckingham

Deepening our Approach

V

CHAPTER TWENTY FOUR

Homeopathic Research

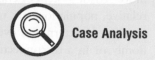

Case Analysis

Iris R. Bell

Introduction by David Owen

"Truth lies in the achievement of a contact with reality – a contact destined to reveal itself by an indefinite range of yet unforeseen consequences"

M Polyani

Different homeopaths will have different reasons to reflect on and study the research and evidence base for homeopathy. All of us owe it to ourselves and our patients:

1. to ask why we might do something
2. to enquire into what others have done and if it worked
3. to monitor the outcomes of our treatments and
4. in the light of this, ask how we might modify what we do.

This, similar to the learning cycle, is the cycle around which we can refine and develop our experience. Much of this text is concerned with only the first step of this cycle and I am indebted to Iris Bell for so comprehensively addressing stage 2 of this. More than that, if the basic principles can be grasped this chapter gives a solid foundation for monitoring the outcome of every patient you treat. There are many diverse ways of enquiring into the homeopathic process and if the most appropriate questions can be asked there are a wealth of meaningful and worthwhile techniques for examining both the art and science of homeopathic practice. Iris has made a formidable start in redressing the skewed and dis-

torted perception that too many in the conventional Western paradigm project onto the evidence base for homeopathy. There are, of course, many arguments that conventional scientists might put up in response; some of these – such as the lack of objective enquiry by homeopaths into what they practice – do have some substance to them.

While qualitative enquiry and research does not necessarily extrapolate (or linearly progress) to quantitative research, it dose nonetheless address many important questions about patients and interventions. If this chapter acts as a reminder to homeopaths that critical and thoughtful enquiry into the homeopathic process is an important responsibility, then it will have served its purpose. If, in addition, it furthers your individual understanding and stimulates an enquiry into how you work and might research the models of health, approaches to treatment and methodologies for prescribing, then it will have served you well. In the evolution of our profession, critical thinking and systematic enquiry have a long tradition and provide us with both an opportunity and a responsibility.

As you read this chapter, you might like to reflect on the different research tools necessary to evaluate the range of outcomes each approach and methodology offer, and on the matrix of different types of research and experience that are most likely to influence your practice of homeopathy. Remember that as you move between the different models of health, different methods of enquiry and research are appropriate. Some models are more open to 'scientific enquiry' with separate objective events that can be measured. Whereas others require a more artistic system of enquiry where objectivity is relative, populations are not distributed according to a fixed pattern and events do not happen randomly or in a disconnected way. Confusing these two leads to the nonsense of *'trying to measure the beauty of a rose with a ruler'* (David Reilly).

Homeopathic Research

This chapter addresses:

- the scope of the types of research relevant to understanding homeopathy
- the complex issues in designing, performing, and interpreting research studies on homeopathy
- emerging theoretical models for elucidating the nature of healing in homeopathy (Mathie 2003, Walach et al 2005).

Researchers consider homeopathy to be one of the leading whole systems of complementary and alternative medicine (CAM), i.e. a complex intervention involving multiple elements in an integrated package of care (e.g. the patient–provider relationship/alliance and the remedy), as contrasted with mainstream pharmaceutical medicine in which the focus is the purified single drug (Ritenbaugh et al 2003, Verhoef et al 2004, 2005). Whole systems of CAM, like homeopathy, also typically generate global and broad multidimensional local outcomes in a patient-centered way (non-specific effects) (Schulman 2004, Oberbaum et al 2005). In contrast, conventional medicine evaluates itself by its singular ligand-receptor/mechanism-specific, disease-centered therapeutic outcomes. Converging evidence also suggests that the advantages of CAM over mainstream medicine may fall particularly in the areas of greater safety and lower cost (van Haselen 2000). Thus, at the outset, assessing homeopathy using conventional drug-oriented efficacy study designs is a poor fit from the perspective of external, ecological validity (Bell 2005a, Jonas 2005).

A core feature of homeopathy is individualised treatment, but conventional drug testing relies upon averaged group effects. Although systematic, homeopathic remedy development (provings) and

clinical practice are inherently qualitative rather than quantitative in their processes. However, relatively little homeopathic research has adapted the available methodologies from qualitative disciplines (Verhoef et al 2002, Bell et al 2003, Thompson 2004). At face value, for instance, the data from homeopathic provings and case-taking interviews involves identification of qualitative patterns rather than simplistic tallies of symptoms (Sherr 1994, Rowe 1998, Sankaran 2005). Consensus panels have emphasised the need to honour the nature of the CAM intervention in study design (Levin et al 1997), but many investigators have failed to do so in testing homeopathic treatment (Bell 2003). The global and multidimensional nature of homeopathic outcomes also points to the likelihood that the mechanisms of action for homeopathic remedies and treatment overall differ from those of pharmaceutical agents (Bellavite & Signorini 2002, Hyland & Lewith 2002, Bellavite 2003).

In turn, such differences should inform the direction of basic and preclinical science studies on the nature of the remedies and their actions. These considerations have led to emerging theories in homeopathy that invoke macro-quantum entanglement of closed systems and complex non-linear dynamical systems and network science models for the nature of healing in homeopathy. Scientists have also pursued basic science research looking for succussion-dependent, persistent changes in the network structure and interactions of solvent (water) molecules (water clusters), rather than molecular properties of the animal, mineral, or plant source molecules in studying the remedies diluted beyond Avogadro's number in potency. Presumably then, remedies would catalyse self-organising changes throughout the body water at the interface with the physical body (Watterson 1991, 1996, 1997). Biofield and/or electromagnetic mechanisms may also help mediate the interface between the remedy and the physical body (Del Giudice 1988, Rubik 2002). However, dissenting opinions question whether or not homeopathy acts by any local (remedy specific) as opposed to non-local effects, or both, in the first place (Walach 2000, Walach et al 2005).

In short, homeopathic research is in its infancy in the development of testable models and appropriate

Deepening our Approach

V

methodological approaches. The field has already encountered serious, albeit overly biased, challenges, such as a controversial meta-analysis (a systematic review of many different studies) of a small number of efficacy studies with good internal but poor external validity (Shang et al 2005), as a result of premature acceptance of the assumptions and methodologies that are better suited for mainstream medical drugs than for homeopathic research.

Overview

Homeopathic research encompasses many different types of investigations, from basic science to preclinical to clinical in nature, as shown in Table 24.1. Jonas proposed that CAM research shift from an evidence hierarchy, in which meta-analyses of randomised controlled trials are at the top of a pyramid, to an evidence house, in which the broad scope of possible study designs are all valued, depending on the nature of the question asked and the information needed (Jonas 2001, 2005). For example, well-done observational or audit studies on effectiveness may be far more relevant to clinical practice than are efficacy studies because they reflect the patient populations who seek homeopathic treatment (Jacobs et al 1998, Honda & Jacobson 2005) and the multiple factors that contribute to outcomes in the real world (Freeman & Sweeeney 2001). Even studies from allopathic medicine increasingly support the

Table 24.1 TYPES OF RESEARCH APPLICABLE TO THE HOMEOPATHIC METHOD

Approach	Potential relevance to homeopathy
Case reports	Expansion of clinically essential information on individualised treatment
Qualitative studies	Design and analysis of provings Description of therapeutic aspects of the homeopathic interview Characterisation of patient and provider experiences of homeopathic care
Observational outcomes studies	Understanding treatment factors and outcomes in the context of real-world practice Quality of life and disease-specific outcomes can be assessed
Health services research studies	Documentation of costs and access to homeopathy in different health care systems
Epidemiological studies	Identification of features of users of homeopathic self-care and practitioner-provided care Evaluation of longitudinal outcomes of persons treated with homeopathy with and without concomitant treatment from conventional and other CAM interventions
Individual difference studies	Determination of personality traits, genetic/biological, life event histories, and environmental factors in differential outcomes in homeopathic treatment Psychophysiological correlates of exceptional, usual, and poor outcomes for individual patients in homeopathic treatment
Preclinical and plant studies	Animal and plant studies and dose-finding studies in human subjects (e.g. is there a difference between LM dosing and C potency dosing?; do sequential potencies have non-linear effects in opposite directions on the same type of organism?) can reveal properties of remedies not otherwise understood as factors in clinical trial studies
Clinical trials	Comparison of effects of verum homeopathic remedy treatment with placebo Comparisons of effects of homeopathic interviews with conventional psychotherapeutic interviews and sham therapy
Meta-analyses	Assessment of combined multiple trials on a given disorder or intervention, with quality ratings of internal validity; limited by biases inherent in the trials chosen for inclusion and quality criteria (meta-analyses do not evaluate external validity of each trial)
Basic science	Determination of physical chemistry and materials science properties of homeopathic remedies in vitro

Deepening our Approach

V

importance of effectiveness rather than efficacy designs for generating clinically meaningful information (Concato et al 2000). The emphasis on individualisation in holistic, holographic and relational methods of homeopathic diagnosis and treatment also suggests the importance of including individual difference research in the total portfolio of studies and in the design of 'group' studies as well.

For meta-analyses of efficacy research, studies based on different models of health (causation and isopathy, local prescribing, totality and constitutional approaches etc.) are usually combined, as are studies that use a single prescription with those using a combination of remedies. This has little defensible rationale other than the lack of sufficient studies in the literature using any one model or clinical approach. Both positive meta-analyses, such as the Linde et al (1997) study that was originally favourable to homeopathy in its conclusions, and negative meta-analyses, such as Shang et al (2005), combined studies from several different types of clinical treatment models and on multiple different diagnoses. While it is usually possible to draw conclusions, it is difficult to draw valid inferences about homeopathy from such heterogeneous datasets.

Methodological shortcomings have plagued basic science studies of homeopathic remedies, though some investigators have proposed standards for minimising factors that confound and contaminate the data (Becker-Witt et al 2003). With their clinical interest in patient-centered individual cases rather than disease-centered group interventions, homeopaths themselves publish and study single case reports far more than do allopaths.

Sceptics of homeopathy periodically publish papers with various methodological flaws that are proclaimed to be the 'final proof' that homeopathy is nothing more than placebo (Lancet 2005). The reality of science is that no one study or published paper is sufficient to dismiss an entire field, despite the wishful biases of some sceptics, whatever the topic. The body of research on homeopathy indicates that homeopathic remedies have properties different from placebos in test tubes and animals (Sukul et al 1986, 1999, 2001, Endler & Schulte 1994, Ruiz & Torres 1997, Schulte & Endler 1998,

Bertani et al 1999, Ruiz-Vega et al 2000, 2002, Bellavite & Signori 2002) and that homeopathic treatment has shown largely beneficial effects on thousands of patients with a variety of allopathic conditions (Goldstein & Glik 1998, Riley et al 2001, Anelli et al 2002, Thompson & Reilly 2002, van Wassenhoven & Ives 2004, Sevar 2005, Spence et al 2005, Witt et al 2005a,b). The data support the concept that homeopathic remedies are not the same as allopathic drugs in terms of actions on disease-specific local mechanisms and that the dynamical effects and neurophysiology of active remedies differ from that of placebo (Hyland & Lewith 2002, Lewith et al 2002, Bell et al 2004c,f). The evidence to date shows that remedies are generally safe, especially in comparison with conventional drugs (Dantas & Rampes 2000, Riley et al 2001, van Wassenhoven & Ives 2004).

The data also suggest, however, that homeopathy, or at least those approaches and methodologies studied, do not work in all cases under all circumstances for many reasons (Frei & Thurneysen 2001, Frei et al 2005) – only some of which have been formally investigated. Furthermore, as in any clinical intervention, placebo effects play a varying role in real-world outcomes (Bonne et al 2003, Bell 2005b, Jacobs et al 2005, Pilkington et al 2005). The evidence implies that certain types of people out of the general population gravitate to homeopathic treatment (Jacobs et al 1998, Honda & Jacobson 2005) and that homeopathy may be more effective for a subset of patients than for all patients with a given allopathic diagnosis (Bell et al 2004c), although studies have not looked at how different groups of patients use different homeopathic approaches. As in most clinical fields (MacPherson et al 2003, Caspi et al 2004, Aikens et al 2005, Hirsh et al 2005), limited data also suggest that the patient–provider relationship (e.g. empathy favouring patient empowerment and self-efficacy) – largely uninvestigated to date for homeopathy (Mercer et al 2002, Jacobs et al 2005, Thompson et al 2005) – plays some therapeutic role apart from that of the remedies in favourable homeopathic outcomes within the clinical setting.

Qualitative Research

Qualitative research is typically focused on words rather than numbers, often using in-depth individual or group interviews, observations of people living in their own real world environments, and/or analysis of archival sources such as those on philosophy, literature, and history. The multiple methods of qualitative research have different purposes, which Tesch (1992) summarised as asking the following three types of questions:

1. What are the characteristics of language itself?
2. Can we discover regularities in human experience?
3. Can we comprehend the meaning of a text or action?

Qualitative research has an established, though undervalued, place in health research, especially in nursing and medical anthropology (Lincoln & Guba 1985, Denzin & Lincoln 2000, Pope & Mays 2000), and to a growing extent in CAM (Verhoef et al 2002, Bell et al 2003, Paterson et al 2003).

In contrast with allopathic medicine, which is mainly quantitative in its orientation, much homeopathic practice is qualitative by nature. The goal of the case-taking is to answer the three types of questions above in understanding the essential dynamic disturbance in the patient as a whole indivisible system (Sherr 1994, 2002). Most successful homeopathic treatment goes far beyond resolution of a chief complaint and does not even hold as a goal suppression of a symptom or disease manifestation. Whether or not they formalise their procedures with qualitative analysis per se, homeopaths routinely use qualitative approaches in provings research and in clinical case-taking and analysis. Thompson (2004) has called for awareness of the potential of qualitative methods to enrich homeopathic research and practice, including in presentation of case reports. An unexplored opportunity is for homeopaths to collaborate with experienced qualitative researchers to improve the data collection and analysis techniques applied to provings and to clinical information gathering and assessment.

As a parallel, research in acupuncture that overlaps with homeopathy in essential philosophical tenets and potential clinical impact (Vithoulkas 1980) has begun to document global and multidimensional changes during treatment. The changes that patients report extend far beyond the disease-centered, single complaint focus of allopathic clinical studies. Rather, acupuncture patients are reporting changes in life style, sense of meaning in life, energy, improvements in symptoms not mentioned originally at intake, and so on (Gould & MacPherson 2001, Paterson & Britten 2003, Schulman 2004). These are also the broad changes that homeopaths reported in a published qualitative study of possible outcomes in patients with chronic diseases on constitutional treatment (Bell et al 2003) (Box 24.1). The multidimensionality of the changes during homeopathic treatment, as well as the global improvements in sense of

---

BOX 24.1
Practitioner Views of Multidimensional Scope of Patient Outcome Categories in Constitutional Homeopathic Treatment for Chronic Diseases (after Bell et al 2003)
- Adaptiveness
- Coping
- Creativity
- Dreams
- Emotional
- Energy
- Freedom/unstuckness
- Life changes
- Life style
- Mental functioning
- Perceptions by others
- Physical generalities
- Physical functioning: specific
- Personal perception
- Recall
- Relationships
- Sleep
- Spiritual function
- Well-being

Deepening our Approach

V

well-being and energy that homeopaths expect to observe in their patients, are often ignored in the design of clinical studies (Oberbaum et al 2005) in favour of the types of narrow, specific outcomes that mainstream conventional medicine expects from its drugs.

In fact, one of the emerging points in homeopathy research is the necessity of re-examining assumptions used in performing allopathically driven studies. Researchers need to ask: 'What is homeopathy?' 'What happens during homeopathic case-taking?' 'What happens during homeopathic treatment?'

When sceptics review homeopathic studies and conclude that homeopathic treatment has non-specific effects, the conclusion is true, in a sense (Walach 2001). The problem lies in the interpretation of the meaning of 'non-specificity'. To mainstream investigators, non-specific effects are undesirable and are a synonym for placebo effects. The reality is that homeopathy is non-specific in its nature (Walach 2000, 2001, Walach & Jonas 2002), and the convergent data suggest that the non-specificity goes beyond placebo effects and reaches to the heart of the therapeutic encounter (see Chapter 25) (Walach 2002, 2003).

Qualitative research offers a way to go back to first steps in the research endeavour and to describe the homeopathic process. Then investigators can proceed to design studies with features that honour the true nature of homeopathy, including its philosophy, medicines, practice, and clinical experiences. Moreover, because of the nature of homeopathy and the insights it offers to different therapeutic approaches, it may be that qualitative research developed this way will play a more important role than quantitative research in advancing not just the field of homeopathy but the broader questions about 'healing' rather than 'curing'. It is the political paradigm (including commercial and professional power issues) that influences, in subtle and at times unconscious ways, conventional medicine's emphasis on quantitative research.

If the aim is to improve clinical practice and patient outcomes then newer qualitative methods may be the best suited; however, scientists are often not objective with regard to new discoveries and theories (Barber 1961).

Observational and Effectiveness Research

Another issue in homeopathic research is that the complex nature of the intervention and the multidimensionality of outcomes fit better with research designs that examine effectiveness in the real world of practice rather than efficacy of isolated interventions and their specific effects on disease. In conventional medicine, effectiveness studies, especially those with a quality of life emphasis, are typically done after, not before, an allopathic drug has undergone extensive testing in efficacy trials.

However, it is becoming clear that the more appropriate sequence of research approaches for whole systems of CAM, which already have histories of hundreds to thousands of years of widespread use, is to study the intact packages of care with large scale observational trials first, then perhaps to dissect their components to understand their relative contributions to the net effects. For homeopathy, the package of care includes at least the homeopathic interview process itself and the alliance between homeopath and patient in addition to the individualised remedy. Some investigators have argued that the package of care also includes the symbolic meaning of the remedy (Walach 2000), apart from any physical agent, as part of a closed, entangled macro-system involving patient, the patient's symptoms, practitioner, remedy, and the remedy's symptoms (Milgrom 2002a,b, 2003a,b, 2004a,b,c,d, 2005, Hyland 2003, Walach 2003, 2005a). It is also becoming clear that the nature of the outcomes is individualised and extends into global and local outcomes far beyond those involved in the presenting complaint of the patient, such as overall well-being, energy, social role functioning, and so on.

Box 24.2 lists observational studies reported on homeopathy. Most of these data converge on the conclusion that the majority of homeopathically treated patients, i.e. 70–80%, experience

BOX 24.2
Representative List of Observational/Audit Studies in Homeopathy
- Anelli et al 2002
- Goldstein and Glik 1998
- Neville-Smith 1999
- Relton et al 2005
- Richardson 2001
- Riley et al 2001
- Sevar 2000
- Sevar 2005
- Spence et al 2005
- Van Wassenhoven and Ives 2004
- Witt 2005
- Witt et al 2005

moderate to substantial improvements in their overall condition and high levels of satisfaction with care. When compared with allopathic drugs, side effect rates appear lower, and patients often – but not always – report the ability to reduce their reliance on conventional drugs. Two retrospective studies (Frenkel & Hermoni 2002, van Wassenhoven & Ives 2004), but not a recent large scale comparative cohort prospective study (Witt et al 2005b), observed substantial cost savings for allopathic drugs in homeopathically-treated patients. In terms of safety, most of the observational studies on homeopathy support the conclusion that side-effects are lower with homeopathic than with allopathic treatment. Future studies should explore the implications of lower side-effects with homeopathy for patient adherence to treatment – a major practical issue for real-world allopathic clinical care of many chronic and acute diseases. These observational trials have occurred in a variety of countries and cultures – from multiple European nations to Germany, Belgium, the UK, and the USA – across which acceptance of homeopathy varies a great deal, perhaps reflecting that the benefits can be seen in a wide range of cultures.

An important methodological point, however, is that observational outcomes have often derived from quality of life ratings and/or global assessments of overall improvement across patients with

a wide range of conventional diagnoses – what conventional researchers would label as 'non-specific' as well as subjective rather than objective in nature. It is usually not possible to determine presence or absence or degree of specific outcomes in allopathically homogeneous sub-samples, e.g. use of rescue medications and number of emergency room visits for uncontrolled asthma breakthroughs, from the observational studies available to date on homeopathy.

While these types of non-specific quality of life outcomes potentially matter a great deal to patients, public policy decision-makers and third-party payers are likely to view an outcome such as a greater sense of well-being as unhelpful or insufficient in deciding whether or not to pay for homeopathic treatment for all patients with a given conventional diagnosis. It is certainly possible to design well-controlled observational studies to examine not only global quality of life outcomes, but also disease-related objective clinical and health services outcomes. Greater clarity by investigators on the purpose of a given study will help guide these types of design choices (Jonas et al 2001, Jonas 2005, Walach et al 2005).

Table 24.2 provides a list of brief subjective outcome measures that may prove useful in assessing global and individualised outcomes in observational studies. You might like to reflect on how you might use such scores to assess and interpret the response of your own patients to homeopathic treatment. They include measures of global change ratings (the Glasgow Homeopathic Hospital Outcome scale on global well-being and chief complaint); global physical health ratings, a predictive factor for morbidity, service utilisation, and even mortality (Idler & Benyamini 1997, Menec et al 1999); individually-described symptoms (the MYMOP) (Paterson 1996); and overall well-being (the AIOS) (Bell et al 2004a). Quality of life scales (such as the SF-36) are commonly used in outcome studies, but are prone to insensitivity to change over time (Kane 1997) and potentially low relevance for patients' values of functionality and symptomatology. Multidimensional quality of life scales for homeopathic outcomes are not as

Deepening our Approach

V

Table 24.2 RATING SCALES OF POTENTIAL RELEVANCE TO HOMEOPATHIC OBSERVATIONAL AND EFFICACY STUDIES THAT CLINICIANS MIGHT FIND USEFUL FOR PROGRESS ASSESSMENTS

Scale	Variable(s)	Reference
Glasgow Homeopathic Hospital Scale	Positive or negative change in overall condition rating	Reilly 1997
Global health rating scale	Physical health rating	Idler & Benyamini 1997
Measure Your Own Medical Outcomes Profile Scale	Leading individual symptoms ratings	Paterson 1996
Arizona Integrative Outcomes Scale	Global well-being (bio-psycho-social-spiritual) visual analogue rating	Bell et al 2004a
Patrick Quality of Life Scale	Satisfaction ratings with multiple dimensions of life, including but not limited to health	Patrick et al 1988
Connor-Davidson Resilience Scale	Resilience to life stressors	Connor et al 2003

yet available, but some scales from the allopathic literature may cover a sufficient scope of change in health- and non-health-related domains to be useful (Patrick et al 1988).

At the same time, differences in the nature of the outcomes assessed in these observational studies versus the much more narrow, disease-focused often singular clinical outcomes in efficacy trials may help explain, in part, the discrepant findings for homeopathy in observational trials (all favourable) and efficacy trials (mixed positive and negative findings). Clinical trials are typically brief, e.g. 8–16 weeks in duration, whereas follow-up periods with observational studies are often measured in many months to years. Homeopaths agree that it can take at least a year or two, or even more, to see marked and lasting changes in persons who initially present with chronic diseases. Modern texts of homeopathy report the expectation that patients will experience global improvements in well-being and energy, for example, before necessarily reporting improvements in physical symptoms (Vithoulkas 1980). Under such circumstances, it is quite possible for short-term studies to find no apparent effect of homeopathic treatment in a given allopathic diagnosis because the symptoms of the presenting disease have not yet changed, even though the patient as a whole is better or symptoms other than the chief com-

plaint have improved. This situation highlights the importance of carefully selecting more than one outcome, based on the nature of homeopathic healing and the constraints of the study design.

Although politically dominant Western medical systems value efficacy studies over effectiveness studies, clinicians and some researchers have begun to point out in the allopathic literature that effectiveness is what matters most in practice to both the provider and the patient (Wolfe 1999) and efficacy outside of a realistic and practical clinical context may mean little. Furthermore, allopathic researchers have looked closely at the quality of information that well-done observational studies, e.g. those with case-control or cohort designs, offer in comparison with efficacy studies (Concato et al 2000, Concato 2004, Concato & Horwitz 2004). The findings are that properly-performed observational studies of real-world practice outcomes generate similarly valid findings to those of efficacy studies that do not inflate the apparent effect size of the intervention.

Efficacy Research and Meta-analyses

Efficacy studies are where conventional medicine places its highest confidence in testing its drugs, and this is the area where homeopathic researchers express their greatest methodological and theoretical concerns (Bell 2005a, Walach et al 2005). Whereas observational and qualitative studies suggest a highly favourable profile of homeopathy in real-world practice, at least for the majority of patients who choose to undergo this form of care, efficacy studies and the meta-analyses that combine these trials are far more mixed and unconvincing in their findings for homeopathy.

Box 24.3 provides a list of conditions for which homeopathically-prepared remedies (serially diluted and succussed) have been tested using efficacy study designs. The mode of prescribing varies a great deal. Overall, the results of such placebo-controlled research are mixed, with both positive and negative evidence for the efficacy of homeopathically prepared remedies. Of significant concern is the fact that, unlike observational trials, the study designs of these efficacy studies often fail to reflect the full range of medical

conditions treated, usual length of treatment for chronic disorders, or the usual homeopathic clinical practices in the community. Only one study, a negative trial of homeopathy in chronic headache, made any attempt to address one major criticism of most efficacy designs, i.e. short study duration, by following patients for up to a year with no emerging evidence of benefit from homeopathy (Walach et al 2000).

For the better-designed efficacy studies, CAM researchers have adopted a dual selection procedure for subject inclusion criteria. That is, investigators first recruit an allopathically homogeneous group of patients who share a given diagnosis, then they assign the patients to treatment by the individualised diagnosis each patient requires within the CAM system (Bell et al 2002b, Bell 2003). Unfortunately, many efficacy studies on homeopathy are flawed by a failure to take the second step or by compromising on the scope of remedy choices. For example, researchers have limited themselves to studies of first aid uses of

---

BOX 24.3

Representative Efficacy Trials in Homeopathy or Isopathy for Conventional Diagnoses*

- Allergies/asthma: Reilly et al 1986, Taylor et al 2000, Lewith et al 2002, White et al 2003, Kim et al 2005
- Arthritis: Gibson et al 1980, Shipley et al 1983, van Haselen et al 2000, Fisher et al 2001
- Attention deficit/hyperactivity disorder: Lamont 1997, Frei et al 2005, Jacobs et al 2005
- Chronic fatigue syndrome, fibromyalgia: Fisher 1989, Bell et al 2004b, Weatherley-Jones et al 2004
- Depression, anxiety: Bonne et al 2003, Katz et al 2005
- Childhood diarrhea: Jacobs et al 1994; 2000, 2003
- Flu: Vickers et al 2004

- Headache: Walach et al 1997, Straumsheim et al 2000
- HIV/AIDS: Rastogi et al 1999
- Premenstrual syndrome: Yakir et al 2001
- Postpartum bleeding: Oberbaum et al 2005
- Otitis media: Harrison et al 1999, Jacobs 2001
- Pruritis in renal dialysis: Cavalcanti et al 2003
- Sequelae of cancer therapies: Balzarini et al 2000, Oberbaum et al 2001, Jacobs 2005, Thompson et al 2005
- Sepsis: Frass et al 2005
- Trauma: Hart et al 1997, Vickers et al 1997, 1998, Ramelet et al 2000, Stevinson 2003
- Traumatic brain injury: Chapman et al 1999
- Vertigo: Weiser et al 1998
- Warts: Kainz et al 1996

*Note that most trials are small sample studies lacking the statistical power to avoid Type II error.

Deepening our Approach

V

remedies such as Arnica in acute injuries (some of which are not the clinical situations in which Arnica would be the first-line choice of experienced homeopaths) or of isopathically-prescribed (albeit homeopathically-prepared) remedies such as dust mite or other allergens in asthma and allergy patients.

Another major problem with the body of efficacy research studies in homeopathy is that investigators have not followed the usual sequence of conventional research from small feasibility and dose-finding (phase I and II) studies to large-scale (phase III) studies on the same allopathic disorder by multiple independent laboratories. Because of funding limitations, the need for individualised treatment, and other factors, homeopathic researchers have never mounted a large scale efficacy trial of homeopathically-prepared remedies prescribed homeopathically, i.e. the Lewith et al (2002) dust mite study in asthmatics was large, but involved isopathic prescribing. For phase I/II efficacy studies, only conditions such as childhood diarrhoea (Jacobs et al 1994, 2000, 2003), attention deficit-hyperactivity disorder (Lamont 1997, Frei & Thurneysen 2001, Frei et al 2005, Jacobs et al 2005) and fibromyalgia (Fisher et al 1989, Bell et al 2004e) have more than one, typically small-sample, study published using individualised remedy selection.

Small feasibility or pilot studies suffer the common risk of being statistically underpowered in sample size to find an effect (if present), i.e. they are prone to false negative errors, in which investigators fail to demonstrate an effect that is actually there. Sceptics are quick to jump to negative conclusions about the value of homeopathy from such negative pilot studies, but doing so is scientifically incorrect. A primary rationale for phase I and II studies is to determine the feasibility of successfully performing the study procedures in a subsequently larger study of appropriate sample size to detect an effect, if present. Aickin (2004) has even proposed an alternative statistical approach to analysing data from these smaller studies using separation tests to determine whether or not there is any value in pursuing further research on a topic, rather than testing the null hypothesis in a methodologically unsound way.

Conditions in which placebo response rates are high in allopathic research studies, such as depression, are particularly prone to false negative errors (Type II error) in small sample research. It simply takes far more subjects in a study than investigators can run within budgetary and resource constraints to test the null hypothesis properly. Of course, a given small sample study might have positive results that proponents of homeopathy will applaud and sceptics ignore. However, when another small sample study turns up negative, the sceptics declare the end of homeopathy (Lancet 2005) and the homeopathic proponents cry foul (Various 2005). This problem has occurred in the study of homeopathy in depression and should serve as a caution to researchers in their selection of clinical conditions and sample size (Bell 2005b, Katz et al 2005, Pilkington et al 2005). Given the politicised context in which homeopathy research usually occurs (Aickin 2005, Various 2005), it is essential for homeopathic researchers and practitioners to recognise and point out the methodological limitations of small sample studies in their field, regardless of the positive or negative implications of the findings.

A number of efficacy studies of proprietary products such as Traumeel or Oscillococcinum have been well done, and sometimes repeated by independent laboratories. However, sceptics increasingly question the reliability of data supported by industry in conventional medicine, an issue that carries over to CAM manufacturers as well. Studies on proprietary products typically only represent the causative and local approaches to treatment found in over-the-counter self-care applications for acute, self-limited problems rather than practitioner-provided care for chronic diseases.

Meta-Analyses

As a result of the limited amount of replication in the literature, meta-analyses of homeopathy have typically relied on combining results of highly disparate clinical trials on different patient populations and clinical practices (Kleijnen et al 1991,

Reilly et al 1994, Linde et al 1997, 1999, Cucherat et al 2000, Ernst 2002, Jacobs et al 2003, Shang et al 2005). The results of the meta-analyses vary, as do the clinical efficacy trials. Many are positive, some are negative. None informs us in a definitive way as to the value of homeopathy for any given patient. As Walach et al (2005) have commented this approach is parallel to asking the question, 'Is conventional medicine a placebo effect?' Bell (2005a) has offered another analogy, i.e. 'does penicillin work for all patients with fevers?' In certain situations, conventional medicines are no better than placebo, or so the evidence suggests, but in other clinical situations, conventional medicines are superior to placebo (Kirsch 2001). It is thus highly premature and methodologically risky to attempt meta-analyses of the homeopathic literature as a whole, without more careful differentiation into better defined questions, clinical subpopulations, and clinical treatments.

A key point about meta-analyses is that they typically rely on a 'quality' rating score for a given study. While such ratings facilitate inter-study comparisons of internal validity issues, none of the ratings used in meta-analyses include weighted items assessing the external validity of the trial. That is, given that the quality of the homeopathy delivered is highly dependent on the ability of the practitioner to establish rapport with the patient and determine the simillimum remedy, were the practitioners qualified and experienced homeopaths? How many practitioners were involved in the trial? Did the fate of homeopathy hang on the skill of one or many providers? Was the treatment delivered in a manner comparable to that of usual clinical practices in the field of homeopathy? Were the outcomes assessed fully representative of the clinical claims in the field? For homeopathy, these outcomes would include global well-being, energy, changes in multiple symptoms in patterns outlined by Hering's Law of Cure, and resolution or improvement in the chief complaint. In summary, the limitations of meta-analytic tools for homeopathy research at the present time render this approach much less useful than it is for conventional drugs.

Individual Differences Research

Homeopathic practitioners often express bewilderment at the failure of efficacy studies to demonstrate what they 'know' to occur everyday in their practices. That is, many patients get better, many times undergoing transformational experiences in every aspect of their lives. Thus far, homeopathic research has not begun to address these widely reported outcomes and phenomena. Yet, the group averages in many studies do not capture the quality of these outcomes. Clearly, the discussion of qualitative and observational methods above should open the door to future studies of exceptional, usual, and poor outcomes in individual patients.

However, there is an intermediate methodological approach for quantitatively-oriented investigators. Researchers can borrow from the individual difference literature in health psychology and behavioural medicine (Neff et al 1983, Owens et al 1999, Bell et al 2004d, Honda & Jacobson 2005), the growing literature on sub-typing patients for triage to optimal treatment programs (Turk 2005), and new trends in epidemiology (Ben-Shlomo & Kuh 2002). Even the cutting-edge research on human genomics and proteomics is beginning to facilitate biological identification of individuals with different genetic polymorphisms and environmental factors in phenotypic expression of genetic potentials (Haley et al 1999, La Du et al 2001). In general, data indicate that even within a given allopathic medical diagnosis, patients fall into different subtypes on the basis of both their psychology and their biology. These baseline individual differences beyond basic demographics may represent some of the different themes, even perhaps miasms, which homeopaths recognise in patients and are important for determining outcomes.

People who find their way to homeopathic treatment may differ from those who do not (Honda & Jacobson 2005), for example, in a national US sample of over 4200 adults, found that persons high on scores for the stable personality trait of openness had an increased odds ratio for using a whole system of CAM such as homeopathy or acupuncture of 3.55

Deepening our Approach

V

(95% confidence interval: 1.33–9.44). A personality trait highly correlated with openness, i.e., absorption, also predicts greater use of CAM in general (Owens et al 1999) and the likelihood of staying with treatment – active or placebo – once patients begin treatment (Bell et al 2004d). Such findings raise the possibility that the patient samples who end up in observational trials of homeopathy are fundamentally different in psychology and behaviour – and perhaps even biology (absorption is a genetically-determined trait (Tellegen et al 1988) – from patient samples who end up in efficacy trials. Such patients have a differential capacity for shifting and focusing attention and its electrophysiological correlates (Davidson et al 1976).

In addition, Honda & Jacobson (2005) also found that individuals who rely on secondary coping strategies involving modifying the self are more likely to use whole systems of CAM such as homeopathy or acupuncture and mind-body interventions than are non-users of those interventions. Notably, persons who rely on primary coping involving changing the environment rather than the self are less likely to use most forms of CAM other than manual manipulation modalities.

Such findings raise the testable hypothesis that persons who participate in observational trials are markedly different from those who do not. The latter patients have chosen to undergo homeopathic treatment, often to pay out of pocket for the care, and may likely be high on trait openness and/or absorption and in secondary control coping strategies. Their biobehavioural characteristics in turn may differ significantly from those patients with an allopathic disease label who end up recruited to an efficacy trial, willing to participate in a double-blind clinical trial costing them nothing. These baseline differences, which are never assessed in most clinical studies, could contribute to the gap between findings from observational versus efficacy designs.

The evidence also suggests that a modified clinical trial design for testing the efficacy of homeopathy might involve recruiting people whose profiles better match those of patients who end up in observational studies. Then the research question is not whether homeopathy is useful for all persons with a given allopathic diagnosis (a broad public health question), but rather whether homeopathy is useful beyond placebo for the subset of the population with both the allopathic diagnosis and the inherent tendency to choose treatments like homeopathy in the first place (a treatment triage question).

Additionally, patients' life experiences can interact with the psychobiological factors intrinsic to the individual to favour expression or non-expression of disease. That is, multiple prospective longitudinal studies have shown that persons with adverse childhood experiences (Felitti et al 1998, Surtees et al 2003), poor nurturing from parents (Russek & Schwartz 1997, Russek et al 1998), and/or adult life traumatic events (Boscarino 1997) are at greater risk of expressing serious chronic diseases later in life. Consequently, the coping abilities of the individual, as emphasised by many different homeopathic teachers, will come into play in influencing the specific individualised remedy choice and the patient's capacity for responding to homeopathic treatment. These types of data from the non-homeopathic world may be crude approximations of conceptual models proposed by contemporary homeopathic thinkers such as Scholten or Sankaran. Both of the latter homeopaths suggest that there is a triangulation between the dynamical life themes of a given remedy family and specific remedy (see Chapter 22) and the quality or nature of the coping strategies that the individual manifests in reacting to life stresses (Scholten 1996, Sankaran 2003).

Conventional epidemiological research is actually beginning to intersect with homeopathy in the sense of a shared interest in understanding multifactorial disease aetiology in individuals. In epidemiology, for example, some researchers are also looking at what they term the 'life course approach to chronic disease epidemiology', i.e. examining the full time-line of effects from bio-psycho-social-behavioural pathways on the evolution of chronic disease over the lifespan (Ben-Shlomo & Kuh 2002). These types of research are highly relevant to the issues that homeopaths consider routinely in their clinical practices, but these are not studies that homeopathic researchers have as yet undertaken. Based on the above considerations, can constitutional homeopathic treatment, for instance, delay the timing, lessen the severity, and/or minimise the complications from a chronic disease that genes and environmental stressors may otherwise predispose an individual to develop? Might groups of homeopathic patients respond to particular homeopathic approaches and prescribers? Epidemiological studies could address such questions.

Basic Science and Preclinical Research

Relatively recently, two different research laboratories have reported replicable findings on homeopathic remedies versus controls, using different technologies. Elia & Niccoli (1999), for example, demonstrated that the addition of an alkaline material to a homeopathically-prepared liquid preparation of a given remedy diluted and succussed beyond the point where statistically there are any atoms of the material present (Avogadro's number) leads nonetheless to the release of excess, calorimetrically-measurable heat compared with controls. They also published evidence that the changes induced in the homeopathically-prepared remedy-solutions may evolve with time, i.e. the remedy ages and generates an even larger capacity for heat release over a period of months (Elia & Niccoli 2004). In a different approach, Rey (2003) found that irradiating a homeopathic remedy solution that has been frozen to an extremely low temperature and then gradually re-warmed leads to the release of excess, measurable light or thermoluminescence.

These research groups both concluded that the release of energy (heat or light) following treatment of the remedy solution by extreme changes in pH or x-ray irradiation suggests a presumptive disruption of some type of ordered structure in the remedy liquid (e.g. water clusters) not present in the plain solvent controls. One working hypothesis is that the experimental procedures disrupt hydrogen bonding patterns between

water solvent molecules that were generated during remedy preparation. Other investigators in the materials science field have pointed out that weak bonding forces such as van der Waals forces could contribute, in addition to any changes in hydrogen bonds, to the ability of water as a solvent to retain information. It is important to note that, in contrast with the sceptics' positions that all solvents are homogeneous in their molecular network structure, the proposed phenomena involve the non-random, heterogeneous network restructuring of the solvent at the nano-level by the process of homeopathic remedy preparation (Roy et al 2005).

The phenomenon of epitaxy, for example, is widely-known in the field of materials science, but not medicine. Epitaxy is the transmission of structural information from the surface (hence epi) of one material (usually a crystalline solid) to another (usually but not always a liquid). Newer technologies such as transmission electron microscopy may assist in evaluating the physical properties of homeopathically-prepared solutions versus remedy-free solvent controls. Thus, the limited theory and evidence on the nature of homeopathic remedies suggests that the focus should remain on changes in the solvent as a function of remedy preparation using specific source molecules, but the key changes may more likely be at the level of dynamical network structures rather than static molecular species.

Although some investigators doubt that basic science will ever demonstrate reproducible local physical properties of homeopathic remedies (Walach et al 2005), the research area of physical chemistry of remedies is still too unexplored to abandon as a viable direction at this time. At some point there must be an interface at the physical plane between the remedy and the human body, even if the process 'begins' at a different, non-local plane of organisation or occurs as an emergent property in the larger system as a network (Barabasi & Bonabeau 2003, Vasquez et al 2004).

Even in mind-body research, for example, there is some translation of an individually salient psychological experience within the psyche into measurable biological events (Phan et al 2003). The argument as to whether consciousness precedes mind, which precedes body, or vice versa is an ageless philosophical debate. Nonetheless, it is possible to measure events when they occur in the physical plane. Because of the obvious likelihood that homeopathically-prepared remedy liquids (water or, more likely, water-alcohol mixtures with silica contaminants) hold some information for the individual patient, continued efforts to understand the physical translation of that information are still reasonable. The possibility of important new discoveries in the area of basic science remains despite many theoretical and practical challenges.

In vitro research with homeopathic remedies also suggests that remedies have effects different from plain solvent controls, but that the effects are less reliably reproducible from trial to trial, for unclear reasons, than are those of molecular-based conventional drugs. Homeopathic phenomena appear to be probabilistic rather than certain at any given time. This observation in itself may offer insights into the nature of homeopathic remedies and how they affect living systems. For example, the multisite European study re-testing the famous Benveniste studies demonstrated that ultradilutions of histamine affect basophil degranulation, but not all the time (Belon et al 2004). Rather, the evidence suggests that the phenomenon occurs more often with remedies than with controls, but not on all trials at all sites. Animal and plant studies have also shown this pattern of demonstrable, but less than reliable and often non-linear, effects (Endler & Schulte 1994, Schulte & Endler 1998, Bellavite & Signorini 2002).

Isopathic treatment is protective against adverse effects of toxic material doses of agents such as arsenic, with treatment by the same, but homeopathically-prepared, material as a remedy in animal models (Datta et al 1999, Mitra et al 1999, Brizzi et al 2000, Kundu et al 2000, Mallick et al 2003). Homeopathically-prepared and isopathically-chosen remedies may also exert a protective effect in animal models of glutamate toxicity in the brain (Jonas et al 2001) or exogenous biological warfare infectious agents (Szeto et al 2004).

This peculiar variability – especially the bidirectional quality of changes (Bertani et al 1999) – in empirical findings that occurs in homeopathy could be the simple result of poor quality control from study to study, or it could be a clue as to the true nature of homeopathic remedies and how they act and interact with living systems. One animal study, for example, supports the core homeopathic concept that remedies can cause symptoms in a healthy individual and cure them in a sick person. That is, the direction of effects of a homeopathically-prepared mineral remedy mixture depended on the state of the animal, i.e. the timing of remedy administration before, during, or after the experimental injury (Bertani et al 1999). As in other areas of homeopathic research, the field is in its earliest development, and much more systematic and hypothesis-driven work is needed.

As in clinical research on homeopathy, basic science and preclinical research also has suffered confusing variability in study quality and outcomes. In basic science studies, careful investigation often reveals that the process of succussion in remedy preparation contributes indeterminate amounts of silica contaminants from the glass containers into the test solution (Walach et al 2005). With the use of proper standardisation of sample preparation and succussed controls for comparison, lessening some of the contaminant issues is possible (Becker-Witt et al 2003, Linde et al 1994). According to newer data from Jonas et al's laboratory using an enzyme model system, the silica itself may contribute, along with the water and alcohol in the solvent, to the effects of the remedies (Walach et al 2005). Nonetheless, certain technical methods from physical chemistry such as NMR (nuclear magnetic resonance) tests have produced disappointing and inconsistent results on the characteristics of homeopathic remedies.

Proposed Scientific Frameworks for Homeopathic Research

Various investigators have offered two different, system-based conceptual models for how homeopathy acts. The first is complex adaptive systems and network theory, and the second is macro-quantum entanglement theory. It is beyond the scope of this chapter to discuss these models in depth. However, they provide promising frameworks for reconciling the conflicting findings in the research literature and for guiding the design of future research studies on homeopathy.

Complex Adaptive Systems

A system is a set of interrelated parts. Complex systems, including living organisms (Bell et al 2002a, Bellavite & Signorini 2002, Hyland & Lewith 2002, Milgrom 2002b, Bellavite 2003, Bell et al 2004b), are those in which the interactions between the parts generate properties of the larger organisational level of scale that are not predicted by understanding the properties of the separate parts. Knowing the behaviour/properties of a liver, a heart, or a brain will never reveal what a living human being can do in terms of behaviours. That is, a person's behaviour is an emergent property of the person as a whole, indivisible system. Complex systems are self-organising; they find some optimal way of organising their parts within the environmental context (fitness landscape) in which they exist. Properties of the global system can have self-similarity at every level of scale, down to the local (parts) level.

This self-similarity concept is parallel to the clinical notion in homeopathy that deep examination of any symptom will reveal the larger disturbance in the person as a whole, for which a single remedy is indicated. As a result, given the interactions between the global and local levels of a system, investigators should be measuring both global and local outcomes, not just specific allopathic drug-relevant outcomes.

Homeopaths also use the self-organisation concept when they apply Hering's Law of Cure to evaluating the nature of patient outcomes (Vithoulkas 1980). Placebo researchers have no predictions about the patterning of shifts within the person as a whole that will occur in the course of treatment, but homeopaths do, i.e. from within outward, from above downward, and in reverse order of appearance of symptoms in time.

Hering's Law of Cure leads to a testable prediction that true homeopathic healing will follow a self-reorganising pattern of the system as a whole, which is not seen with placebo responses. No research to date has looked for such differences, but systems science would predict that Hering's Law of Cure would occur and could be documented.

Networks (e.g. the internet, social networks, etc.) are a type of complex system in which the inter-relationships and interdependencies are the focus of study (Barabasi 2003, Barabasi & Bonabeau 2003, Vasquez et al 2004). Nodes are the points of connection between the parts. Hubs are nodes that have the greatest number of inter-connections. In complementary medicine, the meridians (interconnections) and acupuncture points (hubs and nodes) in acupuncture are an example of understanding the person as an indivisible network system. However, even biochemical pathways organise into networks of relationships. Interestingly, a leading network researcher has pointed out that treatments targeting the hubs of a network should have the biggest impact on the network as a whole. Water is a major hub molecule across most biochemical reactions in the body (Barabasi & Bonabeau 2003). Therefore, network science would lead to testable prediction that modifying the body water (and human beings are made up of 70% or more water) could have system-wide effects on a person. Taken together with the concept of water clusters in the active remedies that retain the information of the source material without the persistence of its physical molecules, the network model for healing in homeopathy points to the body water as a useful starting place for research on the interface between remedies and living systems.

Furthermore, biological systems are generally non-linear, i.e. output is disproportionate to input. In homeopathy, it is obvious that a remedy is a small input whereas the clinical changes reported constitute a large output, i.e. homeopathic effects are inherently non-linear. Non-linear complex systems are also dynamical, i.e. constantly changing. This concept could help us understand the

Deepening our Approach **V**

difficulty in replicating or reproducing the findings from one study to another, as well as from one point in treatment to another. In reality, the person as a living system has moved on dynamically from the starting point at which it encountered a particular remedy and potency in the past. It is therefore not surprising that homeopaths sometimes report a minimal response or even lack of response to the same remedy at some future time when the situation seems close to the original. It is never identical to the original situation because of changes in the state of the person as a dynamical system at the time they take a dose of a remedy. The bidirectional, state-dependent nature of responses to homeopathic remedies are an example of the non-linearity (Bertani et al 1999).

The nature of systems also suggests that homeopathic researchers should be testing the capacity of the system to respond to environmental change or stress, before and after homeopathic treatment. Right now, most investigators settle for measuring static endpoints at rest (as they do in allopathic medical research) that cannot reveal if the system is more resilient when a stressor arises. Yet, clinically, such resilience is something that patients often report. To do fair tests of homeopathy, we need to design research studies that can show what clinicians and patients claim happens during homeopathic treatment. Both self-report rating scales on resilience and systematic controlled tests of psychophysiological recovery after environmental stressors in the laboratory or the field would facilitate evaluation of the resilience hypothesis.

What is the evidence for the non-linear effects of homeopathic remedies in research studies? No studies have explicitly focused on the effects of homeopathy on the dynamics of the individual. However, a relatively recent study of homeopathically-prepared dust mite administered isopathically to adult asthmatics documented relevant findings (Hyland & Lewith 2002, Lewith et al 2002). In this study, active remedy and placebo did not differ in the final values of the clinical endpoints measured. However, throughout the study, the graphs of the outcome measures followed a different pattern for the active remedy in comparison with the placebo. The remedy group fluctuated up and down on the outcomes much more than did the placebo group. Again, even if the isopathic treatment did not differ from placebo at the end, the dynamics of the process did differ. Rather than rejecting homeopathy from a negative isopathy study, perhaps the data can teach researchers more what to study and how to study it.

At a clinical level, homeopaths and patients report that effective constitutional treatment helps patients become *unstuck* from customary dysfunctional ruts or patterns in their lives (Sherr 2002, Bell 2003). This may translate fairly literally into a shift in the non-linear dynamical patterns of the person as a complex system. In systems theory, recurrent but non-identical patterns of motion organise themselves into what are termed 'attractors'. The basic trajectory appears similar during each run of the system, but the system never goes through exactly the same place during the repeated runs. When homeopathic treatment gets a person 'unstuck', it may be that the person's dynamics have shifted from a less healthy attractor pattern into a healthier one. Complex systems can also have critical points at which their dynamics make a qualitative shift into a new pattern, e.g. self-organised criticality, with a possible clinical parallel of 'never well since ... [a flu, a death in the family, an accident, etc.]'. For example, Sherr (1994, 2002) and Sankaran (2002, 2005) have both highlighted the importance of movement, change, and dynamics, i.e. the 'verb of the case' for Sherr or the non-verbal gesture for Sankaran in their respective clinical approaches to determining the correct homeopathic remedy for a patient. Non-linear dynamical analyses of both subjective and objective outcome measures on homeopathic remedies versus placebo may help clarify the relevance of systems models to understanding how remedies might act (Bell et al 2002a).

Macro-Entanglement Theory

A more radical theoretical possibility for using systems models, but also suggested by some of the data in homeopathy, is that the therapeutic process in homeopathy is non-local in nature. That is, in quantum mechanics, there is a peculiar but well-replicated finding of entanglement. Several different theoreticians have proposed that homeopathy acts via a macro-entanglement process (Milgrom 2002a,b, 2003a,b, 2004a,b,c,d, 2005, Hyland 2003, Walach 2002, Walach et al 2004, 2005). In entanglement within a closed system, change in one element is associated instantaneously with change in the other element, independent of distance or time, assuming that one element describes the global and the other element the local features of the system. Walach (2005b) notes that entanglement occurs 'between those local elements of a system that are complementary to the global description or observable of that system'.

Walach has presented some indirectly supporting evidence for a macro-entanglement model of homeopathic remedy actions in his re-analysis of data from a provings study. The usual quantitative statistical analysis of the symptom findings showed no significant difference between active remedy and placebo. However, the symptom patterns in the verum/active and placebo groups were remarkably similar. Without entanglement, Walach asserts that the placebo group should have shown random symptoms, rather than what he found – the placebo group reported the symptom patterns of the active remedy despite the double-blind protocol. Perhaps this also explains the observation that even those given placebo in proving studies generate some symptoms consistent with the proving (see Chapter 2). There are some empirical manoeuvres that might provide further indirect evidence for the macro-entanglement model (Walach 2003). In any event, this theoretical stance would help explain the discrepancy between findings from open observational studies (where entanglement is not likely operative) and closed, placebo-controlled efficacy trials (where entanglement is more likely).

Other Research Issues

Direct studies of the psychotherapeutic effects of the homeopathic interview will be important in coming years. The usual pace of homeopathic sessions is far less frequent than that of conventional psychotherapy. If the patient–provider relationship constitutes a significant aspect of the net clinical benefit seen with homeopathic treatment, then identification and systematisation of the non-remedy components of the intervention would be clinically valuable in themselves in order to facilitate development of more cost-effective delivery methods for psychotherapy. In the clinical realm, there is an obvious need for cross-cultural and health services research studies to determine the generalisability of findings between different countries. Differences in access to homeopathy as a function of health care payment systems and availability of homeopaths, as well as the lay public's familiarity with homeopathy, also merit study. This is a time for exploratory research as much as for confirmatory studies in homeopathy, as investigators begin to map the territory of science and life into which homeopathic phenomena fall.

Summary

In summary, individual differences in preferences and in capacity to respond, together with major methodological concerns about the ecological validity of many efficacy studies in homeopathy, have led to a growing challenge to the usefulness of conventionally-designed randomised controlled trials for testing homeopathy. Increasingly, homeopathic researchers are calling for:
- utilisation of qualitative research methodologies to characterise the nature of the practice and the lived experience of the patients undergoing homeopathy, as a foundation for subsequent patient-centered outcomes studies
- large scale observational studies to document the real-world outcomes of homeopathically-treated patients
- innovative study designs to accommodate the unique features of homeopathy
- applications of scientific constructs from fields outside conventional medicine, such as complex systems and network science, and even from quantum mechanics and entanglement theory.

Deepening our Approach

V

Homeopathy falls under the CAM umbrella of whole systems research, an emerging field that endeavours to go beyond reductionism to study complex packages of care without first dissecting them on the input side, and whole person-level outcomes beyond disease-specific biomarkers on the output side of the treatment process.

In the quest to convince sceptics, homeopaths have ended up accepting the randomised clinical trial efficacy study as the gold standard for their field, as it is for conventional pharmaceutical drugs. Very little research, other than new provings studies, addresses ways to optimise clinical care of homeopathic patients. However, homeopaths know that their remedies are not conventional drugs and likely do not have the same mechanisms of action as drugs. Homeopaths know that the kinds of outcomes that they see in their patients are not specific to the medicine's effects on a drug receptor subtype on a particular cell, but rather are specific to the patient, whose entire clinical picture as a pattern must match the pattern of effects previously seen in provings of the remedy on healthy people. They also know that clinical care is complex, and improving case selection and case management is an aspect of homeopathic treatment that receives relatively little attention in homeopathic education or research.

The limitations of homeopathic research to date stem, in part, from the fact that homeopathy has focused on developing clinicians rather than researchers. Furthermore, the historical political biases against homeopathy make it difficult for academically-inclined medical researchers to pursue a career in the field – both in terms of obtaining external grant funding and of advancing professionally as members of medical school faculties. Publication biases have also affected dissemination of research findings (Caulfield & DeBow 2005). However, an even more salient issue may be that the allopathic drug-based model for medical research is less relevant to homeopathy than it is to pharmaceutical agents. Homeopathy needs a strong scientific framework within which researchers can advance understanding of the field. Using qualitative methods for listening to the practitioners and the patients concerning their experiences of homeopathy and adapting the concepts and quantitative methods of non-linear dynamics rather than static variables as outcomes, are foundational first steps toward developing a true research science for homeopathy.

References

Aickin M 2004 Separation tests for early-phase CAM comparative trials. Evid Based Integ Medicine 1(4):225–231

Aickin M 2005 The end of biomedical journals: there is madness in their methods. J Alt Comp Med 11(5):755–757

Aikens J E, Bingham R, Piette J D 2005 Patient-provider communication and self-care behavior among type 2 diabetes patients. Diabetes Educ 31(5):681–690

Anelli M, Scheepers L, Sermeus G et al 2002 Homeopathy and health related quality of life: a survey in six European countries. Homeopathy 91(1):18–21

Balzarini A, Felisi E, Martini A et al 2000 Efficacy of homeopathic treatment of skin reactions during radiotherapy for breast cancer: a randomised, double-blind clinical trial. Br Homoeopath J 89(1):8–12

Barabasi A L 2003 Linked. How everything is connected to everything else and what it means for business, science, and everyday life. Plume, Cambridge, MA

Barabasi A L, Bonabeau E 2003 Scale-free networks. Sci Am 288(5):60–69

Barber B 1961 Resistance by scientists to scientific discovery. Science 134:596–602

Becker-Witt C, Weibhuhn T E R, Ludtke R, Willich S N 2003 Quality assessment of physical research in homeopathy. J Altern Complement Med 9(1): 113–132

Bell I R 2003 Evidence-based homeopathy: empirical questions and methodological considerations for homeopathic clinical research. Am J Homeopath Med 96 (1):17–31

Bell I R 2005a All evidence is equal, but some evidence is more equal than others: can logic prevail over emotion in the homeopathy debate? J Altern Complement Med 11(5):763–769

Bell I R 2005b Depression research in homeopathy: hopeless or hopeful? Homeopathy 94:141–144

Bell I R, Baldwin C M, Schwartz G E 2002a Translating a nonlinear systems theory model for homeopathy into empirical tests. Altern Ther Health Med 8(3):58–66

Bell I R, Caspi O, Schwartz G E et al 2002b Integrative medicine and systemic outcomes research: issues in the emergence of a new model for primary health care. Arch Intern Med 162(2):133–140

Bell I R, Cunningham V, Caspi O et al 2004a A new global well-being outcomes rating scale for integrative medicine research. BMC Complement Altern Med Jan 15;4:1. http://www.biomedcentral.com/1472-6882/4/1

Bell I R, Koithan M, Gorman M M, Baldwin C M 2003 Homeopathic practitioner views of changes in patients undergoing constitutional treatment for chronic disease. J Altern Complement Med 9(1):39–50

Bell I R, Lewis D A, 2nd, Lewis SE et al 2004b Strength of vital force in classical homeopathy: bio-psycho-social-spiritual correlates within a complex systems context. J Altern Complement Med 10 (1):123–131

Bell I R, Lewis D A, 2nd, Schwartz G E et al 2004c Electroencephalographic cordance patterns distinguish exceptional clinical responders with fibromyalgia to individualized homeopathic medicines. J Altern Complement Med 10 (2):285–299

Bell I R, Lewis D A I, Brooks A J et al 2004d Individual differences in response to randomly-assigned active individualized homeopathic and placebo treatment in fibromyalgia: implications of a double-blind optional crossover design. J Altern Complement Med 10(2): 269–283

Bell I R, Lewis D A I, Brooks A J et al 2004e Improved clinical status in fibromyalgia patients treated with individualized homeopathic remedies versus placebo. Rheumatology 43:577–582

Bell I R, Lewis D A I, Lewis S E et al 2004f Electroencephalographic alpha sensitization in individualized homeopathic treatment of fibromyalgia. Int J Neurosci 114(9):1195–1220

Bellavite P 2003 Complexity science and homeopathy: a synthetic overview. Homeopathy 92(4):203–212

Bellavite P, Signorini A 2002 The emerging science of homeopathy: complexity, biodynamics, and nanopharmacology, 2nd edn. North Atlantic Books, Berkeley

Belon P, Cumps J, Ennis M et al 2004 Histamine dilutions modulate basophil activation. Inflamm Res 53(5):181–188

Ben-Shlomo Y, Kuh, D 2002 A life course approach to chronic disease epidemiology: conceptual models, empirical challenges and interdisciplinary perspectives. Int J Epidemiol 31(2):285–293

Bertani S, Lussignoli S, Andrioli G et al 1999 Dual effects of a homeopathic mineral complex on carrageenan-induced oedema in rats. Br Homoeopath J 88(3):101–105

Bonne O, Shemer Y, Gorali Y et al 2003 A randomized, double-blind, placebo-controlled study of classical homeopathy in generalized anxiety disorder. J Clin Psychiatry 64 (3):282–287

Boscarino J A 1997 Diseases among men 20 years after exposure to severe stress: implications for clinical research and medical care. Psychosom Med 59:605–614

Brizzi M, Nani D, Peruzzi M et al 2000 Statistical analysis of the effect of high dilutions of arsenic in a large dataset from a wheat germination model. Br Homoeopath J 89(2):63–67

Cavalcanti A M, Rocha L M, Carillo R J et al 2003 Effects of homeopathic treatment on pruritus of haemodialysis patients: a randomised placebo-controlled double-blind trial. Homeopathy 92(4):177–181

Caspi O, Koithan M, Criddle M W 2004 Alternative medicine or 'alternative' patients: a qualitative study of patient-oriented decision-making processes with respect to complementary and alternative medicine. Med Decis Making 24(1):64–79

Caulfield T, DeBow S 2005 A systematic review of how homeopathy is represented in conventional and CAM peer reviewed journals. BMC Complement Altern Med 5(1):12

Chapman E H, Weintraub R J, Milburn M A et al 1999. Homeopathic treatment of mild traumatic brain injury: A randomized, double-blind, placebo-controlled clinical trial. J Head Trauma Rehabil 14(6):521–542

Concato J 2004 Observational versus experimental studies: what's the evidence for a hierarchy? NeuroRx 1(3):341–347

Concato J, Horwitz I 2004 Beyond randomised versus observational studies. Lancet 363 (9422):1660–1661

Deepening our Approach

V

Concato J, Shah N, Horwitz R I 2000 Randomized, controlled trials, observational studies, and the hierarchy of research designs. N Engl J Med 342(25):1887–1892

Connor K M, Davidson J R 2003 Development of a new resilience scale: the Conno-Davidson Resilience Scale (CD-RISC). Depression & Anxiety 18(2):76–82

Cucherat M, Haugh M C, Gooch M et al 2000 Evidence of clinical efficacy of homeopathy. A meta-analysis of clinical trials. HMRAG. Homeopathic Medicines Research Advisory Group. Eur J Clin Pharmacol 56(1):27–33

Dantas F, Rampes H 2000 Do homeopathic medicines provoke adverse effects? A systematic review. Br Homoeopath J 89(Suppl 1):S35–38

Datta S, Mallick P, Bukhsh A R 1999 Efficacy of a potentized homoeopathic drug (Arsenicum Album-30) in reducing genotoxic effects produced by arsenic trioxide in mice: II. Comparative efficacy of an antibiotic, actinomycin D alone and in combination with either of two microdoses. Complement Ther Med 7(3):156–163

Davidson R J, Schwartz G E, Rothman L P 1976 Attentional style and the self-regulation of mode-specific attention: an electroencephalograhic study. J Abnorm Psychol 85(6):611–621

Del Giudice E, Doglia S, Milani M, Vitiello G 1988 Structures, correlations, and electromagnetic interactions in living matter: theory and applications. In: Frohlich H (ed) Biological coherence and response to external stimuli. Springer-Verlag, Berlin

Denzin N K, Lincoln Y S (eds) 2000 Handbook of qualitative research, 2nd edn. Sage, Thousand Oaks, CA

Elia V, Niccoli M 1999 Thermodynamics of extremely diluted aqueous solutions. Ann NY Acad Sci 879:241–248

Elia V, Niccoli, M 2004 New physico-chemical properties of extremely diluted aqueous solutions. J Therm Analysis Calorim 75:815–836.

Endler P C, Schulte J (eds) 1994 Ultra high dilution: physiology and physics. Kluwer Academic Publishers, Dordrecht, The Netherlands

Ernst E 2002 A systematic review of systematic reviews of homeopathy. Br J Clin Pharmacol 54(6):577–582

Felitti V J, Anda R F, Nordenberg D et al 1998 Relationship of childhood abuse and household dysfunction to many of the leading causes of death in adults. The adverse childhood experiences (ACE) study [comment]. Am J Prev Med 14(4):245–258

Fisher P, Greenwood A, Huskisson E C, Turner P, Belon P 1989 Effect of homeopathic treatment on fibrositis (primary fibromyalgia). Br Med J 299:365–366

Fisher P, Scott D L 2001 A randomized controlled trial of homeopathy in rheumatoid arthritis. Rheumatol 2001;40(9):1052–1055

Frass M, Linkesch M, Banyai S et al 2005 Adjunctive homeopathic treatment in patients with severe sepsis: a randomized, double-blind, placebo-controlled trial in an intensive care unit. Homeopathy: the Journal of the Faculty of Homeopathy 94(2):75–80

Freeman A C, Sweeney K 2001 Why general practitioners do not implement evidence: qualitative study. Br Med J 323(7321):1100–1102

Frei H, Everts R, von Ammon K et al 2005 Homeopathic treatment of children with attention deficit hyperactivity disorder: a randomised, double blind, placebo controlled crossover trial. Eur J Pediatr 164(12):758–767.

Frei H, Thurneysen A 2001 Treatment for hyperactive children: homeopathy and methylphenidate compared in a family setting. Br Homoeopath J 90(4):183–188

Frenkel M, Hermoni D 2002 Effects of homeopathic intervention on medication consumption in atopic and allergic disorders. Altern Ther Health Med 8(1):76–79

Gibson R G, Gibson S L, MacNeill A D et al 1980 Homoeopathic therapy in rheumatoid arthritis: evaluation by double-blind clinical therapeutic trial. Br J Clin Pharmacol 9(5):453–459

Goldstein M S, Glik D 1998 Use of and satisfaction with homeopathy in a patient population. Altern Ther Health Med 4(2):60–65

Gould A, MacPherson H 2001 Patient perspectives on outcomes after treatment with acupuncture. J Altern Complement Med 7:261–268

Haley R W, Billecke S, La Du B N 1999 Association of low PON1 type Q (type A) arylesterase activity with neurologic symptom complexes in Gulf War veterans. Toxicol Appl Pharmacol 157(3):227–233

Harrison H, Fixsen A, Vickers A 1999 A randomized comparison of homoeopathic and standard care for the treatment of glue ear in children. Complement Ther Med 7(3):132–135

Hart O, Mullee M A, Lewith G et al 1997 Double-blind, placebo-controlled, randomized clinical trial of homoeopathic arnica C30 for pain and infection after total abdominal hysterectomy. J Royal Soc Med 90 (2):73–78

Hirsh A T, Atchison J W, Berger J J et al 2005 Patient satisfaction with treatment for chronic pain: predictors and relationship to compliance. Clin J Pain 21(4): 302–310

Honda K, Jacobson JS 2005 Use of complementary and alternative medicine among United States adults: the influences of personality, coping strategies, and social support. Prev Med 40(1):46–53

Hyland M 2003 Extended network generalized entanglement theory: therapeutic mechanisms, empirical predictions, and investigations. J Altern Complement Med 9(6):919–936

Hyland M E, Lewith G T 2002 Oscillatory effects in a homeopathic clinical trial: an explanation using complexity theory, and implications for clinical practice. Homeopathy 91(3):145–149

Idler E, Benyamini, Y 1997 Self-rated health and mortality: a review of twenty-seven community studies. J Health Soc Behav 38:21–36

Jacobs J, Herman P, Heron K et al 2005 Homeopathy for menopausal symptoms in breast cancer survivors: a preliminary randomized controlled trial. J Altern Complement Med 11(1):21–27

Jacobs J, Chapman E H, Crothers D 1998 Patient characteristics and practice patterns of physicians using homeopathy. Arch Fam Med 7(6):537–540

Jacobs J, Jimenez L M, Gloyd S S et al 1994 Treatment of acute childhood diarrhea with homeopathic medicine: a randomized clinical trial in Nicaragua. Pediatrics 93(5):719–725

Jacobs J, Jimenez L M, Malthouse S et al 2000 Homeopathic treatment of acute childhood diarrhea: results from a clinical trial in Nepal. J Altern Complement Med 6(2):131–139

Jacobs J, Jonas W B, Jimenez P M et al 2003 Homeopathy for childhood diarrhoea: combined results and metaanalysis from three randomized, controlled clinical trials. Pediatr Infect Dis J 22(3):229–234

Jacobs J, Williams A L, Girard C et al 2005 Homeopathy for attention-deficit/hyperactivity disorder: a pilot randomized controlled trial. J Altern Complement Med 11(5):799–806

Jonas W B 2001 The evidence house: how to build an inclusive base for complementary medicine. West J Med 175(2):79–80

Jonas W B 2005 Building an evidence house: challenges and solutions to research in complementary and alternative medicine. Forsch Komplementarmed Klass Naturheilkd 12:159–167

Jonas W, Lin Y, Tortella F 2001 Neuroprotection from glutamate toxicity with ultra-low dose glutamate. Neuroreport 12(2):335–339

Kainz J T, Kozel G, Haidvogl M et al 1996 Homoeopathic versus placebo therapy of children with warts on the hands: a randomized, double-blind clinical trial.[comment]. Dermatol 193(4): 318–320

Kane R L 1997 Understanding health care outcomes research. Aspen, Gaithersburg, MD

Katz T, Fisher P, Katz A et al 2005 The feasibility of a randomised, placebo-controlled clinical trial of homeopathic treatment of depression in general practice. Homeopathy 94(3):145–152

Kim L S, Riedlinger J E, Baldwin C M et al 2005 Treatment of seasonal allergic rhinitis using homeopathic preparation of common allergens in the southwest region of the US: a randomized, controlled clinical trial. Ann Pharmacother 39(4):617–624

Kirsch I S A 2001 Apples, oranges, and placebos: heterogeneity in a meta-analysis of placebo effects. Adv Mind Body Med 17(4):307–309

Kleijnen J, Knipschild P, ter Riet G 1991 Clinical trials of homoeopathy. Br Med J 302(6772):316–323

Kundu S N, Mitra K, Khuda Bukhsh A R 2000 Efficacy of a potentized homeopathic drug (Arsenicum-Aalbum-30) in reducing cytotoxic effects produced by arsenic trioxide in mice: IV. Pathological changes, protein profiles, and content of DNA and RNA. Complement Ther Med 8(3):157–165

La Du B N, Billecke S, Hsu C et al 2001 Serum paraoxonase (PON1) isozymes: the quantitative analysis of isozymes affecting individual sensitivity to environmental chemicals. Drug Metab Dispos 29(4 Pt 2): 566–569

Lamont J 1997 Homeopathic treatment of attention deficit hyperactivity disorder. A controlled study. Br Homoeopath J 86:196–200

Deepening our Approach

V

Lancet 2005 The end of homeopathy. Lancet 366:690

Levin J S, Glass T A, Kushi L H et al 1997 Quantitative methods in research on complementary and alternative medicine. A methodological manifesto. NIH Office of Alternative Medicine. Med Care 35(11):1079–1094

Lewith G T, Watkins A D, Hyland M E et al 2002 Use of ultramolecular potencies of allergen to treat asthmatic people allergic to house dust mite: double blind randomised controlled clinical trial. Br Med J 324(7336):520.

Lincoln Y S, Guba E G 1985 Naturalistic inquiry. Sage, Beverly Hills, CA

Linde K, Clausius, N, Ramirez, G et al 1997 Are the clinical effects of homeopathy placebo effects? A meta-analysis of placebo-controlled trials. Lancet 350:834–843

Linde K, Jonas W B, Melchart D, Worku F, Wagner H, Eitel F 1994 Critical review and meta-analysis of serial agitated dilutions in experimental toxicology. Hum Exp Toxicol 13:481–492

Linde K, Scholz M, Ramirez G et al 1999 Impact of study quality on outcome in placebo-controlled trials of homeopathy [comment]. J Clin Epidemiol 52(7): 631–636

MacPherson H, Mercer S W, Scullion T, Thomas K J 2003 Empathy, enablement, and outcome: an exploratory study on acupuncture patients' perceptions. J Altern Complement Med 9(6):869–876

Mallick P, Chakrabarti M J, Guha B et al 2003 Ameliorating effect of microdoses of a potentized homeopathic drug, Arsenicum Album, on arsenic-induced toxicity in mice. BMC Complement Altern Med Oct 22;3:7 (http://www.biomedcentral.com/1472-6882/3/7)

Mathie R T 2003 The research evidence base for homeopathy: a fresh assessment of the literature. Homeopathy 92:84–91

Menec V H, Chipperfield J G, Perry R P 1999 Self-perceptions of health: a prospective analysis of mortality, control, and health. J Gerontol (Ser B) 54(2):85–93

Mercer S W, Reilly D, Watt G C 2002 The importance of empathy in the enablement of patients attending the Glasgow Homoeopathic Hospital. Br J Gen Pract 52(484):901–905

Milgrom L R 2002a Patient-practitioner-remedy (PPR) entanglement. Part 1: a qualitative, non-local metaphor for homeopathy based on quantum theory. [see comment]. Homeopathy 91(4):239–248

Milgrom L R 2002b Vitalism, complexity, and the concept of spin. Homeopathy 91(1):26–31

Milgrom L R 2003a Patient-practitioner-remedy (PPR) entanglement. Part 2: Extending the metaphor for homeopathy using molecular quantum theory. Homeopathy 92(1):35–43

Milgrom L R 2003b Patient-practitioner-remedy (PPR) entanglement. Part 3. Refining the quantum metaphor for homeopathy. Homeopathy 92(3):152–160

Milgrom L R 2004a Patient-practitioner-remedy (PPR) entanglement. Part 4. Toward classification and unification of the different entanglement models for homeopathy. Homeopathy 93(1):34–42

Milgrom L R 2004b Patient-practitioner-remedy (PPR) entanglement. Part 5. Can homeopathic remedy reactions be outcomes of PPR entanglement? Homeopathy 93(2):94–98

Milgrom L R 2004c Patient-practitioner-remedy (PPR) entanglement. Part 6. Miasms revisited: non-linear quantum theory as a model for the homeopathic process [see comment]. Homeopathy 93(3):154–158

Milgrom L R 2004d Patient-practitioner-remedy (PPR) entanglement. Part 7. A gyroscopic metaphor for the vital force and its use to illustrate some of the empirical laws of homeopathy. Forsch Komplementarmed Klass Naturheilkd 11(4):212–223

Milgrom L R 2005 Patient-practitioner-remedy (PPR) entanglement. Part 8. 'Laser-like' action of the homeopathic therapeutic encounter as predicted by a gyroscopic metaphor for the vital force. Forsch Komplementarmed Klass Naturheilkd 12(4):206–213

Mitra K, Kundu S N, Khuda Bukhsh A R 1999 Efficacy of a potentized homoeopathic drug (Arsenicum Album-30) in reducing toxic effects produced by arsenic trioxide in mice: II. On alterations in body weight, tissue weight and total protein. Complement Therap Med 7(1):24–34

Neff D F, Blanchard E B, Andrasik F 1983 The relationship between capacity for absorption and chronic headache patients' response to relaxation and biofeedback treatment. Biofeedback Self Regul 8:177–183

Oberbaum M, Yaniv I, Ben-Gal Y et al 2001 A randomized, controlled clinical trial of the homeopathic medication TRAUMEEL S in the treatment of chemotherapy-induced stomatitis in children undergoing stem cell transplantation. Cancer 92(3):684–690

Oberbaum M, Singer S R, Vithoulkas G 2005 The colour of the homeopathic improvement: the multidimensional nature of the response to homeopathic therapy. Homeopathy 94(3):196–199

Owens J E, Taylor A G, Degood D 1999 Complementary and alternative medicine and psychologic factors: toward an individual differences model of complementary and alternative medicine use and outcomes. J Altern Complement Med 5(6):529–541

Paterson C 1996 Measuring outcome in primary care: a patient-generated measure, MYMOP, compared to the SF-36 health survey. Br Med J 312:1016–1020

Paterson C, Britten N 2003 Acupuncture for people with chronic illness: combining qualitative and quantitative outcome assessment. J Altern Complement Med 9(5):671–681

Patrick D L, Danis M, Southerland L I, Hong G 1988 Quality of life following intensive care. J Gen Intern Med 3:218–223

Phan K L, Taylor S F, Welsh R C et al 2003 Activation of the medial prefrontal cortex and extended amygdala by individual ratings of emotional arousal: a fMRI study. Biol Psychiatry 53(3):211–215

Pilkington K, Kirkwood G, Rampes H et al 2005 Homeopathy for depression: a systematic review of the research evidence. Homeopathy 94(3):153–163

Pope C, Mays N (eds) 2000 Qualitative research in health care. BMJ Books, London

Ramelet A A, Buchheim G, Lorenz P et al 2000 Homeopathic Arnica in postoperative haematomas: a double-blind study. Dermatol 201(4):347–348

Rastogi D P, Singh V P, Singh V et al 1999 Homeopathy in HIV infection: a trial report of double-blind placebo controlled study. Br Homoeopath J 88(2):49–57

Reilly D 1997 The evidence profile for homeopathy – creating the verification mosaic. Proceedings of an International Conference on Homeopathy: Improving the success of homeopathy: taking the homeopathic knowledge base into the 21st century. pp. 63–70

Reilly D, Taylor M A, Beattie N G et al 1994 Is evidence for homoeopathy reproducible? [see comments]. Lancet 344(8937):1601–1606

Reilly D T, Taylor M A, McSharry C et al 1986 Is homoeopathy a placebo response? Controlled trial of homoeopathic potency, with pollen in hayfever as model. Lancet 2(8512):881–886

Relton C, Weatherley-Jones E 2005 Homeopathy service in a National Health Service community menopause clinic: audit of clinical outcomes. J Br Menopause Soc 11(2):72–73

Rey L 2003 Thermoluminescence of ultra-high dilutions of lithium chloride and sodium chloride. Physica A 323:67–74

Riley D, Fischer M, Singh B et al 2001 Homeopathy and conventional medicine: an outcomes study comparing effectiveness in a primary care setting. J Altern Complement Med 7(2):149–59

Ritenbaugh C, Verhoef M, Fleishman S et al 2003 Whole systems research: a discipline for studying complementary and alternative medicine. Altern Ther Health Med 9(4):32–36

Rowe T 1998 Homeopathic methodology: repertory, case taking, and case analysis. North Atlantic Books, Berkeley

Roy R, Tiller W, Bell I R, Hoover M R 2005 The structure of liquid water: novel insights from materials research and potential relevance to homeopathy. Materials Research Innovation 2005; in press.

Rubik B 2002 The biofield hypothesis: its biophysical basis and role in medicine. J Altern Complement Med 8(6):703–717

Ruiz G, Torres J L 1997 Homeopathic effect on the sleep pattern of rats. Br Homoeopath J 86:201–206

Ruiz-Vega G, Perez-Ordaz L, Proa-Flores P et al 2000 An evaluation of Coffea cruda effect on rats. Br Homoeopath J 89(3):122–126

Ruiz-Vega G, Perez-Ordaz L, Leon-Hueramo O, Cruz-Vazquez E, Sanchez-Diaz N 2002 Comparative effect of Coffea cruda potencies on rats. Homeopathy 91:80–84

Russek L G, Schwartz G E 1997 Perceptions of parental caring predict health status in midlife: a 35-year follow-up of the Harvard Mastery of Stress Study. Psychosom Med 59(2):144–149

Russek L G, Schwartz G E, Bell IR et al 1998 Positive perceptions of parental caring are associated with reduced psychiatric and somatic symptoms. Psychosom Med 60(5):654–657

Deepening our Approach

V

Sankaran R 2002 An insight into plants. Volumes I and II. Homoeopathic Medical Publishers, Mumbai

Sankaran R 2003 Sankaran's schema. Homoeopathic Medical Publishers, Mumbai

Sankaran R 2005 The sensations of homeopathy. Homoeopathic Medical Publishers, Mumbai

Scholten J 1996 Homeopathy and the elements. Stichting, Utrecht

Schulman D 2004 The unexpected outcomes of acupuncture: case reports in support of refocusing research designs. J Altern Complement Med 10(5):785–789

Schulte J, Endler P C (eds) 1998 Fundamental research in ultra high dilution and homoeopathy. Kluwer Academic Publishers, Dordrecht

Sevar R 2005 Audit of outcome in 455 consecutive patients treated with homeopathic medicines. Homeopathy 94:215–221

Shang A, Huwiler-Muntener K, Nartey L et al 2005 Are the clinical effects of homoeopathy placebo effects? Comparative study of placebo-controlled trials of homoeopathy and allopathy. Lancet 366(9487):726–732

Sherr J 1994 The dynamics and methodology of homeopathic provings, 2nd edn. Dynamis Books, Great Malvern, UK

Sherr J 2002 Dynamic materia medica. Syphilis: a study of syphilitic miasm through remedies. Dynamis Books, Great Malvern, UK

Shipley M, Berry H, Broster G et al 1983 Controlled trial of homoeopathic treatment of osteoarthritis. Lancet 1(8316):97–98

Spence D, Thompson E A, Barron S J 2005 Homeopathic treatment for chronic disease: a 6-year university-hospital outpatient observational study. J Altern Complement Med 11(5):793–798

Stevinson C, Devaraj V S, Fountain-Barber A, Hawkins S, Ernst E 2003 Homeopathic arnica for prevention of pain and bruising: randomized placebo-controlled trial in hand surgery. J Royal Soc Med 96:60–65

Straumsheim P, Borchgrevink C, Mowinckel P et al 2000 Homeopathic treatment of migraine: a double blind, placebo controlled trial of 68 patients [see comment]. Br Homoeopath J 89(1):4–7

Sukul A, Sinhabau S P, Sukul N C 1999 Reduction of alcohol induced sleep time in albino mice by potentized Nux vomica prepared with 90% ethanol. Br Homoeopath J 88(2):58–61

Sukul N C, Bala S K, Bhattacharyya B 1986 Prolonged cataleptogenic effects of potentized homoeopathic drugs. Psychopharmacology 89:338–339

Sukul N C, Ghosh S, Sinhababu S P et al 2001 Strychnos nux-vomica extract and its ultra-high dilution reduce voluntary ethanol intake in rats. J Altern Complement Med 7(2):187–193

Surtees P, Wainwright N, Day N et al 2003 Adverse experience in childhood as a developmental risk factor for altered immune status in adulthood. Int J Behav Med 10(3):251–268

Szeto A L, Rollwagen F, Jonas W B 2004 Rapid induction of protective tolerance to potential terrorist agents: a systematic review of low- and ultra-low dose research. [Review] [19 refs]. Homeopathy 93(4):173–178

Taylor M A, Reilly D, Llewellyn-Jones R H et al 2000 Randomised controlled trial of homoeopathy versus placebo in perennial allergic rhinitis with overview of four trial series. BMJ 321(7259):471–476

Tellegen A, Lykken D T, Bouchard T J et al 1988 Personality similarity in twins reared apart and together. J Pers Soc Psychol 54(6):1031–1039

Tesch R 1992 Qualitative research: analysis types and software tools. The Falmer Press, New York

Thompson E A, Oxon B A, Montgomery A, Douglas D, Reilly D 2005 A pilot, randomized, double-blinded, placebo-controlled trial of individualized homeopathy for symptoms of estrogen withdrawal in breast-cancer survivors. J Altern Complement Med 11(1):13–20

Thompson E A, Reilly D 2002 The homeopathic approach to symptom control in the cancer patient: a prospective observational study. Palliat Med 16(3):227–233

Thompson T D 2004 Can the caged bird sing? Reflections on the application of qualitative research methods to case study design in homeopathic medicine. BMC Med Res Methodol 9;4:4 (http://www.biomed-central.com/content/pdf/1471-2288-4-4.pdf)

Turk DC 2005 The potential of treatment matching for subgroups of patients with chronic pain: lumping versus splitting. [Review] [74 refs]. Clin J Pain 21 (1):44–55

van Haselen R 2000 The economic evaluation of complementary medicine: a staged approach at the Royal

Deepening our Approach

V

London Homoeopathic Hospital. Br Homoeopath J 89(Suppl 1):S23–26

van Haselen R A, Fisher P A 2000 A randomized controlled trial comparing topical piroxieam gel with a homeopathic gel in osteoarthritis of the knee. Rheumatol 39(7):714–719

van Wassenhoven M, Ives G 2004 An observational study of patients receiving homeopathic treatment. Homeopathy 93(1):3–11

Various 2005 The homeopathy debate. J Altern Complement Med 11(5):779–785

Vasquez A, Dobrin R, Sergi D et al 2004 The topological relationship between the large-scale attributes and local interaction patterns of complex networks. Proc Natl Acad Sci USA 101(52):17940–17945.

Verhoef M, Lewith G, Ritenbaugh C et al 2004 Whole systems research: moving forward. Focus Altern Complement Ther 9 (2):87–90

Verhoef M J, Casebeer A L, Hilsden R J 2002 Assessing efficacy of complementary medicine: adding qualitative research methods to the 'Gold Standard'. J Altern Complement Med 8(3):275–281

Verhoef M J, Lewith G, Ritenbaugh C, Boon H, Fleishman S, Leis A 2005 Complementary and alternative medicine whole systems research: beyond identification of inadequacies of the RCT. Complement Ther Med 13(3):206–212

Vickers A J, Fisher P, Smith C et al 1997 Homoeopathy for delayed onset muscle soreness: a randomised double blind placebo controlled trial. Br J Sports Med 31 (4):304–307

Vickers A J, Fisher P, Smith C et al 1998 Homeopathic Arnica 30x is ineffective for muscle soreness after long-distance running: a randomized, double-blind, placebo-controlled trial. Clin J Pain 14(3):227–231

Vickers A J, Smith C 2004 Homoeopathic Oscillo-coccinum for preventing and treating influenza and influenza-like syndromes. Cochrane 1:CD001957.

Vithoulkas G 1980 The science of homeopathy. Grove Weidenfeld, New York

Walach H 2000 Magic of signs: a non-local interpretation of homeopathy. Br Homoeopath J 89(3):127–140

Walach H 2001 The efficacy paradox in randomized controlled trials of CAM and elsewhere: beware of the placebo trap. J Altern Complement Med 7(3):213–218

Walach H 2002 What happens in homeopathic remedy provings? Results from a double-blind crossover study of belladonna 30CH and an analysis by grade of membership (GoM). In: Chez R A (ed) Future directions and current issues of research in homeopathy. Samueli Institute, Freiburg, p110–133

Walach H 2003 Entanglement model of homeopathy as an example of generalised entanglement predicted by weak quantum theory. Forsch Komplementarmed Klass Naturheilkd 10(4):192–200

Walach H 2005a Entangled – and tied in knots! Practical consequences of an entanglement model for homeopathic research and practice. [Review] [20 refs]. Homeopathy 94(2):96–99

Walach H 2005b Generalized entanglement: a new theoretical model for understanding the effects of complementary and alternative medicine. J Altern Complement Med 11(3):549–559

Walach H, Jonas W B 2002 Homeopathy. In: Lewith G, Jonas W B, Walach H (eds) Clinical research in complementary therapies. Churchill Livingstone, Edinburgh, p 229–246

Walach H, Haeusler W, Lowes T et al 1997 Classical homeopathic treatment of chronic headaches. Cephalalgia 17(2):119–126; discussion 01

Walach H, Jonas W B, Ives J, Van Wijk R, Weingartner O 2005 Research on homeopathy: state of the art. J Altern Complement Med 11(5):813–829

Walach H, Lowes T, Mussbach D et al 2000 The long-term effects of homeopathic treatment of chronic headaches: 1 year follow up. Cephalalgia 20(9):835–837

Walach H, Sherr J, Schneider R et al 2004 Homeopathic proving symptoms: result of a local, non-local, or placebo process? A blinded, placebo-controlled pilot study [see comment]. Homeopathy 93(4):179–185

Watterson J G 1991 The interaction of water and proteins in cellular function. Prog Mol Subcell Biol 12:113–134

Watterson J G 1996 Water clusters: pixels of life. In: Hameroff S R, Kaszniak A W, Scott A C (eds) Toward a science of consciousness. The First Tucson Discussions and Debates. MIT Press, Cambridge, MA, p 397–405

Watterson J G 1997 The pressure pixel – unit of life? Biosystems 41(3):141–152

Weatherley-Jones E, Nicholl J P, Thomas K J et al 2004 A randomised, controlled triple-blind trial of the

Deepening our Approach

V

efficacy of homeopathic treatment for chronic fatigue syndrome. J Psychosomat Res 56:189–197

Weiser M, Strosser W, Klein P 1998 Homeopathic vs conventional treatment of vertigo: a randomized double-blind controlled clinical study. Arch Otolaryngol Head Neck Surg 124(8):879–885

White A, Slade P, Hunt C et al 2003 Individualised homeopathy as an adjunct in the treatment of childhood asthma: a randomised placebo controlled trial. Thorax 58(4):317–321

Witt C, Keil T, Selim D et al 2005a Outcome and costs of homoeopathic and conventional treatment strategies: a comparative cohort study in patients with chronic disorders. Complement Ther Med 13(2):79–86

Witt C M, Luedtke R, Baur R, Willich S N 2005b Homeopathic medical practice: long-term results of a cohort study with 3981 patients. BMC Public Health Nov 3;5:115

Wolfe F 1999 Critical issues in longitudinal and observational studies: purpose, short versus long term, selection of study instruments, methods, outcomes, and biases. J Rheumatol 26(2):469–472.

Yakir M, Kreitler S, Brzezinski A et al 2001 Effects of homeopathic treatment in women with premenstrual syndrome: a pilot study.[see comment]. Br Homoeopath J 90(3):148–153

CHAPTER TWENTY FIVE

The Therapeutic Encounter and Supervisory Relationship

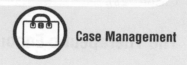 Case Management

David Owen

Introduction

The homeopathic relationship is built up through many layers of communication between patient and homeopath (see Chapters 3, 8, 13). This relationship is in its own way therapeutic and is an integral part of the homeopathic process (see Chapter 23). Being clear and making explicit the therapeutic agreement is a vital part not just of developing and deepening this relationship but also of using this relationship to help the patient. This agreement or 'contract' includes how information from the case is used, the boundaries of the relationship, what is expected or provided by each party, and at what points the treatment is to be reviewed and ended. These are essential components of a reliable and beneficial therapeutic encounter. The therapeutic encounter fundamentally alters not just what is perceived homeopathically but provides non-remedy specific effects (including placebo effects) with the potential to summate or deplete the specific treatment effects.

Recognising the importance of, and at times difficulties in, the therapeutic relationship and encounter raise important questions for the practising homeopath, such as:

- How to both invite and yet be protected from patient's projections?
- How to enable patients to reveal their inner nature without pushing too hard or inappropriately?
- What support (personal, practice and professional) is required?

- How does the homeopath establish and obtain this support?
- How do you develop the practical experience and competence to work with increasingly complex, confused and hidden cases?
- How do you work with the subtle patterns (themes) and projections (onto and by you) that are an important part of managing the patient and yourself?

These are challenges facing many of the healing professions and homeopaths are no exception. To work with projection in an effective and sustainable way you need to pay attention not just to the application of the homeopathic process but also to your own state. It requires the ability to observe the homeopathic relationship clearly – to use 'super...vision'. At different times you may need additional support, training, resources and opportunity to reflect. Supervision is one way of providing these reference points to the homeopath. It is well developed in the psychological and social work professions and we in the homeopathic profession can learn much from their models and experiences of supervision. These include sharing and exploring cases with colleagues (peer supervision), with a more experienced prescriber (facilitated supervision), or alone through reflection (self supervision). Not only do these processes enable the patient's treatment to be reflected on carefully, but also the very issues that are confusing or hidden are frequently mirrored onto and can then be explored in the supervision process, through what is known as 'parallel process' (see Chapter 28).

The Therapeutic Encounter

Balancing the process of the consultation and the task of finding a remedy is the art of the therapeutic relationship. Rapport, empathy and the therapeutic agreement are informed by qualities of authenticity, honesty and compassion. These in turn are informed by non-judgemental acceptance and unconditional positive regard of the patient (Rogers 1971, Kaplan 2001).

The consultation can be thought of as moving through several stages (Box 25.1) where each connects to the next, and the whole process may be repeated several times. In practice these are not separate or sequential steps but part of a flowing and evolving process. Establishing rapport and empathy enables the patient – it includes agreeing on the aims of treatment and our various roles as a homeopath. Care, compassion and establishing consent lead to greater revelation and focusing the case. When received in a non-judgemental way it allows greater honesty and a sense of what is truly important to the patient to surface. This is reinforced and made safer by naming and clarifying what is and what is not expected to happen – what we might call the boundaries. As this happens, what at first appears as a case made up of disparate pieces of information starts to converge; over the consultation, or several consultations, a

congruent whole emerges. When this happens you start to gather a clear sense of what is happening in the case and hopefully start to see a single coherent wholeness to the case. Reaching this point allows you to encounter the patient in a way that will both facilitate the matching of a deep-acting remedy and offer the opportunity to reflect this 'wholeness' back to the patient.

What you, as a homeopath, set out to achieve will be influenced by the models of health through which you predominately see a case. It may not be the same in each case or for each homeopath. How we work will be determined by the implicit and explicit therapeutic agreement. Our ability to form and develop an agreement with the patient on why we are there and what we are doing will determine how we practice. The roles we play may include witness, confidante, remedy seeker, carer, healer, physician, etc. – each will influence how the consultation and therapeutic relationship unfolds. Even in our role to find the simillimum there will be sub-roles determined by the approach to treatment and methodologies we are working with. It is important not just to be competent in a number of roles but to be able to articulate them, negotiate, and agree what most appropriately meets a patient's needs – which is not always the same as what the patient at first wants!

Rapport, Empathy and Enablement

The homeopath's ability to empathise with the patient is a major factor in establishing rapport. This stems from a synchronous trust and confidence between the homeopath and patient – lack of trust, fear of failure, disapproval or judgment undermine this confidence. Typically the patient may feel at risk if they perceive that you are not sincere and professional, and you may be defensive if there is an unfair risk of criticism, litigation or being taken advantage of.

Rapport is the 'coming alongside' of the patient and homeopath, accompanied by awareness and shared understanding of each other and of what each can expect from the other. If rapport is coming alongside, then 'enablement' is the extent that the patient is able to move together with

---

BOX 25.1

Stages of the Therapeutic Relationship

1. Rapport, empathy and enablement
2. Therapeutic agreement and contracting
3. Care, compassion and consent
4. Deepening the case
5. Non-judgemental acceptance
6. Authenticity, honesty and boundaries
7. Congruence
8. Reflecting back to the patient and selecting a remedy

Deepening our approach

the practitioner in a therapeutic direction, and is a significant factor in having a positive outcome of treatment (Mercer et al 2001, 2002). Rapport, empathy and enablement (see also Chapter 28) in a homeopathic consultation require realistic levels of confidence in each other. This balance is easier to achieve if the homeopath and patient both feel they have adequate time, agreement on what they are doing, and realistic expectations.

The Therapeutic Agreement

At some point in the consultation the patient has to revisit the past and glimpse the future, entertaining both the reality of being ill and the possibility of being well.

The therapeutic agreement between patient and homeopath provides the 'ground rules' about the consultation and treatment process. It may develop gradually and informally at the beginning of a consultation and becomes more detailed and formal as the consultation progresses. It may be referred to as the therapeutic contract and includes information about the practice and procedures followed. Practitioners vary in how much are unspoken assumptions and how much are recorded; often it is a verbal agreement, although aspects may be written in practice information or recorded in the notes.

As the consultation progresses the agreement may include a discussion about the different approaches to treatment possible and the likely outcomes, including the need for follow-up. It will address things like the patient who wants a cure without addressing the cause and what the homeopath feels unable to provide, e.g. an obese patient might want to lose weight without wanting to make any change to their diet but needing some specific nutritional advice. The contract may also address issues about compliance, what to do if there is a reaction to treatment or treatment is discontinued, and when and how the patient should contact the homeopath if an urgent problem arises. There is no harm in patients being sceptical about what homeopathic treatment might offer, but where this exists it is tremendously helpful for it to be made explicit, so that appropriate discussion and explanation can be offered. It is failure to establish a clear agreement that is the cause of most dissatisfaction for patients and homeopaths.

The checklist in Box 25.2 shows some of the factors to consider when developing a dynamic and evolving therapeutic agreement. Some of these are more straightforward than others and some patients and homeopaths will find it more important to agree certain points than others. Even in a simple case, if the task, expectation and process are clear, treatment is easier. In more complex cases, an established contract makes it easier to focus the consultation and, if necessary, to explicitly modify or alter it at a later date. Exploring the agreement may reveal aspects of the case that are not otherwise offered in the consultation. It can help to reflect on what the patient is frightened or wary of contracting for, and what the patient imagines might happen but will not ask the homeopath about.

It may help to consider separately those parts of the agreement that cover issues like confidentiality, cost of treatment, the number and duration of consultations and interval between them, communication with third parties, and what happens if things go wrong or if the expectations of either party aren't met. Having a formal complaints procedure for patients to follow is an important way of ensuring the patient is 'heard' – and you and your practice learn from any mistakes.

Getting the Agreement Right

It is not uncommon for someone to arrange an appointment for someone else – maybe for a child, for a husband, wife or partner, or for an animal in a veterinary practice. In these cases it is important to be clear about what contract you have with whom. In some consultations there can be more than one contract at play – conflicts will arise when these two contracts give rise to different expectations, as Jonathan's case illustrates. It is important that whether and how other people are influenced by or influence the treatment is clarified in the consultation. These others may be employers, family or friends, and may be actively involved or not.

Deepening our approach

V

BOX 25.2
Some Factors to Consider When Developing a Dynamic and Evolving Therapeutic Agreement

About the Consultation

- Availability of appointment – how patients can go about making an appointment and changing it
- Time keeping, arriving and ending on time
- Confidentiality
- Duration of consultation and duration of treatment
- Regularity of appointments
- What does the history entail, what areas are you going to talk about?
- Will you see a patient alone or with a partner, a parent or other?

About the treatment

- Details of consultation times, duration and an outline of what a consultation involves
- Times when you are available to be contacted
- Are life style changes necessary and expected?
- What does the patient want to happen?
- What is the homeopath's expected response to treatment? Is it the same as the patient's?
- An explanation of why aggravations are sometimes necessary and what they mean
- Incorporating other treatment strategies. What about conventional treatments, and other complementary treatments?
- How will complaints be dealt with and by whom?

About the Management

- Patient's and their families' choice of approach and expectations

- Experience and competence of the practitioner
- How to deal with complaints or broken contracts
- What support of colleagues and professional body does the homeopath have?
- How to handle seeing other therapists and communication between you, the patient and them
- How will we know when the patient is better and how will we know if they are not? It is important to contract with patients to let you know if they discontinue treatment, and preferably why. It is not uncommon for patients (especially those with acute and simple conditions) to 'not want to bother you' once they are 'better'

About the Contract

- What has been agreed from both the patient's and the homeopath's perspective
- How is it agreed and recorded – verbal or written?
- How does it protect the patient and homeopath from dependency and being taken advantage of?
- When during treatment does the contract need revisiting?
- How might each consultation have its own goals and how do these tie in with overall treatment goals?
- Are confidentiality and consent clear?

CASE STUDY 25.1

Jonathan, aged 10 months, was brought for homeopathic treatment by his mother, Sue. He would not easily go to sleep, woke at nights and wouldn't settle unless he came into his parents' bed. Sue was in a lot of distress about Jonathan's sleep pattern, partly because she was worried about what was going on and was very tired herself. Jonathan appeared untroubled by his not sleeping but was waking up hungry and wanted breast feeding. Once Sue had a chance to talk about her concerns, which included some ambivalence about stopping breast feeding, the contracts relating to both Jonathan's and Sue's needs were clearer. A remedy was prescribed for Sue and some general advice on feeding given.

Deepening our approach

V

CASE STUDY 25.2

Mark presented with a right-sided 'frozen shoulder' that he thought was caused by tennis. When he spoke about work, where he felt criticised, he clenched his right hand and pushed it into the palm of his left hand with a screwing movement. When invited to talk about his feelings about work he was at first reluctant. When he was made aware of the importance of how he felt and the homeopath 'mirrored' the hand movements he was making while talking, the consultation moved on to explore his feelings of resentment.

CASE STUDY 25.3

Paul has indigestion due in part to a poor diet; he feels unable to contract to change his diet but is prepared to look at why he eats so many stimulant foods (coffee, spicy and sugary). After acute treatment for his indigestion, taking into account his desire for stimulants, he returns wanting to prevent further attacks and now feels better able to change his diet.

CASE STUDY 25.4

Jill, age 46, has anxiety and panic attacks, but enjoys the attention from her husband, doctor and therapists because of it. When she explored her need for attention she realised it related to a deep fear of being alone that tied in with her children leaving home.

In some cases, the patient will see the illness at one level, while the treatment requires an understanding of the illness at a different level. The patient who understands the different approaches to the treatment of their case may become happy to treat at a deeper level, as Mark's case illustrates.

When establishing a contract, a patient may wish to be rid of a symptom but be reluctant to modify their life style – even if it is the causative factor. The limitation of treatment needs to be explained and the contract may need to be modified to support the patient with their symptoms or to help minimise the damage of the causative factor. As Paul's case shows, some patients are reluctant or feel unable to change their life style or life situation – sometimes patients need to be sufficiently ill before they will make these changes, with others the homeopath works to these limitations hoping in time to treat more deeply. Often, experience of a positive response to limited treatment, and the change in well-being that accompanies it, will encourage the insight and willingness to address these health needs more comprehensively.

Some illnesses provide secondary gains for the patient, who may then wish to contract to remove the presenting problem while wanting to maintain the secondary gains, as Jill's case illustrates.

Care, Compassion and Consent

What the patient believes they have agreed to with the homeopath forms the basis of their consent for treatment. The extent to which the homeopath informs the patient about what is likely to happen and what might possibly happen governs the extent to which the consent is 'informed'. Ultimately the exact outcome cannot be known beforehand and so consent can never be fully informed. What we can share are the qualities and values of the treatment process and the direction treatment is aimed in. The agreement fosters the goodwill between the patient and homeopath that helps develop trust and rapport. It allows the patient to be clear about what to expect from the homeopath, and what the homeopath expects from the patient. Ultimately all freely given consent is dependant on trust and goodwill.

Communicating the impression of the case and the plan of treatment back to the patient lays the foundation for the patient to understand the possible reactions to treatment and, as far as possible, to consent to the treatment.

Deepening our approach

V

Deepening the Case and Non-Judgemental Acceptance

'The perpetrator is a victim of a victim.'

It is helpful in the planning stage to clarify with the patient what they believe the aim of the treatment to be. Understandably they may wish simply to be rid of the symptom, but the reality is that a new state of health may be needed which will have implications above and beyond the simple removal of symptoms. This process may itself deepen the case.

Some aspects of the therapeutic agreement are easy to establish – where the consultations will be held, how long they will last, how much they will cost, etc.; some, such as how the homeopath will respond if working at the limits of their experience or competence, are more difficult. Other aspects of behaviour such as honesty, confidentiality, openness, goodwill, and non-judgemental attitudes may be established as part of rapport or as part of a professional code of practice (see Chapter 30).

All patients arrive at a homeopathic consultation with some belief about what will happen and how. It can be helpful at the beginning of each follow-up to refresh your memory of the agreement with the patient. It can set the direction and tone of the consultation, deepen rapport, and address problems before they become too serious. At the end of a consultation modifying if necessary and restating the agreement can act as a summary of what has happened 'so far', clarify any communication needed with third parties (e.g. other carers or family), and both set up the next consultation and establish what support the patient may need between consultations.

The patient may desire a very clear outcome – understanding this is an important part of understanding the patient. It may or may not be what the homeopath wants to contract to do. The greater a patient's expectations then the greater the patient's fear of them not being met or fear of being judged or rejected – allowing these issues to surface deepens the case. For example, the patient may present seeking relief from diarrhoea, but won't tell you that it is linked to a state of anxiety

or perpetual anticipation of 'being found out', as might be seen in a Lycopodium patient. At other times they may acknowledge anxiety but not think that you want or are able to help. In these cases they won't 'contract' to work with their anxiety – to find out why the anxiety is there and so reveal which anxiety remedy they might need. This will relatively mask or confuse a case.

Authenticity, Honesty and Boundaries

In some cases 'curative' treatment might only be able to achieve so much at one time. At a certain point in the treatment a patient may change from 'curative' to 'supportive' treatment, to maintain an improvement or reduce deterioration from an ongoing disease process. These are both aspects of the 'healing' role of the homeopath – the patient will go through phases where supportive or maintenance treatment is more relevant than curative treatmentenance.

Boundaries

For the contract to become clear then the relationship between the homeopath and patient needs also to be clear. One important aspect of this relationship is expressed in terms of social and professional boundaries. Establishing boundaries includes discussion of confidentiality, who else the patient consults with, notification and correspondence with other health care professionals, access out of hours, and what happens if you know or meet the patient in other settings. In more difficult cases awareness of and maintaining boundaries become an important way of identifying and managing projection (see Chapter 23). Contracting is one way of moving from working to an unconscious agenda to working with a clearer, more purposeful, agreement.

Reflecting Back to the Patient and Selecting a Remedy

In many ways our professional lives are a series of therapeutic encounters. It is through these separate encounters that we help patients to express what is, for them, struggling to emerge. Our work is in facilitating this revelation – allowing the patient to move towards who they really are and to balancing what is inside with what is outside. Like a gardener, we help reveal the beauty and balance in a situation; our intentions, like the idealised picture that a gardener may hold, will shape and inform our work. This is why respect for others and a freedom from the need to 'work our own stuff out' is so important.

If you only work with patients you like and easily understand you are unlikely to really challenge yourself or face what you are unfamiliar with. Encountering what is deep inside a patient requires a freedom from expectation of what you will find and a freedom from avoiding what you don't want to see. If you solely 'hunt the remedy' then you will limit what you can find.

We see that a dynamic and healing contact between you and your patients requires an awareness of and connection to yourself, an openness to receive what and who the patient is, and an ability to express this both in the homeopathic relationship and through the homeopathic remedies.

REFLECTION POINT
- How clearly do you agree aims of treatment with a patient? If you were a patient consulting with yourself what would you like agreed?
- Are there some patients that you find it especially easy or hard to develop a rapport with? Why is this and how might you address this?
- Write a guide for treatment that all patients can be given and a checklist of points you might like to cover when making a therapeutic agreement.

Supervision – Super...Vision

'A *formal process of professional support and learning which enables individual practitioners to develop knowledge and competence, assume responsibility for their own practice and enhance consumer protection and safety of care in complex clinical situations. It is central to the process of learning, to the scope of the expansion of practice and should be seen as a means of encouraging self assessment and analytical and reflective skills'*

A Vision for the Future, 1993

'*Supervision: A Quality of looking without attachment, fear or favour at "what is". Over view. The meta commentary, "observing I" ...aspirational and 'good enough'...It begins with embodiment – being present to experience.'*

Sheila Ryan, 2004

There are many ways you might get support and resources to deal with cases. In a developmental and training sense you may find your teachers will observe your work, or you may have opportunities for apprenticeship, or a more or less formal mentorship. Your needs will change as you gain experience – different individuals, groups and organisations will provide different things at different times. The desire and need to 'get better' at what we do needs to be balanced with 'being good enough' at what we do. This is reflected in the journey from student to novice, to apprentice, to mentee, to independence, to teacher and mentor.

Aspects of ourselves will always be hidden or unconscious, however expert we become, and there will be situations where we have to face our limits and the unknown. It is not a question of training to reach a point where we might be all things to all patients – rather it is recognising that we all, at times, require ongoing support, development and education. When important issues remain unconscious and give rise to problems they must be allowed to surface or they will leak out onto colleagues, family and back to your patients. For this reason we all require opportunities for support, reflection and (lifelong) learning. Individuals from some health professions seem reluctant to recognise this, perhaps reflecting their 'buying into' the illusion of omnipotence, where nothing is left in the unconscious.

As the homeopath treats more complex and hidden cases, seeking to know the deeper aspects of a patient's case, so the homeopathic relationship – the dynamic between the patient and homeopath seen through the lens of the remedies – becomes more central in the healing process. To keep the homeopathic relationships focused and clear, attention needs to be paid to any areas of difficulty. The quote below is from a member of a homeopathic supervision group:

'A supervision group gives me the opportunity to study my cases and reflect deeply while presenting them to others. The group provides peer feedback and support and poses questions I need to consider. Areas of my work that require deeper study and change are highlighted. So much is about my attitudes and awareness – when these are transformed my way of working and my effectiveness are also transformed. It takes courage to show my work with honesty – the highs and the lows. The validation and acceptance from the group is liberating. The reminders of my purpose are inspiring. The combined wisdom and guidance of the group clarify my direction. The dynamics of the group provide the shift and movement forward of my journey of personal development.

'The group gently illuminates my blind spots and monitors my safety and the safety of my patients. The added advantage of group supervision is the opportunity to witness how others are working and to learn from their success and failure. The common experience that bonds the members of the supervision group encourages deeper processing of my difficulties in the safety of friends and colleagues who really listen and understand. I tend to lack confidence in my ability and approach the group with feelings of inadequacy. However, I am swiftly put at ease by expert facilitation. I liken the encouragement I receive to the best effects of the homeopathic remedy. It really does have the wow factor! So that my indwelling reason-gifted mind can freely employ this living healthy instrument for the higher purpose of my existence.'

Even in cases that are not confused or hidden it is important to have a place where one can feel supported, can benefit from the experience of others (education), and can develop homeopathic knowledge. It is important for each of these three aspects (support, education and development) to be addressed. At a personal level the homeopath has to be educated to learn the information and apply the technique, supported in coming to terms with what is not known (and the feelings this brings), and helped to develop a personal style of working.

Supervision happens in three main settings – as part of personal reflection (self supervision), as part of a group or one-to-one with a colleague or supervisor.

Self Supervision

'When treatment difficulties arise which a therapist cannot resolve the therapist develops unconscious identification with his patient. Unable to verbalise these indications they become enacted.'

Sachs & Shapiro (1976)

Personal reflection is a cornerstone to homeopathic practice, which is one reason why reflection has been encouraged throughout this book. To be able to observe and reflect on something that happened or is happening is an important part of clinical practice. Box 25.3 suggests some questions you can ask yourself after a 'difficult consultation'; with experience you will be able to reflect on these during a consultation.

Consider how you might feed back the results into the consultation, taking into account how the patient might be feeling. It can help to consider a range of possible responses available to you in any

---

BOX 25.3
Self-Supervision Questions
- What did I feel at this point?
- What was I thinking?
- What bodily sensations did I have?
- What was most obvious thing I didn't notice?
- What would I rather have done?
- What problems or risks were there if I had done things differently?
- What sort of person does the patient see me as?
- How does this episode remind me of past situations?
- What is my fantasy (delusion) about the situation and what am I fearful of?
- When else have I had this feeling?
- What am I expecting to learn from this situation?
- How can I acknowledge the patient for the opportunities this difficulty gives me?

situation. For example, you might give yourself three options about what to do next – they may range from the safe and sensible, to 'thinking outside the box' and imagining a more extreme possibility. Sometimes, when re-examined, the extreme ideas actually provide quite practical and useful strategies.

Peer Supervision

'When the therapist does not understand the meaning of a patient's enactment he conveys the meaning to his supervisor by a parallel enactment.'

Interpretation of Freud

When a case is discussed in supervision, aspects of it – particularly those that are unresolved in the consultation – come alive. Issues that cause difficulty or which are hidden in the consultation may be enacted; peers can observe this and comment on the dynamic. For many practitioners this peer supervision gives support and allows sharing of issues, but if it lacks formality, safety or clarity it can avoid exploring and revealing each other's blind spots. It can easily default to sharing successes and 'miracle cases' – and the hiding away in the collective unconscious of the difficult cases.

Facilitated Supervision

'Emotions experienced by a supervisor, including even his private subjective fantasy experiences and his personal feelings about the supervisee, often provide valuable clarification in processes currently characterising the relationship between the supervisee and the patient.'

H Searles (1955)

When we start to talk about a patient we spontaneously bring to the surface the feelings that have been projected onto us and that we have accepted (often unconsciously) from that patient. These issues will be mirrored in the relationship with the supervisor, who will aim to observe the unconscious, unacknowledged behaviour in the supervisee. An experienced supervisor will not only reflect the content of the consultation and strategies and interventions used by the homeo-

path, but will be able to reflect back to the supervisee something of their own internal processes and patterns. It enables you to gain insight into assumptions and biases in the way you work and allows your projections and unresolved feelings to be played out, identified and explored in a safe but conscious way.

Facilitated supervision can also be the place to 'try out' different approaches and interventions, particularly the more extreme of the range of options mentioned in self supervision. Once you are comfortable using something in a supported setting and have received feedback on it, it is often possible to use it during a consultation.

Styles of Supervision

Without supervision, do not be surprised if your mistakes keep repeating themselves.

There are many different styles of supervision that lend themselves to different settings, issues, supervisors and supervisees. They range from the informal 'chat' about a case to a formal structure applied rigorously. It may take place 'between consultations' or in a dedicated session that may be a one-off or regular meeting. It may be organised individually or established as part of a 'network' of advanced teaching and professional development that may or may not be linked to revalidation or appraisal. Supervision may or may not be a requirement to practice or be monitored by an educational, representative or regulatory body.

In addition to the different styles of receiving or giving supervision there are a variety of models or structures. Most models seeks to understand the therapeutic relationship and intervention through a series of processes or stages – such as identifying restorative, formative and normative elements (Proctor 1987), that mirrored earlier work looking at support, education and management (Kadushin 1976). A process model of supervision I have found most helpful, and have most experience in as supervisee and supervisor, is the seven-eyed model of supervision (Hawkins & Shohet 2000).

Deepening our approach

V

349

The Seven-Eyed Model of Supervision

Supervision is helpfully understood by thinking of it in terms of the worlds of the patient, homeopath and supervisor. Figure 25.1 is a model of supervision showing the focus of supervision for patient, homeopath and supervisor, and from the perspective of the homeopathic relationship and the supervisory relationship.

Level 1 examines the patient's presentation; level 2 reflects on the treatment given. In level 3 the homeopath's relationship to the patient is examined. These first three levels are informed by what has happened in the homeopathic consultation.

Level 4 invites the homeopath to explore their own internal process. What do they notice when they recount the case and what do they feel towards the patient? Level 5 looks at what is brought in parallel into the supervision session, what is enacted when talking about the case. Level 6 is the supervisor's own internal process. Levels 4 to 6 focus on and are informed by what happens in the supervision session. Level 7 focuses on the context in which both the treatment and supervision are taking place.

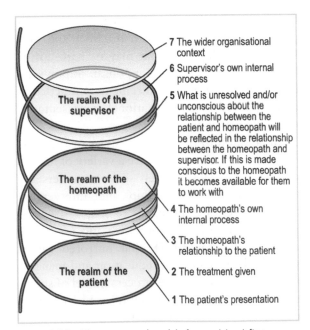

Figure 25.1   The seven-eyed model of supervision (after Hawkins and Shohet 2000)

7 The wider organisational context

6 Supervisor's own internal process

5 What is unresolved and/or unconscious about the relationship between the patient and homeopath will be reflected in the relationship between the homeopath and supervisor. If this is made conscious to the homeopath it becomes available for them to work with

4 The homeopath's own internal process

3 The homeopath's relationship to the patient

2 The treatment given

1 The patient's presentation

The realm of the supervisor

The realm of the homeopath

The realm of the patient

Supervision happens in a broad context of practice that includes explicit and implicit norms of professional behaviour, codes of practice, organisational and management issues – part of the supervisor's agreement with the supervisee is to clarify their importance and the extent to which these are included. When supervision is provided as a practice management or professional organisation tool it can lead to revealing inconsistencies and conflicts between personal, practice and organisational priorities. Although supervision is usually driven by, and centred on, personal and practice issues it also informs and is informed by the professional organisations the homeopath works within (see Chapter 28). The different 'eyes' or 'plains of focus' within this model of supervision inform an understanding of the therapeutic encounter, so are discussed more fully.

Level 1

On many occasions when reflecting on a case it is apparent that there just wasn't enough detail present to provide the information necessary to make an accurate prescription. Something needed to happen to 'bring the patient into the room'. The content of the consultation, when reflected on in supervision, is frequently much greater than first appreciated. It includes information about how the patient dressed, moved, sat, how exactly they looked, and how this changed as they talked about their symptoms. By inviting homeopaths to sit, walk, talk, or move like the patient insights are gained to how the patient might be feeling and what they are communicating – revealing, for instance, an apparently masked case.

Level 2

It is not uncommon to find that highly competent homeopaths appear far from competent when discussing a difficult case in supervision. When they have seen no clear strategy or intervention indicated they often fall back on old patterns of intervention, rather than recognise why they find this case difficult. Reflecting on what 'buttons' have been pushed by a patient and what you would really like to do or say to the patient can sometimes offer new possibilities.

Deepening our approach

Levels 3 and 4

Clues to projection taking place are when the consultation suddenly becomes emotionally charged or contracted boundaries are broken. Level 3 focuses on the homeopath's relationship to the patient and the conscious and unconscious interventions. It is here that the patient's possible projections are often revealed and their transference clarified. Sometimes looking back at a case it is seen very differently, hence the value not just of thinking back to the case but also of videos of consultations and detailed analyses of both the obvious case and also the smallest nuances of the patient and homeopath.

Exploring how the homeopath and patient interact can be helped by imagining the consultation as a 'documentary' or as if a 'fly-on-the-wall' camera is observing it. What would it look like, how would you feel watching it and what would you suggest to someone else in the same situation? Indeed, inviting the homeopath to observe their own internal process frequently sheds light on what is being projected onto the homeopath and their reciprocal projections (see Chapter 23). The physical sensations and the feelings the homeopath has both during the consultation and also in supervision reveal the deepest projections that contribute most to cases appearing confused and hidden.

One of the benefits of taking part in supervision, even while relatively new to practice, is that it helps develop an awareness of projection in others and thence in you.

Level 5

What is mirrored in the supervision often reveals those things that have been transferred, often unconsciously, by the patient onto the homeopath. Dealing with this projection is an essential part of maintaining one's focus and clarity.

Level 6

The supervisor's own internal process (including emotions and sensations) will, if made conscious, reflect (and possibly clarify) what is happening to the supervisee. At this level the supervisor/supervisee and supervisor/patient relationships are both important. How the supervisor reacts to what they perceive and feel in supervision gives valuable information. However, if it remains unresolved, the supervisor will need to address it in his own supervision.

Level 7

The supervisor may have a responsibility to an employing or professional community. Balancing this responsibility to the responsibility to the supervisee and the patient is one that needs continual monitoring so that the interests of all parties are protected and served. It is through the ears and voices of the supervisors that our professional bodies can develop and evolve.

REFLECTION POINT

- Think of the most common difficult situation you find yourself in as a homeopath. Go through the self-supervision exercises in Box 25.3. What are the factors in you that 'invite' this difficulty? What is your attraction to and avoidance of working with this issue in facilitated supervision? What does this tell you about this issue?
- Why do you think some health carers have a resistance to obtaining and using supervision?
- Remember – over time patients who get better will be discharged, while those that are difficult may keep returning!

Summary

Being clear on the factors that determine the therapeutic agreement, and how these influence the consultation and therapeutic encounter, can guide how you both take and receive the case. Uncertainty about the therapeutic agreement, the boundaries, the expectations and the projections causes many of the difficulties homeopaths experience when managing cases. By exploring and understanding the factors that shape and influence the agreement and encounter it is possible to undertake, explore, make sense of and help situations and patients that otherwise would be at best untreatable by you and at worst harmful to you.

Deepening our approach

V

Developing and extending your competence, while at the same time paying attention to the day-to-day 'housekeeping' that being a practitioner requires, is all part of supervision. The importance of the projection (both from the patient to the homeopath and from the homeopath to the patient) enacted in the relationship between the homeopath and the supervisor and the supervisor and the homeopath is vital to working with more challenging confused and hidden cases.

Acknowledgement

Robin Shohet and the centre for staff team development.

References

Fowler J 1996 The organisation of clinical supervision within the nursing profession. J Adv Nursing 23: 471–478

Hawkins P, Shohet R 2000 Supervision in the helping professions, 2nd edn. Open University Press, Buckingham

Kadushin A 1976 Supervision in social work. Columbia University Press, New York.

Kaplan B 2001 The homeopathic conversation. Natural Medicine Press, London

Mercer S W, Watt G C, Reilly D 2001 Empathy is important for enablement. Br Med J 322:865

Mercer S W Reilly D, Watt G C M 2002 The importance of empathy in the enablement of patients attending the Glasgow Homeopathic Hospital. Br J Gen Pract 52:901–905

Proctor B 1987 Supervision: a co-operative exercise in accountability. In: Marken M, Payne M (eds) Enabling and ensuring. Supervision in practice. National Youth Bureau, Leicester

Rogers C R 1973 On encounter groups. Pernguin, Harmondsworth

Ryan S 2004 Vital Practice, the homeopathic and supervisory way. Sea change, Portland

Sachs D M, Shapiro S H 1976 On parallel processes in therapy and teaching. Psychoanal Q 45(3):394–415

Searles H F 1955 The informational value of the supervisor's emotional experiences in psychiatry. Psychiatry 18:135–146

Shohet R 2005 Passionate medicine – making the transition from conventional medicine to homeopathy. Jessica Kingsley, London

Bibliography

Freeman R 1998 Mentoring in general practice. Butterworth-Heinemann, Oxford

Ryan S 2004 Vital practice. Sea Change, Portland, UK

A Vision for the Future 1993 Department of Health, London

Deepening our approach

V

CHAPTER TWENTY SIX

Holographic and Relational Models of Health

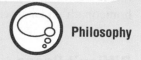 **Philosophy**

David Owen

Introduction

There is no such thing as perfect health, just good enough health.

Having explored in previous sections the rationale for causation, local, totality and constitutional approaches to treatment, it is now important to return to thematic and reflective approaches. These have been described in previous chapters and have been found to work well in cases that are otherwise confused or hidden. When the holographic and relational models of health that underlie them are understood, the homeopath is more likely to be able to use thematic and reflective approaches and 'make them your own'. They bring with them slightly different ways of studying the materia medica, a different emphasis in the case, different methods of analysis and different management issues – each of which is described in subsequent chapters in this section.

While approaches to health and illness based on causal and holistic perspectives are well established, the holographic and relational views are less well described. The description of the holographic and relational models of health, the approach to treatment they bring, and the methodology for prescribing they offer are therefore offered more tentatively. They are separate and distinct but are presented together for reasons of space and because both are informed primarily by the homeopathic relationship. Considering them together also offers us the opportunity to explore how the different models, approaches and methodologies present in this textbook are part of a spectrum, often needing to be integrated for the optimum management of the patient.

The holographic model recognises that any part (of the whole) reflects the whole. So facets of a case or remedy tell us something about the patterns running throughout and reflect something of the whole case or remedy. The patterns we observe running through a case or remedy will be influenced by our own state.

Working with the holographic and relational models uses the 'state of the homeopath' and relies on the insight you have into your own norms. This raises important questions about self awareness and development as part of a homeopath's training. As a relationship is often communicated by feeling, it is frequently the feelings in the patient and homeopath that reveal the consistent themes in a confused case and the dynamic of the hidden case. For this reason, emotional intelligence is explored further in this chapter.

To help understanding difficult cases and why the approaches presented here are so important we start by exploring further what makes a case appear confused or hidden. This leads on to the broader cultural context that influences our work, especially the collective unconscious and cultural suppression (linked to society and hereditary predisposition) that is developed later in this section. The confused and hidden cases in any population tell the homeopath about the health of that population. And while the most usual contract for the homeopath is with an individual patient, we also play an important role in the health of a population (see 'Public health homeopath' in Chapter 30).

Difficult Cases

Difficult cases are difficult to see clearly – it follows that these are difficult to manage. Cases that do not respond easily and quickly to treatment and cannot be seen clearly in the causal biological or holistic models of health are often confused or poorly expressed (hidden). These unclear and shadowy aspects of the confused and hidden case are detected by the way they are projected on to the things around the patient (see Chapter 23). Even if you choose not to work this way, it is important to know about it as negative feelings can be 'dumped' by the patient on those around them – including the homeopath. If you are unaware of this you may project back to the patient and/or become drained and feel manipulated. Paradoxically, there is often a form of collusion when this happens, with each 'blaming' the other – often preventing you or the patient from seeing and addressing what is going on.

Once the case is accepted as confused or hidden you may feel a lessening of the pressure to get the simillimum in one consultation as it may require a phase of clarifying the case. There may be no single well indicated remedy or a number of partially indicated remedies. You may have to accept that the case will only become clear over a period of treatment and that it is not necessary, or indeed possible, to see the whole case from the outset.

Understanding why cases are confused and hidden, and how the holographic and relational models make working with these easier, is an important part of increasing the number and difficulty of cases that you can treat effectively. Initially you may only explore the holographic or relational model when a detailed case history and analysis fails to point to the totality or constitutional remedy. In time you may find these approaches becoming the foundation of a reliable and repeatable approach to treatment. As confused and hidden cases often reflect a deep sus-

ceptibility and the potential to get symptoms in the future, illnesses the patient would otherwise have been expected to get may be prevented.

The Holographic Model

'…the classical contrast between the solid particles and the space surrounding them is completely overcome. The quantum field is seen as the fundamental physical entity; the continuous medium which is present everywhere in space. Particles are merely local condensations of the field; concentrations which come and go, thereby losing their individual character and dissolving into the underlying field.'

Fritjof Capra 1975

A natural progression from the holistic model, where one symptom cannot change without affecting all aspects of the case, is to see each symptom that an individual expresses as containing and reflecting aspects of the whole case. The way in which each symptom expresses one facet of the whole pattern is similar to the way every piece of a hologram holds the whole picture, and the genetic code in one cell holds the information for the whole individual. This principle is observed and used in many diagnostic systems (including reflexology, auricular acupuncture, and tongue or iris diagnosis) where one part of the body is related to others. If any one symptom could be understood in its entirety it would explain the whole case. Understanding the pattern (also called the essence or theme) that lies behind the symptoms of an otherwise confused case reveals something more fundamental that often runs through several layers of the case.

Several different themes may run through a case but the most central themes run deepest and link many symptoms. The most consistent or deepest theme is sometimes referred to as the most central, fundamental or essence. They express themselves in the local, mental and general symptoms of the case and the remedy. The more central (or universal) the theme to the patient the more important it is to match it to the theme running through the remedy. Matching these themes is the basis of essence and thematic prescribing and in confused cases these more central themes provide reliable information to prescribe on.

The different themes we are able to recognise, and 'make sense of' depends on how we interpret our world. By studying the themes of the materia medica and by creating a map from cross referencing themes of different remedies we can be helped to recognise different patterns that run through cases. We may categorise them in many different ways, examples include using yin and yang, the three kingdoms, four humours, five elements, seven rays, twelve star signs, etc. Similarly we may use three, five or any number of miasms to reflect susceptibility and themes that run through a case or remedy picture. In different cultures, the miasmatic influences an individual is subject to may be slightly different. In cultures where thrush or glandular fever are more common, or have been suppressed more than ringworm or malaria, it may be more relevant to work with the former rather than the latter miasmatic groups. However, there are connections and similarities to miasmatic groups in different cultures – reflecting illnesses that we are all susceptible to and identifying common threads and miasms that run through the materia medica is expedient. Remember, miasms will evolve as different illnesses occur and are suppressed.

REFLECTION POINT

- Rather than themes determining how a patient (or remedy) expresses themselves in different situations, consider instead that patients (and remedies) 'seek out' particular situations where these themes *can* express themselves. How might a patient with a theme of being accident-prone seek out situations where accidents are more likely?

Confused Cases

In a complex case the picture may have many aspects compared to a simple case, but 'what you see is what you get' (see Fig 10.2). In a confused case the symptoms appear muddled because one set of symptoms overlies another. They have a number of layers – some of which might be clearly visible, others not. Figure 26.1 illustrates the comparison between confused and hidden cases. In a confused case the picture presented in the totality does not reveal an accurate reflection of the hierarchy and depth of the case. The deeper symptoms are not the most noticeable and the patient may be unconscious of them.

In the same way as there is a continuum of cases running through the complex, confused and hidden, so it can help to think of consciousness and unconsciousness not so much as black and white as a scale of greyness. In confused cases some symptoms may be unconscious but easier to bring to the surface; other features may be deeply unconscious and the patient may deny or rationalise them. In hidden cases there is often more that is deeply, even instinctually and culturally, unconscious.

Understanding confused cases is possible from themes that express themselves in the presenting symptoms. But if these have been suppressed then the expression may be in other areas of the case, such as childhood illnesses or family history. There may be several stages to treating these confused cases; each stage may reveal new symptoms as the picture is clarified. If deeper symptoms surface then new themes may emerge.

As a symptom moves inwards to a deeper level (due to suppression), the outer expression becomes a less accurate reflection of what is really happening to the individual. The extent to which suppression disturbs the body's ability to react to a stimulus depends on the extent to which the suppression can produce a new pattern of symptoms (or illness). This new pattern has its own themes that reflect the cause of the suppression – setting up patterns or layers of illness such as, for example, the steroid, the Prozac, the antibiotic, the alcohol layer. These layers distort and confuse the picture and may need removing before deeper aspects of the case can be seen. Each layer may need to be removed before other layers become visible. This may be achieved just by removing the suppressive agent or may require treatment based on what can be seen – and may include isopathic

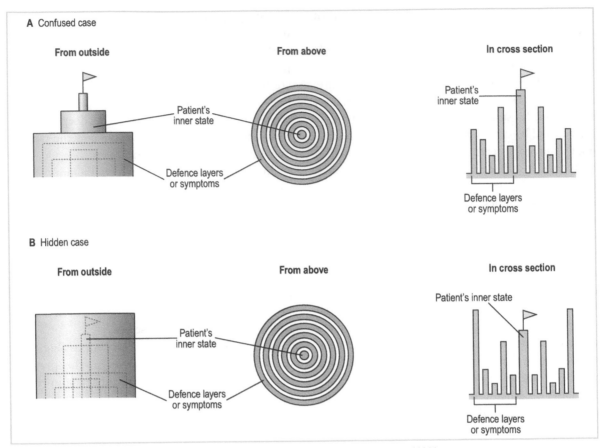

A Confused case

B Hidden case

Figure 26.1   Figurative comparison of a complex, confused and hidden case

and organ-based prescribing to reduce a particular wall and see a deeper layer.

Walls and Layers

As suppression increases so the case becomes less transparent, as if a wall is built around the patient (Fig. 26.1). Like all walls it keeps some things inside (and hidden) and other things outside. As cases get more confused and hidden, yet more walls hide and confuse increasing proportions of the case. Working with these cases is a matter of gradually removing one wall after another. In many cases it can be hard to tell just how many layers or walls there are. In these cases it is difficult for the patient and homeopath to know exactly how much treatment is going to be required as it depends on what surfaces.

Sometimes just removing one wall is enough for the patient to start improving, particularly when those factors that led to the construction of the wall are no longer present. Of course the protective role of the wall should be noted and (like the benefits of secondary gain) taken into account in patient management. Treatment does not necessarily entail the dismantling of all these walls but can involve enabling the homeopath to see through 'windows' in the walls and the patient to move through 'doors' in them at the appropriate stage of treatment. Dismantling the wall before the patient has managed to make changes to the situation in which they needed to develop their walls is akin to de-compensating the patient. In different situations different aspects of a case are expressed – it is possible to imagine situations where a patient would develop a wall for protection, as Fran's case illustrates.

It can help to think of each symptom, like a wall, as having four aspects: the theme itself [hardness], the two sides of the wall (one the active protection it offers the patient [brittle], one the passive block to the patient's free and healthy expression [broken]), and finally the patient's compensated behaviour or view of the situation from behind the wall [cautious, safe]. A theme or pattern running through a case may include symptoms in the active, passive, or compensated form. So a confused case with a theme such as hardness may have some symptoms showing brittleness (active), others appear broken or snapped (passive), and some an avoidance or cautiousness even to the point of softness (compensation). This explains why in some confused cases there are paradoxical co-existing or alternating symptoms (Saine 2000)

that appear like two or more illnesses but in fact are one and the same – even if no single anatomical or pathological disease entity can be identified as underlying or explaining all the symptoms.

Essence and Themes

'The human soul responds to the processes and substances of our world with myth, legend and poetic imagery and these can be understood as the revelation of the higher reality lying latent, like a sleeping princess, within the natural phenomena. They constitute, one might also say, a homeopathic proving in a very clear and heightened form … In contemplating these images and symbols we may be led deeper into the hidden genius of the substance and its remedial actions than by confining our attention strictly to the realm of material effects and the rubrics of official provings.'

Ralph Twentyman

CASE STUDY 26.1

Fran, age 49, presented with a multi-system connective tissue disease that included rheumatoid symptoms. She talked of how hard it was being ill. Over the first two consultations she glimpsed for the first time that all had not been well as a young child. She realised a series of difficult and bullying relationships reflected the physical and emotional abuse she saw her mother suffer from at the hands of her father. She felt she had to 'walk on egg shells' or else he'd go for her. This left her understandably cautious about revealing her feelings. Once she found she could talk about this without being criticised, she started to reframe her view of her parents' relationship and behaviour and was also able to start talking about her own history of broken relationships. She had to feel very 'secure' and 'safe' with her homeopath before she could fully open the door to her emotional pain. As she revealed more, including her anger with her mother for putting up with the abuse, so deeper-acting remedies could be prescribed. Only then did her presenting symptoms significantly improve.

The essence is the single central pattern of information that expresses itself in any symptom of a remedy or case. In practice one consistent pattern or essence is not always recognisable; instead the pattern observed in the case and remedy can be understood in terms of a number of different themes. For example, in the remedy Nitric acid there is an essence of 'dissatisfaction', but there are also the themes that run through the Nitricum and Acid remedies of 'sensitivity' and 'weakness to respond' – together contributing to its unique expression of dissatisfaction. Each remedy may have several themes, not all of which have to be observed in the same patient at the same time, to the same degree. In many confused cases the deepest aspects are projected (or leak out) in the consultation without necessarily being consciously named by the patient. They may be reflected in the words used or movements made, the sensation or 'feelings' they experience, or those they generate or stimulate in you.

In less well-known remedies only some themes are clear and how the themes come together to form an essence is uncertain. Themes may appear contradictory, for example, a Natrum muriaticum patient is sensitive but by appearing withdrawn and introverted may appear at first glance as 'thick skinned or indifferent'. Understanding the themes expressed in a remedy often helps the homeopath to extrapolate and interpret the remedies in situations that are very different from the original provings. While this brings certain risks until provings are repeated in contemporary situations, it does allow us to open up the materia medica to situations patients are in now.

REFLECTION

- Suppression is a major cause of symptoms moving to a deeper 'layer'. The suppression of eczema often precedes the onset of asthma. I invite you to reflect on the possibility that it is the suppression of illness rather than the disease itself that sets up a miasm – so it is the suppression of syphilis that set up the syphilitic miasm.
- How does a miasm compare to the walls or layers around the patient in Figure 26.1?
- Given their importance, can you name the main themes and essence of the main miasms (see Chapter 17)?
- Looking at Figure 26.1 how might different consultations reveal different views of the same patient and how will you know when you are really seeing the centre of the case?

The Relational Model

The relationship between the patient and their world (including the homeopath) reveals the themes at play in the patient; what happens to the homeopath in the homeopathic relationship can reflect the patient's state. The more 'intense' the experience or stronger the feelings in the homeopath, the more likely it represents something of importance to the case. It is particularly useful when the case is otherwise masked or hidden, as such cases invariably project more on to their situation and those around them. Thus the greater the problems for the homeopath if they are not effectively integrated into the consultation and management of the case (see Chapter 23). These projections are most often sensitively communicated and most easily detected by 'feeling'. The use of emotional intelligence enables

the homeopath to work 'relationally', adding what is to many a new dimension to the understanding of patients and remedies.

Identifying and matching the patient's emotional state to the 'feeling' state of remedies requires emotional awareness and the ability to communicate emotionally. It is important to stress that while this is most easily perceived as a psychological interaction, what is expressed psychologically mirrors what is present at a somatic level. The homeopath (and patients) working with confused and hidden cases must be prepared to work as much with the psychological realm of illness as the somatic. If one was to work with these cases using the model of aetiology then it would be fair to say that many difficult cases, and multi-system long-standing chronic illnesses, have an emotional cause. That is to say, at the time when a patient is developing their first symptoms or shortly before, there has been a significant change in their emotional state. It is not uncommon to see patients whose symptoms flow from bereavements, rejections, abuses, promotions or failings. The emotional reaction to these events is a more subtle, individual way of understanding the trigger than the event itself. Unfortunately suppression and lack of comprehensive emotional pictures of the remedies make the aetiological model poorly suited to these cases.

A frequent cause of cases being hidden is that the symptoms fail to fully reflect the susceptibility. It may be that the illness has become overly functional or structural, or because the homeopath is unable to see the case clearly. Frequently these two problems go together to give what are known as 'one-sided' illnesses, where significant parts of the totality are unconscious to the patient or unseen by the homeopath. The susceptibility may be further challenged and the case masked by deteriorating disease, maintaining causes, insufficient vitality, inherited predisposition or cultural suppression. In practice these often happen together and may be the result of an untreated or suppressed confused case, congenital disease or as a result of an unrecognised illness (often a culturally endemic disease).

Many homeopaths are informed by their relationship with the patient, even if they do not use it explicitly. It is my observation that many practitioners who describe themselves as working 'intuitively' (Brien 2004) are in fact manifesting many aspects of working relationally. How you feel in a consultation can guide you to the deepest aspects of the patient's case, correlate with the patient's remedy state, and be a reliable pointer towards the simillimum. Put simply – what happens to you, especially the feelings you experience, can help choose a remedy.

Different homeopaths experience different feelings in response to patients fitting a particular remedy. For example, an Arsenicum album patient will generate specific feelings that may be different for each homeopath depending on their state. If the homeopath himself is in an Arsenicum album state those feelings are likely to be very different to those they would experience if they were in a Phosphorus state.

To use this approach requires a steadiness and insight into your own state. Learning the emotional reaction you have to different remedies is part of developing a 'living materia medica' – a natural extension of essence and thematic prescribing. The attuned homeopath will be interested in how patients in different remedy states can make them feel – producing changes in their own feelings or subtle physical signs, such as a prickling up the spine, a catch in their own voice or throat, a misuse of a certain word or a certain feeling arising when the patient is talking about a particular issue.

In order to work reliably in this way with a high level of competence the homeopath needs to be aware of and develop a language for their own and others' emotional state; to be able to invite, identify, communicate and work with emotions and behaviours that are the result of projection. It requires awareness of how different feelings relate to each other and the patient's state. For example, after a significant loss such as a bereavement a patient will often go through phases of grieving (Kubler-Ross 1970) that very roughly can be described as denial, sadness, anger, heightened sensitivity to further loss, and resolution. Patients may cycle through these phases over days or many years and can get 'stuck' in any of them. These different phases correlate with different remedy pictures – patients in each give quite a different feeling.

Emotional Intelligence

'We promise according to our hopes and perform according to our fears'.

Francois Duc de la Rochefoucauld

Emotional intelligence is an important attribute if we are to function supportively in, and sustain, any emotional relationship. It is important when working in any model of health or using any approach to treatment – but it is particularly important when working predominantly in the relational model or using the reflective approach. It is important in establishing empathy, especially if working with confused and hidden cases. It is distinct from academic intelligence – which is about ordering, sorting, measuring and comparing pieces of information. The intellectual and emotional intelligences involve the activity of different parts of the brain. The intellectual activity is sited predominantly in the neo-cortex, emotional intelligence in the sub-cortex. Different hemispheres of the brain are more active in one form of intelligence than another, with left brain activity equating to academic intelligence and right brain activity relating to emotional intelligence. Some individuals are more left-brain dominant and others more right-brain dominant.

Some authors have attempted to differentiate this intelligence in relation to gender, describing emotional intelligence as more feminine and academic intelligence as more masculine. Most researchers in the field report that men and women are equally able to use either or both intelligences – their dominant style will depend on their background and upbringing (Goleman 1995). Factors that are important in developing and using emotional intelligence include personal and social competences; these are not developed as a result of learning facts but are a vital part of entering into a therapeutic relationship as a health professional. They contribute hugely to your 'self awareness', self-confidence, self-control and personal motivation – without them you risk damaging yourself and the patient.

REFLECTION POINT

- You might like to reflect about what in your training is specifically helping you develop these skills. Likewise I suggest you score out of ten how aware you are of others feelings, concerns, needs and wants (empathy); and also your more general social skills, including your communication skills, the range of people you have an easy rapport with and your ability to influence and enable others.

Empathy

'Mortals can keep no secrets. If their lips are silent, they gossip with their fingertips; betrayal forces its way through every pore.'

S Freud

Empathy (see Chapters 13 & 23) is an awareness of others' feelings, needs and concerns. It is the way we connect with each other emotionally. It is known that a good level of empathy enables rapport and that it depends not only on our self-awareness but also on the cultural, social and personal relationship that exists between individuals. Empathy enables patients to acknowledge, work with and, in time, express their underlying feelings – which can in its own right be a healing process.

Developing Empathy

The ability to work with empathy is related to the awareness of how your own feelings can be affected by others and others' feelings affected by yours. High levels of empathy often give confidence to deal with situations where there are high levels of challenge and risk. Although aspects of empathy are certainly influenced by family history and early experience, all homeopaths should be able, through experience and personal development, to work reliably and meaningfully with their and other's emotions. Box 26.1 details aspects of emotional communication that are particularly helpful when working relationally.

BOX 26.1
Aspects of Emotional Communication That are Particularly Helpful When Working Relationally
- Ability to express feelings
- Ability to make observations related to feelings and to check out the observations with the patient
- Ability to discuss and contract with a patient about working with feelings
- Ability to model working with feelings and inspire others to work with feelings
- Ability to trust feelings
- Ability to use feelings in balance with goals and outcomes
- Ability to support patients to become emotionally competent
- Ability to ask for support
- Ability to work with negative and suppressed feelings without becoming trapped in these feelings
- Ability to be aware when patients are projecting feelings on to you and when you are counter-projecting feelings back to them
- Ability to be honest about feelings

Emotions as Part of the Totality

The patient's emotional state is connected to all other aspects of their totality. So too is the homeopath's emotional state connected to what is going on for them physically and psychologically. It is possible that small body movements, phrases and facial movements of the homeopath and patient will influence and reflect the emotional state. Patient and homeopath behaviour, including body position, where they look, how they move etc., offer insight into what is happening in the patient. This does not preclude there being changes in other areas of the body and mind that may include subtle shifts of 'energy' that are currently not directly measurable. Perhaps the small movements that influence the swing of a pendulum or changes in pressure of electrical connections (and therefore current flow) lie behind some of the 'subtle' techniques such as

Dowsing, Radionics, Emanometer (Boyd 1923), Vega, bioelectrical, kinesiology, etc. – used by some to reflect what is happening to the patient.

The Hidden/One-Sided Case (Organon, Paras 172, 190)

We learn more from our difficult cases than our easy ones. They teach us about our therapy, our self and our world.

Some serious diseases first emerge with no apparent or gradual build up of symptoms, e.g. the sudden onset of heart disease, cancers, schizophrenia, multiple sclerosis, epilepsy, and alcohol and drug abuse. These hidden, or one-sided, diseases are usually disorders of function and structure – where the disorder is not expressed fully, or at all, in the realm of sensation. In most of these a complete case with local, mental and general symptoms is absent; the patient attends with their presenting symptoms and not a lot else. There may be an absence of any history of acute illnesses and the sense of being 'stuck' in a certain situation or life style. By the time these problems present to the homeopath they are often quite advanced (as Peter's case illustrates) and may even be life threatening.

Hidden cases range from those that are slightly obscured (but in which a careful history may reveal some features), to those where all the details of the symptoms are swamped by a single prominent symptom. It is as if the patient's 'normal behaviour' is not recognisable as symptoms. Sometimes an illness may present as one-sided, when the case is presented on the patient's behalf by a third party, such as a parent or pet owner.

In hidden cases prescribing may be based non-specifically on the presenting symptom (local prescribing) but this rarely gives marked or permanent results. Or it can be based on subtler indications of the case – where treatment and support over some time may reveal the deeper aspects. It may take some time before a complete case emerges – and even then it may be confused. In these patients an initial response to treatment with an acute illness, aggravation or return of old (often forgotten) symptoms, giving more prescribing information, is a positive response.

In Peter's case, after receiving local treatment (Crataegus) his blood pressure improved slightly but at follow-up he was frustrated that he was not 'better'. He spoke of his frustration about his homeopathic treatment and wanted to know when he would be better. The homeopath felt a little 'bullied' and realised that this might be how the patient felt. When the patient was asked if he was ever bullied he at first denied it and then admitted it was a recurring pattern – running from childhood, through several jobs and in his first marriage. He 'always felt put upon'. He made a significant improvement after Lycopodium 10M.

Figure 26.1 illustrates a hidden case where a 'wall' masks what is happening. Sometimes all that can be seen is the mask. The more the homeopath buys into the same walls and defences as the patient, the harder it is to see through them or 'see over the wall' to view the case more clearly.

Patients are frequently unaware of symptoms of sensation and feeling, especially when they are 'somatised' into symptoms of function and structure. Revealing the sensation and feeling is one way of 'seeing into' the hidden case. The homeopath who is able to draw out the sensation and feeling by, for example, 'matching and enacting' (see Chapters 13, 23) may be able to unmask them. In the same way as a garage mechanic may detect early problems with a car,

---

CASE STUDY 26.2

Peter, age 54, a financial director, presented with marked hypertension. It was detected at an insurance medical and he is 'otherwise 100% well'. On investigation he is found to have early coronary artery disease. He works long hours and may be made redundant in the near future. He knows many people in this position. He remarried 5 years ago and does not see his first wife; he sees his children occasionally. He has no fears, has no temperature preference and eats what ever he is offered. He says there are no symptoms.

so a homeopath may detect illness before the patient is aware of it. This is one of the benefits of regular 'check ups' and is why the homeopath's role is as much to prevent more serious illness as to treat it when it's there. Good rapport, psychological awareness and perceptive case work is necessary to identify and treat these issues while they manifest as subtle changes of sensation and feeling – and before they present with functional disturbance and structural damage. Many patients benefit from improved long-term health and reduction of chronic illness when they have had homeopathic treatment over some time. This long-term benefit is often not assessed when evaluating the benefits of homeopathy (see Chapter 24).

Cultural Predisposition

The feelings and sensations that patients put up with, or are unconscious of, are often those prevalent in their family, community or culture. They do not stand out and are often not considered pathological until the disease is expressed in a functional or structural way. So, for example, in Peter's case the feeling of being 'put upon' was one that he assumed (possibly correctly but not healthily) many business executives felt and 'came with the territory'.

As the homeopath, if you unconsciously accept cultural norms you may find it hard to see when these are contributing to illness. For example, in patients with the 'C' type personality that are prone to cancer (see Chapter 17) there is a strong sense of duty and responsibility. If the homeopath unconsciously 'buys into' the same sense of duty and responsibility, they (like many others) will struggle to recognise it – perhaps until the structural changes of cancer are manifest. In different cultures the difficulty in expressing some symptoms and the prevalence of others (often particularly of sensation and feeling) is a form of cultural palliation, and 'susceptibility'. Understanding the culture that you and your patients are part of will often shed light on the one-sided and hidden illnesses you are likely to see.

The more people in a population suffer from a particular one-sided illness, the more it points to a cultural predisposition and suppression that individuals in the culture face. In our current Western culture, heart disease frequently relates to unresolved issues about relationship, control and power. The prevalence of cancer corresponds to issues around excessive growth, overburdening responsibility and duty. As homeopaths we can have a role in helping a culture, community or family to learn from the illnesses they are prone to, especially those of the one-sided/hidden type (see 'Herd immunity', Chapter 18).

Inherited Disease

While simple and even complex cases can be understood in terms of the symptom, personal susceptibility and suppression, the more confused and hidden cases need to have their cultural and inherited factors considered (see Chapter 28). One-sided illness is an issue not just for the patient but also their community, culture and generation. One view of hidden cases is that they represent illnesses incompletely dealt with in the parents' generation; conversely, how illness is treated in today's patients will determine the illnesses that are hidden in future generations.

There is a spectrum of inherited influence in patients' histories, ranging from their appearance through a slight predisposition to full blown congenital disease. The degree of influence correlates with how strongly miasmatic tendencies are expressed in the individual. They are most marked when structural, but can also manifest on the level of sensation and function. The less structural, the more reversible the predisposition is likely to be – and the more preventable and treatable inherited illness is. Some susceptibility is normal; each of us will have resistance to some illness at the expense of susceptibility to others.

Homeopathy, through the treatment of inherited susceptibility and miasms, along with the reduction of cultural suppression, has huge scope in preventing and minimising inherited diseases. Untreated inherited susceptibility will be passed on to future generations.

The Personal and Collective Unconscious

'In the time span of a century, after centuries of enquiry the concept of the unconscious psyche was realised and eventually established by these physicians. Although this vital realization has been made available to all, it has not yet been integrated into consciousness by the medical profession in general.'

A Maguire (2004)

In psychology, patterns of behaviour are explained through the idea of complexes and archetypes. The work of Jung, amongst others, provides the homeopath with a model for exploring the personal unconscious, so important in confused cases, and a way of understanding the collective unconscious, a large part of hidden cases. Understanding the remedies as containing or representing information that can be matched to the patient's personal and collective unconscious is an important part of working with otherwise confused and hidden cases.

Jung developed the idea of 'complexes' that are groups of ideas (or aspects of the individual) bound together by a single emotional charge. While the content of these complexes is often unconscious to the individual, they cause the individual, in different situations, to be susceptible to and experience specific feelings. If a homeopath is able to identify a particularly strong or unusual feeling or emotion in a patient, then it may reveal important aspects of the patient (complexes) that can be matched to remedies that cause a similar emotional charge. In this way complexes may be compared to themes running through a patient's case.

Figure 26.2 illustrates the patient's personal conscious as being informed by their personal unconscious, which in turn is informed by the collective unconscious. The patient's conscious self is what a patient perceives of themselves reflected through thoughts and symptoms. The personal unconscious is composed of a number of complexes and the emotional charge that goes with these is reflected in the feelings of the patient. The collective unconscious has a number of 'patterns' or archetypes that are common between different people. These archetypes are both influenced by different situations and influence the situations the individual seeks out or creates. The main themes (including the miasms) observed in the case represent fundamental patterns and relationships

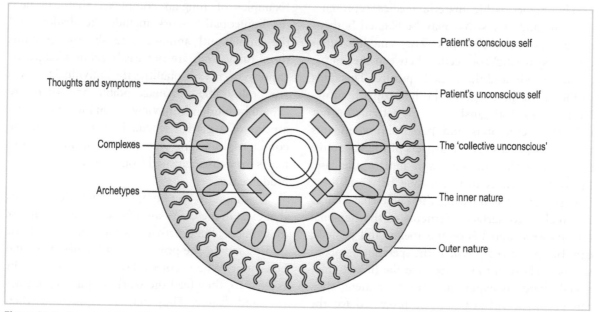

Figure 26.2 Representation of the patient's conscious self, informed by the personal and collective unconscious

between the archetypes and determine the shared behaviour and experiences of different races and cultures. It is interesting to consider how this is also reflected in the unconscious of non-human animals (see Chapter 18), with some themes running (like remedies) through all life forms, and all aspects of our 'world'.

Different cultures recognise and name archetypes differently. They may be represented as an aspect of the divine (Aphrodite), a star sign (Virgo), or as a type of behaviour (playboy, hero, healer, warrior etc). Each of us has our own different balance of complexes and archetypes. Complexes are likely to be more 'individual' and so approximate to a more individual remedy state. Archetypes often relate to states that are shared or found in particular groups of people or at particular times of life. This explains why some remedy states present at particular life stages or in particular situations patients find themselves in, such as the Pulsatilla and Calcaria child, the Sepia mother, or the Natrum muriaticum widow. For this reason understanding the 'typical' remedy states of different stages of life can help in understanding the remedies that are frequently helpful to patients at that stage of life and in recognising the truly unique qualities of a case.

The homeopathic materia medica represents concepts and states that may be likened both to complexes and archetypes. The remedies often offer a 'symbolic' connection between the source of the remedy and the remedy picture. This adds to the subtle language of the homeopath, allowing them to distinguish between patients on not only their conscious and personal unconscious symptoms but also those aspects of the collective unconscious that influence and 'initiate' the case. In confused cases distinguishing between these is important; by allowing the emotional charge and feeling to surface, elements of the personal unconscious, and hence the theme and remedy, can be perceived. When the personal unconscious is allowed to surface, and the linked emotional charge is experienced in the patient, then this emotion will not only be projected for the homeopath to detect but also cause a response in

the homeopath. The response in the homeopath reveals aspects of the collective unconscious that are important in the hidden case.

By exploring the emotional charge in the homeopath – and how this connects to the dominant archetypes in the patient – the patient's state and, indirectly, the remedy can be explored.

An individual's personal unconscious connects to and reflects the collective unconscious of which they are part. The more accurately the deepest inner state of the patient matches the collective unconscious, the better adjusted or more 'normal' they are considered. This 'normality' is in turn expressed in each culture's 'collective unconscious', through the myths, fables and fairy stories that are embedded in that culture. Frequently we can see remedy pictures run through these archetypes, e.g. the fairy princess (Phosphorous); the washerwoman (Sepia); the knight in shining armour (Aurum or Patina); Cinderella (Pulsatilla), etc. Some archetypes are more common in particular cultures and are represented by the polychrest remedies of that culture – these remedies are frequently indicated and touch many aspects of both the patient's case and the collective unconscious.

Psychological Complexes

Examples of Jungian complexes that can help the homeopath's work include the shadow and the anima and animus. The shadow contains those things that are not easily acknowledged or expressed – mainly qualities the individual believes are undesirable or unacceptable and therefore should be hidden from view. It can influence many aspects of a patient's behaviour and health; the conscious disguising or witholding of information needs to be distinguished from truly unconsciously hidden cases.

The anima is the complex of female qualities that exist in men. The animus is the male complex in women. They provide a valuable model for understanding the power and influence of sexual behaviour. When projected onto those the patient is close to, they feed the world of passion, attraction and dislike. They may be suppressed when the expression of a feeling is taboo, leading to sexual shame and guilt (given the historic cultural sexual repression, it is not a coincidence that two of the three core miasms are related to sexually transmitted disease). They may then connect to the shadow to be 'enacted' – leading to abhorrent sexual behaviour such as masochism and sadism.

Understanding the influences of a patient's personal and collective unconscious can greatly help in explaining patterns of behaviour and symptoms that would otherwise appear confused. Using psychological models that enable the homeopath to perceive what is otherwise masked is an important part of working with hidden cases.

Archetypes and Symbols

'It is not uncommon to find a "mirror that breaks, or a picture that falls, when a death occurs; or minor but unexplained breakages in a house where someone is passing through an emotional crisis".'

C Jung

Archetypes are often related to objects that have a 'symbolic connection' to the ideas they represent. To the homeopath these symbols can be intimately related to a patient's remedy state (objects, acts, thoughts, feelings or situations) and include the source material of the remedy itself. How the patient relates to these symbols, even (or especially) unconsciously, provides important information about the patient (and the remedy).

Some archetypes reflect qualities about how we experience, or operate in, the world. We can use these to communicate complex ideas about each other and ourselves – so we might talk about the 'angelic' child or the 'ratty' child. When patients enact these archetypes it is understandable that they generate feelings in us; recognising these can often reveal otherwise hidden aspects of a case.

Fundamental Essence

Some psychological complexes and archetypes are so dominant in a particular cultural group of patients that they represent an essence and a corresponding remedy that runs through many patients. For example, in England many patients internalise their grief, especially the sadness of loss – the so-called 'stiff upper lip'. Many patients present aspects of this essence and it is easy to see aspects of the remedies that have this theme, such as Natrum muriaticum. These remedies need to be particularly well known so that they are appropriately prescribed.

In any culture, family, stage of life, or even species in veterinary practice, understanding the common complexes and archetypes, essence and themes helps understand those confused and hidden cases. Many of the polychrests have well described fundamental essences with common pictures that present in different environments or stages of life, e.g. Sepia in downtrodden women or at 'hormonal' times. Learning these is an important part of deepening the homeopathic materia medica.

Some circumstances of life are more favourable to patients with particular complexes or archetypes. In the same way, in some situations a particular remedy type may function well. To be a successful popular musician will require a different remedy profile from being a librarian. Each remedy will fit a certain situation, but health requires the ability to function in changing environments. In some ways being in a particular situation 'brings out' the corresponding remedy (Cicchetti 1993).

REFLECTION POINT
- How might dreams of an object or symbol point to a remedy or group of remedies? After a homeopathic prescription how might dreams be affected? To what extent is a changing environment important to you; how is your vitality influenced by change and how does it relate to creativity? How much does studying different remedy pictures facilitate a good case history?
- In what way might Jungian complexes relate to different thematic and miasmatic states?
- How does an understanding of archetypes, complexes and symbols linked to 'the snake' help you explain or remember common features of the remedy Lachesis?

Summary

This chapter has brought us back to the central idea of there being different models of health through which the homeopath can view people. Homeopathy bridges many different systems of health and borrows from many empirical systems – but has resisted claiming its own diagnostic model. While conventional diagnosis partially serves the pathogenic and biological models of health, the ideas of psychotherapy inform the understanding of more complex and difficult cases. Psychotherapeutic concepts offer much towards an understanding of the holistic, holographic and relational models. Confused and hidden cases offer the greatest challenge to homeopaths and the rest of this section looks at these in more detail, building on the concepts introduced here – including the importance of situational, emotional and 'living' materia medica; and the role of the homeopath in managing cultural and inherited factors in individual and groups of patients.

References

Boyd W E 1923 Emanometer. Br Homoeopath J 13:55

Brien S, Prescott P, Owen D, Lewith G 2004 How do homeopaths make decisions? Homeopathy 93(3): 125–131

Capra F 1975 The tao of physics. Shambhala Publications, Boulder

Cicchetti J 2003 Dreams, symbols and homeopathy, archetypal dimensions of healing. North Atlantic Books, Berkeley

Goleman D 1995 Emotional intelligence. Bantam Books, New York

Jung C G 1979 Man and his symbols. Aldus Press, London

Kubler-Ross E 1970 On death and dying. Tavistock Press, London

Maguire A 2004 Skin disease: a message from the. Free Association Books, London

Saine A 2000 The method II. Lutra Services, Eindhoven

Bibliography

Carlyon J 2003 Understanding homeopathy. Helios Homeopathy, Tunbridge

Dossey L 1982 Space, time and medicine. Shambhala Publications, Boulder

Jung C 1970 Collected works. Routledge and Kegan Paul, London

Schadde A 1995 Intuition, and dream-work. Am Homeopath 2:100–104

Shore J 1999 The kingdoms in homeopathy: a practical technique for everyday consulting. J Am Inst Homeopath 92(4):236–242

Twentyman R 2004 Medicine, mythology and spirituality. Sophia Books, Forest Row

Whitmont E 1980 Psyche and substance, essays on homeopathy in the light of Jungian psychology. North Atlantic Books, Berkeley

CHAPTER TWENTY SEVEN

Emotional and Living Materia Medica

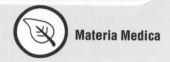

David Owen

'To know that what is impenetrable to us really exists, manifesting itself as the highest wisdom and the most radiant beauty which our dull faculties can comprehend only in the most primitive, symbolic form – this knowledge, this feeling, is at the centre of true religiousness.'

Albert Einstein

Introduction

Dealing with more difficult cases requires a deeper understanding of the patient, ourself and the remedies. Lack of understanding of any of these three factors can, alone or in combination, cause a case to be difficult. In this chapter we will continue to develop the way remedies may be understood. As deeper illness is treated it does, however, become increasingly difficult to view the materia medica in isolation. This chapter looks at how knowledge of the materia medica grows from experience and how remedies frequently relate to and follow each other. It explores the importance of the emotions and being 'sensitive' to the remedies to develop an emotional and 'living' materia medica; and discusses how this process relates to the homeopath's own development.

Ultimately the difficult case is just where the homeopath, patient and remedy do not fit neatly together. Confused cases have many layers, each partially visible, but if a remedy is found that covers all the parts that are visible the case starts to become less confused. A hidden case has important aspects masked, but if the homeopath is sensitive to other key information in the patient and

can match this closely to a remedy the case starts to become less hidden. Broadening our knowledge of a wider range of medicines and developing a deeper understanding of medicines we may already know helps 'make sense' of more cases. While an understanding of the miasmatic constellations and the family map of remedies are essential tools in this process, different homeopaths find a number of ways to build both the breadth and the depth of their materia medica knowledge.

Experience of observing closely when a remedy has acted is a major factor not only of consolidating knowledge but also extending your understanding. When this is shared and confirmed in the homeopathic community, as with the maps of the different kingdoms and families, it leads to a wisdom that the homeopathic profession as a whole can access. Ultimately the practice of homeopathy is not just a technique, or a skill in applying a technique, but a body of shared knowledge constantly evolving. This includes a relevant and effective materia medica that is dynamically related to the skills of consulting, analysing and managing patients. It reveals an interconnected and overlapping materia medica where not only are the unique qualities of individual remedies important, but also those features that run, like threads, through several related remedies. These insights are central to the differential diagnosis of remedies.

Just as emotion is an important component of a patient's case, so is the emotional picture of the remedies important. Appreciation of this requires an emotional intelligence and competence in the homeopath in order to develop an 'emotional materia medica'. The realisation and understanding that certain remedies can generate certain feelings in you is the basis of a 'living materia medica'. To move from the formal teaching of remedy types to the personal knowledge of remedies frequently involves a shift in your perspective, which requires support. If you choose to engage with this process I would advise you to identify a trainer, mentor or supervisor who can help.

Thematic Approaches to the Materia Medica

If all we have is a hammer then everything looks suspiciously like a nail.

The more remedies available and the more information available about each remedy, the greater the potential for the individualisation of each patient to their simillimum. Recording this information in a way that can easily be used and shared is a very real challenge to the homeopath. Seeing patterns to the proving, toxicological and clinical symptoms is a way of extending and remembering the large amounts of data about each remedy available to us. It also allows one symptom to reveal a pattern running through the whole picture. Some patterns or themes (see Chapters 21, 22) run like a thread through several remedies, shedding light on how one remedy is related to another. As much of this information comes from clinical experience some is better validated than others and there are issues about the reliability of the information. This is another area where personal experience and the ability to judge the reliability of your own observations are important.

As with all methodologies prescribing thematically depends on the information in the case and remedy being matched accurately. The greater the number of areas of the case and remedy that match, the more likely the remedy will act. If themes in the remedy cover several 'angles' or themes in a case, then it is more likely to be accurate. Figure 27.1 represents how different themes

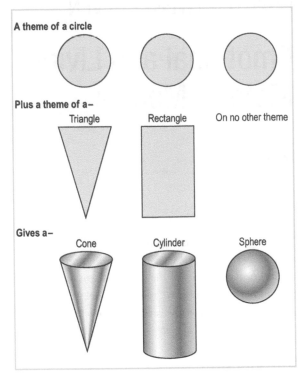

Figure 27.1   How themes build a picture

can build an overall picture. The theme of a circle might represent a cylinder, a cone or a sphere, as all resemble a circle from one view. From another angle or with the addition of another theme they are less likely to be confused. We might, for example, describe the essence of a cylinder as having the theme of both a sphere and a rectangle, the essence of a cone as having the theme of a circle and a triangle. When studying remedies thematically it is the combination of themes that make a remedy unique – what is not there is as important as what is there. For example, if a circle has no other theme it must have an essence of a sphere.

Themes in Remedies

'…*When a person presents a peculiar symptom, a dream, a modality, or an experience, clearly, intensely and spontaneously: find it directly in the materia medica or repertory; see the feeling it creates and connect it with the overall case; it is directly connected to the source of the remedy. Any marked thing can be understood in this way.'*

Rajan Sankaran

At different times in each patient different themes of a remedy are dominant and expressed. These can be thought of as representing the 'life cycle' of each remedy. In some patients the theme expressed most strongly will depend on the disease process, in others it relates to the stage of life they are in. A remedy may have several different themes that themselves are related and a patient may express these in different ways, e.g. the theme of heightened sensitivity in Causticum may first show as being impressionable, but later as worn out. Sepia (Box 27.1) illustrates the way different themes can express themselves differently at different times.

Building up the different themes and their expression in a remedy will benefit from having observed a number of different patients at different stages of life and with different illnesses. It also helps to know how related remedies express their themes – the picture may also be reflected in the way the source material of the remedy is expressed in myths, and cultural and other uses and applications. This information is added to information from provings, toxicology and clinical experience.

Changing Miasms

We have already touched on miasms and their deep connection to the themes that run through cases and remedies (see Chapters 14, 17, 22). Miasmatic states develop not only because of the diseases suffered and suppressed within a population but also due to other more subtle forms of suppression and changes in susceptibility in a population. It is why some cultures are more prone to certain miasms than others. So, for example, the Tubercular miasm relates not just to the suppression of tuberculosis (TB) but also to the prevalence of TB within cattle. This correlates with the major industrialisation of agriculture, where ceaselessly wandering animals have been confined to limited areas and subject to agricultural husbandry and breeding procedures that do not always have the animals' best interests foremost in consideration. The miasms each culture is particularly prone to will be reflected in all expressions of that culture and will change not just as disease patterns change but as that culture alters. In this way the art, music, architecture, values of a culture all reflect and inform the miasmatic status.

BOX 27.1

Sepia

A patient needing Sepia may at puberty be concerned about body image, after pregnancy have difficulty bonding to their child, at the menopause feel 'fagged' out.

For Sepia, made from the ink of the cuttlefish, the underlying issue is reconciling the male aspects of their nature. This is often more difficult for a woman, so Sepia is more commonly indicated in women. It can show itself in a number of ways including the 'worn out washer woman' who becomes a burnt-out and exhausted type and eventually survives because she becomes 'too tired to feel'.

Second, some Sepia patients escape into a complaining nature, where the world is never right but in which they are fatalistic and do nothing about it.

Third, and I believe we are seeing more of this now because of our cultural and social values, is the individual who seeks to survive by detaching themselves from many 'feminine' aspects of their lives and throwing themselves instead into a few other areas of life – whether business pursuits or very focused physical endeavours. This latter picture is often seen in women who deny their femininity and project themselves into activities that take them away from sexual intimacy or family life to succeed. It includes some individuals who find a 'community' or 'monastic life' eases the reconciliation of the anima or animus.

Different 'Maps' of the Remedies

Identifying themes that relate to the kingdoms, families and miasmatic groups to which remedies belong is one way of 'mapping the territory' of remedies (see Chapter 22). There are other ways, too, of identifying and ordering themes. Other systems and models by which we interpret and order our environment often inform these. Understanding the remedies as they relate to the different elements of fire, earth, water and air is one example. Another is the use of colour. Yet another uses the astrological zodiac or phases of the moon. In each of these models different themes can be found in the materia medica to order and structure the diverse information the remedies represent. A detailed evaluation of the pros and cons of these various ways of characterising remedies is beyond the scope of this book, but you are likely to come across them in your studies. Where these reveal or help you recall thematic connections they will usefully serve your own appreciation of and practical use of the materia medica in a thematic way. However, it is unrealistic and idealistic to expect one way of looking at and comparing themes in remedies to suit all homeopaths or every remedy ('Other relationships of remedies', see p. 377).

REFLECTION POINT

- Reflect on the connection and symmetry between illness, the environment and the theory of miasms. What new miasms do you see developing now or in the future? What remedies might these relate too?
- Reflect on a new or emerging illness. How does this illness relate to changes in the environment and/or even behaviour?

Emotional Materia Medica

Emotion is frequently connected to the expression of deep symptoms and can easily communicate itself to the receptive homeopath. Frequently a feeling in the patient – such as unexpressed anxiety, sadness, irritation, loneliness, jealousy, envy etc. – can point to an important symptom and theme in the patient. These feelings not only

help us to navigate through a case (revealing the patient's totality and constitution on a subtler, deeper level), but also add qualitatively and quantitatively to how different parts of a confused case can be connected through a theme or pattern.

Working emotionally, both with cases and with remedies, enables many facets of a big picture with a vast amount of information to very quickly be connected and communicated. The emotional materia medica seeks to understand the key important feelings in a remedy, often connected to important themes. ('Feelings' in this book is used to refer to 'the emotions', not the perception or sensation of touch – although the connection between the two reveals a coherence in patient and remedy between the sensations experienced and the emotional state. One informs the other.)

Often it is the strongest feelings that relate to the deepest themes – these are the feelings we see expressed time and again in the remedy's materia medica and in the cases of patients of these 'remedy types'. It is no coincidence that when a patient talks about how a symptom 'feels' they often move from describing a sensation with words like 'it feels like...', 'it is as if...' and 'its quality is...' to expressing an emotion with words like 'I feel...', 'I am...' (see Lucinda's case).

CASE STUDY 27.1

Lucinda, aged 34, presented with severe varicose veins and she had put up for years with severe symptoms of premenstrual tension and diarrhoea. Asked to describe how her veins felt, she said: 'they are irritating and feel as if they are going to explode'. She then went on to talk about her own irritability, anger and frustration, saying, 'I'm angry and ready to explode'. She put this down to her stressful job where over several years she had competed with colleagues for promotion. Despite her irritability she 'really wants to be liked'. When she said this she was near to tears. Inviting her to stay with her feelings she talked for the 'first time in ages' about her adoption and her feeling with her adoptive parents that 'they might send me back if I'm not good enough'. She says 'I'm fighting to stay on top of it all'. This started to make sense of her competitive nature and what might otherwise be a confused picture. She responded well to Nux Vomica, a remedy state often established in children when there is a relative absence of daily affection with a need to compete. It is a state that can easily be generated in those who feel they have to compete for affection – a not uncommon 'boarding school' remedy.

Reflective Approaches to the Living Materia Medica

Knowing yourself is the key to understanding the living materia medica.

'Living materia medica' is about 'how it feels to be this remedy'. It frequently involves the homeopath's reflection on their emotional reaction to a patient needing a particular remedy. It is generated in response to what is projected by the patient and/ or by what the homeopath projects reciprocally to the patient (see Chapter 23). It is especially useful when contrary feelings are expressed by the patient (confused) and when the patient finds it hard to reveal deeper aspects of the case (hidden).

As one might expect, there is a spectrum between the confused expression of the symptoms in one or two aspects of the case on one hand and the almost totally hidden case on the other. There is accordingly a spectrum of approaches one might use in confused and hidden cases. It is a simplification to say that all confused cases benefit from thematic prescribing and knowledge of the 'emotional' materia medica, or that all hidden cases benefit from relational prescribing relying on the 'living' materia medica picture. In practice both the emotional picture of the patient and the living reaction of the homeopath are intimately related and often perceived together – in the same way as both are intimately related to the totality, constitution, local symptoms and causes to which they are susceptible. Which is most useful is a mat-

ter of where the case is expressed, and how the homeopath is attuned to the case and their knowledge of the remedies. It is as if each new aspect of a remedy builds on the previous pictures you have learnt, moving from what has caused a remedy state, right through to what a remedy state can cause in you!

When we develop our living materia medica it is informed by our own sensitivity. How we feel will inform how we relate to a patient; each remedy will feel slightly different and generate a different feeling in us. However, for a particular homeopath the feeling we experience with a patient suiting a particular remedy is relatively consistent, as long as the homeopath's state is relatively consistent. To work this way reliably the homeopath needs to be aware of their own emotional make-up, which will be influenced by their own health.

Importance of the Homeopath's Own Well-Being

The patients whom homeopaths find hardest (usually the most confusing and hidden) are often mirrored in the remedies that are least well known or those we most need to study. This is true not just for the community of homeopaths and the remedies we need to develop but also for us individually. We will find it hardest to recognise the remedies that we are relatively blind to – these are likely to be the remedies we, personally and culturally, are most likely to need ourselves. Remember – there is a connection between you, the patients you attract and the culture that patients and you live in.

Perhaps in the same way as an Aurum (gold) patient will seek to keep gold or the equivalent as money and external markings of their value around them, we as homeopaths must be alert to the risk of dependency on what we receive through the projections of our patients. If we are unable to recognise cases they perhaps represent features of our own remedies.

The preparation and protection that allows us to be sensitive to the patient's remedy state is important. It includes being well; having sufficient time, good boundaries, support and supervision with difficult cases; and the ability to recognise the features that belong to the patient and those that belong to you.

Studying Emotional and Living Materia Medica

The teaching of materia medica is like breathing life into substances, bringing them alive.

Reading the materia medica introduces us at the simplest level to remedies and the sensations, feelings and signs that each might have. How you feel reading the remedy and reflecting on what 'life is like' for this patient type is an important part of knowing the remedy. When a remedy is well taught it brings to life aspects of the remedy, and can through the projection that takes place create a similar, if mild, state in the student. The emotional state generated is, in fact, the projected remedy state acting in the homeopath. When treating a patient in a remedy state it brings that state forward in the homeopath, as if the patient's remedy is 'proved' on us. If you spend enough time with a Sepia patient it will elicit first your reaction to Sepia qualities, and then start to set up Sepia qualities in you. This principle underlies how people 'rub off' on one another, how pets and owners, parents and children often grow in likeness and share qualities of the same (or closely related) remedies.

In addition to the keynotes, modalities, generals and mentals as reported in a variety of materia medicas, your own personal materia medica will include an awareness of the themes and emotional states that commonly occur in those remedies in different situations. It will give an idea of patients, friends or characters in books or films that suit this remedy, and how these make you feel, and will include your own clinical experience. It will be an evolving dynamic record of a personal 'living' materia medica.

Positive and Negative Features

As symptoms are usually presented as something the patient wants to be rid of, most materia medica are presented as the negative or unwanted symptoms. Each remedy picture also has an equally positive side. The ambition of Nux Vomica can be the seeking of approval and affection – and when

channelled in a balanced way can be very healthy for a business. The loyalty of the Aurum patient is second to none. The determination of Calcarea carbonica will carry through projects that would otherwise never be finished. While these features can all be problematic in some settings, in others they are strengths. These strengths are just as important in pointing to an indicated remedy, but are often not well represented in the materia medica. A living, personal materia medica looks at the jobs different remedies excel at, the sort of partner or parent they are, etc. Every remedy has positive attributes that compensate the negative and when treated these positive states are not lost but rather a better balance is achieved.

There are many examples of exciting and evocative writers revealing the themes of the remedy pictures. The challenge for us when we are privileged to work with these and difficult cases is to gain a greater personal insight not only to the case but also into the remedies and ourselves. With this personal development allied to a personal materia medica many confused cases become clearer and hidden cases more visible.

REFLECTION POINT

- Think of a remedy that you know well. What would it be like to live your life as that remedy, what sort of clothes would you like to buy, how would you socialise and work, and what would you do well and what sort of situations might trigger you becoming ill?
- Think of a remedy you find hard to recognise, learn or prescribe. What personal and/or cultural blind spots might this represent?

Related Remedies

Remedies do not act in isolation from the patient state or the homeopath's state. Remedies can be understood by understanding their relationship to each other.

Understanding how remedies relate to each other is an important part of the overall management of patients – especially when a series of remedies is necessary to help the patient to complete recovery, and to offer comparisons of remedies that should be considered in a differential diagnosis. Recognising the relationships of one remedy to another facilitates working with patients over a period of time, extending both the breadth and depth of materia medica. This is especially useful when working with differential diagnosis if a full remedy picture is not known. Given the absence of well documented information about the holographic and relational picture of remedies (especially less well known remedies) it is of particular importance when using thematic and reflective approaches to treatment. In the new and emerging materia medicas, looking at remedies in families, it is particularly helpful and compliments what we know of the remedies from provings and other sources.

Sometimes just considering the related remedies will raise angles to the case history or case analysis that might otherwise not have been thought of. Patients who are keen and ready to understand their own case better may find it helpful to read some materia medica themselves. Indeed, if used cautiously patients can make clear and helpful distinctions between remedies in their differential diagnosis and between related remedies.

When making a second prescription, if a remedy isn't a recognised complementary remedy but the indications for it are clear, then you should not hold back from prescribing it. If it is listed as an antidote or inimical remedy then it may cause you to take a second look at the indications for it. Remedy relationships can be used as one of the features pointing towards or away from the simillimum – but not as a sole pointer to a prescription (Rehman 2004).

Many remedy relationships have been confirmed clinically over time; some of the different relationships are described below. Some materia medicas give lists of remedies that follow one another well, and other relationships of remedies as part of the materia medica (Gibson Miller 1993). Some repertories list the relationship of remedies – using these in case analyses can provide relative inclusion and exclusion information. Boenninghausen drew up a list of remedy affinities, which he also referred to as concordances.

Remedies that Follow Well

Homeopaths have historically noted how some remedies follow others frequently and effectively; they perhaps reflect the common levels of frequent pictures observed in cases. This can help when deciding between several partially indicated remedies. At all follow-up consultations new observations about the patient, and any partial obstacle to cure, must be taken into account before looking at a new remedy. It is dangerous to use 'follows well' as a short cut, because although a related remedy might be partially indicated there may well be others that are better suited.

Most lists of remedies that follow well are lists of remedies that follow the main remedy well. But in some materia medicas, for example Clarke's, there is a list of remedies that the named remedy will frequently follow. Often the remedies in both categories are the same, and looking at the themes in the different remedies can give insight into a theme running through a remedy picture. Just to confuse matters, however, remedies that follow well sometimes also appear in the antidoting remedy sections. But it is possible for a remedy in one situation to complete the cure that another remedy has begun, while in another situation the same remedy might antidote the first remedy.

Complementary Remedies

A subset of those remedies that follow well will be directly complementary to the action of the previously acted or partially acted remedy. Sometimes these are called 'synergistic', as using one remedy after the other gives a better effect than using either remedy on its own. Frequently complementary remedies are deeper acting remedies that are better known, so it may just be that they can be matched at a deeper level. In many cases complementary remedies are the acute or chronic of each other. For example, Natrum muriaticum is complementary to Bryonia; it will often complete the action and deal with the underlying chronic predisposition to the acute conditions that Bryonia cases present. It does not mean that all acute Bryonia cases will have an underlying state that fits one of the complementary remedies; rather, the complementary remedies are slightly more likely to be needed and should be considered when looking at the chronic treatment of a Bryonia state, although, of course, Bryonia might be the remedy that fits the case at the deepest level, or that represents the most fundamental layer. One remedy may have more than one acute and chronic complement, e.g. Natrum muriaticum is also a 'chronic' of Ignatia and of Apis mel.

Sometimes complementary remedies share similar symptomatology. In confused and hidden cases where the deeper aspects of the case are not clear, the complementary remedies can hint at or point towards a possible underlying state of the patient, and allow this to be explored.

When reading the materia medica of complementary remedies and those that follow well, it is often possible to identify shared themes or patterns that run through the related remedies. It is common for these shared patterns also to run through botanical, mineral or zoological families of remedies, and to run through other remedies related to the same miasm. Identifying the miasmatic tendencies in a case can help point towards complementary and remedies that follow well. For example, in an allergic case that fitted Phosphorous partially, there were several traits of the tubercular miasm; when other remedies in the tubercular miasm were considered a stronger case for Silica could be made.

Collaterals

Collaterals are remedies that have a similar picture but are not necessarily complementary or following well, such as Mercurius and Kali iodatum, Cina and Chamomilla. These comparisons can, however, be useful in the differential diagnosis of cases (Sankaran 1975). They sometimes include remedies belonging to the same family (Arnica and Bellis perennis) or one remedy source containing high levels of another (Colocynthis and Magnesia phosphorica or Sepia having Phosphorous and Sulphur in it).

For some remedies there are collateral relationships between the three different kingdoms: animal, vegetable or mineral – sometimes referred to as 'analogues', e.g. Ignatia as the plant analogue of Natrum muriaticum, Aluminium as the mineral analogue of Lycopodium. Interestingly, the mineral analysis of Lycopodium shows it as containing high levels of Aluminium. It is worth reflecting on the overlap of themes between the kingdoms – that in one way all plant remedies will express part of the picture of their constituent minerals, and that all animal remedies reflect the plants they or their prey have eaten.

Certainly it is possible to see a simple theme or axis running through remedies made from the elements and to gradually discover more different but interconnecting themes in the salts, plants and animals. In confused cases, as the remedy picture becomes clearer the number of axes or themes running through the case often reduce, at times correlating with the remedy moving from animal to plant, to mineral salts, to elemental remedies. This might be behind Hahnemann's observation that many cases end up needing Sulphur.

Cycles of Remedies

There is often a natural cycle of states that people will flow through in different situations, one naturally flowing into another. Related remedies can reflect this cycle. So in grieving Ignatia often precedes Staphisagria, which precedes Natrum muriaticum – correlating to the stages of denial, anger and sadness in the grieving process. Some cases move through these cycles a number of times, giving a spiral or helical relationship of remedies. It is important to understand these remedy relationships as they tell us about the way cases often unfold. One of the ways we can make sense of complex and hidden cases is through an observation of the spiral of symptoms that manifest over a long period of time.

Few homeopaths would use this cycle or order in the absence of clear indications, or hesitate to go against the order in the presence of clear indications to the contrary. They can, however, be useful both to illustrate how themes often develop and unfold in patients (and therefore need to be reversed), and also as pointers to how several remedies are often indicated as part of a curative process. Examples of these cycles of remedies are given in Box 27.2.

Frequently Observed Cycles of Remedies
- Calc., Lyc., Sulph
- Nux-v., Sep., Psor.
- Bell., Merc., Hep.
- All-c., Phos., Sul.
- Puls., Sil., Fl-ac.
- Sulph., Sars., Sep.
- Caust., Coloc., Staph.
- Ars., Thuj., Tarent
- Berb., Nux-v., Sars.
- Ign., Nat-m., Sep.
- Bell., Nux-v., Sars.
- Acon., Spong., Hep.

Antidotes

Remedies may be antidoted by other remedies (see Chapters 15, 16). It is possible that the benefits of one remedy will be partially lost if followed by an antidoting remedy. Others suggest that using a homeopathic antidote for an aggravation caused by a remedy can resolve the aggravation without stopping the healing process (see Chapter 15). My experience is that if a deeper picture is revealed after one remedy, the next remedy can be given with no worry about antidoting. If on the other hand a remedy acts partially but no deeper picture is seen, then prescribing on the remaining symptoms (if just as superficial as those treated by the previous remedy) it is likely, if the second remedy acts, to lead to a loss of the partial response to the previous remedy. Knowing the antidotes to a remedy reinforces the need to make sure a follow-up prescription is only given when a deeper picture is obtained. Some remedies have many reported antidotes, others only few.

Incompatible or Inimical Remedies

Incompatible or inimical remedies are those that are recommended not to be prescribed in succession. However, it is quite possible to see a patient at follow-up or to re-take a case and to see a remedy that previously was not visible. In this case, knowing that it was inimical to a previously indi-

cated remedy would not be a contraindication. Prescribing an incompatible or inimical remedy at the same level as a previous remedy can cause the case to become more confused and hidden. Take the example of an eczema case where Apis mel has acted partially. If Rhus toxicodendron is then used when the case is no clearer at a deeper level, the Apis symptoms often return or the case generally gets more confused. There are many other suggested incompatible or inimical remedies observed by different authors, but they should not stop a prescription if a remedy picture is clear and seen deeply. If, however, two incompatible or inimical remedies are equally indicated in a case, often a deeper level of understanding will reveal which of them is best suited, or another layer of the case may be seen pointing to a different remedy.

Other Relationships of Remedies

There are, of course, many other ways of noting and using remedy relationships in prescribing. Different homeopaths and different schools of homeopathy have their favourites. Some will cross reference to other health care systems (e.g. the five element theory), others to ways of understanding the body (e.g. the chakras). Each in their own way is an attempt to see the patterns in an otherwise difficult case and to see relationships between remedies and sometimes indicate other remedies that would otherwise not be considered. These systems are outside the scope of this text, although you are advised to look into some of them as they can provide helpful pointers and management approaches, particularly in confused and hidden cases. One such system is the bowel nosodes that I have found useful in managing cases where several remedies appear equally indicated or where there is a lack of reliable symptoms (Paterson 1950).

New Remedies

As you seek to work with more confused and hidden cases you will discover a tension between expanding the breadth of your materia medica by learning new remedies and exploring in greater depth the remedies you already know. Both are important and can be combined – but the exact balance is a matter of individual choice and may well evolve and change during your career.

Reframing the 'Living Materia Medica'

'We don't do homeopathy, but we co-operate with the process of homeopathy.'

Anne Clover

As patients' understanding of 'the self' has evolved, so too have their expectations about health. Homeopathy has reacted to this by deepening the way we understand our remedies through the development of holographic and relational models of health. In the art of homeopathy while remedies might traditionally have been thought of as the colours on the homeopath's palette, they can also now be thought of as a 'living installation'. The voice, actions, even the intentions of the artist while at work, influence how the art is conveyed and seen. Seeing the remedies as part of a living, evolving materia medica is one of the greatest tools you have to counter the relatively limited and fixed perspective that causes cases to appear difficult or even incurable when they are just many layered (confused) or hard to see (masked and hidden).

What Can Be a Remedy?

In the same way as no two patients are identical, so no two patients will present exactly the same need. If we take everything in the universe as represented by a point, then the information of that point is unique. Possibly each point could be a remedy. For example, a remedy may at a subtle level be influenced not just by its plant, animal or mineral origin but also by where it was obtained, the time it was collected, perhaps even the intention of those who prepared it. As remedies are understood as more energetic than matter so it becomes easier to recognise how remedies may be made from electricity, moonlight, colours or sounds – the so-called imponderables. These present challenges of standardisation and have not always been proved fully, but remedies such as

that made from magnetism have been used since the time of Hahnemann.

The extension of the materia medica into new remedies and the understanding of old remedies in new ways is connected to our ability to use this information. The extension of the homeopathic art from the grossest causes and symptoms into the deepest aspects of a patient's psyche requires an understanding of the materia medica from the most material of effects to the subtlest influences.

Sometimes new remedies bring with them an appreciation of subtle points of difference in established remedies that would not be distinguished otherwise. For example the remedy Lac caninum from dog's milk has been used for many years. Proving of other animal milks has revealed important and subtle differences between these remedy pictures and provided a new comprehension of the thematic and reflective aspects of Lac caninum.

New remedies often fill important gaps in the materia medica. For example, when we consider grief remedies there appears a group of patients that seem to be grieving something internal, something that may never have happened externally to them. Ignatia helps this grief but it may only seem to act at a superficial level. The proving of Cygnus olor, the swan, has shown a remedy that can often act in this type of grief much more deeply.

How Information on New Remedies Is Obtained

The student homeopath should be aware that not all sources of information about remedies are equivalent. Some authors, for example, recount dream provings or meditative provings (see Chapter 2). Some include the effect of the proving on those around the prover. This innovative type of proving is regarded with suspicion by more traditional homeopaths, but as long as the source of the information is given for any proving data, the practitioner can decide on its usefulness and reliability. Some repertories and materia medica now indicate the origin of each piece of information.

If we return to the idea of illness (or remedy state) as lacking certain information (see Chapter

6) then patients may either seek to manipulate their situation in a certain way, so they can function in it with the information they have or seek to draw the information to themselves in some way. This may be why patients are drawn to certain plants, minerals and animals that relate to their remedy – the Aurum case drawn to gold, the Sepia patient who may love the colour sepia, the Coffea patient craving coffee. As we broaden our understanding of the remedies we begin to recognise that all the information in a remedy picture can be interpreted as a pattern or essence – every aspect of the environment that a patient in a remedy state lives in reflects something of the remedy state. This tradition of seeing a connection between our environment and the remedies we might need runs through many indigenous medical systems, from herbal cures to shamanic healing. The greater the affinity for that substance in ourselves or in our culture, the more likely it is to be useful as a remedy.

Remedy and What Is Absent

By considering susceptibility to illness as being similar to lacking certain information, then we can see health as being the presence of all the necessary information. A remedy state can therefore be thought of as having all the information 'minus' that which is lacking. I invite you to consider that a remedy state might be helpfully understood as, on a subtle level, having all the other remedies except for the remedy needed. This is the same as when we see a colour – what in fact we are seeing is the visual spectrum without that colour (the colour is actually absorbed and all the other wavelengths reflected). Maybe in the same way as when we see the colour red we see all the other colours because red has been absorbed, when we see the remedy Pulsatilla it is because Pulsatilla is held in the patient and we are seeing everything but the Pulsatilla-ness.

Health, then, is a combination of the information from all the remedies necessary in a particular situation. This would be consistent with the idea that when we recognise something in others it is because there is some recognition of it in ourselves. We cannot see in others what we cannot recognise in ourselves. In practice, we recognise in patients remedy states that we in some way know ourselves. When we study we merely connect to what is already inside us, we rediscover things. Hence the feeling of discovery mingled with familiarity when learning new remedies – but also the potential for inaccurate perceptions if working with remedy states we are unconscious or unfamiliar with.

If we consistently find it hard to recognise a remedy, then we should reflect on what we may not be seeing in ourselves. These 'blind spots' can often be detected when sharing difficult cases with colleagues and provide opportunities for the homeopath to develop. In some ways it is possible to see the difficult patient as representing something the homeopath needs to recognise, and the same difficulty may be drawn to you repeatedly until it is recognised.

Remedies as Vectors

One way to think about the remedies is as an information vector, each with their own uniqueness represented by the ability to move a case a certain distance in a particular direction. Figure 27.2(a) illustrates a remedy as a vector that is capable of

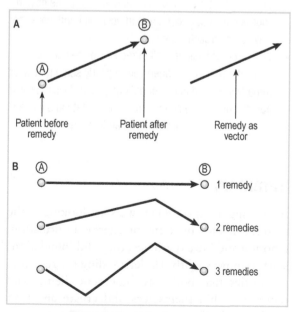

Figure 27.2 Remedies as vectors

'moving' a patient from state A to state B. Figure 27.2(b) illustrates how one, two or three vectors might combine in moving a patient in a particular direction for a particular distance, from A to B.

A further development of this model is that the vector representing a remedy may differ depending on the potency. In a higher potency the vector might be thought of as longer and thinner (needing to be more accurate), in a low potency as shorter and broader (with a wider range of action). High potencies are sometimes thought of as 'rifle shots' compared to the 'shot gun' of a low potency. Lower potencies may also need repeating several times to 'go as far' as a single high potency remedy.

REFLECTION POINT

- What is the most useful way for you to develop your knowledge of emotional and living materia medica? What can you do to extend your theoretical knowledge of the remedies so that you start to understand how those remedy types might relate to you and how they make you feel?
- Reflect again on how remedies can bring out a remedy state in you when you are taught them and study them (remember that in a healthy state we might contain all the remedies). How does studying the remedies help in your personal development and how will it influence the way you approach cases?
- When you consistently fail to recognise the need for a particular remedy, or when you regularly see a particular remedy indicated in lots of patients, what does it tell you about your relationship to that remedy state and indeed your own remedy? How will you address this?

Summary

As we might expect when we start looking at the materia medica in terms of energy, information, emotion and life experience, the solid foundations start to move slightly. Understanding the remedies as entities that both have coherent themes and patterns within themselves and create an effect on those who perceive them is part of developing an emotional and living materia medica. That, in turn, makes the remedies more personal. It raises many interesting and important questions for us and invites a reinvestigation of basic homeopathic principles.

Remedies can have both a material effect and a subtle effect – understanding the remedies in the different models of health can help in separating, in understanding and in learning their broadest picture. Of course, in one way this separation is artificial and each aspect of a remedy manifest in one model of health parallels the others.

It is an exciting time to be studying homeopathy and materia medica, so we must be aware of how our own state will colour our objectivity. There are many ways of developing and extending your understanding to help you explore and extend the materia medica – not only for your own practice but also for the profession of homeopathy as a whole.

Working with confused and hidden cases helps in seeing the remedies as dynamic, feeling and 'living' entities. Supervised clinical practice and sitting in with experienced homeopaths are important experiences for developing your knowledge; as is your gradual introduction to managing increasingly confused and hidden cases.

By knowing the remedies in more detail and in a broader range, it is surprising how often a difficult case that would otherwise be confused or hidden reveals itself simply as a multi-layered case. If one layer is taken at a time the confusion in the eyes of the beholder can diminish. When you can perceive the case sensitively, and incorporate your own reaction to the patient as a living materia medica, the hidden case can be unveiled. Understanding our materia medica in new ways opens up a case that would otherwise be impossible to treat – and would in the past have been called incurable.

References

Gibson Miller R 1993 Relationships of remedies. Homoeopathic Publishing Company, London

Paterson E 1950 The bowel nosodes. Br Homoeopath J XL No3 July

Rehman A 2004 Encyclopaedia of remedy relationships in homeopathy. Thieme, Stuttgart

Sankaran P 1975 The clinical relationship of homeopathic remedies. Homoeopathic Medical Publishers, Bombay

Bibliography

Bailey P M 1995 Homeopathic psychology. North Atlantic Books, Berkeley

Clover A 1990 Homeopathy reconsidered – a new look at Hahnemann's Organon. Victor Gollanz, London

Coulter C R 1986 Portraits of homeopathic medicines, vols I and II. North Atlantic Books, Berkeley

Henrrick N 1998 Animal mind, human voices. Hahnemann Clinic Publishing, Nevada City

Sankaran R 2002 An insight into plants, vol I and II. Homoeopathic Medical Publishers, Mumbai

Scholten J 1993 Homeopathy and minerals. Stichting, Alonnissos, Utrecht

Scholten J 1996 Homeopathy and the elements. Stichting, Alonnissos, Utrecht

Shore J 2004 Birds: homeopathic remedies from the avian realm. Homeopathy West, Berkeley

Vithoulkas G 1980 The science of homeopathy. Grove Press, New York

Vithoulkas G 1988 Essence of materia medica (Indian edition). B Jain, New Delhi

Zaren A 1993, 1994 Core elements of the materia medica of the mind. Ulrich Burgdorf Publishing, Gottingen

CHAPTER TWENTY EIGHT

Understanding the Dynamic of Confused and Hidden Cases

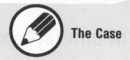

David Owen

'The meeting of two personalities is like the contact of two chemical substances: if there is any reaction, both are transformed.'

C G Jung

Introduction

Complex cases that do not heal (especially if the cause is maintained or symptoms suppressed) gradually become more deep-seated. As the case goes deeper it often appears more confused. As less and less reliable and individualising information is expressed it becomes hidden. As the case is internalised it moves into the deepest realm of the individual, leading eventually to functional and structural symptoms. If, in turn, the symptoms are suppressed, then new susceptibility patterns are set up – leading eventually to hereditary predisposition in subsequent generations (see Chapters 15, 17).

Patients view and shape their environment according to their state, including the treatment and even the homeopath they choose. Every aspect of the patient's life situation reflects something of them. In any family, community, tribe or race the values and behaviours projected by its members will determine what that group considers normal. From this perspective of normality those illnesses that have contributed most to the unconscious norms will be least apparent and most hidden. When the actual case is confused or hidden from the homeopath then we must look at our patients in new ways to notice such things and work with their cases.

What is not said becomes more important, as does the influence of the patient's family, community and culture. The limitations of our perception due to our own bias and attitudes shape what we perceive and how clearly we see the patient (see Chapter 23). Understanding ourselves is a prerequisite to understanding our patients. Confused and hidden cases provide the homeopath with the opportunity to understand the case (and ourselves) in a dynamic way. This explains the patient in terms of themes, layers and projection – where what happens in one area of the case 'holographically' reveals the underlying patterns in the case and where what is projected, reflects what is masked.

Exploring the deeper aspects of patients' cases in this way leads naturally to an exploration of our own nature. The influence of what is projected on to you, and those things you are unconscious of in yourself, will colour what you see and how you act. How we manage ourselves and our own health is vital to working well and sustainably. Your ongoing education, support and development opportunities are all vital to working competently and successfully (see Chapter 25). While your early training will be focused predominately on your personal knowledge and skills (and attitudes), as you start managing more difficult cases the context in which you practice becomes increasingly important. As we take up a place alongside others working with the health of the individual, and have insights to share and learn from in the communities we serve, so the organisational structures we operate in and the professional bodies we belong to become increasingly important.

The Difficult Case

'I have often been asked to prescribe in cases where the symptomatology was beautifully presented but not an idea could be drawn from it to betray the state of the patient ... The case is incurable until it can be taken in a manner to present what is true of the patient.'

J Kent, *Lesser Writings*

In an ideal world all homeopaths would be able to decode the pattern of illness in all cases. The reality is that some homeopaths see some cases more clearly than others and what is difficult to treat in one approach is easier with another. Any cases will be difficult if you do not know the remedy or how to find it, and these cases will present your greatest challenges and biggest opportunities. Of course what can start out seeming to be a simple or complex case may transpire, as new information emerges or as the case changes, to be a confused or hidden case. The experienced homeopath will move between different models of health to understand the case and seamlessly 'blend' approaches to treatment and methods of prescribing to find the simillimum. But it is important to recognise that while each prescription represents a point in the treatment process that may be curative in practice, more difficult cases need to be understood and allowed to reveal themselves over time – and may need a sequence of remedies that each move the case in a healing direction.

If we know just a few common remedies, then any cases that present outside the pattern of these remedies will be difficult. Expanding your knowledge of the materia medica is the starting point for working with those cases where the picture and its evolution are perfectly clear, but you just do not know the corresponding remedy picture. When there is no confusion or 'hidden-ness' but you just do not know the materia medica needed then it is just a matter of studying harder. In patients where the case history has been incompletely taken, then it is just a matter of re-taking the case. When you are not able to tell several possible similar remedies apart, it is just a matter of giving the analyses more time and comparing the differential materia medicas. In many cases that at first appear challenging, it is just a matter of lack of materia medica knowledge, incomplete case-taking or inaccurate case analyses.

In other cases that appear difficult it is because the homeopath's or patient's expectations are unrealistic. You may just be working outside of your competence zone. A complex case may just take time to respond or have a number of levels of symptoms that each need treating in turn. These are fundamentally different from confused cases, where what is happening in the different layers of the case distorts what can be seen, and from hidden cases, where much of the case exists in the unconscious. Now and again after proving or learning new remedies it is possible to see what would otherwise be confused cases as just complex ones, where a single totality encompasses all of the otherwise confusing layers in the case.

When there are several diverse symptoms that fit no clear totality, then it is often possible to see a theme or pattern running through the symptoms that reveal several layers of the case. It may be necessary to treat these layers one at a time, allowing the patient to gradually get more in touch with the deeper aspects. Often it is through enquiring about a patient's sensory aspect of a symptom that the patient's emotional feelings and the deepest patterns in the case are revealed, as Beryl's case illustrates (Case Study 28.1).

Ironically, once the deepest theme running through a confused case is seen, or what is being projected in a hidden case is revealed, the case is no longer so confused or hidden – although it may take some time to clear completely. Put simply, the confused and hidden case is an internalisation of the illness – the initial job of the homeopath is to let it surface. This sometimes requires a cautious reduction of the suppressive or palliative treatment to see what symptoms emerge. While there is a continuum between the complex, confused and hidden case, it is helpful to think of them in different ways as they each require a slightly different orientation to the case and a slightly different focus of the treatment. However, the factors relevant to each impinge on the other and it is helpful to build up your competence gradually, dealing with increasingly confused and hidden cases as you become more experienced.

Untangling the Confused Case

Understanding the patient must come before deciding the remedy.

In confused cases there are many symptoms that have no clear pattern or appear to lack a clear hierarchy. Sometimes the different symptoms will include contradictory qualities and modalities – in

> ### CASE STUDY 28.1
> Beryl, age 68, presented with difficulty sleeping, general tiredness, multiple joint pains and increasing anxiety since her hip replacement (after she had tripped on an uneven pavement and fractured the hip) 6 years previously. She had been on sleeping pills for 6 years. She had a lot of pain that necessitated walking with a stick and was using regular anti-inflammatories that gave her indigestion, that was in turn being treated with drugs. When asked to describe the pain she was unable to describe it accurately – as if she was reluctant to get in touch with it. She responded initially to Aconite 30 and Valerian tincture that helped her anxiety and sleeping.
>
> At follow-up she was able to reduce her sleeping pills. At a subsequent visit, when she was invited to think about the sensation and feeling in her leg, she described it as feeling like the leg might break again at any time, 'as if it were made of glass'. She became fearful while talking and said that since her fall she had been 'worried about everything', 'obsessive about the smallest thing'. Silica was prescribed cautiously (due to its reputation for exuding foreign bodies); over several months her symptoms and general health improved and she reduced her drug treatment.

the same way as several different sounds made at the same time create a confused noise or one sound is 'drowned out'. If the sound can be understood as coming from several different individuals or instruments, then a pattern behind the confusion may be seen and heard. In a confused case there are several levels of symptoms and layers of themes that need to be teased out. Recognising these different layers and levels is like recognising the different instruments and the different strands (harmonic motifs) that might run through an orchestral piece. If you can only recognise one instrument or strand, appreciation of the music will be more difficult.

Occasionally one remedy that fits a particular theme will cure the case and go straight to the centre. Initially each layer may appear unrelated, but a carefully taken case can sometimes reveal an obvious and clear pattern. In looking for 'the centre of the case' homeopaths aim to get to the heart of the matter – the fundamental source of the disturbance in each individual patient. In confused cases the centre of the case may just not be visible but the intention is still to perceive the case as deeply as possible. What may appear at one consultation as the centre of the case may, in fact, be covering a deeper level of disturbance. During a period of treatment things that were initially unconscious or not apparent at all may surface.

Themes are expressed and noticed in a number of ways. They may run through the case as specific or similar words, phrases, movements or sounds that the patient uses a great deal. For example, in a case requiring the remedy Secale (from a mould), the words blast, stink and rotten appear. A Phosphorous patient might use visual, insightful and 'sensitive' words and expressions. These themes are increasingly represented in the thematic materia medicas (see Chapters 22, 27) and emerging from searching the materia medica, made easier by computers (see Chapter 19) and from clinical experience. As more homeopaths work this way so the detail in the remedy, and case pictures that can be used this way, are increasingly being recorded. As little known remedies become better known, so we find that they do, in fact, cover many cases in which we would otherwise be unable to see a simillimum.

The 'Common Thread'

In the holographic model of health every aspect of the patient and their interactions tells us something of their real nature. The homeopath is part of the tapestry on which the patient plays out and projects their themes. The pattern underlying the themes represents a thread that connects the themes, but also can be thought of as a connection between the internal themes and every part of a person's external life. It is these we are referring to when we talk of 'cutting the ties', 'no strings attached' and being 'tied down'. The themes can be thought of as having at least two threads, both a unique sensation (feeling or essence) and also a 'verb' or 'pace' (order or mode). When working thematically (the level of the vital sensation in Sankaran's hierarchy see page 69 and Chapter 22) we match the case to the materia medica not just on the qualities of the sensation but also the order or pace with which it is expressed. These two qualities reflect the two axis of family and miasm used for classification of remedies in Chapter 22. Sensation and emotional feelings are like two sides of the same thing. As the sensation becomes more vital to the patient so the emotional feeling connected with it and released when discussing it becomes more central to the case. As the symptoms sink into the more functional and structural aspects of the case, so the sensations become more difficult to elucidate. At the same time the emotional feelings become more ingrained and projected by the patient, offering opportunities to perceive the case. As this happens patients increasingly projecting their symptoms onto their world including the homeopath causing greater and greater transference and counter-transference. Generally as cases get more deep-seated so understanding the feeling and the projection gets more important.

Periodic Disease and Symptoms

Some confused cases are due to periodic symptoms, where symptoms come and go depending on the situation the patient is in at the time. This relationship between the situation and the patient's symptoms is vital to understanding confused cases. For example, someone who is expansive will be fine while they can continue to expand and flow in their life, but if they are in a contracted or constrained life situation, perhaps from poverty, then they will get ill. Here the 'activation from poverty' is an important symptom. Someone who is very self-contained will be fine while they are in an environment that allows them to remain sheltered and protected, but when they are vulnerable or required to be expansive they may get ill – so they may have aggravation from or fear of crowds. Due to the speed at which patients' lives can change, symptoms can be confused because patients may move rapidly, and quite profoundly, from one situation to another.

Part of managing these cases is to gather information about how they function in different situations. For a patient who avoids a certain situation (palliation) that would otherwise cause symptoms, the homeopath can invite the patient to imagine they are in that situation. For example, a patient with a fear of heights could be asked to imagine they are in a high place and to explore how that feels both as a sensation and an emotion. Taking the complex case is both about establishing the deepest themes and about those that run most broadly. Hence we talk of layers that intertwine through a confused case, rather than merely levels of symptoms (see Chapter 6).

Suppression

The more suppression there has been, the more layers there are likely to be – and the more confused the case is likely to be. There is a significant difference between taking the case of a child who manifests a chronic symptom and has had no suppressive treatment compared with one who has had much suppressive treatment. Equally, there is much difference between treating chronic symptoms in someone with a healthy, balanced family history, compared with someone with strong miasmatic taints.

Frequently those symptoms and syndromes that have received the least suppressive treatment give the least confused picture. This is why in patients presenting physical symptoms that have been treated allopathically or antipathically it is often in the psychological sphere that the case is clearest (including the emotional feeling). For those presenting psychologically and who have been suppressed by psychiatric drugs the physical symptoms may be the clearest indicator (including the physical feeling or sensation). Inviting the patient to discuss symptoms in areas of the case that 'do not bother' them often requires a greater degree of explanation and an openness to see the broader implications of homeopathic treatment – as does recognising the need to sometimes reduce drug treatments to establish a clear picture.

Deepening the Case

'A sigh might tell you more about the deeper aspects of the patient (and the patients willingness to go deeper) than any words.'

The importance of good rapport and empathy, allowing the case to be discussed at a greater depth, has already been discussed but presents particular challenges in confused and hidden cases (see Chapters 13, 25)

As the carer demonstrates their ability to 'hold' the patient's distress and symptoms, so more is able to surface – sometimes including problems and symptoms the patient did not initially intend to reveal, or indeed was not conscious of. If empathy is high, then the patient is more likely to feel able to both 'get in touch with' and share distressing and deep-seated symptoms. This revealing of deeper information may be enough to clarify a confused case. While this deepening of the case can shed light and clarify a confused case, it can also sometimes lead to deeper aspects emerging that seem paradoxical and can make a case more confused. As cases unfold we may therefore see confused cases becoming clearer and complex cases appearing to become confused. A patient might at different times move through the different types of case – even moving backwards and forwards as deeper issues are revealed and healing at different levels takes place.

For example, a patient may present with a simple case of diarrhoea, but a deeper more complex case with allergies, familial susceptibility and

other symptoms may emerge in the consultation. A choice then has to be made, with the patient, on the focus of the case and treatment. Initial treatment might focus on the diarrhoea, or on the totality, or explore the themes in the case that perhaps connect with deeper issues the patient wants help with. If a deeper picture is to be explored the case may need to be re-taken. The hope is that after treatment the patient will have undergone transformative healing at a much deeper level than they ever intended when they first sought help for their diarrhoea.

Retaking the Case

We only understand the remedies as well as we understand our patients, and vice-versa.

Each model of health presents a slightly different view of the optimum consultation. Seeking the themes and sensations in a case or even recognising and processing the projections going on will require a different focus from seeking the 'cause' or 'presenting symptom', or even the 'totality' and its hierarchy. As the case unfolds within a consultation, or at different consultations, choices about where it is going and on what it is focusing are constantly taking place in the homeopath and patient. Many of these flow naturally, some (e.g. whether the case needs to be re-taken) are more conscious decisions.

Re-taking the case allows new information to emerge, and may bring out qualitatively different information from the previous case. Moving from one model of health to another when seeking to understand a case can mean changing and blending different consulting styles. When a patient is seen by two different homeopaths it is not uncommon in more confused and hidden cases for quite a different case to emerge. A practitioner using a thematic approach can often 'make sense' of a case that a practitioner using a symptomatic, or even totality, approach would find impossible. In the confused case a thematic approach may be curative or clarify the case so that after several layers have been peeled away a new simillimum based on the totality, or even on a presenting symptom, causation, or mix of these can be perceived.

At times the contrast between the different case histories that may be elicited from a patient can be extreme – this fact itself sheds light on what is happening in the case. A good prescription based on a theme or miasm may mean a confused case that seems to be 'all over the place' re-presents with great clarity. Remember, re-taking a case not only informs us about the new state of the patient, but can also be used to inform, educate and develop our knowledge of a remedy that has acted. Hence your study of materia medica goes hand-in-hand with your case experience. In some cases retaking the case suggests different remedies that can 'unlock' a stuck case, as Linda's case illustrates (Case Study 28.2).

CASE STUDY 28.2

Linda presented with a persistent skin rash and had been seen by two previous homeopaths over a number of years. She had responded to both Phosphorous and Lachesis in the past but presented in a Pulsatilla state with strong features of the other two remedies. It was agreed that at the next consultation the case would be re-taken and the psychological themes particularly explored. She spoke spontaneously about her psychic and emotional sensitivity as a child. When her brother had been ill she had been the one that had been expected to take responsibility for caring for him. As she describes this, her shoulders sagged and she grimaced. The homeopath could feel the sense of weight on her shoulders. Linda felt responsible for keeping everything together in the family and felt deep resentment about it, which was mirrored in her deep resentment about her skin – 'Why me?'. After Staphisagria, based on this theme and several keynotes, she reported it 'gave me more energy'. She developed two new keynotes of Phosphorous that then acted more deeply than before.

Using the Emotions

Perceiving emotions means knowing your own emotions as well as those you are observing.

Everything the patient 'brings with them' to the consultation is of relevance; not only are all the physical senses important to the homeopath but also the 'emotional sensitivity'. Often the deepest themes in a case connect to the emotions the patient feels – this, in turn, connects with the emotion the homeopath feels. Hence the importance of asking the patient not only 'what is the sensation' of a symptom, but also 'how does it feel' emotionally when they have this sensation. Reflecting on the physical sensations you have while taking a case and on how you feel emotionally can guide the case, especially when working relationally.

Remember – the deeper the theme runs in a case then either the stronger the expressed symptom or the more the projection that takes place. The stronger the projection the stronger the emotional feeling. Experience of interacting with patients and noting the sensations and feelings is one of the most important parts of the training of the homeopath who wants to work with confused cases. Often a consultation only gets going when tears or laughter are expressed; when they emerge, they are often defining points in the case history. The release of emotion often coincides with the best time to glimpse the patient's projections.

Common Pitfalls In Confused Cases

It is often not easy, in practice, to work with confused cases. There can be elements of both the complex case (a lot of diverse information) and elements of the hidden case (important symptoms often masked). Some of the common difficulties that arise are noted in Box 28.1.

REFLECTION POINT
- Reflect on how you identify and approach confused cases. What aspects of working with confused cases (Box 28.1) do you find hardest and how might you address each of these in your own practice?

BOX 28.1

Common Pitfalls in Confused Cases
- Viewing the case too pathologically or too psychologically
- Thinking all complex cases are confused
- Failure to agree with the patient what has to be treated and how you will treat it
- Trying too hard to be objective – leading to blind spots (failure to be present) and unconscious judgements
- Unable to re-take the case with 'fresh eyes' because of an inability to leave past impressions behind
- Failure to identify patients' projections and work with feelings; often due to uncertainty or discomfort
- Being too comfortable or too uncomfortable in the case, not 'sitting with' or 'holding' the 'creative tension' required
- Failing to get support or supervision
- Allowing the patient to 'tell their story' without inviting them to 'be in it'

Revealing the Hidden Case

Invariably the hardest part of seeing a difficult case is seeing those parts that the patient doesn't want or can't show. To touch a patient's vulnerability you need to be vulnerable yourself. Being vulnerable means getting to know yourself – but to be vulnerable you will need support.

Understanding what is going on in a case has to precede treatment. Frequently in a hidden case, the illness is projected on to one small area of the person's life or body (one-sided disease). As the symptoms go deeper it is not uncommon for them to get harder to understand. Either symptoms get more 'personal' and harder for some patients to communicate or they can slip into the unconscious – making it hard for the patient to even recognise them. A patient may start off by saying, 'I'm normal in every way, but...' or 'this lump just came up' or 'I'm completely OK'. In each case an invitation to reveal more may be met with a quizzical, almost shocked, look. In other hidden cases

it is the homeopath who is unconscious of what is being expressed in a case.

The Apparently Hidden Case

A common cause for a case to appear hidden is failure to communicate clearly, such as a young child being unable to communicate their modalities. A patient may be reluctant to reveal information because they do not feel safe to do so, or because they don't understand you need to know more. For example, a patient on benefit or claiming compensation may think that if they reveal emotional or personality symptoms it may undermine their sick role status. These patients might need reassurance through a clear agreement, e.g. assumptions the homeopath takes for granted about confidentiality may need to be made explicit. Another patient may play down their symptoms, talking about a 'touch of flu,' or mask their unhealthy complexion using cosmetics.

These apparently hidden cases can often be addressed by carefully 'setting the scene' for the consultation, including contracting clearly. Sometimes the patient has so adapted to their state, or adapted their situation to their state, that they cannot describe symptoms. It is as if the whole case, except for the one-sided symptom, has been palliated. In these cases it can help to invite the patient to imagine what they would be like in different settings or if they didn't have the symptom. Although less reliable, the answer to a question about 'how might you react if...?' is better than no answer at all to the question 'how did you react when...?'. When exploring the possibilities in a case, aspects of the apparently hidden case can be revealed. What is not there can be as informative as what is there. The detective type role of the homeopath is like that of Sherlock Holmes who solved a case by reflecting on 'the dog that did not bark' (in Sir Arthur Conan Doyle's short story 'Silver Blaze').

It is possible that some aspects of a case may be hidden while others are part of a simple case. For example, a patient with heavy periods may not reveal her changed sex drive or other symptoms she feels embarrassed about or does not think are relevant. In many such cases just deepening rapport over time and using all available information sources can reveal what was otherwise hidden. For this reason I refer to them as 'apparently hidden' – using the case-taking and receiving techniques covered previously they can usually be revealed.

REFLECTION POINT

- Reflecting on your learning style (see Chapter 12) can you see what types of patients you might most easily communicate with to reveal their case and those that might find working with your 'default style' the hardest?

True Hidden (Or One-Sided) Cases

While improving communication can reveal some hidden symptoms, others are not communicated because the patient or homeopath is unconscious of them. The unconscious symptoms that hold the key to understanding the case are hidden – and these are the 'true hidden' (or 'one-sided') cases that are the focus of this chapter. Due to the symmetry between the patient's emotional, intellectual and physical symptoms, if the case is unconscious or hidden in one of these it may be more available in another. This requires the homeopath to be able to communicate effectively intellectually, emotionally and by close physical observation and examination. It can help to separate those symptoms that the patient is unable to show, possibly because they are unconscious of them and those the homeopath is unable to perceive or see because the homeopath fails to recognise them. In practice the two are interconnected and often go together – reflecting the cultural blind spots, illnesses and susceptibilities that the patient and homeopath are subject to.

The skill of the homeopath in masked and hidden cases is to judge the right time to examine the 'hidden-ness' and the right intervention to make. The time to consider making an intervention in the case is usually when the energy in the case is becoming stuck. The patient may be 'retreating' into minutiae or repeating a pattern that has been repeated several times before; the homeopath will feel things are going in circles without deepening (Kaplan 2001).

When a symptom is unnoticed by the patient it represents a sort of shadow side that the patient is unconscious of. When it is are not noticed by the homeopath, it may be because it corresponds to an aspect of the homeopath's own personal or collective unconscious.

Parallel Process

'Parallel processes are complex, interlocking systems. Resistances, stalemates and impasses occurring at an unconscious level are communicated by enactment. The enactment when brought into awareness is a way of identifying or resolving the stuckness which is then re-enacted in the reverse direction.'

Gediman & Wolkenfeld (1980)

Parallel process is one of the richest tools the homeopath has available for finding out and exploring, through 'correspondence', what is hidden in the patient and homeopath's personal or collective unconscious. It uses the fact that when one thing changes it affects other things; and if change in one of these is not consciously recognised it is often possible to see the change through parallel changes that can be recognised.

We find that when issues are not made conscious, but are masked or hidden, they are acted out through the behaviour of the individual or the society of which they are a part. This is why case-taking must take account of where patients live, and the families and the culture they belong to. Understanding how one thing projects onto other areas, through a corresponding or 'parallel' process (even if a patient or homeopath is unconscious of it), plays a vital role in understanding hidden cases. It is also one way of explaining how personal behaviour, attitudes and health influence cultural and social norms, including the socialisation and normalisation of behaviour, and vice versa.

Aspects of the patient that are 'in conflict' and have been unresolved for years are often hidden and may instead be reflected in parallel conflict in other relationships – sometimes with parents, friends or lovers and at other times with the homeopath. Inviting the patient to explore tensions and conflicts in their relationships, including with you, reveals much about the inner tension they carry. One technique useful to identify or explore this is to ask the patient to talk to you as if you were the parent, sibling or partner. I have found this 'role play' at times allows a huge shift in an otherwise confused or hidden case.

It is the pressure to 'belong' that unites people with similarities and enables cultures to operate collectively. While this has obvious strengths in relation to the stability of a culture there are potential hazards, particularly in regard to the health of the individual. It explains why certain cultures are susceptible to certain illnesses and epidemics. In this way the illnesses that individuals within a culture are susceptible to tell us about the strains and changes that culture as well as the individual are facing – or need to face.

Casting the net, Catching the Symptoms

Your house, garage, car and clothing, the books, television, films and jokes you like and dislike, all say something about you.

Everything a patient tells you reveals something about them. If you cannot glimpse the themes and symptoms you may notice the 'unconscious shadow' of the patient. The shadow, and those parts that cannot be named, may point to those areas that have been hidden the longest. The patient may need time and encouragement to notice their dreams, to explore their personal relationships or their childhood history. Some patients find that an exercise to complete between appointments allows things to surface that remain hidden when the patient feels scrutinised in the consultation. This 'home work' is a reminder that treatment is a process that continues between consultations and prescriptions of remedies.

Remember that patients may reveal non-verbally what is not being said. They may move their body in a certain way, become restless, even tap or hit parts of their body. Whenever a physical sensation is expressed as a functional or structural disturbance it is a form of somatisation. They may cry or laugh, and they may withdraw into previous familiar feelings or situations. The skill of the homeopath is in judging the right time to offer any intervention, as well as offering the right

intervention. You may have to resist the tendency to intervene until you are clear which is the right intervention to make – just as it is best to wait until you are clear which is the right remedy to give.

The use of free association (see Chapter 13), asking the patient to say the first word that comes to mind in response to your choice of word, can express the hidden aspects of the mental picture. For example, you might ask the patient to say the first thing they think of when you say 'black' or 'home'. Using drawings and doodles can also help to bring out what is otherwise hidden. For example, a patient who suffered from cancer found it hard to talk about herself. She is an artist and paints with 'a mathematical theme' and precision – discussing this she was able to talk about her 'issue with structure' and 'fear of losing control'.

Common Pitfalls in Hidden Cases

It is a challenge working with hidden cases but recognising something is missing is the first step. Consultations which use the relational model of health reach out to connect both the patient and you in a much deeper way than in other models. It is as if we not only invite the patient to go on a walk to meet their fears, delusions and dreams but we also go on the walk with them – being prepared to meet not just their fears, delusions and dreams as aspects of their unconscious but our own as well. We work together to recreate, in a more conscious way, what is already there but is hidden in the case. We navigate through the projection of symptoms in order see where they are unconsciously enacted, to witness them and observe their effect on us. Some of the common difficulties that arise are noted in Box 28.2.

REFLECTION POINT
- How easily do you engage with patients whose cases are partially or completely hidden? Looking at Box 28.2, what might you do when working with hidden cases to see the case more clearly and to 'protect' yourself? What does the incidence of heart disease and cancer in Western society say about that society?

BOX 28.2
Common Pitfalls in Hidden Cases

- Not recognising or learning from our mistakes but repeating them
- Identifying 'why you?, why this?, why now?' for the patient but not for yourself
- Failure to establish clear boundaries, so getting 'sucked into' the case
- Failure to persist when the patient or yourself feels discomfort
- Missing or ignoring off-hand or off-the-cuff remarks
- Failure to connect and to work 'relationally'
- Having inadequate time to take or reflect on the case
- Lack of support for your own vulnerability
- Failure to set up adequate supervision
- Over-identification with our need to heal, leading to striving too hard to 'fix' patients rather than helping patients to help themselves
- Allowing patients to become overly critical or overly idealistic towards you – both of which reduce your ability to be objective and to be self-aware
- Confusing wants and needs, requests and demands

Managing Yourself

Life and living are the best therapy.

At the end of each episode of treatment you might like to reflect on the lessons you have learnt about the patient, the illness, the remedy, yourself and the culture you are working in. It should not be surprising if you find certain recurrent difficulties or find a particular sort of case or patient difficult. The nature of our work is that those who get better no longer need to see us, while those that don't continue to attend. This, combined with more difficult cases often seeking out homeopaths who are more experienced, means that over time you are likely to be working with a growing proportion of difficult cases. It is important not just for your patients but also for your own well-being to manage this. It may

be that you have to take more cases to supervision, you need to identify those cases that need referral, or that you ensure you are clear about those patients who you are supporting and maintaining and not expecting more. There will be times when you will need treatment yourself. It can be both difficult to ask for help, and difficult to help yourself. In difficult cases due to projection it can be hard to maintain a healthy balance between subjective and objective views of yourself. It is therefore prudent to establish clear avenues of support and, if necessary, treatment, before you need them.

Be Realistic

An established and experienced family doctor was troubled by homeopathy because he felt it implied everything he had been doing up until now must have been wrong.

Different treatments, such as other complementary and conventional medical approaches, each have their own expectations. Encouraging patients to make clear choices informed by what they can expect from each is an important part of any patient's treatment. Being secure about what the patients can expect from the treatments we suggest, and the patients' ability to make informed choices about their treatment, is important. If we cannot do this we are likely to be intolerant of other health care systems, the patients who use them and even other homeopaths who work differently from us. We need to inform practitioners of other health care systems about what we do and why – so that they can see where homeopathic treatment interfaces with their own and which outcomes are likely from which treatment. If we can explain what we do and how it relates to other therapies, we are much more likely to help in the overall development of health care models that can integrate different treatment modalities. No one therapeutic system meets all of a patient's needs all the time.

Each model of health, approach to treatment and methodology has its limitations. Between them, most cases can be understood and a plan of treatment formulated. Only rarely is a case untreatable – but the possible outcome of treatment needs to be realistically assessed. In some conditions, such as some patients with degenerative and metastatic illnesses, the structural damage cannot be reversed – although the disease process may be slowed down. In some cases the focus of treatment may be the control of a particular symptom, even if the overall disease process is not significantly altered. In these cases the patient and homeopath need to be clear on what they agree to treat, especially when other treatment modalities that may alter the picture are being used alongside homeopathy. For example, a patient with metastatic illness receiving chemotherapy and radiotherapy may want help to tolerate these – so focusing on cause and local effects may point to the necessary remedy. The most frustrating and difficult cases are often those where you and the patient have different and/or unrealistic expectations.

Know When to Rest and When to Get Help

Many patients with difficult cases seek only relief from their worst symptoms. Treatment might give this relief, only to reveal other symptoms that you believe require treating. It may be that these symptoms represent a deeper aspect of the case that, if untreated, means relapse is more likely. Equally, in the homeopath's mind the relief might be only partial and, without consolidating treatment, likely to relapse. You and the patient must agree on what to do when these points are reached and it helps to be clear on the options at this time. It is helpful to clarify with the patient when the aim of treatment is curative and when maintenance or prevention of deterioration is the aim.

In confused and hidden case it is often appropriate and realistic to have phases of treatment that just aim to maintain an improvement or allow a case to become clear. This may go on for some time until the case is clear, or until the patient or you are ready to tackle other aspects of the case. When you have worked hard with a patient to obtain an improvement it is reasonable to want to see it maintained. As a general rule if symptoms have not gone completely, relapse will occur at some time if no maintenance treatment is offered. As part of any maintenance treatment follow-up appointments help to identify the earliest signs that the patient is relapsing and allow for repeat treatment if necessary.

There are many other practitioners and homeopaths available to the patient – and many supervisors available to you. Knowing when to make use of them to support the patient or yourself is important. A patient may reach a point where they are partially better but need, for example, to change their diet or look at a relationship they are in before they are ready to work at a deeper level. Being clear which phase the management is in, and what other treatments the patient is using, is important both for you and the patient.

Endings

At the point when the patient will remain well (unless there is new causation) and may be discharged, it is worth reflecting with the patient what has been achieved and how they will monitor their health, how the patient's life has changed, and what further support they might need. For example, with life style or dietary change, how will the patient know if there is a relapse? What feedback does the patient have to offer on the treatment and your practice? While some patients choose to use homeopathy to actively maintain health, many realistically only seek help when their illness prevents them from doing something they want or when symptoms become too uncomfortable. By giving patients warning of the ending, it allows them to work through any important or unresolved issues relating to their treatment. Often when patients are warned that a course of treatment is coming to an end then issues surface that they might want help with but have not previously asked about. Frequently these are deeper issues and problems that may have been quite longstanding. For some patients ending treatment without due care is experienced as a withdrawal of support or even a 'rejection'.

REFLECTION POINT

- If you find you are frequently in a difficult situation or have difficult feelings I invite you to reflect on why this might be so. By working through these difficulties we can develop as homeopaths and extend our competence.

- It is interesting to ponder to what extent the issues we face in practice reflect the issues we need to address for ourselves. Perhaps the patient is not just the 'bringer of the difficult case' but also the bringer of our opportunity for our own personal and professional development?

Practice and Professional Organisation Issues

Much that is taught can be learnt but only a fraction of what can be learnt is taught. To practise health it helps to be healthy, to have a healthy practice and to belong to a healthy organisation.

In difficult cases much of the picture is informed by the environment and situation the patient chooses to live and the family, community and culture they belong to. It therefore should come as no surprise to you – if you understand the idea of parallel process and holism – to realise that when managing difficult cases it is not just the personal issues relating to a patient's case and analysis that present a challenge. They are also reflected in what we find difficult to structure and organise in our practices and the political and cultural issues professional organisations are likely to struggle with.

These are as much aspects of our work that need support as our individual patient work. It is an important part of our education, especially in managing difficult cases, to address practice and organisational issues such as time keeping, financial management, clinical governance, working with other health professionals and ethical guidelines. Equally, while it is easy to see how personal development is linked to your training, the development of your practice and the contribution you can make to the development of your professional organisation are important parts of being a homeopath. Although many of the issues that you as a student might want to address relate to your personal understanding and prescribing of homeopathy, as you start to see more patients so the practice and organisational issues emerge.

The reverse is also true, in that if you create a difficult practice or professional tensions it will make more cases appear difficult. Such things as having enough time; being valued or paid enough; being liked or disliked; being able to share your work, relating to colleagues or staff; feeling you belong balanced by enough autonomy; and feeling your professional body is connected, relevant, supportive and developing, are all important in seeing cases clearly. To be aware of the breadth of issues that affect how you see and manage cases, it helps to think about the different development, support and education challenges that regularly occur in the personal, practice and professional organisations areas of your work. This is illustrated in Table 28.1, which draws on just some of the issues that regularly arise in supervision and can each influence how you work (Owen 2002).

Table 28.1 EXAMPLES OF FACTORS TO CONSIDER IN YOUR WORK AS A HOMEOPATH

	Education	Support	Development
Personal	Being told new information. Learning from successes and mistakes	Being heard. Coming to terms with what you do not know	Having your case taken. Changing views, e.g. what health and illness are
Practice	Clinical governance. Understanding different styles of case work.	Practice problems. Finding your own style. Having others around you to support your work	Reflecting on difficult cases. Continued professional development (CPD). Competence. Finding a career path.
Professional Organisational	Establishing best practice. Codes of practice. Population issues, e.g. vaccination policy	Finding a role model or mentor. Sense of belonging	Examining critical events. Relation to other organisations, government and public heath

In the same way as it is possible to see illness as something that is essential in a dynamic and changing world – not the opposite of health, but an integral and necessary part of being 'healthy' – then at a practice level the challenges and difficulties we encounter inform the development of a rewarding, sustainable and 'healthy practice'. At an organisational level, the differences and tensions that are acted out by the different communities and schools of homeopathy parallel and inform fundamental and important questions our community needs to reflect on if it is to respond to new challenges in a healthy manner. In the same way as symptoms are necessary for health, so difference and diversity are necessary for strength and stability.

How you work through these issues appears to be a personal choice but will often be strongly influenced by parallel issues in your practice and profession. It is not surprising, therefore, to see the values that run through the relationship between homeopaths and their patients being reflected in their practices and professional organisations. Problems that are identified in the personal, practice or profession are likely to be reflected in each other. Dysfunction in an organisation will affect members of that organisation and vice versa. Given their expertise with individual patients, it is surprising to me how few homeopaths use homeopathic principles in the understanding or running of their practices and the organisations they are part of.

Projection of unresolved and unconscious issues, parallel expression in groups, and projective identification can all shed light on 'the case' – whether an ill patient, a failing practice or dysfunctional organisation. For example, projection in an organisation is often used to displace negativity onto a susceptible person – making the individual a scapegoat and giving the organisation the illusion of power, cohesion and control that lasts until either the scapegoat is ejected, the scapegoat declines to carry those feelings, or the organisation becomes conscious of what it is doing and decides to change. Homeopathic principles and techniques of mirroring back using like to treat like can have a powerful effect on an organisation as much as on an individual. For example if you are in a meeting that is exhibiting many Lycopodium features, you might try interacting as a Lycopodium type would.

There are, of course, many situations that are difficult to teach about in textbooks or the classroom. This is why careful supervision, mentoring and practice-based teaching are so helpful. The individuals providing such services to you should be in a good position to help you observe the issues that are common to those starting in practice and identify problems that you are particularly susceptible to. A supervisor makes these issues available for you to consciously explore and learn from, rather than allowing them to be submerged and re-enacted indefinitely. Supervision can play an important, I would say transformative role, in the development of your practice and ideally is informed by and feeds back to the professional organisations you belong to.

Different Practice Settings

When starting in homeopathic practice it is important to realise that different practice settings have inherent limitations. So, for example, general practitioners who use homeopathy often complain about being constrained by the time limits of their consultation. You can use homeopathy effectively in these situations, but the models with which you are able to perceive the case have to be carefully focussed. You may have to adjust your way of working so that you build up a case picture over a number of visits, perhaps with the benefit of knowing other family members and the home environment. Ultimately the structure and organisation of your practice will reflect how you can work and what you are realistically able to achieve.

Summary

As you can see, in understanding confused and hidden cases, the dividing lines between the case history, the materia medica, the case analysis and the actual prescription are becoming blurred. While to understand homeopathy as a science we need to keep things separate – so keeping it measurable and able to be analysed – to work with homeopathy as an art we are required to see the interconnections and be aware of where the issues run together and how treatment is a process. We confront our limitations when working with difficult cases and therefore learn more from cases that appear confused or hidden than we do from our easier ones. Ultimately, our difficult cases give us something that allows us to understand others – and ourselves – better.

References

Gediman H K, Wolkenfeld F 1980 The parallelism phenomenon in psychoanalysis and supervision: its reconsideration as a triadic system. Psychoanal Q 49(2):234–255

Kaplan B 2001 The homeopathic conversation. Natural Medicine Press, London

Owen D 2002 Learning experiences – what works for postgraduates. Homeopathy 91(2):95–98

Bibliography

Hawkins P, Shohet R 2000 Supervision in the helping professions, 2nd edn. Open University Press, Buckingham

Morrissey J, Tribe R 2001 Process in supervision. Counsell Psychol Q 14(2):103–110

CHAPTER TWENTY NINE

Approaches to Treating Confused and Hidden Cases

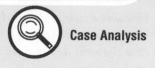 **Case Analysis**

David Owen

'Health exists when there is a perfect harmony between soul and mind; this harmony alone must be obtained before cure can be accomplished.'

Dr Edward Bach

Introduction

Homeopaths working with confused or hidden cases draw on information about the remedies and the case from every possible source. Using this disparate information we practice our art and apply our science to achieve a rational, replicable and curative approach to treatment. As more patients use suppressive treatments and live longer in a rapidly changing culture, more confused and hidden cases develop. Combined with patients' increased expectations of well-being – meaning not just an absence of morbid pathology, but a positive sense of physical, intellectual and emotional balance – this will lead to an inevitable increase in the number of difficult cases that will present to us for treatment.

In this chapter the different methodologies, management strategies and issues raised by managing confused and hidden cases are explored. The essence, thematic and reflective approaches that relate to the holographic and relational models of health are considered in more detail – each bringing their own management issues. In practice several approaches to treatment are frequently combined and, unless the analysis strategies used and your expectations of a particular treatment are clarified, it makes interpreting the action of a remedy used more difficult, leading to the not infrequent 'spoiling' of cases.

While several homeopaths may reach the same or similar conclusions about a simple (or even complex) case, there are often several different strategies for the management of confused and hidden cases. The remedy eventually selected depends on many factors, including the 'pros and cons' of each methodology, your practice situation, the patient's expectations and your agreement with them, your knowledge of the materia medica, perception of the case and experience of the different approaches. Why you use some remedies more than others, and why some cases are hard for you but not necessarily hard for another homeopath, are important questions to reflect on. It is both liberating and frightening to explore the uncertainty that there might not be one 'best' way to treat a patient; rather there may be a choice of ways for you to treat this patient in this setting at this time!

Rarely will one remedy bring the most hidden and confused case all the way back to health. Over time, as treatment of a difficult case unfolds, different approaches may be used at different stages. Hidden and confused cases move to complex cases and become gradually less complex and eventually simple. If this is possible in some cases it raises important questions as to whether it is possible in all cases – if so, perhaps there are no 'incurable cases'.

Essence and Thematic Approaches

One day a case and remedy may be unclear to you; you go out of the room briefly or come back to the case the next day and the case and remedy needed at that moment is clear.

In confused cases several patterns of symptoms can be understood as a series of themes. These themes may intertwine like strands in a rope to give a single essence or be composed of different themes that are mixed together and appear superimposed one on top of another through a series of layers. The different themes (strands) run between different levels of symptoms in a case and connect these horizontal levels by vertical themes which often provide a way of integrating many different parts of the case or contradictory aspects into a coherent whole. So a patient with a single or predominant essence of blandness running through all physical, mental and emotional expressions of the case will point to the essence of the remedy Graphites. A patient with a theme of anticipatory anxiety can indicate several Carbon remedies; if they also have this theme running deeper – perhaps as a fear of something awful happening – it may again point to Graphites. The methodology used is to match a patient's picture or 'pathograph' (Swayne 1998) to the picture or 'monograph' of the remedy picture. If all the themes in a case match a single remedy the case often becomes clear. If several different themes run in contrasting directions or point to several different remedies, then the case often appears confused.

Thematic Analysis and Treatment Strategies

Thematic analysis therefore goes through several stages – matching what features of the case are thematically connected to what other features of the case, then deciding which themes are most important or central to the case, then matching the most important themes to a remedy. Identifying the themes is an important part of the case and the analysis. A confused case often has several different themes that do not point to a single remedy. This recognition that a case that fits a clear pattern may be partially covered by several remedies leads to looking more closely at the materia medica of all the remedies in the 'differential diagnosis'.

If one remedy clearly covers the majority of the themes in a case it may be 'good enough'. Even if it does not cure it will reveal more and deeper aspects of the case, allowing a better prescription to be made. It may also reveal new information that invites a different model, approach or methodology that in turn points to a different remedy. When looking at the themes in a case where there is no clear simillimum several strategies are useful:

- You may choose a remedy partially indicated in several models or approaches. For example, if several remedies of the Ranunculacae family are partially indicated thematically but there was a traumatic aetiology, then Arnica might be selected.

- You may take into account confirmatory and exclusion symptoms and themes to both promote and demote a possible remedy in your analyses. What might at first appear as minor or less prominent symptoms or themes can become very significant in choosing one remedy over another one.

- You may choose a remedy that fits the most or strongest themes and it is possible to weight and score themes in a similar way that symptoms are scored. It is possible to collate all the aspects of the case that relate to each theme, and to effectively consider them like one 'combined rubric'. These different combined rubrics can then be analysed to see which remedies and groups of remedies have the themes. In effect the themes, each of which might include several rubrics, are being analysed rather than the individual symptoms (see Chapter 19).

- You may choose a remedy that best represents the themes that run most broadly through the physical, mental and emotional layers of the case. For example, the theme irritability could include mental and emotional irritability but if tissue sensitivity/irritability was also seen this theme would be considered more strongly.

• You may weight the theme that runs (or appears to run) most deeply, or has been there the longest.

In practice (as with repertorisation) a combination of these different strategies is used, taking into account how well known the remedies being considered are and where and how easily information about the themes of those remedies can be obtained. It is not uncommon for a confused case that falls between several remedies to match another, sometime related, possibly little known, remedy that allows many of the themes to be integrated in a single remedy picture. Many of the polychrests have clear essences and thematic pictures built up from provings and clinical experience but the thematic picture of less well used remedies is understandably slower to develop, although this has changed over the last few years with the introduction of materia medica by family and kingdom. Although some homeopaths feel that until these pictures are validated by provings, they are not reliable. The researchers and writers who actively endeavour to clarify these pictures are owed a debt of thanks by all homeopaths. The profession is at a time of huge growth which needs to be supported by a sound development of the resources available. If homeopaths can develop new thematic materia medica knowledge reliably it will greatly help the management of difficult cases. Remember that while an essence or theme may belong to a single remedy it may also be in common within a family or group of remedies (see Chapter 22).

Suppression of Themes

Suppressive treatments often change the active expression of a symptom. A suppressed symptom may come out in a deeper way or become a passive or compensated manifestation of the original symptom, sometimes these determine the adverse effects or toxic effects of the suppressive drug (in their own way a type of proving). This change in the original symptom expression along with new symptoms from medication often adds to the confusion in a case.

In confused cases where adverse effects impose another symptom level over the case it can be necessary to remove this lesional level before the deeper levels of the case can be seen more clearly. Sometimes a thematic remedy can run through even the suppressed level, i.e. the remedy that matches the susceptibility of the patient determines how and to what suppressive drugs they will react. There are two reasons why conventional drugs provide important remedy pictures – one is that they represent levels of illness that overlie suppressed cases, the other is that those drugs that have most toxicity and side effects often match patients' susceptibility.

Some conventional drugs are likely to owe some of their effectiveness to working homeopathically (or isopathically) – e.g. lithium, gold, adrenaline, desensitisation and even some vaccinations – but the doses that are used and the failure to match them accurately to the patient can cause frequent unwanted effects. It is therefore not surprising that the side-effect profile of drugs often reflects their homeopathic remedy picture and that many conventional medicines used historically are today deep-acting homeopathic remedies, such as Mercury, Gold, Belladonna and Digitalis. To manage a patient's confused case it helps to be competent to monitor their conventional medication and to understand the lesional level set up by these drugs, as in Sam's case. These deep cases obviously need careful consideration and contracting that may include liaising with other carers of the patient. Remember, when conventional medicines

CASE STUDY 29.1

Sam had been on a mix of sleeping tablets and tranquilisers for 50 years and his case was multilayered and confused. By reducing his tranquiliser and prescribing it in potency, deeper aspects of a case emerged – including dreams about an episode in the war when he had to kill someone by hand. He was enabled to stop the tranquilisers and worked through the withdrawal effects more speedily than (it is likely) he otherwise would have. A strong feeling of remorse that he had not previously been aware of emerged, with a clear remedy indicated. He slept well after this and his many symptoms all eased.

work powerfully, with adverse effects, it means that they are acting in a sensitive individual. It is common to find patients who have avoided much allopathic and antipathic dosing are more sensitive as provers and may react more sensitively to allopathic and antipathic drugs.

Due to the nature of confused and hidden cases, even when you feel you have a good match of remedy to case, it is quite likely that after treatment or over time new information will emerge that points to a different remedy at a subsequent re-taking of the case. Homeopaths differ in the extent that they use successive remedies to 'clarify or clear' the case or where they wait until the picture is completely clear before they prescribe. One way to think of hidden cases is that they have become 'frozen in time'. It is as if the disease process has led to, or required, the individual to become solidified in other ways; to freeze or fix the illness in one particular aspect of themselves. When these cases are carefully managed they begin to thaw and issues and symptoms begin to surface in other aspects. At first the patient is likely to be more bothered by these new symptoms than by those that had been 'frozen'.

Miasmatic Prescribing

Miasms and miasmatic prescribing have been covered in Chapter 17. However, there are several important considerations when thinking about miasms and thematic prescribing, as there are two groups of remedies that can be indicated by the miasmatic theme running through a case. First, when a miasmatic theme is particularly strong in the absence of other clear themes the nosode of that miasm may be specifically indicated, e.g. Medorrhinum for Sycosis. Second, the miasmatic theme may indicate or favour one of the already partially indicated remedies that have an affinity to (or belong to) a miasmatic group. Some examples of miasmatic themes and remedies and how they can be used are given below.

1. A miasmatic remedy may be used for a specific layer that confuses or hides the case. It may be for the deepest 'visible' layer of a case, sometimes referred to

as a fundamental layer – although once removed a deeper layer may become apparent. Not only might the 'miasmatic layer' obscure the case, but also it can actually block the case from responding, as in Jill's case. Any layer can block a clear picture and/or a remedy acting. Sometimes these layers can have a specific trigger, e.g. after vaccination or an illness, as Peter's case illustrates.

CASE STUDY 29.2

Jill, 35, presented with postnatal depression. She had put on weight, lost her libido and felt detached from her child. There was a previous history of menstrual problems, and her appearance and confirmatory craving for vinegar indicated Sepia. This gave a transitory improvement in mood but she had become colder and tired. After a time with no improvement she was prescribed Psorinum for the miasmatic layer of under-activity, flatness and its correlation of Sepia. After Psorinum she became warmer, had more energy and felt a little better. At a subsequent consultation she was able to talk about her own childhood and her feelings of loss when her parents separated – she had previously avoided this. She was prescribed Sepia again and this substantially helped the case.

CASE STUDY 29.3

Peter, age 35, presented with post-viral fatigue with onset after vaccination to Hepatitis B. He failed to respond to a totality and constitutional approach and so a treatment based on causation from the vaccination was considered. This causation was considered alongside his 'miasmatic' susceptibility to the aetiological agent. After treatment isopathically with a nosode of Hepatitis B 30c split dose, new symptoms developed that indicated a remedy that acted deeply.

2. The miasm may describe a theme that runs through several layers in the case, e.g. the general under-activity of Psorinum might be seen in many symptoms, even though other remedies are each partially indicated, as in John's case.

3. Each miasmatic remedy also has a remedy picture in its own right and can be prescribed on this alone – although in practice it is usually supported by trends from that miasm running through the case. The case of Joanna illustrates this.

CASE STUDY 29.4

John, age 48, had chronic skin problems and Sulphur, Calcarea carbonica and Lycopodium were each partly indicated. Sulphur was, on balance, best indicated although his profound chilliness and food preferences relatively contraindicated this. He was prescribed Psorinum as it covered several features connecting different layers of the case. He got a significant aggravation of the skin and a clearer psychological and physical picture of Lycopodium emerged that later acted deeply.

CASE STUDY 29.5

Joanna, a 16 year old girl, was brought to me by her parents. She had several episodes of binge drinking, had twice taken an overdose and had a history of cutting herself. She bites her nails, is emaciated, self-critical and feels she is a disappointment to herself and her parents. She comments: 'I want to make them pay, they will be sorry when I am gone'. She is cold, chilly and craves coffee. The keynotes along with the theme of failure, despair and flatness led to a prescription of Psorinum that gave significant benefit.

Reflective Approaches to Managing Otherwise Hidden Cases

Before embarking on the management of the truly hidden case it is important to remind ourselves that symptoms might be expressed as active, passive or compensated (see Chapter 14). The active symptom might be difficult to see but if the passive and compensated state is visible this may give the best indication of the remedy. In cases where symptoms are there but are mostly passive or compensated, they can be difficult to draw out and see, hence they are often only 'apparent' one-sided cases.

In cases that are 'truly' hidden all the symptoms, except for just one or two major or common symptoms, are masked. Once you recognise this you can shape the consultation and explore the strategies to reveal the hidden case accordingly. By registering this you become more aware of other information offered by the patient including projection.

CASE STUDY 29.6

Mark, age 57, presented with angina that was being treated conventionally; he had common angina modalities but otherwise appeared asymptomatic. Describing his angina he used a clenched fist and hit his chest. Mirroring this movement back to him led to him discussing how he felt 'thumped in the chest' and 'winded'. He went on to describe a feeling that he had lost his freedom and whenever he 'metaphorically' stood up to these feelings he was 'hit in the chest' and 'knocked down'. The homeopath who presented this case in supervision was able to describe his own feeling of being trapped by this case and a wish to escape – in supervision he explored what this meant for him and how he could feel free to enquire about this. At follow-up Mark talked freely about how he used to use recreational drugs and had never felt free since. This theme contributed to selecting the remedy that greatly reduced the frequency of his angina attacks.

CASE STUDY 29.7

Catherine, age 38, had interstitial cystitis but with few modalities. She had not responded to local treatment. There was no clear totality or themes. Whenever the case history got close to anything other than the presenting symptom, Catherine started talking about other people's problems, which she worries about. The homeopath reported in supervision that the patient is 'frustrating'. She makes the homeopath feel 'manipulated' and she holds back from talking about herself. At a subsequent follow-up when Catherine is asked about her interest in helping others and the homeopath is guided by their own frustration, Catherine offers that she finds it hard to ask for help herself. Others had hurt her in the past. She has suppressed her anger towards those that hurt her because she felt vulnerable; she talks about her inner 'excruciating' hurt and 'stifling' rage. The theme of hurt and vulnerability was compensated by her wish to 'throw' herself in to help others. A fuller but confused picture emerged. After a partial response to Staphisagria a clearer picture emerged and she was more able to talk about herself – although it took six months before her presenting complaint improved significantly.

Remember, when important aspects of the case are masked or hidden they must always show themselves in some other way – most often through somatisation (see Chapter 15) and projection, often a form of compensation (see Chapter 23). It is perhaps not surprising, then, that the most hidden cases are also those with the most structural or life-threatening illnesses and that have the strongest projections and/or generate the strongest counter-projections in us, as Mark's case illustrates.

When you are conscious and able to reflect on what is happening 'in relationship' with the patient and appreciate the remedies as 'living materia medica' you can match otherwise hidden cases. Cases and remedies have both positive and negative attributes and will respond in a different and dynamic way in different situations and to different homeopaths. As you increasingly understand yourself and reliably appreciate how patients in different remedy states make you feel you can use this to much effect, as Catherine's case illustrates. I suspect this is behind much of what is called 'experience'.

Managing Confused and Hidden Cases

There are two parts to analysing difficult cases. First, different approaches and methodologies give a number of possible remedies in the differential diagnosis. The second part of analysing the case is deciding between these possible remedies. The two stages of finding the remedy are like tuning a radio – the first stage, often using the repertory, is like roughly tuning in to the close remedies; the second stage, of differentiating remedies in the differential diagnosis, often using the materia medica, is like fine tuning to the exact frequency. However, at the heart of managing confused and hidden cases is realising that cases take time to unmask and clear – the management is a process not a single intervention.

There are two main implications – first, it is unlikely a single prescription will 'help' the patient back to full health; second, that your responsibility for a patient extends beyond just a single consultation and intervention. When working with confused and hidden cases it is helpful to aspire to find a single remedy that fits the case most closely at that time but at the same time to realise that a series of remedies are likely to be needed as the case unfolds (see Chapters 15, 30). Sometimes those different remedies can be glimpsed at an earlier consultation. When just one remedy is seen then it can be an indicator that the case is no longer masked or confused.

Commonly in confused cases different methodologies indicate different remedies – some homeopaths will use more than one remedy together or in close succession (e.g. in veterinary prescribing, Chapter 18). For example, a child who has long-standing and suppressed eczema may receive a miasmatic or thematic remedy in high potency, say a 200C split dose. But if a local remedy is also indicated it may be prescribed as a low potency either orally, as a 12C daily, or as a local cream. Different homeopaths like to separate out each course of treatment in different ways, both by time and by potency. The main considerations are the extent to which one remedy may block the action of another, the need to get a local improvement before the patient (or parent) agrees to working at a deeper level, and the extent to which other suppressive medication would be used if local treatment was not given. Although ideally a single remedy would be used to cover the whole case, in practice the patient may benefit from both a deeper-acting remedy and one that helps manage local symptoms so they can reduce or stop allopathic drugs.

In confused cases treatment can be like untangling a knot or tangle of kite string – if you just pull the end the knot gets tighter. Treatment must often loosen the string first so that the tangle can be seen clearly. In hidden cases, where the cause of the tangle is invisible, treatment is like following one end to free the string, while keeping an eye on the whole mess as it becomes apparent. Often hidden cases have to move through a stage where they appear confused (with several symptom complexes and themes at different layers) before a complex case (where a totality and/or a constitution can be seen clearly) emerges.

REFLECTION POINT

- In managing confused and hidden cases there are many different factors that affect how confused or hidden the case is. Reflect and revise how the patient's illness, family and culture; the patient–homeopath relationship; and the homeopath's knowledge, experience, practice set-up and professional culture can each affect how clearly a case is seen.

Low Vitality

The masks and walls that an individual creates around them, that to a greater or lesser extent both protect and hide them, each draw on the vitality to be sustained. Consequently, it is not surprising that in deeply hidden and confused cases, which have often been developing over a long time, the vitality is often low and the case appears quite stuck.

Even slightly unmasking the case increases the patient's vitality and may be enough to generate new and clear old symptoms. The bigger the mask then the more it 'protects' – but the more vitality it takes to maintain it. The homeopath often has to balance when to lift the mask so that the case can be manifest more clearly without removing the vital protection (decompensating the case) that can lead to the patient give up on treatment. Choosing when to unmask a case is influenced by the therapeutic relationship and agreement (see Chapters 23, 25), including the patient's choice, the symptoms that are apparent, the amount of suppression, the support available to the patient and homeopath, and the homeopath's competence in terms of ability, knowledge and experience.

In some masked cases simple life style changes can support the patient and help increase the vitality, so making it easier to reveal the case in a gentle and caring way. For example, in patients with cancer, juice diets, nutritional supplements and psychological support can all help a clearer, less masked, picture emerge without the patient feeling blamed or guilty or disempowered. If the vitality is very low in debilitated patients, then remedies may initially need to be given in low potency and suppressive and palliative treatment change gradually. But if the vitality is adequate the deep-seated case that is revealed behind the mask benefits from high potencies. I have found it helpful in hidden cases with much structural damage, but that have adequate vitality to use 200c plussing potencies (Ramakrishnan & Coulter 2001) (see Chapter 20).

Psychiatric Illness

Psychological symptoms can be considered like any other symptoms. The suppression of symptoms may hide or confuse the case and adds to the tendency of many patients to withhold symptoms to which they feel a stigma is attached. It is interesting to reflect on how the hidden nature of some symptoms mirrors how society seeks to hide away, institutionalise and avoid these symptoms. Severe depression, psychosis, schizophrenia and organic brain disease can all present as seriously masked and hidden cases. Unmasking these, especially those on much allopathic medication, is difficult to manage in an outpatient setting – intensive monitoring and residential support is often required. Without the benefit of hospital care in a collaborative context the most deep-seated of cases are effectively incurable.

Awareness and Longstanding Illness

Treatment of longstanding conditions often leads to a rebalancing of what is conscious and what is unconscious to the patient. The state that initially arose, perhaps as an adaptive defence, can gradually be changed and replaced by a more appropriate state. This parallel between health and awareness is sometimes used by those seeking a greater awareness of self. Each new state involves the revelation (unmasking) of information that may point to a new remedy. As the patient moves through different states of health, so they may need support to adjust to their health state and 'connect to' a sociably acceptable version of reality that incorporates a new sense of self, taking into account what has been revealed. This takes place through changes, sometimes dramatic ones in the perception and interpretation of reality. It may include changes in how they see others and how others see them and how they interface with their life situation, as well as the symptoms they express. In this way patients move gradually through states that might be equated to stages of health that interface with the patient's awareness (Laing 1990). Jenny's case illustrates this.

This journey into a new state of health can lead to an extreme change of awareness – the deeper the illness the greater the shift, i.e. it is often greatest when treating hidden and confused cases. These changes may require your time and support as much as finding a remedy. In a small way the same re-adjustment to normality happens with each journey into wellness. Perhaps this is why the role of healer has often been closely associated with such roles as spiritual and religious advisors in communities.

CASE STUDY 29.8

Jenny, age 27, presented with psychotic symptoms following recreational drug use. Much of the case was at first hidden. After homeopathic treatment based on a potency of the hallucinogenic drug she had used, her psychosis improved slightly and she gained a number of insights into herself following the remedy and consultation. Her new view of herself enabled her to explore her jealousy with her sister and mother that, with a local symptom, pointed to Lachesis. Some time after this she spoke about unresolved issues with her father, around whom she felt anxious. She was able to express her anxiety and to speak about why she had attracted and put up with rather abusive relationships. She developed food cravings of Calcarea carbonica that she remembered having as a child and responded deeply to this remedy.

Hereditary Factors and Congenital Illness

The susceptibility (including hereditary and congenital) of today and how it is managed will influence the susceptibility (including hereditary and congenital) of tomorrow.

In hereditary and congenital illnesses the homeopath is interested in the susceptibility that one generation 'bequeaths' to another (see Chapters 13 & 17). While the illness symptoms are clear, other aspects of the case are often hidden – perhaps because the illness or susceptibility has always been present and the psychological and physiological adjustment to it has always been there or has developed unconsciously. Hereditary illnesses often appear intractable, fixed and incurable, as the maintaining cause is considered to be the genetic information that is immutable. However, the expression of any genetic susceptibility can be influenced by homeopathic treatment, although this is often symptomatic. For example, many Down's children appear to have fewer infections and less severe symptoms when successfully treated homeopathically.

Although difficult to evaluate, it appears that by treating the parents before or during pregnancy illnesses that might otherwise be expected can be reduced. For example, allergic illness often has a hereditary element that appears to be preventable. On the same basis a young child or baby can be treated using information from the case of the parents. If miasmatic susceptibility is treated it can reduce the expression of inherited susceptibility and reverse the trend of hereditary predisposition and susceptibility over generations – thus decreasing the risk to future generations

The genetic code of one generation is shaped by the health of previous generations. The environmental factors we set up for ourselves are also influenced by our genetic make-up. So these two are artificially separated and it is more useful to consider them as an inseparable connection that binds the genetic predisposition of one generation to the environmental exposure of another generation. As one of the major influences on predisposition in one generation is the suppression experienced by previous generations, then the main groups of susceptibility that we see in individuals are related to common diseases that have been suppressed in previous generations. The symptom patterns and diseases that we are exposed to now and that are suppressed will establish the miasms of the future; this is not just genetically mediated but is transmitted by social, cultural and environmental influences.

Relating in the Different Models of Health

Each model leads to a slightly different style of the relationship between you and the patient; each style communicates slightly different information. The way the patient and homeopath relate to each other is influenced by the balance of listening, inviting, clarifying, questioning, summarising, suggesting and advising that takes place in the consultation. You might like to reflect on which of these are more suited to the relationship in each model of health. And to reflect on the different levels of control and dependence using each might bring. So while quite a questioning style might reveal what a patient did to 'cause' the illness, it

may also appear like you have the answer – a more inviting style might allow you and the patient to explore what projections are taking place but may invite unwanted projections.

Combining Different Approaches

How much time and energy do you spend trying to make sure things don't get worse versus making things better?

Many different factors influence a person's health. They include physical factors that are inherited (vascular, immunological, anatomical) and acquired (infection, environment), and physiological factors that are situational (light, diet, exercise, relaxation) and cultural (sanitation, work, habitation). These may all reveal different priorities and attitudes to treatment. The patient, their family, different health carers and government may each have different priorities – not just with respect to what models of health are in fashion or dominant, but when to use different treatment modalities (conventional or complementary). In most patients the homeopathic remedy is just one step in a treatment that not only might use several remedies but also involve many factors that influence our health in a matrix of interconnecting processes. The homeopath attempting to focus only on 'their bit of the puzzle' and who thinks 'the right remedy will cure everything' risks being idealised by patients and falling into the trap of feeling they have the answer to every problem – both are frequently observed in health professionals.

Idealisation occurs because of a patient's wishes to locate all the answers to their health needs in someone who can help them, rather than accept uncertainty about the answers or their responsibility to find them. It is a type of projective identification (see Chapter 23). It is not uncommon for patients to identify with their doctor or homeopath, claiming they have power and influence that exceeds their role. When patients project high expectations the homeopath can be tempted to buy into this idealisation, feeling special or privileged and thinking 'Oh yes, I'm the best', or 'I can cure this'. It sometimes is accompanied by the giving of gifts. It is easy to accept the patient's sincere need of help, especially if no-one else has been able to help, but it is important to recognise our own place in the patient's care.

By helping patients get *themselves* better we step back from the 'divine role' and instead apply our knowledge to help patients heal themselves. If we are not in touch with our own humility about what we can and cannot do, we can start to think we have the answer to every problem – often accompanied by a need for perfection and called 'omnipotence' by psychotherapists. The idealisation we invite from patients when we project omnipotence at first can make the patient secure and trusting. But it is a precursor for the patient feeling their health is not their responsibility – and when treatment fails their (often high) expectations, that the homeopath is to blame. When prevalent in a health care profession it is accompanied by passive aggression and a litigious culture of blame. The omnipotence we briefly feel from a patient's idealisation is, of course, a precursor to feelings of not measuring up, failure, disappointment and, for many, the need to work harder until they are exhausted.

This 'wounded and hurting healer' is an all too common state for all health care professionals, and homeopaths are no exception. The practitioner goes from one 'success' to another, relying on the next patient to praise them for getting them better and to renew their fading ideal picture of themselves. This gradually increases their expectations of what they should be able to do and the failure they feel if they don't achieve it. It is reflected in 'flipping' between feelings of power and powerlessness, being needed and being alone, feeling important and feeling ignored. These are dangerous feelings that can lead some therapists into unexplained depression and even suicidal states – one reason, perhaps, for high rates of suicide in health professionals.

As you might expect, the tendency to idealise others and to invite idealisation go together. It is therefore a dangerous sign for a student of homeopathy to idealise any one teacher and for any teacher to receive unchecked a student's idealisation. The real insights that teachers give and can be respected for are the revealing of what students can connect to as their own inner truth. By idealising a

teacher you risk demoting your own inner wisdom, blocking your own creativity and feeding a low opinion of yourself. This low opinion leads to the need to promote teachers, over-identify with the need to do better and attract idealisation. Another symptom of idealisation is, I believe, only focusing on teaching and sharing successful cases. For many homeopaths talking about those cases they find difficult or where expectations were not met is a vital step in their balancing being a good homeopath with aspiring to be the best homeopath.

Idealisation and a sense of omnipotence are common in many health professions, perhaps reflecting the therapist's own pain and need for healing. It is important for preventing and managing these and other projections that time is made to process them. It is why supervision and attention to your own health is necessary not just for your patient's best treatment but also for your own well-being. Paying attention to the health of our profession provides a place where what is hidden and compensated for can be seen and addressed, for the benefit of all.

Step-by-Step Approach to Treatment

Once it is accepted that the management of a difficult case may take several stages, that may include different remedies or the same remedy several times, it is clear that the treatment process involves several steps. Deciding when a remedy has fully acted and when and whether another treatment is indicated occupies as much of the analyses of more complex, confused and hidden cases as deciding what the next remedy could be. These steps are illustrated in Figure 29.1 and build on the ideas of remedies as a vector (see Fig 27.2).

If the overall treatment process requires moving the case from A to B it may be possible with:

1. a single remedy (that may need repeating) or
2. moving through several layers as a confused case becomes clear or
3. several consultations and remedies may be needed to clarify the case or
4. initial treatment might seem to move the case away from the desired outcome, this may be a stage in revealing the case.

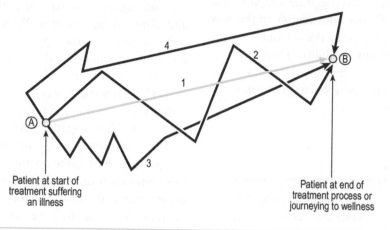

1. One remedy may be sufficient to take the patient to a complete cure to move them from A to B. The more difficult the case, the less likely this is to happen and the longer it is going to take to resolve.

2. Representing several remedies each moving the case on partially. The remedy may be prescribed for different reasons according to different models, approaches and methodologies in each case. Its is likely that as the case progresses, new information will surface, representing the deeper aspects of the case. Some remedies frequently follow others.

3. In some cases, a number of remedies may only move the case on slightly until the picture is clear enough to find a remedy that can act more deeply. This can be the case in hidden cases where initial remedies can be as much about revealing the case as finding the true simillimum for the deeper case.

4. Some remedies may initially move the case in the wrong direction. It is then a matter of retaking the case, in an attempt to move the case in the right direction.

Patient at start of treatment suffering an illness

Patient at end of treatment process or journeying to wellness

Figure 29.1 A step-by-step approach to treatment

Different approaches and methodologies might be needed at each stage. For example, a patient with a confused case of respiratory disease may become clearer after an organ remedy that supports the lungs (see Chapter 15). A hidden case of heart disease may benefit from remedies that support the heart while the case is being revealed or indeed if no therapeutic agreement exists to work at a deeper level. This may be because the patient is reluctant to reveal deeper aspects of the case or the homeopath does not feel experienced enough or is not in an appropriate setting with the time or support necessary.

Using too Many Remedies or 'Over Dosing'

When a number of remedies are used in succession there are several possible effects. As we have illustrated above the case may gradually be revealed and a curative response followed. It is also possible that a remedy that covers the case incompletely may distort the case picture, perhaps by removing or reducing symptoms that could help point to the true simillimum.

In some cases that have received many remedies it is as if the case becomes more confused, possibly including a shift in the patient's susceptibility. I have previously invited you to reflect on the homeopathic remedies as having an information quality. If a healthy person is thought to have a certain resistance or susceptibility determined by the 'information' they have at their disposal it raises important questions as to what the effect on an individual is when new information is added.

There are potentially an infinite number of possible situations a patient could be exposed to that would require an infinite amount of information to cope with. It is reasonable to consider that the overall capacity of the individual for different pieces of information is limited. If each piece of information represents something that the patient is resistant to, then perhaps the flip side of this is that each also gives a reciprocal susceptibility.

Perhaps the information an individual needs can sometimes be obtained from the situation they are in. Is this why poisons and antidotes, like nettles and dock leaves, are often found near to each other? If the homeopathic remedies are another way of providing this information (there is no reason why they cannot have a material action as well), then if remedies keep getting added it may be at the expense of other information. In this way 'over medication' may be to the detriment of the individual's overall susceptibility. This may also explain why sensitivities and allergies may occur when the patient is in a new situation or following drug treatment (or vaccination).

REFLECTION POINT

* Reflect on a recent patient whose management you found difficult. Were you clear about your impression of the case, and did you plan their treatment taking into account that it might take several treatments? Did the patient clearly understand the plan of treatment? Were the patient's feelings communicated clearly, and were you able to get in touch with your own feelings? In experiencing the case as 'difficult', what feelings arose from this and how did they help or hinder you as the homeopath?

Summary

Confused and hidden cases make up a significant proportion of the chronic illnesses that patients present to homeopaths. As thematic and reflective approaches are used to treat these cases, so they become clearer and the opportunities for working with multilayered and hidden cases increase. Managing these cases brings opportunities and challenges not just for the patient but also for the homeopath's personal, practice and professional development.

As an artist will blend together different colours – so, in practice, the homeopath will blend together different methodologies to manage patients. There are many different combinations of approaches and methodologies, each with a different likelihood of success in different circumstances, and each suiting different patients, different situations and different homeopaths. With experience, you will develop your own preferred styles of working, remembering that if one approach does not suit there are other models and approaches that may. There is not one way of 'doing homeopathy', rather there are many ways of 'co-operating with patients and homeopathic principles'.

Difficult cases provide opportunities not just for patients and homeopaths, they also enable the homeopath to start exploring the health of a community and population for present and future generations – ideas that are developed in the next chapter.

References

Laing R D 1990 The politics of experience *and* The bird of paradise. Penguin, London

Ramakrishnan A, Coulter C 2001 Homeopathic approach to cancer. Quality Medical Publishing, St Louis

Swayne J 1998 Homeopathic method. Churchill Livingstone, Edinburgh

Bibliography

Hahnemann S 1835 trans Tafel L 1896 The chronic diseases, their specific nature and homoeopathic treatment, 2 vols. Boericke & Tafel, Philadelphia. Reprinted 1998. Homoeopathic Book Service, Sittingbourne

CHAPTER THIRTY

Managing the Bigger Picture

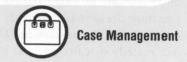

Case Management

David Owen

'As our institutions are so are our people.'

JH Allen

Introduction

In this chapter we re-examine the management of those cases that at first appear difficult. We explore integrating different therapies and different homeopathic approaches, and reflect on illness from the broader perspective of public health. For many difficult cases there is not one answer or one protocol that must be followed, rather there are a number of strategies that you might use to manage difficult cases – using the models and approaches so far described. It may at first seem a weakness in the science of homeopathy that there is no one answer but the art of homeopathy has evolved in a number of ways and can be integrated with other therapies to suit the illnesses, patients and communities it serves. Not all patients (or homeopaths) agree on the outcome they want or on how far they want any treatment to go – it may range from treating an episode of acute illness, to relieving a symptom, to removing every symptom, to preventing an illness, to having a 'positive sense of well-being', to being able to maintain wellness in different situations.

As treatment unfolds the agreement between homeopath and patient on what is being treated, and how, is likely to change. As a result what is 'best practice', and what is required to practise it, is going to be subject to change and your competences to deliver it need constant monitoring. In the attempt to provide the best care, homeopaths have developed a number of ways of working with remedies including using mixtures of rem-edies, combining with other treatments and using machines to help indicate the treatment. Some of these are described below.

The practice of medicine always takes place within a cultural context, which is influenced by the family, community, national, racial and 'world' view of that time. Our own practices and professional organisations will not only shape how we practice but also will determine how easily what we do sits within these different views at any time. We have already touched on the role of the homeopath in treating illnesses that affect the health of the communities we live in and in determining the burden of inherited illness and the well-being of our children's children. It is interesting to reflect on the dual role of the homeopath – not only treating an individual but also serving society and influencing 'public health'. This dual role can at times be the cause of some conflict and tension and so warrants further discussion. It reintroduces the idea that illness may not only reflect the imbalance between an individual and their situation but between a population and its environment.

Integrating Different Models and Treatments

Until a patient has learnt what they have to from an illness it should not be a surprise if they are difficult to manage or if it reoccurs.

At times different approaches will simultaneously indicate different remedies – in these cases you must decide which remedy and approach best fits the overall management. The ideal of finding one remedy that fits the case in all the models of health is rarely achieved but will, if there are no obstacles to cure or maintaining causes, give a good prognosis. A case is difficult to manage because the case is unclear or is hard to analyse, often due to lack of time or the remedy not being known in the appropriate models of health. In practice, over a period of time deepening and revealing the case makes the patient's case more visible, allows analyses using the totality and constitution, and allows obstacles to cure (and maintaining causes) to be identified and treated.

Treating the Inner and Outer Manifestations of the Case

In confused cases it is not uncommon to observe that the outer case, consisting of local symptoms, and the inner case, reflecting themes running more deeply, at first appears at odds; and, depending on the approaches used, different remedies may be indicated. What this means for many difficult cases is that the homeopath has to approach the case from either the outer manifestations of the illness or the inner susceptibility of the patient. In an attempt to do both some homeopaths use both a local prescription and a partially suited constitutional, thematic (including miasmatic) or relational one. These are usually given in different potencies – lower potencies for the local and higher for the susceptibility. The aim is to both relieve local symptoms and establish a clearer case.

As the case becomes clearer it often becomes possible to see one remedy that matches both the outer and inner aspects of the case – where the inner and outer aspects mirror each other and the totality and constitution clearly and accurately reflect the patient's true state. Such a remedy acts reliably and deeply and while most homeopaths would give this remedy in single high potency, others will repeat regularly at high potency and some will accompany this with the same remedy in lower potency on a daily or weekly basis – perhaps working on the more material and structural components of the illness.

The danger in treating before the case is completely clear is that treatment may alter the expression of symptoms in a way that further confuses the case, leading to prescriptions that may give short-term benefit but fail to act deeply. While to the homeopath it is obvious that until the deeper level is dealt with the superficial level won't resolve on any permanent basis, the patient may require some symptomatic relief before they reveal the centre of the case.

If a patient has distressing, even if superficial, symptoms they may feel a need for some local treatment and symptom relief. This can put the homeopath in a difficult position if they feel the symptoms are just an expression of a deeper state. Much of the art of managing confused and hidden cases is balancing these two aspects – drawing on the skills of the homeopath to relieve immediate suffering and to treat the 'inner state'.

Some homeopaths require the patient to take no symptomatic treatment. Unfortunately this means some patients are reluctant to be treated homeopathically. Some homeopaths prefer that patients use 'local' natural remedies, including herbal remedies and low potency prescribing, to support and control those symptoms. Other homeopaths recommend allopathic and antipathic (conventional) drugs and treatments if symptoms need treating. For a patient to follow what may be a lengthy course of treatment it may be necessary to allow patients to experience initial tangible benefits, albeit sometimes superficial ones, while the deeper case is gradually unfolding. In patients who are initially reluctant to work at a deeper level, the homeopath may choose to meet the need to reduce the most superficial symptoms while gradually making the patient more aware of the deeper underlying aspects of their illness.

Homeopaths who use remedies on the one hand to fit more superficial levels, while on the other hand prescribing for the deeper levels, sometimes refer this as 'inter-current' prescribing. This is also used to treat acute conditions that occur while a chronic is being managed – but taking care that any inter-current acute is recognised if it is a healing reaction and is not suppressed to the detriment of the patient. Knowing when to leave an inter-current acute alone, and when and how to support the patient in recovering from such an acute, is often difficult and benefits from the experience of knowing how different remedies in different potencies act. The point at which an inter-current acute needs treating and how it is managed will often play a large part in how successfully you manage more difficult cases. Remember that many patients might also receive or try other treatments for symptoms that emerge during treatment – these will alter what you see and how the case progresses. Knowing something of these other treatments is an important adjunct to your homeopathic knowledge.

By now you will appreciate the tension between two schools of thought. One extreme is represented by homeopaths who feel that if no common remedy covers all the predominant themes and symptoms, or reflects all the qualities of the inside and outside of the case, it is best to re-take the case and re-study the materia medica until a best-fit remedy can be prescribed. Once prescribed, no inter-current treatment should be given. This approach is sometimes referred to as 'unicist' prescribing. At the other extreme are homeopaths that might use several remedies concurrently – sometimes referred to as 'pluralist' prescribing. Remedies may be used in a specific order to cover different aspects of the case in turn or, in some schools, mixed together in the same preparation – sometimes referred to as a complex prescription.

Interconnection of Different Models of Health and Approaches to Treatment

However you choose to work it is important to reflect on why you choose to work in one way and not another, and on the strengths and weaknesses of your management. It will be influenced by many factors, including the context and culture you are working in. As such it is informative to be aware of our homeopathy history (Campbell 1984), how different medical systems have evolved and intertwine (Sutherland 1920), and to be aware of the political implications (Coulter 1981) that implicitly or explicitly affect your choice. Homeopaths working in a particular way are likely to gain more

experience in this way and to attract patients who want to work that way – leading to different 'schools of thinking' that without an understanding of why different strategies exist can become dogmatic and inflexible.

While I have depicted a hierarchy and structure to the different models of health starting with causation and ending with relational, in practice, each of the models of health can be observed to be at play in all of the others. The cause does not happen independently from the effect or the susceptibility – nor is it unaffected by the observer and the relationship in which the cause is observed. It is helpful to think about each model of health as containing aspects of all of the others. While we can study each model or approach or methodology separately it is important to realise their connectedness. For example, causation does not only happen in the realm of individuals with respect to their situation. It also happens in relation to their ancestors through inheritance, through their family, through acquired and learned behaviour, through their community and culture. These causes all influence the symptoms, the susceptibility, the themes and relationships of the patient.

Mixtures of Remedies

Figure 30.1 revisits the idea of remedies as vectors (see Chapter 27). When remedies are combined they might set up a third remedy, perhaps with recognisable aspects of the component remedies. However, if that combination remedy has not been proved, unique symptoms specific to that mixture will not be known and how the component parts might interfere with each other is unknown – making it difficult to interpret the outcome. The information in a remedy may be better understood like a sound wave that, when combined with another sound wave, creates a new wave form and sound contributed to by the parts.

Single or 'unicist' prescribing uses one prescription of a single remedy at a time. It is usually not repeated or changed until specifically indicated. Complex prescriptions may be combinations of any number of remedies, sometimes including herbal and nutritional supplements. An example of a complex

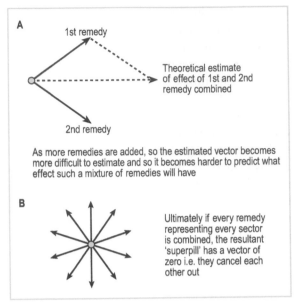

Figure 30.1   The effect of combining remedies

is the combination of Ruta grav, Rhus tox and Arnica in a remedy for painful joints. An example of pluralist prescribing is a patient with a chest infection receiving initially a miasmatic prescription of Tuberculinium bovinum followed closely by a local remedy of Rumex crispus.

In one way all remedies are mixtures of component parts, whether of atomic components, different atoms, salts or ingredients. A plant remedy may be thought of as containing a number of mineral salts, and remedies from animal sources often have themes that run through the plant remedies. However, when each individual remedy is proved, it always has aspects of its own unique picture. While a case may have indications for several closely matched remedies, and each cover aspects of the case, only one will fit it most closely. If one remedy that covers the case is not found, then different schools of homeopaths respond differently. Some use inter-current remedies to cover the component parts, some may combine different remedies, and some will use a remedy to seek to clear the case. Others will wait and re-take the case or study the materia medica until they identify one clear remedy – possibly considering the case incurable if one cannot be found. Each

approach provides opportunities and has limitations. Those favouring unicist prescriptions sometimes report that when many remedies have been used in close succession the case is more confused – sometimes referred to as 'spoilt cases'.

One of the criticisms of mixtures is that when two apparently similar remedies are mixed together the resultant remedy may act unpredictably. This seems to be particularly true the higher the potency of the remedies mixed. Perhaps this is why it is more common to see low potencies and herbal medicines used together than high potency medicines. In any mixture or combination if the indication for each constituent part is known it is easier to see how those components might cover different aspects of the case and to interpret the response to treatment. This is qualitatively quite different from using a mixture based on just pathology without knowing why each component is indicated or how it might shift the case.

If all mixtures were an addition of the qualities of one remedy to another, with nothing lost, then one pill with all the remedies in it would cover all cases (Fig 30.1b). Consider how many remedies combined in one pill might be drawn as a vector – effectively they would 'cancel' each other out. The important issues that you will need to address about each prescription have been covered previously but the points in Box 30.1 are to allow you to reflect on and revise these. It is for each homeopath to decide practically what best suits their patient and themselves, based on the principles you are using, the therapeutic agreement and your level of competence and confidence.

Generally, and understandably, it will be easier for homeopaths to reach a consensus on the management of simple cases – as cases get more difficult so there will be greater variation in practice. Different homeopaths will, depending on their knowledge, experience and preference, use different models, approaches and methodologies. Being explicit about them, and recording them clearly in the notes when you record the impression, plan and prescription, along with establishing how you monitor the outcome, will help you (when you review a case) to repeat your successes and explore different management strategies in those that do not initially respond.

BOX 30.1
Issues to Address With Each Prescription

- What type of case are you treating?
- What model of health and approach to treatment are you using?
- Have you a therapeutic agreement that you and the patient are happy with?
- Does this prescription reflect the depth of causation, the level of the symptoms, the breadth of the totality, the layers of the essence and/or intensity of the projection?
- Are there confirmatory or exclusion factors?
- How reliable is the prescription?
- What methodology are you using and what is your confidence in the prescription?
- When to prescribe and when not to
- What advice to give about inter-current treatments
- When to follow up the patient
- How changes will be elicited and monitored
- Is there a risk of an aggravation?

- What support and information does the patient need?
- What potency and frequency of administration is needed?
- When will you know if you need to change the prescription?
- What is the patient's vitality like?
- How will you manage relapses?
- If using several remedies, what are the indications, instructions and potential interactions for each?
- How will you know when to seek supervision?
- If the patient's symptoms are relieved, will they have made a transition to a better state of health?
- When would you consider you have done all you can for a patient?
- How will you discharge a patient; and will they need, or will you offer, long-term support or 'health maintenance'?

Integrating Different Types of Treatment

As some patients are increasingly seeking a positive state of health and are increasingly wary of suppressing symptoms, so they are pursuing an increasingly varied range of complementary treatments. In order to integrate these treatments and to manage patients who are using them at the same time as receiving homeopathy, it is important to be familiar with their basic principles and where, particularly, they interface with homeopathy. It can help to identify those that influence health in different ways. You might find it helpful to consider them in terms of whether they work predominantly on susceptibility, vitality or life style (as illustrated in the boat analogy in Figure 6.1).

If you read through the case of Susan you may recognise a variety of non-homeopathic interventions that might be used in addition to the conventional treatment she received. Each different

indication might, like a homeopathic approach, have certain key points to recommend it. For example, if her headaches were worse from moving the head into certain positions or if there was restricted movement of the neck, then manipulation of the neck would be relatively more important to consider. If she had tenderness over acupuncture points, this might indicate she was likely to respond to this treatment. In addition, a case could be made for herbal treatment based on possible hormonal imbalance – especially if, say, her headaches had been much better in pregnancy. Further dietary work might have helped her, including further food exclusion – as might 'naturopathic' advice from fasting to 'detox' and 'cleansing' programs. Her own initial reluctance to look at psychotherapeutic approaches might be considered either a contraindication or an indication that she needed this! In practice you are often in the position of having to

413

advise patients who might benefit from several possible interventions. At times it is necessary to 'blend' these together into a coherent integrated package. Of course in many cases the patient's case can be understood as a number of interconnecting events or factors. So a headache might affect posture, ongoing pain make the patient depressed, a depressed and tense patient might be more likely to have an accident and develop a whip-lash, etc. Where a particular therapist intervenes will depend on their training and the patient's choice but in more difficult cases intervening in several ways with several therapeutic tools can often get results more quickly, that hold for longer and sometimes in cases that will not respond to a single intervention.

CASE STUDY 30.1

Susan, aged 56, has had headaches (worse over the last 8 eight years) since she was 12. Some pain is present over the eyes most of the time, although this gets very much worse approximately twice a week for six hours. The worst pain is usually unilateral, spreading from the occiput to the forehead. It is a sharp, stabbing pain.

Modalities

Initially the headaches came monthly and were relieved with aspirin. In her 20s migraine was diagnosed and she was given medication that helped for a few months, after which the pain returned and was worse. Headaches relieved in the past when coming off cheese, coffee and fatty foods. She is currently trying to keep these to a minimum. Worse from bright lights and damp weather; better from local pressure and warmth

Past Medical History

Susan fell off a horse aged 11. She was driving when involved in a road traffic accident aged 47. Her granddaughter, a passenger in the car, was injured. This has left unresolved issues between her and her daughter. She describes her menopause as 'horrific', although it was relieved by hormone replacement therapy that she stopped three months ago. She had a gall bladder operation aged 46.

Symptoms Review

Constipated all her life. Bowels open once or twice a week. Hay fever since children were born.

Medication

Currently on Pizotifen and Cafergot. In the past has used Sumatriptan, which helped initially.

Social History

Parents separated when she was a child. After road traffic accident lost contact with her daughter. Her husband has a busy job as a university lecturer and has raised blood pressure.

Dietary Factors

Likes fruit, dairy products. Dislikes fish.

Family History

Mother had migraines, maternal grandmother died of tuberculosis, daughter used to suffer from asthma, eczema and hay fever.

General Symptoms

Hot and perspires easily.

Temperament

Susan is unable to 'show feelings' but very sensitive. Previously she changed her family doctor when he suggested counselling. She says she is a 'loner, particularly if I'm feeling ill, when I just want to be left alone'. Her husband says she's a perfectionist. She enjoys playing the piano and music makes her feel better. She belongs to the church, which is her 'main comfort in life'.

Susan was initially treated on a totality picture with essence and keynotes informed by the repertorisation. It pointed to Natrum muriaticum, prescribed as a 200c split dose (two doses one that night and the other next morning). At follow-up Susan is slightly more engaging and (either because of the remedy, improved rapport or both) is able to talk about 'periods of depression' that she gets; her headaches are unchanged. She feels 'responsible' for her parent's separation and finds herself thinking about this often, especially on 'rainy days'. She is prescribed Natrum sulphuricum 200c split dose, partly on the new information but also because there are several pointers to both Sulphur and Natrum muriaticum and the aetiology of head injury, for which Natrum sulphuricum is well indicated. She returns after a month 'much much better'. Susan is seen after three months and has come off all conventional drugs and started to go to a counsellor with her husband.

As with other cases presented in this book only key extracts are offered to illustrate the learning points. In Susan's case the time-line is important in revealing aetiology and the effect of suppressive medication that was probably responsible for turning an occasional acute picture into a permanent chronic one. Indeed, overuse of analgesics is well recognised for changing an occasional acute headache to a frequent chronic one and I suspect this suppression happens in many other conditions.

Modifying the Patient's Situation

While case-taking reveals the relationship between a patient and their life situation, both its role in their condition and as a potential obstacle to cure, it does not necessarily do anything to change that situation. However, a slight shift of emphasis in the case-taking can help patients make clear links between their symptoms and facilitate a change in life style. In the holistic model it may help patients understand their susceptibility; in the holographic and relational models it may help them become conscious of aspects of themselves and aware of how they project themselves and how others might project onto them – an insightful and powerfully therapeutic process.

In a way every illness offers the patient an opportunity to notice and change themselves and their situation in some way – in the same way as ecological problems provide important lessons and opportunities about (and for) environmental change. Homeopathy has a long tradition of working alongside interventions suggested to modify a patient's life style, whether it be dietary advice, advice on exercise, removing potentially harmful chemical factors, or reducing negative psychological factors, including stress management, hypnosis, relationship counselling and other interventions that can break damaging psychological patterns.

I have found many patients where a remedy becomes clear or a well indicated remedy acts much deeper (when maintaining causes and obstacles to cure are removed or reduced) by using the additional support and advice from other complementary medicines. Identifying colleagues that can give this advice, and who themselves understand the homeopathic process, is an invaluable resource. For example, I have found acupuncturists and reflexologists able to guide and inform about 'organ damage' and the monitoring of outcome in severely handicapped patients who have difficult communicating verbally.

In many cases of advanced disease, such as metastatic disease, I find it helpful to be explicit to the patient about the role of different interventions. While the homeopathic treatment frequently enables (and is enabled by) the other interventions the patient is making, it also requires careful interpretation so that the contribution of each intervention can be understood. It does, however (unless you make the interventions yourself), require the ability to work with and communicate with a variety of professions – sometimes using diverse concepts, language and models of health.

I find it helps patients with advanced disease to plan such integrated care by thinking of the components of the care like the four sides of a square. This can be drawn out for the patient in order to remember how different interventions may help and to see how different aspects of their care connect. On one side are the vitality treatments that include the homeopathic prescription. On the second are the 'structural and bio-mechanical treatments' that include assessment of the musculoskeletal system and often include advice on environment and life style. The third side is 'functional', where important bodily functions and organs can be supported using herbal remedies (or homeopathic mother tinctures) and nutritional products. The fourth side is the psychological advice and support that can help the patient. In some cases a homeopathic remedy might act more deeply and 'hold' for longer if other treatments are integrated into the patient's care.

In some cases it is appropriate and helpful to name a fifth aspect (that I sometimes draw as the top of a pyramid running up from the four-sided square). This reflects the spiritual or religious dimension that may be addressed by the patient in many ways – including healing, pastoral care, prayer, meditation, etc. So, for example, a patient with advanced cancer may receive advice from a number of sources – on homeopathic treatment, on diet and nutritional supplementation, on organ support (particularly liver) and on psychological support (such visualisation or relaxation techniques). Each side may include a review of their conventional medical treatment. The spiritual dimension is helpfully named for many patients, especially when death is near, to connect their healing journey with their spiritual one. A fear of death in both the patient and homeopath, reflecting the fear in society, is one of the major obstacles to seeing the case when managing severe illness. Clarifying for yourself, and understanding for others, what life and death mean is a precursor to seeing these cases more clearly (Levine 1987).

A 'homeopathic' treatment that requires particular mention in the treatment of cancer is Iscador, made from mistletoe. It can provide both material organ support for the patient and a direct benefit for the vitality, leading to increased survival times (Leroi 1962, 1965). Iscador is an example of a remedy prepared in a similar way to homeopathic remedies but used traditionally through a related school of thought and practice called Anthroposophy.

There are many other systems of medicine in which remedies are prepared in a similar way to homeopathic remedies, such as the tissue salts, that you may be interested in – or that patients may expect you to know something about.

The Homeopath as a Machine

The subtle appreciation of illness from a homeopath's perspective is often inadequately expressed by a gross conventional diagnosis. But integrating psychotherapeutic models to understand the patient's mental state and to describe the homeopathic relationship provides a sensitive tool to describe the individual. However – as you are finding – this requires substantial reflection, development and support. It is therefore not surprising that (like many health care professionals) homeopaths and patients are drawn to diagnostic and treatment tools as a channel, or even an alternative, to exploring and expressing their own sensitivity and influence. Many homeopaths and patients are drawn to forms of diagnosis (whether dowsing, bio-electronic techniques, applied kinesiology or others) in an attempt to perceive more easily, reliably or deeply.

Although some practitioners use these techniques successfully, I see little reason why any machine or gadget might reveal anything more useful for the careful selection of a remedy than can be achieved by the homeopath interacting with the patient in a dynamic way. The ability to stay alert to your own movement, phrases, body language and feelings, and to perceive and monitor their significance in relation to the patient and their case, is your own instrument. When you are actively and consciously in a consultation the homeopathic relationship is a powerful part of not just selecting and advising a treatment but of the healing process itself.

When machines and instruments are used to select a course of treatment without a clear understanding of the case (whether you use conventional investigations, bio-electrical, dowsing or indiscriminate repertorisation), the case perceived is going to be limited by the sensitivity of the machine employed. All machines bypass aspects of human sensitivity and reason, risking the relationship that is the fundamental difference between being a technician and a homeopath. While machines can help to gain a snapshot image of part of the whole, they risk perpetrating the myth of the case as a series of disconnected parts – and the illusion that treatments (often multiple when prescribed using these machines) which attempt to correct a range of disconnected abnormal results will bring health. More dangerously, as with any tests, they can raise inappropriate concerns leading to irrelevant treatments – and taking the patient away from the true opportunity they have to heal.

REFLECTION POINT

- To what extent do you feel it is true that a patient can only suffer one illness at a time? A number of different styles of working, ways of prescribing and issues that relate to the integration of homeopathy in difficult cases have been described. How aware of developing your own preferences are you and what has most influenced these?

- Before embarking on the management of severe, life-threatening and terminal illnesses, it is important to have reflected on the place of palliation, healing and cure. Palliation has already been discussed and may prevent the full expression of an illness. Healing is a process that takes place over time. Cure is a place or state where the organism is balanced. Reflect on the role of each and when each is appropriate as a goal of treatment – how might management be difficult if you and a patient have different aims?

Cultural Issues and Public Health?

'Establishing connections with others is not merely a matter of participating in a particular pattern of personalities. It is a matter of realising our nature. If we adopt a style of aloneness in our relations with others, we contradict a fundamental life process; we defy the bio-dance, the ebbing and flowing pattern that connects, without which life would cease.'

L Dossey (1982)

If health is the ability to maintain the integrity of the organism in new situations and facing new challenges, then illness is an inevitable side effect of growth and change. When healthy we have the ability to accept, invite or take on greater changes in our environment. The healthier we are, the more we are able to explore different life styles and accommodate to different situations. This is true for individuals and communities – even populations. The health of one affects the health of the others. An individual's susceptibility, resistance and immunity is directly linked to the susceptibility, resistance and immunity of the whole population. The homeopath, like all health carers, has a role in society and public health by identifying environmental triggers and causes of illness and promoting healthy life styles. Indirectly we also have a role in identifying how the illnesses patients suffer from now will contribute to the susceptibility of future generations – and how correct treatment can reduce this susceptibility reflected in inherited predisposition.

While the patients we treat focus on individual care, our practices provide care in a community and our professional organisations should have a voice and role in the health of the population, ensuring that the broadest perspectives that homeopathy offers about health are communicated effectively. For example, amongst the growing numbers of patients with a susceptibility to heart disease, there are frequently psychological issues around stressful and difficult relationships that are increasingly recognised as contributing to heart disease. The homeopathic community, through working with patients, is one of the professional groups most aware of the broader issues related to these frequently masked and hidden cases, and could champion social change to address this in the population. The deepest illnesses and the most hidden cases often reveal a great deal about the culture the patient is in – offering important public health insights.

One issue that often reoccurs for homeopaths is the tension between 'belonging' to a community and being on 'the edge' of a community. As a therapist you provide something of a conduit for both individuals and communities. You both have to belong to know what it is like to experience and share what is taking place, but at times you have to operate outside of it. It is not always easy to be free from the bias and hidden and unconscious influences that a community chooses – belonging to strong professional organisations can support you and in some ways compensate for this.

Cultural Illness

Traits and issues that are poorly expressed or dealt with in society may explain why certain symptoms go unnoticed or unacknowledged by some patients and therapists. This is a major contributor to hidden cases that often present with the most serious of illnesses. By developing and challenging attitudes to health, the homeopath, in the best tradition of scientists and artists, invites the population to reflect on what it believes and express what it feels.

Although we focus our treatment on individuals, the treatment can also have a dynamic effect on those around them. It is interesting that often a 'stuck' case can shift when other members of the family receive treatment. Just as an ill person can affect those around them so can a healthy person – health is as 'infectious' as illness! In this context, and as a profession, we have a responsibility as homeopaths not only to heal our patients but also to try and heal our health care system.

Teaching of Homeopathy

Ideas are developed in a symbiotic way between an individual's personal insights, their practice and their professional culture. So in homeopathy the ideas and teachings that evolve depend on and belong equally to the individuals who articulate them, the patients and colleagues that are part of their practice, and the homeopathic profession past and present. The knowledge of any individual must always be seen in the context of the wisdom of the community as a whole. It seems to me that while there is no doubt about the transformative role some individuals bring to our understanding, there are ideas that are expressed synchronously through several different teachers

at the same time and many insights occur because change in one thing allows us to see other things differently. There are times when it is right for 'ideas to emerge'.

It is an important responsibility of our professional bodies to ensure that the role and value of the homeopathic community they represent is recognised. The knowledge resides not only in a few individuals but also within our profession. The checks and balances that our professional bodies offer can help in validating emerging ideas and reinterpretations of observation.

REFLECTION POINT

- To what extent do you think the sum of illnesses in a community defines that community's well-being? To what extent do you feel you have a responsibility to a community as well as individual patients? Is it likely to be easier or harder to see confused and hidden cases and to identify the projection in patients from a similar cultural background to yourself?

Summary

In this chapter we have looked at the wider context of homeopathy, how the different ways of prescribing connect, and how homeopathy can integrate with other treatments. We have named but a few of the many interventions that you and your patients might try to integrate. Each, like homeopathy, has their own system and knowledge – part of the management of any difficult case is realising how different pieces of advice and advisors can work together.

Given the importance of the context in which we work and the situation any patient is in, I have discussed some of the community and cultural factors that influence our work. Realising the importance of this to our health, the health of our patients, and the health of future generations raises many questions – I hope those questions, like others that this book has asked you to reflect on will contribute to the foundation of your practice in homeopathy.

Conclusion

The last patient will never be healed.

In this book I have set out to describe a structure that I have found useful in understanding and applying a series of views (or models) of health, approaches to the treatment of illness, and methods of prescribing remedies. These have helped me to co-ordinate the many different ways homeopathy can be used and to manage patients in a rational and repeatable way. It is important to me that you realise it is my intention for you to take from this framework only what is useful to find your own styles of working. My wish is that the book may inspire you to find the balance of art and science that suits you, to actively and enthusiastically enquire into the mystery our patients so generously bring to us, to courageously apply that enquiry to your own self, and to record and share your successes and – perhaps more importantly – what appear to be your failures.

At all times remember the importance of experience in your training and development – not only the experience of present and past teachers but also your own. When what you have been taught (including what is written here) is not consistently borne out by your experience, then I invite you to take it as an opportunity to explore and elucidate the homeopathic principles underlying them for yourself. In training, it can appear that you are showered with a variety of ideas, styles and advice – if this book enables you to integrate just some of this knowledge it will have served you well. Once you start in practice you can often feel quite alone with the suffering that presents to you on a daily basis. When you feel isolated I hope this book will provide some common ground and a basis of respect between yourself and a wide range of colleagues from whom you can receive and to who you may offer support.

Many homeopaths appear to fail to establish a practice that matches their initial ideals – often seeing few patients or struggling to make ends meet. By returning to the principles and practice detailed in this book I believe you will find different and relevant ways to engage with patients and build your practice. For those who have been in practice for some time it can appear that there is no clear direction or path to follow, no best way to practice – at times it can feel like crossing a wilderness! Hopefully this book will have helped you identify some key tools to seeing the uniqueness of each patient and to find a new direction for your work – to move out of the wilderness. If you have reflected on and clarified the central homeopathic principles that are true to you, then this book will have served you well.

To my experienced colleagues I offer this book as a collection of ideas, some of which you will be familiar with, some of which you will easily agree with and which may serve to make you feel less alone. If there are some you are unfamiliar with, then I am pleased to have shared a little of how I see things – but I remain enthusiastic and eager to hear of your experience and insights that I am currently unfamiliar with. If there are ideas you do not agree with but if reading this book helps clarify and strengthen your own views, then I encourage you to share them.

I hope you have reflected a great deal while studying this book. Although each model is described separately I believe we are all influenced by each of them, to some extent, in every encounter. Determining and shaping every encounter is our ability to be in a relationship; our ability to relate to others is shaped by our awareness of ourselves. We cannot but be influenced by cause and effect, susceptibility and the total expression of those we are in contact with, the patterns we recognise or how they resonate with our own, the projections we are influenced by and the way they are reflected in us. If we do not consciously attend to how each of these affects us we will remain unconsciously influenced by them.

I encourage you to do all you can to be aware of the personal, practice and professional reference points that reflect and influence our attitude and state of mind. Once aware of these, they can operate at all times, and in any situation, to help you perceive yourself and others clearly. Understanding the homeopathic relationship is at the heart of understanding how our unconscious needs, fears, delusions and desires are expressed – and central to perceiving the case without becoming stuck in it. For me, the more difficult the case, the more that can be learnt from it, but also the more important it is to have a place and context to re-examine that case so that you can explore other ways of working with that patient, identifying the projection and clarifying what at first is not obvious. I wish you well in finding both small groups of colleagues and the individual supervisors and mentors who will help you with this.

This book has attempted to present a structure that will help you practice homeopathy. It has invited reflection in your learning, pointed out the development that is enmeshed in your training, and encouraged you to establish the support necessary to tackle difficult cases and learn from the experience. There is much that is theoretical, but it is informed by the experience of my colleagues and myself. One thing is certain, in the future – and perhaps very rapidly – a number of the premises explored in this book will be outdated. It is not that the truths we work from change, rather that our perspectives of them do. Disease is changing and the challenges the homeopath faces now are very different from those even 50 years ago. We are fortunate to have a diligently recorded homeopathic legacy of much wisdom and experience. How we take this forward is our responsibility and while the attitudes and practice described in this book represent my current clinical experience, the practice of homeopathy has a

long tradition of teachers evolving their thoughts and appearing to change their mind. I will be honoured if you permit me the same opportunity.

References

Campbell A 1984 The two faces of homeopathy. Jill Norman and Hale, London

Coulter H L 1973–1977 Divided legacy; a history of the schism in medical thought, 3 vols, 1994 vol 4. Wehawker Press and North Atlantic Books, Berkeley

Dossey L 1982 Space, time and medicine. Shambala Publications, Boston

Leroi A 1962 Progress in iscador therapy of malignant tumours (I – Brain and Skin). Br Homoeopath J 51(1):31–37, 176–185

Leroi A 1965 Iscador therapy of cancer. Br Homoeopath J 54(1):27–35

Sutherland J P 1920 The idealism of homeopathy. John Bale, Sons & Danielsson, London

Levine S 1987 Healing into life and death. Gateway, Bath

Bibliography

Kent J T 1929 Lectures on homeopathic philosophy. Ehrhart & Karl, Chicago IL. Reprinted 1981 North Atlantic Books, Berkeley Lecture 37

Cicchetti J 1993 Dreams, symbols and homeopathy. North Atlantic Books, Berkeley

INDEX

CPI Antony Rowe
Eastbourne, UK
June 03, 2024